OXFORD SPECIALIST HANDBOOK OF
Forensic Psychiatry

T0202387

OXFORD SPECIALIST HANDBOOK OF
Forensic Psychiatry

SECOND EDITION

Nigel Eastman

Emeritus Professor of Law and Ethics in Psychiatry
St George's, University of London
Honorary Consultant Forensic Psychiatrist
South West London & St George's Mental Health NHS Trust

Gwen Adshead

Consultant Forensic Psychiatrist and Psychotherapist
Broadmoor Hospital

Simone Fox

Consultant Clinical and Forensic Psychologist
South London and Maudsley NHS Foundation Trust

Richard Latham

Consultant Forensic Psychiatrist
East London NHS Foundation Trust

Seán Whyte

Consultant Forensic Psychiatrist and Clinical Director
South-West London & St George's Mental Health NHS Trust
Visiting Senior Lecturer, Institute of Psychiatry, Psychology &
Neuroscience, King's College London

Hannah Kate Williams

Specialty Registrar in Forensic Psychiatry & Medical Psychotherapy
South-West London & St George's Mental Health NHS Trust

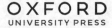

OXFORD
UNIVERSITY PRESS

OXFORD
UNIVERSITY PRESS

Great Clarendon Street, Oxford, OX2 6DP,
United Kingdom

Oxford University Press is a department of the University of Oxford.
It furthers the University's objective of excellence in research, scholarship,
and education by publishing worldwide. Oxford is a registered trade mark of
Oxford University Press in the UK and in certain other countries

Published in the United States of America by Oxford University Press
198 Madison Avenue, New York, NY 10016, United States of America

British Library Cataloguing in Publication Data
Data available

Library of Congress Control Number is on file at the Library of Congress

ISBN 978–0–19–882558–6

DOI: 10.1093/med/9780198825586.001.0001

Printed in the UK by
Ashford Colour Press Ltd, Gosport, Hampshire

Preface

The *preface* to the first edition of the handbook offered justification for addressing its 'psychiatry and law interface', alongside clinical forensic psychiatry, based upon the fact that UK practice of forensic psychiatry had, by 2012, substantially moved on from its largely clinical service roots. So that 'forensic psychiatry' had become, and now firmly is, concerned with *both* the clinical discipline of assessing and treating mentally disordered offenders *and* the meeting of law and all psychiatry, within the academic discipline of 'psycho-legal studies'. Hence, now a significant proportion of higher trainee forensic psychiatrists not only train in their clinical speciality but also undertake some form of legal training, most commonly an LLM in Mental Health Law; based upon recognition that clinical forensic psychiatry cannot be practised effectively, or ethically, without a real understanding of how psychiatry and law relate to one to the other (and often 'don't'). Whilst some higher training schemes have developed 'psycho-legal workshops', which aim to offer 'quasi experience' at the interface between clinical psychiatry and law. And, most notably, the GMC New Curriculum for Forensic Psychiatry includes the express requirement for forensic trainees (surely also seniors) of gaining both 'knowledge' of a wide range of relevant law and also 'capabilities' that are not only clinical but also 'clinico-legal'.

This second edition of the handbook is published alongside its companion volume, the *Oxford Casebook of Forensic Psychiatry*. This offers a wide range of 'case problems' across both 'clinical forensic psychiatry' and 'law and psychiatry', as well as some related separate advisory text on 'decision-making techniques' and 'critiquing paradigms for decisions taken'; with cross referencing into this new edition of the handbook to enable the reader to find information relevant to each case. It is also presented in a fashion that allows for psychiatrists from other Commonwealth common law jurisdictions to import their own particular law into the cases.

The necessity of understanding 'law and psychiatry' is not limited to those who practice the designated speciality of forensic psychiatry. It applies to *all* psychiatrists who are regulated by, operate within, or make use of law. And this is emphasised by the advancing scope and complexity of mental health and mental capacity legislation, and their interface; making increasingly 'technical' satisfying the duty of all psychiatrists not only to treat their patients well clinically but also to pay proper regard to their civil rights. The three domestic jurisdictions, plus the RoI, reflect each nation's different emphasis on individual freedom, paternalism, legalism, and public protection. So that, whilst their various mental health laws remain true to many of the principles of the first very early Mental Health Acts, particularly medical dominance within the legal process, the details have diverged in the four jurisdictions. So that we lay out a detailed comparison of each of the four jurisdiction's law in regard to treatment of both mental and physical conditions; including for Northern Ireland the new 'fusion' legislation expressed by the MCA(NI) Act 2016, due soon to come into force. Notably, the UK government has very recently published, post the Wessely Review, a White Paper for its intended new Mental Health Act for England and Wales.

It is also not possible for criminal lawyers effectively to represent or prosecute someone with a mental disorder, or for any civil lawyer to deal properly with a litigant in any legal context involving psychiatric evidence, without a real understanding of both the nature of psychiatry and of its interface with law. Hence, this handbook remains distinct from others in the OUP series in addressing not one discipline but two, and the relationship between them. As such it is intended therefore not only for trainees and senior practitioners in forensic psychiatry, indeed all psychiatry, but also for all lawyers who need to understand psychiatric concepts and thinking, and how they relate to law and legal process.

The justification for a second edition of the handbook lies not only in its 'companion' relationship with the *Oxford Casebook* but also in the substantial legal, research, clinical, and service developments that have occurred since publication of the first edition.

The first edition was published very soon after the partial defences to murder had been reformed in England and Wales, based upon the recommendation of Law Commission that particularly 'diminished responsibility' should be made much more congruent with psychiatry. With the implication also that there should be less room for jury decision-making not properly underpinned by expert evidence. However, in a number of important cases the Court of Appeal has been highly resistant to this change, and effectively has dragged the law back towards its perhaps natural, and more comfortable, incongruence with medicine, expressed in reiteration of the traditional 'primacy', even 'exclusivity', of the jury, so as to render the practical impact of the reform minimal. We also further describe developments in the law of insanity, automatism, and intoxication, as well as in regard to 'joint enterprise'; with an update also on the law of self-defence in Irish law. And there is new law in England and Wales on both 'coercive control' and 'slavery'. We have also updated our treatment of safeguarding in light of its new statutory basis. In regard to civil rights, there is new law on 'deprivation of liberty safeguards', and the boundary between applying the MHA and MCA, and on Article 2 of the ECHR, plus further developed extradition case law. We also now give law relating to the regulation of medical practice, including expert witness practice, enhanced space.

The Sentencing Council helpfully published in 2020 *Sentencing Offenders with Mental Disorders, Developmental Disorders, or Neurological Impairments*. Although this emphasises 'culpability' over 'safety', including perhaps privileging 'hybrid orders' over 'hospital orders'. The *Guidance* not only requires expert witnesses to offer reports written in its terms, but also presents ethical challenges to such experts. It also has potential implications for services.

In line with our intention to render both the handbook and the casebook further applicable to non-UK common law jurisdictions in the Commonwealth, this edition also deals with the death-penalty and related capital jurisdiction practice.

Relevant epidemiological knowledge has advanced a good deal since the first edition was published, particularly expressed through a number of well-designed systematic reviews which allow us to be better able to quantify the magnitude by which various mental disorders affect the risk of violence, and, perhaps more importantly, to examine hypotheses about how much other factors such as socioeconomic status, family environment, and substance misuse do (or do not) explain away increased risks of violence for some mental disorders. For this reason, the clinical pages have changed substantially, with updated epidemiological data and with many questions posed in the first edition now answered, on occasion leading to new understanding that contradicts what was common understanding at the time of publication of the first edition. We have also included reference to recent research about the effectiveness of various treatment programmes discussed in the first edition, for example sex offender programmes, whilst highlighting some gaps upon which the next generation of researchers might focus their efforts. Forensic psychotherapy was inadequately dealt with in the first edition, and we hope that we have now rectified this.

Clinically we have enhanced our treatment, in relation to offending, of developmental disorders, including autism, ADHD, and intellectual disability; neuroscience; dementia; traumatic brain injury; genetic disorders; and sexsomnias. We have also included more about marginalised groups, with new pages on ethnicity, transgender issues, and old age psychiatry within forensic psychiatry. Of particular importance, we have now given more space to physical health in secure forensic settings, given the vexed problem of weighing risk management against causing iatrogenic disease. Whilst we have brought together and updated topics previously scattered throughout the first edition. We also have added new topics, including 'radicalisation' and its relationship with mental disorder (if any), given expansion of the government's Prevent and Channel anti-radicalisation programmes into health and social services; plus new drugs of misuse, including 'legal highs'; and 'gangs'.

The issue of 'integrated' versus 'parallel' service provision has now largely been settled in favour of extending specialist service provision into the community (perhaps logically so, in that assessing and managing risk is the more difficult in that context). Alongside some geographically proximate comprehensive forensic mental health services seeking efficiencies and economies of scale by forming 'service partnerships'. Whilst, in regard to the issue of 'prison versus hospital' service provision for offenders with severe personality disorder, DSPD within hospital has been abandoned, in favour of an OPD pathway favouring prison, with some medium secure and very limited high secure provision. We have also now included information about new assessment tools, both in regard to appropriate secure placement of patients and in regard to sexual offenders with intellectual disability.

As regards diagnostic aids, DSM-IV has become -5, and ICD has become 11, and we of have course taken account of this. Although, to economise on space, this edition now refers the reader to those volumes, or to the *Handbook of General Psychiatry*, for detailed description of categories, rather than reproducing them within the handbook. Both DSM-5 and ICD11 are referred to in the book, but with a focus primarily on DSM-5.

We hope that this new edition of the handbook will make a further contribution to enhanced understanding and enjoyment of the ethical practice of forensic psychiatry, and to the practice of lawyers who have to deal with mentally disordered individuals subject to criminal or civil law.

NE
GA
SF
RL
SW
HKW
London
August 2021

Acknowledgements

In compiling and writing this handbook we have benefited from the hard work and good advice of a considerable number of our colleagues and friends, and from the support of our families and employers. We would like to thank in particular the following psychiatrists, psychologists, barristers, solicitors, judges, academics, and other colleagues for their support and for giving of their time so freely to comment upon drafts of parts of the handbook, and to suggest corrections and improvements:

Dr Ali Ajaz
Ms Jo Bownas
Dr Bee Brockman
Mr Michael Botham
Mr Chris Butterfield
Dr Bernard Chin
Ms Emma Chandra
Prof John Crichton
Dr Hannah Crisford
Dr Rachel Daly
Prof Kimberlie Dean
Dr Mayura Deshpande
Dr Claire Dimond
Dr Bridget Dolan QC
Ms Lorna Downing
Dr Simon Duff
Ms Mhairi Fleming
Dr Alasdair Forrest
Dr Rachel Gibbons
Dr Emily Glorney
Dr Adrian Grounds
Prof Gisli Gudjonsson
Dr Az Hakeem
Dr Nick Hallett
Ms Stephanie Harrison QC
Mr Anthony Haycroft
Dr Eleanor Hind
Dr Nick Hindley
Ms Julia Houston
Prof Harry Kennedy
Prof Michael Kopelman
Dr Sanya Krijes
Ms Julia Krish
Dr Tina Irani
Dr Sarah Mackenzie Ross
Ms Heldi McCaskill
Prof Amina Memon
Prof Gill Mezey

Dr Anna Motz
Dr Catherine Penny
Prof Derek Perkins
Dr Danny Riordan
Mr Mark Simpson
Dr Andrew Smith
Dr Huw Stone
Dr Derek Tracey
Prof Birgit Völlm
Ms Connie Wernham
Mrs Lisa Whyte
Mr Brian Williams
Dr David Alun Williams
Prof Huw Williams

We would also like to thank trainees from the South London Higher Training Scheme in Forensic Psychiatry who read some parts of the handbook alongside 'test-using' cases in the companion *Oxford Casebook of Forensic Psychiatry*; also Rachel Goldsworthy, Lauren Tiley, and Pete Stevenson at OUP for their advice, support, patience, and hospitality.

Contents

Abbreviations

5HT	5-Hydroxy Tryptamine (also known as serotonin)	BPD	Borderline Personality Disorder
AA	Alcoholics Anonymous	BPSD	Behavioural and Psychological Symptoms of Dementia
ABC	Antecedents, Behaviours, Consequences	CAF	Common Assessment Framework
ABH	Actual Bodily Harm	CAMHS	Child & Adolescent Mental Health Services
ABI	Acquired Brain Injury	CARATS	Counselling, Assessment, Referral, Advice, and Throughcare Services
AC	Approved Clinician (E&W)		
ACCT	Assessment, Care in Custody, and Teamwork		
ACE	Adverse Childhood Experiences	CAT	Cognitive Analytic Therapy
		CBT	Cognitive-Behavioural Therapy
ACS	Abel Cognitions Scale	CCE	Child Criminal Exploitation
ADHD	Attention Deficit Hyperactivity Disorder	CCG	Clinical Commissioning Group (England)
ADMCA	Assisted Decision-Making (Capacity) Act 2015 (RoI)	CCRC	Criminal Cases Review Commission (UK)
AMCP	Approved Mental Capacity Professional (E&W)	CD	Clinical Director/Conditional Discharge/Conduct Disorder
AMHP	Approved Mental Health Professional (E&W)	CE	of the Common Era (equivalent to AD, Anno Domini)
AMP	Approved Medical Practitioner (Scotland)		
AOT	Assertive Outreach Team	CFT	Community Forensic Team
AP	Approved Premises	CHAT	Comprehensive Health Assessment Tool
APA	American Psychiatric Association	CID	Criminal Investigation Department
ART	Aggression Replacement Training	CJD	Creutzfeld-Jacob Disease
		CJS	Criminal Justice System
ASBO	Antisocial Behaviour Order	CLIA	Criminal Law (Insanity) Act 2006 (RoI)
ASD	Autistic Spectrum Disorder		
ASPD	Antisocial Personality Disorder	CMHT	Community Mental Health Team
ASR	Annual Statutory Report		
ASSET	Assessment Tool (used by YOTs)	CoP	Court of Protection (E&W)
		Coru	'Fair', the Health & Care Professional Regulator (RoI)
ASW	Approved Social Worker (NI)		
AWIA	Adults With Incapacity (Scotland) Act 2000	CPA	Care Programme Approach (E&W), Continuing Power of Attorney (Scotland)
BAME	Black, Asian, and Minority Ethnic	CPD	Continuing Professional Development
BCE	Before the Common Era (equivalent to BC, Before Christ)	CPN	Community Psychiatric Nurse
		CPS	Crown Prosecution Service (E&W)
BCS	British Crime Survey	CPSA	Criminal Procedure (Scotland) Act 1995
BMI	body mass index		

CQC	Care Quality Commission (England)
CRPD	UN Convention on the Rights of Persons with Disabilities
CSA	Child Sexual Abuse
CSE	Child Sexual Exploitation
CSO	Community Support Officer
CT	Computed Tomography
CTO	Community (E&W)/ Compulsory Treatment Order (Scotland)
CU	Callous-Unemotional
DA	Dopamine, or Dopaminergic
DBS	Deep Brain Stimulation
DBT	Dialectical Behaviour Therapy
DHSC	Department of Health & Social Care (E&W)
DoJ	Department of Justice (RoI)
DoL	deprivation of liberty
DoLS	Deprivation of Liberty Safeguards (E&W)
DMP	Designated Medical Practitioner (Scotland)
DPP	Director of Public Prosecutions
DSM-5	APA *Diagnostic and Statistical Manual*, 5th Edition
DSPD	Dangerous & Severely Personality Disordered
DTO	Detention and Training Order (E&W)
DVLA	Driver and Vehicle Licensing Agency (UK)
DVPO	Domestic Violence Prevention Order (UK)
ECG	Electrocardiogram
ECHR	European Convention on Human Rights & Fundamental Freedoms
ECtHR	European Court of Human Rights
ECT	Electroconvulsive Therapy
EDR	Expected Date of Release
EEG	Electroencephalogram
EGVE	Ending Gang Violence and Exploitation
EIS/T	Early Intervention (in psychosis) Service/Team
EMDR	Eye Movement Desensitisation Reprogramming
EPA	Enduring Power of Attorney (RoI)
EPSE	Extra-pyramidal Side Effects
EQUIP	Equipping Peers to Help One Another
ERASOR	Estimate of Risk of Adolescent Sexual Offence Recidivism
ETS	Enhanced Thinking Skills
EU	European Union
EUPD	emotionally unstable personality disorder
E&W	England & Wales
EWO	Education Welfare Officer
FASD	Foetal Alcohol Spectrum Disorder
FBI	Federal Bureau of Investigation (US)
FCAMHS	Forensic CAMHS
FFT	Functional Family Therapy
FIPP	Firesetting Intervention Programme for Prisoners
FME	Forensic Medical Examiner (formerly known as police surgeon)
FMHU	Forensic Mental Health Unit
fMRI	Functional Magnetic Resonance Imaging
FRQ	Forensic Restrictiveness Questionnaire
FSH	Follicle-Stimulating Hormone
FTTMH	First Tier Tribunal (Mental Health) (E&W)
GAD	Generalised Anxiety Disorder
GBH	Grievous Bodily Harm
GCS	Glasgow Coma Scale
GMC	General Medical Council (UK)
GnRH	gonadotrophin releasing hormone
GP	General Practitioner
GRC	Gender Recognition Certificate
HCA	Health Care Assistants
HCP	Health Care Professional
HCPC	Health & Care Professions Council (UK)
HCPTS	Health & Care Professions Tribunal Service (UK)
HCR20	Historical, Clinical & Risk Management 20-Item Scale
HIW	Healthcare Inspectorate Wales
HLA	human leukocyte antigen
HMP	Her Majesty's Prison
HMPPS	Her Majesty's Prison and Probation Services

HMRC	Her Majesty's Revenue and Customs		LPS	Liberty Protection Safeguards (E&W)
HoNOS	Health of the Nation Outcome Scale		LREC	Local Research Ethics Committee (UK)
HR	Human Resources		LSU	Low Secure Unit
HSE	Health Service Executive (Ireland)		MACI	Millon Adolescent Clinical Inventory
IAPT	Improving Access to Psychological Therapies		MAO	Monoamine Oxidase (MAOA, type A; MAOB, type B)
ID	Intellectual Disability		MAPPA	Multi-Agency Public Protection Arrangements (E&W, Scotland)
ICD11	WHO *International Classification of Diseases*, 11th Edition		MAPPP	Multi-Agency Public Protection Panel
ICJ	International Court of Justice, The Hague		MARAC	Multi-Agency Risk Assessment Conferences
ICS	Integrated Care System (UK)/ Indefinite Custodial Sentence (NI), Indeterminate Custodial Sentences		MASH	Multi-Agency Safeguarding Hub
			MBT	Mentalisation-Based Therapy
IM	Impression Management		MC	Medical Council (RoI)
IMCA	Independent Mental Capacity Advocate (E&W)		MCA	Mental Capacity Act 2005 (E&W)
IMHA	Independent Mental Health Advocate (E&W)		MCANI	Mental Capacity Act (Northern Ireland) 2016
IMR	Inmate Medical Record (in prison)		MDO	Mentally Disordered Offender
			MDT	multidisciplinary team
IPP	Indeterminate sentence of imprisonment for Public Protection		MHA	Mental Health Act (E&W 1983; RoI 2001)
IPS	Individual Placement and Support		MHC	Mental Health Commission (NI, RoI)
IPT	Interpersonal Therapy		MHCTA	Mental Health (Care and Treatment) (Scotland) Act 2003
IPV	Intimate Partner Violence			
IQ	Intelligence Quotient		MHNIO	Mental Health (Northern Ireland) Order 1986
IRA	Irish Republican Army			
IRMS	Integrated Risk Management Services		MHO	Mental Health Officer (Scotland; a social worker)
IRRMS	Intensive Risk and Rehabilitation Managements Services		MHRT	Mental Health Review Tribunal (NI, RoI)
ISSP	Intensive Supervision and Surveillance Programme		MHT	Mental Health Tribunal (Scotland)
IT	Information Technology		MHU	Mental Health Unit (of the Ministry of Justice, E&W)
JP	Justice of the Peace		MI	Motivational Interviewing (or Mental Illness)
LA	Local Authority			
LALY	Liberty-Adjusted Life Year		MoCA	Model of Creative Ability
LD	Learning Disability		MoHO	Model of Human Occupation
LED	Licence Expiry Date		MoJ	Ministry of Justice
LH	Luteinising Hormone		MPCS	MacArthur Perceived Coercion Scale
LHB	Local Health Board (Wales)		MPTS	Medical Practitioners Tribunal Service (UK)
LPA	Lasting Power of Attorney (E&W)			

MREC	Multi-centre Research Ethics Committee (UK)	PCSO	Police Community Support Officer
MRI	(Structural) Magnetic Resonance Imaging	PD	Personality Disorder
MST	Multi-Systemic Therapy	PDS	Paulhus Deception Scale
MSU	Medium Secure Unit	PED	Parole Eligibility Date
MWC	Mental Welfare Commission (Scotland)	PET	Positron Emission Tomography
NA	Narcotics Anonymous (or Noradrenaline)	PICU	Psychiatric Intensive Care Unit
		PIPE	Psychologically Informed Prison Environment
NAPO	National Association of Probation Officers (E&W)	PPANI	Public Protection Arrangements for Northern Ireland (cf. MAPPA)
NCA	National Crime Agency		
NCISS	National Council of Investigation and Security Services (US)	PPD	Paranoid Personality Disorder
		PPG	Penile Plethysmograph
NDD	neurodevelopmental disorder	PREM	Patient-Related Experience Measure
NFA	No Fixed Abode/No Further Action	PRN	Pro Re Nata (as required)
NHS	National Health Service (UK)	PROM	Patient-Related Outcome Measure
NI	Northern Ireland		
NICE	National Institute of Health and Clinical Excellence (UK)	PSA	Professional Standards Authority
		PSR	Presentence Report
NIMHE	National Institute for Mental Health (England)	PTSD	Posttraumatic Stress Disorder
		QALY	Quality-Adjusted Life Year
NMBI	Nursing & Midwifery Board of Ireland (RoI)	QTc	Q-T interval (corrected for heart rate)
NMC	Nursing & Midwifery Council (UK)	RA	Responsible Authority
		RC	Responsible Clinician (E&W)
NPD	Non-Parole Date	RCPsych	Royal College of Psychiatrists (UK)
NPS	National Probation Service (E&W)	RDS	Research Development and Statistics
OASys	Offender Assessment System		
OCD	Obsessive-Compulsive Disorder	REBT	Rational emotive behavior therapy
		REC	Research Ethics Committee
ODD	Oppositional Defiant Disorder	RoI	Republic of Ireland
OLR	Order for Lifelong Restriction	RMA	Risk Management Authority (Scotland)
ONS	Office for National Statistics (UK)	RMO	Responsible Medical Officer (Scotland, NI)
ONSET	An Assessment Tool Used by YOTs	RMP	Registered Medical Practitioner
OPD	Offender with Personality Disorder	R&R	Reasoning & Rehabilitation programme
OT	Occupational Therapy		
PACE	Police and Criminal Evidence Act 1984 (E&W) / Order 1989 (NI)	RSA	Road Safety Authority (RoI)
		RSU	Regional Secure Unit (may comprise both MSU and LSU)
PCC	Police & Crime Commissioner		
PCL-R / -YV	Psychopathy Checklist (Revised / Youth Version)	RSVP	Risk of Sexual Violence Protocol
PCN	Primary Care Network (England)		

SAMM	Support After Murder and Manslaughter		TC	Therapeutic Community
SAVRY	Structured Assessment of Violence Risk in Youth		TCO	Threat Control Override
			TD	Tardive Dyskinesia (Persistent Oro-facial Dyskinesia)
SCPO	Serious Crime Prevention Order (UK)		TDCS	Transcranial Direct Current Stimulation
SDE	Self-Deceptive Enhancement		TOMM	Test of Memory Malingering
SED	Sentence Expiry Date		TPIM	Terrorism Prevention and Investigation Measure (UK)
SFT	Schema-Focused Therapy			
SHPO	Sexual Harm Prevention Order (UK)		TWOC	Taking (a Vehicle) Without Consent
SIFA	Screening Interview for Adolescents		UK	United Kingdom
			UN	United Nations
SMI	Severe (and enduring) Mental Illness		US	United States (of America)
			VAF	Vulnerability Assessment Framework
SNASA	Salford Needs Assessment Schedule for Adolescents		VBP	Values-Based Practice
SOAD	Second Opinion Appointed Doctor		VOO	Violent Offender Order (UK)
			VRAG	violence risk appraisal guide
SOAP	Sex Offender Assessment Pack		WEMSS	Women's Enhanced Medium Secure Service (E&W)
SOTP	Sex Offender Treatment Programme			
			WHO	World Health Organisation
SPECT	Single Photon Emission Computed Tomography		WMA	World Medical Association
SPR	Scope of Parental Responsibility		WPA	Welfare Power of Attorney (Scotland)/World Psychiatric Association
SQIFA	Screening Questionnaire Interview for Adolescents		YISP	Youth Inclusion and Support Panel
STC	Secure Training Centre		YJA/B	Youth Justice Agency (NI) / Board (E&W)
STEPPS	Systems Training for Emotional Predictability and Problem Solving		YJS	Youth Justice System (cf. CJS)
			YOI	Young Offender Institution
SVP	sexually violent predator		YOT	Youth Offending Team
TBI	Traumatic Brain Injury		YRO	Youth Rehabilitation Order
TBS	Terbeschikkingsteling (Dutch system similar to DSPD)			

Part I

Introduction to the handbook

Chapter 1

Introduction to the handbook

Welcome

We hope you enjoy this second edition of the *Oxford Specialist Handbook of Forensic Psychiatry*; we have enjoyed writing it. Whether you are an established psychiatrist brushing up on the <u>Pritchard criteria</u> (p.602) before entering the witness box, a trainee psychiatrist drafting your first <u>risk assessment</u> (p.164) or a lawyer looking for guidance on the likely quality of a psychiatric <u>expert witness</u> (pp.654–659), we hope you will find it a useful and reassuring pocket guide.

The model of the handbook is unchanged. However, it is now accompanied by a companion volume, the *Oxford Casebook of Forensic Psychiatry*, intended to give practical decision making guidance on the use of the information set out in the handbook.

Forensic psychiatry, which expresses a domain of medical jurisprudence, comprises offending behaviour in mental disorder (clinical forensic psychiatry), plus law in relation to all psychiatry (legal psychiatry): it is an 'interface' discipline. The handbook and casebook aim to be equally useful to clinicians, lawyers, and judges operating on either side of that interface.

No page covers a topic comprehensively, as this would lead to vast duplication, with the same points being raised on many different pages to which they are relevant. Instead, we have cross-referenced between pages.

We have used the following conventions throughout the handbook:

• Abbreviations are used wherever you would encounter them in clinical or legal practice. You can find a list of abbreviations on p.viii.
• We indicate cross-referenced topics by underlining, followed by the page number in brackets (e.g. <u>functional psychosis</u>, p.72).
• Diagnostic terms are those of the <u>DSM-5</u> (p.144) except where otherwise specified.

We have relied heavily on the work of a large number of other authors in the compilation of this handbook, without space for detailed referencing. We thank them all, and acknowledge their copyright in their work. That said, any errors or omissions are our responsibility alone. If you would like to give us feedback, correct a mistake, or make a suggestion, you can do so at www.oup.com/uk/academic/ohfeedback.

A note on jurisdictions

Law and aspects of legal systems relevant to the forensic psychiatrist differ from one country to another. Our primary focus is on the three UK jurisdictions (England & Wales, Scotland, and Northern Ireland), plus the Republic of Ireland (RoI). However, the companion casebook is, by its design, capable, we hope, of use across a wide range of Commonwealth and other <u>common law</u> (p.368) jurisdictions.

Using this handbook

Currency of the law

Organization of the handbook

Our approach to the law

Using this handbook

Our philosophy

This book is for everyone who is interested in, or encounters practitioners of, forensic psychiatry and related disciplines. It focuses on the relationship between psychiatry and law, and the clinical practices that underpin it.

We aim to enable readers to find out some of the key facts and issues within a given topic simply, rapidly, and in an easily digestible form. The handbook therefore promotes brevity and ease of reference, at the expense of detail, and with some over-simplification. For example, the prevalence figures for the mental disorders listed on pages 72 to 119 are derived from a variety of studies that use different definitions of the disorders in question, occasionally use different prevalence periods (although it is usually one year), and cover different populations.

Organisation of the handbook

The handbook is divided into four main parts (II to V), which are intended to be complementary in presenting both clinical forensic psychiatry and legal psychiatry. We have used detailed cross-referencing of topics.

A clinician dealing with a man exhibiting personality disorder (PD) might begin by looking at pages within Part II dealing with the clinical assessment and treatment of PD and its behavioural manifestations from a specific forensic perspective, then be cross-referred to pages in Part IV for information about a criminal charge and process faced by their patient, and then refer to Part V for information about legal tests to which PD might be relevant. They might later wish to seek guidance in Part III on how they might ethically decide whether to recommend treatment in hospital, in the knowledge that the risk assessment could be used by the court instead as a basis for the imposition of indeterminate penal sentencing.

A lawyer dealing with the same man, as a defendant, might look for guidance in understanding the clinical concepts in the psychiatrist's court report, or the risk assessment offered to the court, within Part II, and then be referred to pages in Part V, concerning the court report and how it might be probed in cross-examination.

Our approach to the law

Although we have written extensively about many areas of law in the handbook, we have self-consciously not tried to write a legal textbook. The aim of the handbook is to summarise and describe areas of law of relevance to the <u>interface between law and psychiatry</u> (p.351). This necessarily implies that we do not always write in the technically precise manner of legal texts. However, by sometimes adopting a different approach we hope that the handbook will be of use to both medical and legal experts, from their different sides of the frontier. Where we refer to a legal case its citation appears either immediately within the text or, if the case is either particularly important or the relationship between its clinical psychiatric aspects and legal issues is of particular interest, then both the citation and a summary of its facts and legal analysis appear within the appendix, Legal Cases.

One of the difficulties of writing a handbook of psychiatry and law is that fact and opinion in both fields is changing rapidly, particularly in the UK and Ireland, in the early years of the twenty-first century. We have tried to ensure that we have reflected accurately the position in the four jurisdictions of the UK and Ireland as of mid-2020, and have referred to impending changes where appropriate.

Clinical forensic psychiatry and legal psychiatry

Clinical forensic psychiatry is concerned with the assessment and treatment of mental disorder where it appears to be associated with offending behaviour. A clear understanding of law is therefore necessary in order to practise clinically. For example, it is not possible to transfer your patient out of the criminal justice system into hospital, or to write a report to aid your client in compensation proceedings, without knowledge of the relevant law.

Legal psychiatry comprises all law relating to mental disorder and its treatment and care. The relationship between psychiatry and the law is bilateral, including the giving of psychiatric evidence in a wide variety of civil and criminal legal contexts, and the use of law for clinical purposes and for the regulation of clinical practice.

Why all psychiatry is forensic psychiatry

All psychiatrists must be acquainted with those areas of law that bear directly on treating and managing their patients. These include mental health and mental capacity law (pp.462–545), the law and procedures relating to public protection (p.592, p.252, pp.296–301) and report-writing (pp.678–710) for courts and mental health tribunals. Psychiatrists do not need to become 'quasi-lawyers', but they do need to be 'frontier' professionals capable of recognising and understanding legal questions, knowing how to prepare evidence relevant to those questions, and being capable of understanding how lawyers and courts reason and make decisions.

Tensions between law and psychiatry

The purposes of a discipline and the interests of its practitioners determine the constructs it uses. Constructs in psychiatry are determined by its pursuit of human welfare, including through understanding disorder in order to reverse or manage it, or its effects. By contrast, law pursues abstract justice, though it may sometimes involve balancing the welfare of different parties against one another, or against societal welfare.[1]

Even within one discipline, different branches often give rise to different approaches to determining constructs. For example, since criminal law is concerned with culpability (p.354), its definitions of *mental disorder* are characteristically tight, and address justice, not human welfare. By contrast, the constructs utilised in sentencing, often focused upon determining the degree of culpability, or relating to public protection, are more loosely defined. In turn, these differ from the constructs of aetiology and treatment used in Medicine and Psychology.

The balance struck between patient welfare and public protection is bound to differ between mental health professionals and legal agencies. Psychiatry and law address related concerns with potentially different values (pp.281–291). Negotiating the interface (p.358) between the two is both difficult and crucially important.

---

1 Justice from the perspective of the individual (i.e. proportionality, p.355, or 'just deserts'). There are other meanings to *justice*—see the discussion on p.352 and elsewhere.

Forensic services and teams

Criminal justice and court services

Almost any professional group can offer forensic testimony. There are forensic entomologists and forensic accountants, as well as forensic pathologists. Psychologists and psychiatrists who give expert testimony act as 'forensic' professionals, regardless of their clinical practice.

Clinical mental health services for offenders may be offered by general psychiatrists, rehabilitation psychiatrists, substance misuse services or any psychiatrist working in a secure setting or court diversion service (p.268).

Mental health services in prison

British and Irish prisons receive mental health inreach services (p.270), provided in the UK by the NHS, and usually comprising community psychiatric nurses and visiting psychiatrists, often with a dedicated healthcare centre. Prisons may also ask for opinions from the catchment area psychiatrist (typically a general psychiatrist working in psychiatric intensive care, or a forensic psychiatrist if secure hospital treatment is thought necessary).

In addition to the psychiatric services into prisons, many prisons also retain their own psychology service staffed by forensic psychologists.

Secure psychiatric services

The professionals who work in secure mental health services (p.258) include the same disciplines expected in any mental health service, although often in greater abundance. Some secure services will also employ forensic psychologists because of their expertise in offender management programmes. Generally, however, the distinguishing feature of any 'forensic' mental health professional is that they have experience of working with severely mentally disordered men and women, usually with long and/or significant histories of violence, and often in long-stay residential care.

Specific staff groups found in forensic multidisciplinary teams

Most clinical forensic MDTs consist of psychiatrists, psychologists, nurses, occupational therapists, social workers, and sometimes a creative/forensic psychotherapist (e.g. music/drama and/or arts therapist).

Forensic psychiatrists are psychiatrists with further higher training in the subspecialty of forensic psychiatry. Typically, though not always, they chair or lead MDTs. They often hold legal responsibility for the patient as responsible clinician or responsible medical officer (RMO, p.468). They will be supported by a specialist **pharmacist**.

Clinical psychologists working in forensic settings have undertaken general training in Clinical Psychology to doctorate level. Within forensic services they usually have expertise in risk assessment, and the use of specialist psychological tools and treatment programmes that involve psychological techniques such as cognitive and behavioural therapies (p.206). Psychology services also include assistant psychologists who are professionals, who typically have an undergraduate degree but have not yet gained a place on a clinical training course, and/or trainee psychologists, who are currently completing the doctoral course.

Forensic psychologists are, by training, quite distinct from clinical psychologists, typically having a master's degree in their subject. They usually address offending behaviour, often not in the context of mental disorder. Hence, they often carry out risk assessments and oversee the <u>psychological treatment programme for offenders</u> (p.220), particularly in prisons. They may or may not have general mental health experience.

The <u>nurses</u> (p.224) in forensic mental health services have different roles depending on the service setting. **Qualified nurses** have a specialist mental health nursing qualification and manage the more junior nursing staff. **Health care assistants** may be unqualified; **associate practitioners** may have an undergraduate degree (such as in Psychology) and basic nursing training. Community teams include nurses whose role is to make good therapeutic relationships with patients, and act in liaison between the patient, the patient's carers and the rest of the MDT. In secure residential settings, nurses also take the lead responsibility for <u>relational security</u> (p.224), together with specialist security staff who manage <u>physical</u> and <u>procedural security</u> (p.190). They may have the best understanding of patients' mental state and thought patterns; they are also subject to the greatest stress and anxiety in the MDT because of their prolonged close patient contact.

The **occupational therapist** (p.228) is trained to understand the effects of mental disorder on work and creative function, and to offer interventions that promote recovery. They typically work closely with both psychologists and nursing staff, especially in inpatient settings.

The **social worker** (p.226) in a forensic MDT may or may not have specialist forensic experience. They typically have a degree in social work; then acquire mental health experience.

Forensic psychotherapists are trained <u>psychotherapists</u> (p.204) who have specialised in working with mentally disordered offenders. They may or may not be medically qualified. They may work in specialist services or provide consultation and supervision for forensic multidisciplinary teams. They may deliver individual or group interventions. There are few such posts in the UK; emphasising the need for forensic psychiatrists to develop some psychotherapeutic skills.

Probation officers (p.584) may be involved in supervision of mentally disordered offenders in the community, usually in collaboration with mental health professionals. Interventions may include measures aimed at risk reduction and rehabilitation. They also take on particular roles with sex offenders, and commonly co-ordinate sex offender interventions, sometimes with mental health service involvement. They may work jointly with forensic psychiatrists in the production of presentence reports.

Criminologists study crime and criminals, and do not, in the UK or RoI, have direct involvement in the care of mentally disordered offenders. The impact of criminological research is, however, widespread and seen throughout this handbook, since many mentally disordered offenders are driven to offend not only in the context of their mental disorder but also by criminogenic factors.

Who became the forensic psychiatrists?

The modern forensic psychiatrist combines up to three historical roles: the physician tending the mentally unwell, the superintendent of the asylum, and the expert witness to the court. Each of the three has its own origins.

Physicians

Physicians—appliers of specialised knowledge in order to treat the sick, distinct from a religious role of ministering to the sick—can be recognised as long ago as Egypt in the twenty-seventh century BCE. A theme common to early medicine across many cultures, including Europe, India, China, and the Islamic world, is that physicians dealt only with physical health: mental ill-health was not seen as a 'medical' problem at all, but rather as a personal, family one, mostly dealt with informally by extended family networks (except for people who were rich or of high social status, who could afford personal physicians to treat their mental illnesses). Only with the beginning of the industrial era in the West from the eighteenth century onwards, and the associated dislocation of families and disruption of kinship networks, did mental illness become a social problem requiring the intervention of specialised social actors and social institutions.

Asylum superintendents

People with mental illness who were poor or of low social status were committed to lunatic asylums, which were originally nonmedical institutions. Over time these went from being progressive institutions that aimed to offer a human sanctuary to the distressed, to overcrowded 'bins' whose chief aim was the removal of the obviously mentally ill from the streets. Treatment was rarely available. Each asylum was presided over by a superintendent, who might or might not be medically qualified, but even if so, did not treat inmates personally, but merely oversaw the unqualified 'lunatic attendants'. Nineteenth-century asylums in the UK included those developed specifically to deal with the 'criminally insane', first at the Bethlem Hospital and then Broadmoor Hospital, built for the purpose.

Psychiatrists

With the dissemination in the early twentieth century of new scientific (or sometimes pseudo-scientific) developments—such as Kraepelin's identification and classification of psychotic disorders, Charcot's research on hypnosis and hysteria and Freud's establishment of psychoanalysis—practitioners of psychiatry, who now had an institutional home in the asylums, were recognised as a single profession with a specialised body of knowledge. Psychiatrists, now so called, edged out office-based neurologists from the treatment of mental illness.

Psychiatry consolidated its professional position during the twentieth century, with armies turning to it after the First and Second World Wars to treat their 'shell-shocked' soldiers (which led to the development of group therapy, p.214), and with the discovery of antipsychotics (p.200)—which presaged the ascendancy of biological psychiatry and the side-lining of psychoanalysis. During the latter half of the century, psychiatric subspecialties developed alongside the biological/psychoanalytic division, such as child psychiatry, liaison psychiatry (providing advice and psychiatric care to patients of other medical specialties), and community psychiatry.

Forensic psychiatrists

The forensic subspecialty was a relatively late arrival, separating from mainstream general psychiatry largely because of two developments, one institutional and one ethical. In the UK, although there had been an isolated body of (with hindsight) recognisably 'forensic' practitioners in prisons and the special hospitals (p.258), the development of the regional secure units (RSUs, p.258) from the 1980s onwards led to the establishment of a group of psychiatrists with a distinctively different role (i.e. caring for patients detained in a secure hospital environment, or in prison), who were numerous enough to develop their own subprofessional identity and their own Faculty of the Royal College of Psychiatrists. In a very different vein, and partly to sidestep any perceived compromise of their ethical position as doctors (p.298), many psychiatrists in the USA who had traditionally concentrated on assessment of defendants or litigants for the courts, rather than treating patients, redesignated themselves as 'forensicists' and sought separate recognition in the American Academy of Psychiatry and Law. Thus, somewhat divergent ethical and clinical traditions of forensic psychiatry were established in the USA and Europe, according to whether the doctor's primary duty was seen as being to the patient or to the State via aiding the administration of justice or public protection.

Expert witnesses

The role of the expert witness (p.652) can be traced back to the Roman Empire, with courts accepting evidence from physicians, amongst others. However, as dealing with mental illness was not yet seen as part of medicine, judges and juries regarded themselves as competent to decide questions of insanity. Only in the nineteenth century, as asylums spread and those administering them came to be seen as experts, did courts begin to defer to psychiatric expert witnesses.

History & future of forensic psychiatry

The origins of what are now called forensic psychiatric services are found first in the provision of secure residential care for people with mental illnesses who committed serious offences and second in concerns about the mental health of prisoners.

Madness has been seen to be associated with unpredictable violence since Roman times. However, until the nineteenth century, families were largely responsible for the care of their dangerous relatives. Long before the emergence of forensic psychiatrists (p.13), special facilities were created to manage mentally disordered offenders. Chiefly because of the effects of the Criminal Lunatics Act 1800 (p.462), two new wings of Bethlem Hospital were opened in 1816 to accommodate high-risk patients who needed long-term supervision in a secure setting. In 1853, Broadmoor Hospital (p.258) was built to accommodate overcrowding in the Bethlem units, three years after the Central Mental Hospital in Ireland, which took offenders as well as other patients.

People with mental illness who offend

In Victorian times, mental health care focused on 'asylum', indefinite residential detention safe from the rest of society. It was envisaged that patients would live in the hospitals for the rest of their lives, meaning many of the early residents of Broadmoor Hospital would not now be seen as needing high secure care. The concept of different levels of security need arose in the wake of the closure of the county asylums, and increasing understanding of mental disorders as being treatable.

After the opening of two further high secure hospitals in England in the twentieth century, plus the State Hospital in Scotland, there was, much later, the development of RSUs (p.258) in the UK, as recommended by the Butler inquiry (p.780) in 1974; it and other contemporaneous reports also recommended increased provision for prisoners with mental health needs, women patients, offender patients from different ethnic backgrounds and offenders with PD, plus court diversion (p.268).

Mentally disordered men and women in hospitals who posed a risk to others were managed exclusively by general psychiatrists until the subspecialty of forensic psychiatry emerged in the 1970s. Thereafter, forensic psychiatrists took over the management of higher-risk patients, whilst leaving general psychiatrists to care for a large number of patients who still posed a significant risk of harm to others.

Prisoners with mental health needs

Professional concerns about the risk posed by the mentally disordered proceeded in parallel with public health concerns about the mental wellbeing of prisoners. Prisoners who became mentally ill in prison (or were ill on arrival) needed to be transferred to psychiatric services secure enough to prevent most escapes. In part, the development of secure mental health services was driven by the results of epidemiological studies that showed very high levels of mental illness and PD in prisons, most notably the ONS studies (p.781).

Serendipity and disaster

The development of services for people who commit crimes whilst mentally disordered has often occurred in response to high-profile 'disasters', and associated public anxiety about the risk of violence that those with mental disorders may pose—rather than rational <u>needs assessment</u> (p.276). However, most people with mental disorder do not commit violent crimes (see p.44), and most prisoners who need mental health services are serving sentences for nonviolent offences.

A good example of how service development can be driven by publicity rather than evidence-based policy was the development of the former <u>DSPD services</u> (p.781) in E&W. Over £140 million was spent developing services for the needs of 2,000 men who were thought to be at especially high risk of violence. However, the programme was inefficient, and much less effective in risk reduction than community substance misuse and rehabilitation programmes. The hospital DSPD programme has been scrapped, in favour of the offender personality disorder pathway, which includes some hospital, but predominantly prison, provision.

The future of forensic psychiatry

The debate at the time of the Butler report about making prisons therapeutic institutions was rapidly won by those in favour of creating separate secure hospitals instead. The debate then shifted to the extent to which the secure hospitals and forensic psychiatrists should be separate from general psychiatric hospitals and psychiatrists. Initially, there was almost complete separation in the UK, and forensic institutions grew to consume almost 15% of all NHS funding for mental health, despite treating fewer than 0.1% of the patients receiving mental health care from the NHS.

This situation was clearly unsustainable both financially and ethically (as it led to a sense that all the 'bad objects' were somewhere else), and there has been gradual reintegration of forensic services, and forensic patients, into mainstream psychiatry. This has had the beneficial effect of spreading some forensic expertise into general psychiatry, with risk assessment and legal knowledge being particular examples. However, complete integration would likely be unsustainable: medical services overall tend to become more rather than less specialised because research consistently shows that the best outcomes of complex interventions are obtained by practitioners who practise it frequently rather than only occasionally.

Part II

Clinical forensic psychiatry

Clinical and social aspects of crime

Crime to the forensic psychiatrist

Forensic psychiatry and crime

Forensic psychiatrists are generally referred a subgroup of criminal offenders, for either of two reasons:

Concerns that the offender is mentally disordered
- Where an alleged or convicted offender has a history of mental illness.
- Before trial (p.566), where mental disorder may be a ground for diversion (p.268) on bail or while on remand.
- At sentencing (pp.442–444), when a treatment order (pp.500–502) is considered.
- While an offender is serving a sentence, especially in prison (p.270).
- After an offender has been released and is under supervision.

Concerns that the offence is unusual and odd
- Crimes involving great or unusual cruelty to the victim.
- Crimes committed by someone unusual, such as a child or elderly person.
- When a defence team hopes that a psychological explanation may appeal to a jury or judge, and affect the likelihood of conviction (p.407) or be taken in mitigation (p.638) of the offence.
- When the prosecution think that psychological or psychiatric testimony may properly lead to an extended (pp.442, 448) or indeterminate sentence (p.449) on risk grounds.

General psychiatric colleagues may also seek advice where a patient's mental disorder poses a risk of harm to others, and treatment may reduce their risk of offending.

Conflicts and confusions

Forensic psychiatrists may disagree on their role in the criminal justice system (pp.8 298):
- Some argue that their predominant role is to **diagnose and treat mental disorders**, and only address risk of offending if it is functionally linked to mental disorder.
- Others argue that their role is to **assist in the psychological explanation** of serious crimes, and if possible to **reduce the risk of reoffending** by whatever means, including nontherapeutic means.

Each position raises its own problems for the profession and for the individual practitioner because the association between mental disorder and violence (p.44) is not straightforward nor, usually, can the violence be managed (p.240) solely by addressing the mental disorder; because British (or at least English) society in particular expects forensic psychiatrists to contribute to public protection (p.592) and because there are unavoidable ethical role conflicts (pp.298, 314, 318) between being a doctor and working with the criminal justice system. Each strand of opinion resolves these conflicts in its own way.

Violence, crime, and mental disorder

<u>Crime statistics</u> (p.22) provide a picture of criminal rule-breaking behaviour. The commonest type of criminal rule-breaking is theft and other types of acquisitive offences. Only 20% of recorded crime involves physical violence, and only a minority of those offences will cause serious physical harm.

Debate continues as to whether violence is uncommon but normal behaviour (given its occurrence in all human societies) or whether it is an abnormal behaviour arising from at least an unusual mental state (given its comparative rarity as a form of social rule-breaking). Whichever view is taken, there is good quality evidence that some mental disorders can be a <u>risk factor for violence</u> (pp.166, 180), usually in combination with other risk factors.

Prevalence and measurement of crime

There are several difficulties in establishing how rates of crime differ, either between different regions or in one place over time. Court records and rates of conviction and imprisonment are of some use, but the most reliable and commonly cited measures are national and international police records of crime (e.g. the European Sourcebook) and household surveys of victimisation (e.g. the British Crime Survey (BCS)). See Box 2.1

> ### Box 2.1 Sources of comparative crime statistics
> British Crime Survey
> US National Crime Survey
> European Sourcebook of Crime & Criminal Justice Statistics
> Home Office Research Development & Statistics publications
> UN International Crime Victims Survey
> US Department of Justice World Factbook of Criminal Justice Systems

These measures give an indication of the frequency of specific crimes and, if the crimes are repeated, the measures can be used to estimate trends over time.

For example, the 2019-20 BCS shows that the proportion of people who were a victim of violent crimes was 1.6% in E&W, compared to 3% in 2007-8. More generally, it shows that total crime in all the UK nations, which rose inexorably throughout the twentieth century, has fallen steadily from 1996 to the present. In RoI, by contrast, rates of violent crime have risen between 2010 and 2020, when over 2% of adults were victims of violence.

Comparative prevalence figures for different countries can be found on pages for individual crimes (e.g. homicide, p.46; stalking, p.52; and sexual assault, p.56). Some broad international patterns, all expressed as rates per 100,000 citizens per year, include:

- The clear gap in crime rates between continental European countries and the 'Anglosphere' (USA, UK, Canada, Australia, and New Zealand) that existed ten years ago has vanished: the former range from 21.6 (Switzerland) to 47.3 (France); the latter from 40.6 (Canada) to 47.7 (USA).
- The UK rate on the same survey is 44.5; RoI's 45.7, and Sweden's surprisingly 47.4.
- The USA, Russia, and many Eastern European countries have higher rates of murder (5.0–8.2) than Australia, New Zealand, the UK, and other Western European countries (0.7–1.2).
- El Salvador has the world's highest murder rate (52.0); all of the top-ten countries are in Central and South America, with the exception of South Africa (36.4).
- Property offences such as burglary show a very different pattern from violent offences, with for example the rate in otherwise peaceful New Zealand (1353.6) being vastly higher than that in Eastern Europe and Slovakia (83.0).
- In general, Middle Eastern and other Islamic countries report lower rates of most crimes than Western or former Eastern Bloc countries.

- Finland arrests or cautions more of its population (8233.9) than Anglosphere countries (USA 3152.3, New Zealand 2045.5, and Canada 2751.1); other European countries tend to have even lower rates.

The data from which such interpretations are made are not perfect. Problems with official figures include:

- Misleading and internationally inconsistent definitions of crimes (e.g. rape, p.56, includes consensual sex with a minor in the USA, whereas in E&W this is a different crime: see p.58).
- Reported crime statistics can be inflated by multiple charges arising from the same instance of crime, especially in property offences.
- Crimes may not be reported to the police. In 2017–18, only 11% of violent crimes in E&W led to criminal charges. Under-reporting may be influenced by local culture and expectations (e.g. a man may not report domestic violence by his wife, fearing stigma, or if reported, it may not be recognised as 'domestic violence' but categorised differently).
- Changes in the reporting and recording of crimes may lead to a misleading impression of increasing crime. For example, from 2015 to 2017 in the UK, the rate of police-recorded sexual offences and violent crimes more than doubled. However, this trend was not seen in the BCS.
- The statistics are typically collected for political reasons (e.g. to assess the performance of the police service), not to describe social reality in a neutral fashion.
- They are not a complete record of criminal offences known to the authorities. For example, in E&W some include 'Notifiable offences' (those tried in a Crown Court, p.384) but not 'Summary offences' (those dealt with by lower courts).
- There are changes over time in what is counted for the purposes of inclusion into the official records.

Victimisation surveys attempt to overcome these difficulties: typically surveys of a randomly selected representative group conducted by a neutral organisation. Their own limitations include:

- Omission of crimes without identifiable victims (e.g. fare evasion, drug possession) or where victims cannot be surveyed (e.g. children).
- Recall and response biases determined by surveyed victims (e.g. greater chances of remembering more traumatic crimes, or middle-class respondents might classify some acts as crimes that working class respondents might regard as noncriminal behaviour).

Both sets of figures, some sociologists aver, cannot ever be reliable because whatever their source they rely on someone interpreting and classifying a series of events, and this process of the construction of meaning is inevitably determined as much by social structures, ideologies, and values as by anything intrinsic to the events themselves.

Psychology & philosophy of volition

Philosophy of volition

In *Nicomachean Ethics*, Aristotle argued that people are not responsible for actions they have not freely chosen. This argument has continued to be the basis for attributing criminal responsibility: essentially, you are only responsible for actions that are under your **volition** (from the Latin, *Volo*, meaning 'I want', i.e. that you have freely chosen with knowledge of the meaning and possible consequences).

Philosophical debates often address the extent to which people feel compelled to do actions they do not really intend or whether you can be responsible for actions with unintended and unforeseen consequences. You may be less to blame if you can show that you did not intend the outcome of your choices or you intended some positive outcome (e.g. in palliative care when giving high-dose opiate medication that may relieve pain but also hasten death).

Another philosophical debate involves the question of whether humans are free to make choices. Some philosophers argue that all events (including mental events) are caused by what preceded them, and, therefore, free will does not exist or is an illusion. There are strong counter-arguments against this position: philosophers and lawyers have argued that free will, responsibility, and determinism are metaphysical concepts that cannot be proved through science. The law exists independent of scientific data to regulate relationships between individuals, and the assumption of freely made choices is crucial to social contracts and civic trust.

Neuropsychology of volition

Neuroscientists have attempted to study free will, using neuroimaging to identify parts of the brain activated when people make choices. The orbitofrontal cortex is differentially activated depending on whether the choice-maker feels that they are making a free choice, and neuronal activity takes place before the choice-maker is aware of making a choice. Whether this means that the choice was truly 'free' depends upon whether the subconscious parts of the mind involved are regarded as part of the 'self' that is making the choice.

It is often assumed that people choose actions rationally so as to maximise the probability of achieving their 'best possible goals'. However, studies suggest that humans use differing systems for analysing choices[1] and are influenced by many factors that are not always conscious or based on unbiased appraisal of evidence.

It has been hypothesised by Damasio and others that, whereas long-term goals are selected consciously and through intellectual processes, emotional processing is essential to volition, and that it is this discrepancy that explains the common experience of repeatedly choosing something that conflicts with one's goals (e.g. overeating when trying to lose weight, smoking cigarettes when trying to quit or shopping for luxuries despite wishing to pay off a large overdraft).

1 Collectively known as 'system one' in the work by Kahnemann and others, drawn on elsewhere in the handbook, as opposed to the conscious, rational but slow 'system two'.

Disorders affecting volition

Disorders that damage frontal lobe structures can influence volition (e.g. dementias, p.116). Disorders of movement (e.g. Parkinson's disease) can also affect volition, as can acute intoxication with substances such as cannabis. Schizophrenia (p.73) can also cause a state of avolition, typically with flattened affect. Disorders of volition may also affect the sense of identity (e.g. brain damage rarely affecting sense of ownership of the body).

Addiction (p.76) is not usually seen as a disorder of volition but rather loss of self-regulation and impairment of control. There is research interest into addiction neuropsychology and the relevance of limbic system neurotransmitter function.

Legal and moral responsibility

Assignment of criminal responsibility often rests on an assessment of defendants' volition (i.e. on how, not why, they chose to act).[2] Choices can include choosing to do nothing (e.g. in crimes of omission, p.400); therefore, being reckless (p.403) or negligent (p.403) can represent choices as much as an intention (p.402) to commit an offence.

In moral philosophy, knowledge of an action's wrongness is required for it to be morally blameworthy. In contrast, it is a principle of law that ignorance of the law cannot excuse wrongdoing (see pp.400–413). The law ignores the question of whether the individual had the capacity to take into account the wrongness of the action, and with the exception of children (p.406), holds individuals responsible even if they lacked a capacity for moral reasoning (unless they have other deficits of mental function that render them unfit to plead, p.602). This reflects the different, although overlapping, social functions of law and morality (p.352).

Personal beliefs and professional opinion

Professionals' views about volition and free will may affect how they approach criminal responsibility. Those with a strong belief that neuroscience explains all mental function may take a determinist view that people with mental disorders are not responsible for their actions. Professionals who place a high value on personal autonomy may be more inclined to keep the question of responsibility open, even in cases where people have active symptoms. These views also have influence on risk assessment and management. Practitioners should be aware of their own views, or values, and how they may influence the objectivity of their opinion (p.675).

2 Except in offences of strict liability (p.405).

What is violence?

Violence differs from aggression and anger: the former causes physical harm; the latter psychological or no harm. Not all angry people are aggressive, and regulated aggression is a key part of some sports. All violence has the potential to become severe, but in most countries, severe or fatal violence is a comparatively rare form of crime (see p.22).

Violence risk depends upon the presence of a number of factors operating in combination (as in a bicycle lock). Some violence risk factors are common (e.g. being male, young, and misusing substances). Less-common risk factors include antisocial attitudes and a paranoid mental state. Many individuals may have two or three risk factors but may never be violent, unless or until further risk factors are added.

Definitions

- *Aggression* is intentionally intimidating or gaining advantage over another, without necessarily involving physical injury.
- *Violence* involves using physical force against another person, causing harm.
- *Criminal violence* involves directly injurious behaviour which is against the law, such as <u>sexual offences</u> (pp.418) and <u>arson</u> (p.422).

Instrumental (proactive) violence is for attaining a goal (e.g. armed robbery). It is usually planned and comparatively affectless. The exception is *sadistic violence*, where controlling the victim excites the perpetrator (especially inflicting humiliation); sexual arousal may be present.

Expressive (reactive) violence is usually accompanied by strong affects, particularly hostility, fear, grief or anger. The violence communicates these feelings to the victim, and the perpetrator may not recognise the harm caused. It may be impulsive or planned, and is more likely with substance misuse.

The relational context of violence

The contexts in which men, women, and children become a victim of violence tend to differ in terms of the relationship with the perpetrator.

- **No relationship: violence against strangers**. It is rare for perpetrators to be strangers to their victims. Such violence is more likely to be instrumental and/or political. In the absence of these motives, those who attack strangers are likely to suffer from mental illness, often of a paranoid nature. Males are more at risk of attack by a stranger than women. A minority of child sex offenders target children unknown to them. Stalking perpetrators may target strangers because they 'feel' they know them through a fantasised relationship.
- **Current intimate relationships**. Of victims 60%–70% of victims of violence are known to their abuser, most commonly parents, children, siblings or partners. This is especially true for mentally disordered offenders: 90% of victims are known and usually within the family setting. Domestic violence makes other kinds of violence, such as child abuse and neglect, more likely. The violence is often integral to the relationship and feelings of dependency and need. In the UK, one in four women and one in seven men experience domestic violence. Women's injury rates are higher, and they are five times more likely than men to

suffer sexual attacks. Domestic violence involves a complex relationship between control and dependency (economic or emotional) making it difficult for victims to leave.

- **Former intimate relationships**. Relationship breakdown is a potent trigger for violence. Many victims report that violence escalates when they attempt to end the relationship. Ending the relationship with a perpetrator of violence may lead to stalking (p.52), which significantly increases the risk of serious violence. In one community study, relationship breakdown predicted violence over the following year.
- **Child abuse and neglect**. About one hundred children are killed yearly in E&W, 80% by those in a parental role. Infants younger than one year old are most at risk. Fatal assaults are often preceded by child abuse and neglect; about 10%–16% of children experience abuse or neglect, which carries a significant mortality rate. Sudden fatal assaults on children may be precipitated by crying, especially in young perpetrators with their own histories of childhood adversity. About 11% of women and 3% of men in the UK experience childhood sexual abuse, most commonly in homes with domestic violence or childhood physical abuse. Childhood maltreatment (especially neglect and physical abuse) doubles the odds of violence in adulthood. Witnessing family violence and substance abuse are major risk factors for later interpersonal violence and mental health problems.

Social factors in crime and violence

Criminology explores theories of why crime occurs. There are a range of explanatory models within the discipline: some focus on individual risk factors (such as mental health); others on social factors such as poverty and class. These different models have different policy implications. A more robust approach emphasises the interaction of individual, cultural, and social risk factors, and has been influential in the development of actuarial risk assessment (p.166). Commonly identified factors include:

Economic and health factors

(see also p.36)
- Poverty
- Unemployment
- Chronic physical or mental illness

Familial factors

- Childhood adversity including physical abuse and neglect by carers, parental poor care and harshness, parental criminality, substance misuse, and mental disorder
- High conflict, intra-family violence
- Large family size (associated with neglect and poverty)

Peer factors

- Antisocial peers and little contact with pro-social peers
- Gang membership (p.38)

Educational factors

- Low educational ability
- Low academic attainment
- Lack of parental involvement
- Truancy
- Weak school structure or chaotic environment

Societal factors

- Inequality of income and social status
- Poor access to, or low perceived value of, education
- Poor housing
- Prejudice, on grounds of race, poverty, and geography
- Poor family and community support
- Lack of community cohesion and leadership

Social factors in crime prevention

Many governments attempt to reduce crime rates by tackling the social and economic problems listed above, in the hope that this will lead people who might otherwise have committed crime to engage in more pro-social behaviour, such as obtaining a job and paying taxes. (This makes a particular assumption about criminals' motivation for committing crime.)

Such governments have therefore directed resources towards improving public housing, increasing access to education, expanding social services, and improving local health services, amongst other measures. Some studies have found an apparent resultant reduction in crime rates, but the picture is complex: for example, a reduction in one form of crime (e.g. joyriding, p.428) may occur at the same time as a rise in another form (e.g. robbery, p.426); moreover, the effect of the public spending directed this way may be impossible to disentangle from simultaneous changes in other socioeconomic factors, such as a boom or bust, or increased rates of mobile phone possession amongst school-age children. The same problem plagues assessment of the impact of changes to law and policing: for example, stringent gun control in the UK may have increased knife use in gang violence. These individual, or social, criminogenic factors may appear unrelated to mental disorder, but some (like childhood adversity and social isolation) increase the risk of both mental disorder and criminality, making it difficult to tease out the association between mental disorder and crime (p.44).

Neurobiology of violence

Neurobiological explanations for crime and violence have been studied since Lombroso in the eighteenth century.[3] Violent behaviour is understood to have polygenic influences, with antisocial behaviour being about 50% heritable.

Developments in structural and functional brain imaging have supported studies exploring neurobiology of offenders. Functional neuroimaging examines the brain in activity; PET and SPECT studies estimate metabolism rate in different brain areas. fMRI scans show live responses of the brain in response to stimuli. Most studies compare offenders (usually volunteers from the prison population) with either nonoffenders or nonviolent offenders. Many studies have identified unusual brain activity in violent offenders compared to others; typically, in the amygdala, orbitofrontal cortex, and mesolimbic system.

However, prison studies are problematic because they may be biased in terms of who becomes imprisoned, and of those, who volunteers. Scanning is expensive so sample sizes are small. Statistical power is limited by the behaviour's low base rate. The studies assume that the violence is a homogenous action with the same meaning for every offender; yet the offender who kills his wife in a jealous rage may be very different from the offender who kills a shopkeeper during a robbery, but both may be included in an MRI study of murderers.

Evidence from neuroimaging studies

Several studies focus on offenders with psychopathy (p.90) and antisocial personality disorder (p.82). Abnormality of amygdala and hippocampal function may explain restricted emotional responses to distress and failure to learn by experience. Structural abnormalities in the main white matter tract connecting the amygdala with the orbitofrontal cortex, the uncinate fasciculus, have also been associated with psychopathy. Studies of prefrontal cortex function suggest that these groups may lack impulse control and be socially disinhibited, similar to people with traumatic brain injury (p.112).

However, it is not known how many people commit similar crimes without these traits; nor how many people have these traits but do not commit violence offences. Those in prison or secure care represent a subgroup of offenders who may be especially vulnerable, perhaps because of childhood trauma causing these neural abnormalities.

Genetic and related neuroendocrine studies

Meta-analysis of twin and adoption studies suggests that around 40% of the variability in antisocial behaviour between individuals is explained by genetic factors. Whilst there is increasing evidence that genetic and environmental factors interact with respect to antisocial behaviour, some types of antisocial behaviour appear to be more heritable than others (e.g., children with 'callous-unemotional' (CU) traits). Genetically mediated deficiencies in MAOA activity have been associated with increased levels of violence and

---

3 Lombroso established classical criminology, and averred that criminality was inherited and could be detected through physical defects.

aggression, leading to at least one successful claim that an alleged murderer should be acquitted on the grounds of his low levels of MAOA. Moreover, MAOA activity seems to mediate experiences of childhood abuse and mal-treatment, such that children with high MAOA levels are less likely to display antisocial behaviour when older than are similarly abused children with low MAOA levels.

In mice, the targeted disruption of certain genes has been associated with aggressive behaviour; many such genes have a role in brain development and the function of neurotransmitter systems implicated in aggression (e.g. neuronal nitric oxide synthase and the serotonergic system).

People with CU traits also show endocrine abnormalities, including per-sistently low levels of cortisol (a hormone involved in responding to stress). Low cortisol, and decreased cortisol response to stress appear to be re-lated to cold, unemotional violence (of the sort committed by people with psychopathy), whereas serotonergic dysfunction appears to be associated with emotional, explosive violence.

The evidence from human studies suggests that testosterone has a role in social dominance, but is less clear regarding its role in aggression.

Neurodevelopment and psychopathy

Children with significant CU traits and adults with psychopathy are less able to recognise facial emotional expressions, especially fearful expressions, and they have reduced physiological and behavioural responses to such ex-pressions observed in others. The deficit may be partly attentional: children with CU traits fail to concentrate on the eyes when looking at faces, and telling them to look in the eyes before responding improves their accuracy. It has been hypothesised that a failure from birth to attend specifically to the eyes may impair attachment and bonding with the parent, thereby impairing emotional development.

The amygdala is known to be involved in the processing of emotional stimuli, particularly stimuli indicating fear and submission, and adults with psychopathy show reduced amygdala activation to facial recognition stimuli compared to controls. It is also involved in stimulus-reinforcement learning, and impairment of this function may explain why adults exhibiting psychop-athy find it difficult to learn from punishment or other negative outcomes.

Medicolegal implications

These findings are sometimes cited to argue that perpetrators of serious violence are born with irreversibly abnormal brains. However, some per-petrators of violence do not have abnormal brains, and some people with abnormal brains are never violent. Current evidence does not allow a move from correlation to cause, and even if all violent offenders were shown to have these abnormalities, there would still be legal debates about how the courts should deal with them. Great caution should be exercised in making inferences about criminal responsibility (p.406) and agency (p.407) from neurobiological results.

Adverse childhood experiences

Adverse childhood experiences (ACEs) have been recognised as risk factors for adult physical and mental health problems for many years. They include:

- parental mental illness or substance misuse,
- parental violence,
- exposure to poverty,
- having an incarcerated parent,
- emotional abuse,
- physical abuse,
- sexual abuse, and
- neglect.

The WHO supports the study of ACEs internationally, and publishes a standard measure that can be used for population studies, to inform public health strategies.

Prevalence of adverse childhood experiences

A number of international studies have found that the prevalence of people who suffered four or more kinds of ACE is about 10%. Much higher rates are found in forensic populations: for instance, 46% of prisoners in one Welsh prison in 2019 had experienced four or more kinds of ACE; and 80% had experienced at least one, nearly three times the population baseline. A Norwegian study of female prisoners found that 34% had experienced five or more ACEs. Studies of both male and female sex offenders in the USA also found that very few had experienced no adversity, and nearly half had experienced four or more ACEs.

Impacts of adverse childhood experiences

Individuals who are exposed to four or more kinds of ACE are at considerably increased risk of developing significant physical ill-health and problems such as substance misuse, mood disorders, and self-harming behaviours.

Exposure to childhood adversity is also associated with violent offending. Two US studies have indicated that the risk of violence increases with every additional ACE. One of these studies compared one-off violent offenders with those who had committed multiple violent offences and found higher ACE scores in the latter group.

The mechanisms by which exposure to early childhood adversity and increased violence risk in adulthood are not yet clear, but the relationship is not likely to be directly causal. The ACE score is a proxy for the experience of chronically high levels of stress, which may impact the development of the immune system and of the hypothalamic-pituitary-adrenal axis, with implications for arousal and affect regulation. Exposure to multiple ACEs is hypothesised to affect the development of neuronal networks in the orbitofrontal cortex and between this part of the brain and the amygdala.

The main implication for forensic psychiatry is the importance of taking a detailed history and examining sources such as GP or social care records. It may be especially important to enquire about frightening experiences in childhood such as physical abuse, and recalled memories of parental mental health and substance misuse. It appears that the combination of multiple ACEs is predictive of risk, not exposure to single kinds of maltreatment such as sexual abuse.

Unconscious factors in violence

Attachment and violence

Unconscious factors in violence

Research into child development suggests that early childhood attachment experiences are retained in the mind as unconscious **working models** of relationships in adulthood. These models are particularly activated at times of stress and give rise to <u>defence mechanisms</u> (p.212): habitual responses which occur in reaction to conscious stressors, like painful feelings or unconscious reminders of unresolved distress. People are often unaware of the defences they use, particularly those that are immature and dysfunctional, such as <u>denial</u> (p.212). Mature defences include humour and sublimation (e.g. choosing to exercise rather than break something when angry); immature defences typically involve reality distortion. Everyone uses immature defences at times, but they are especially common amongst people with <u>personality disorder</u> (p.78).

Violent offenders use more reality-distorting defences than the general population. Their use may explain apparently meaningless violence, such as attacks on strangers or severe self-harm. **Projection** may be a particularly risky mental mechanism for violence commission, as shown in Table 2.1.

Table 2.1 Projection and violence

Ordinary projection	Projection and violence	Mechanism
A is overweight and dieting. She says she feels disgust when she sees B, who is also overweight. The disgust with B is also A's self-disgust projected onto B.	C was severely abused as a child. He manages his distress and fear by denying it. He is convicted of child cruelty after a violent assault on his baby son when he cries.	Unbearably painful feelings and thoughts are denied in self-experience, but perceived in others. Some people can care for their distress when projected into others; violent offenders tend to attack their vulnerability, shame, and neediness when they perceive it in others.

Attachment and violence

Exposure to three or more <u>ACEs</u> (p.32) prevents the formation of secure attachments and leads to working models of relationships that are insecure and disorganised. People with disorganised attachments are more likely to have clinical psychiatric disorders, and to use reality-distorting defences. <u>Splitting</u> (p.312) is often found in disorganised attachment and leads to others being either idealised (wholly good) or denigrated (wholly bad). This defence often leads to professional disputes within mental health care and services.

A meta-analysis of studies of insecure attachment found that it was a risk factor for violence. This may be because most violence takes place in the context of relationships that are under strain in some way. People with secure attachment systems can tolerate the stress of relationship breakdown or loss without becoming psychotic or violent (or both); in contrast, relational stress or disruption is a potent risk factor for violence in people with insecure attachment systems, especially those with disorganised attachment who may both fear abandonment and seek to reject people they are close to. They may experience care as smothering or control, but experience any kind of distance as rejection generating fear, helplessness, and anger, leading to an unstable mental oscillation which is sometimes called the **core complex**.[4] Sadomasochistic violence involves a more strongly competing fear of abandonment, meaning that violence towards the other person is not aimed at their removal but rather keeping them under control so that they can move neither too close nor too far away.

Attachment systems also affect relationships between mental health professionals and their patients. It is not unusual for patients to project onto professionals attributes of early attachment figures (**transference**); the professionals' emotional reaction in response may reflect this (**countertransference**). For example, if a patient idealises their doctor, they may like the patient and see them as 'well'—and fail to perceive how the patient denigrates the nursing staff, and acts out cruelly towards them. Reflective practice sessions (p.309) allow teams to notice and think about such dynamics and may generate hypotheses about how unconscious mechanisms are at play when the patient is violent.

---

4 A psychoanalytic theory developed by Melvin Glasser, former Chair of the Portman Clinic: a universal developmental stage of separation and individuation, featuring simultaneous anxieties about engulfment by, and abandonment by, the primary caregiver. Adverse childhood experiences can lead to failure to develop past the stage, so that the core complex persists into adulthood.

Crime and violence from a developmental perspective

Persistence and desistance

Younger age and being male are strongly associated with criminal behaviour. However, the majority of young offenders desist from crime as they get older; and it is highly unusual for people to start offending in their forties or fifties. The reasons for both desistance and persistence are complex, involving social, cultural, and historical factors, plus interactions between developing individuals and their environment.

Protective factors (causing desistance) include being first-born, small family size, being an active and affectionate infant, resilient temperament, high IQ, positive disposition, and receiving large amounts of attention from caregivers and social bonding.

The likelihood of violent offending is increased with every additional risk factor in a child's early life. Socioeconomic deprivation and child-rearing factors (such as low family income and poor parental supervision) are more important for females, whereas parental characteristics matter more for males.

Offending in children under age twelve years

In the UK, few children under the age of twelve years exhibit sufficiently serious rule-breaking or aggression to warrant prosecution. Severe cruelty or violence by children younger than age 10–12 year is rare, and nearly always associated with having been maltreated. Developmental psychologists have emphasised that brain development continues into the third decade of life, especially in the frontal cortex—making <u>ages of criminal responsibility</u> of age 10–18 year years (p.406) appear arbitrary and 'unjust'.

Offending during adolescence

During adolescence, more than half of boys and a third of girls commit an offence, although they may not be prosecuted. The rate rises to a peak at age fifteen for girls and eighteen for boys. Much of it comprises <u>status offences</u> (p.428) that can only be committed by children, such as underage sex or truancy.[5] By age seventeen for girls, and age twenty-one for boys, offending behaviour ceases for all but a small minority.

Offence type progresses with increasing age; with those aged twelve to thirteen tending to commit <u>criminal damage</u> (p.422) and minor <u>assaults</u> (p.416); those aged fifteen to sixteen, <u>theft</u> (p.426) and similar property offences; and those aged eighteen to twenty-one, drug offences and vehicle offences.

<u>Sexual offending</u> (p.418) may emerge in adolescence, associated with the onset of puberty and interaction with other risk factors for antisocial behaviour. A subgroup of adolescent sex offenders will persist into adulthood.

---

5 Although only the adolescent can 'commit' truancy, it is actually their parent or guardian who commits the offence of failing to secure their regular attendance at school.

Adolescence-limited and life course–persistent violence

Persistent childhood aggression predicts both delinquency and conduct problems in adolescence across different cultures. There are two distinct developmental trajectories in relation to both antisocial behaviour and violence:

- In the **adolescence-limited** group, the violence and antisocial behaviour starts early in adolescence (around age twelve), peaks around age 15–16, and disappears almost entirely by age twenty-one, and is influenced by social processes and deviant peer groups.
- In the **life course–persistent** group the rate of violence and antisocial behaviour rises steadily until the midtwenties, then declines slowly and falls to a low level only in the midforties. These offenders account for a disproportionate number of serious crimes of violence. A subgroup have callous and unemotional traits (p.31), linked with the later emergence of psychopathy (p.90); the remainder have higher levels of anxiety and lower IQs, and are likely to develop ASPD (p.82).

Adult-onset offending

One-quarter of first-time convictions occur in offenders aged thirty years or older (though some may have been criminally active but not detected). First-time offending in an otherwise pro-social adult should raise questions about the onset of serious mental illness and/or that some neuropsychiatric condition has contributed to offending risk.[6]

Older adult offenders

The number of older offenders is rising, mostly because of increased healthy life expectancy. Another factor is the conviction of older adults for 'cold cases' detected by new technologies, particularly involving DNA detection, and prosecutions for historic sexual offences.[7]

New offending behaviour in people older than fifty is still rare: physical causes of any new and unusual offending behaviour should be investigated. For instance, the first signs of a dementing process may be disinhibition, hostility, and physical violence to family members, or inappropriate or deviant sexual behaviour.

---

6 However, note there is a high prevalence of minor brain damage in prisoners overall.

7 This, combined with a tendency to longer prison sentences (p.448) in the UK, has led to vastly greater numbers of elderly people in the prison population.

Gang crime

Involvement with deviant peers is the most proximate influence determining the onset of antisocial behaviour, including its escalation to violence. In North America two-thirds of seriously violent youths are gang members. In the UK, 1% of adolescents are thought to be members of an organised street gang, rising to as many as 20% of black male adolescents in some deprived areas of London. While only a minority of individuals are involved with gangs, gang violence accounts for a significant amount of violence by men in their late teens and early twenties, especially severe violence involving weapons.

Preventing gang-related violence is a major cross-government priority in E&W, and a number of government programmes are in place, including the Ending Gang Violence and Exploitation programme. Scottish policies have resulted in an 81% fall in those younger than eighteen convicted of handling an offensive weapon, although the threat from gangs continues. In NI, the Democratic Unionist Party asserted in 2014 that there were more than 140 gangs with different religious and partisan affiliations in the province.

Gangs and illicit drug economies

International data on homicide rates shows that the illicit drugs trade is a major risk factor for fatal violence. Although within the UK the overall prevalence of illicit drug use has decreased over the last twenty years, there have been shifts in the way in which illicit substances are marketed and traded that may have contributed to an increase in gang-related violence. For example, since 2014 there has been a significant increase in the use of crack cocaine, and the development of comparatively sophisticated drug trafficking gangs operating a business model dependent upon the exploitation of vulnerable children and adults. There are reports that vulnerable young people can be groomed and trafficked to participate in the illicit drugs trade, which increases the risk that they will be victims of violence. The term '**cuckooing**' has been used to describe when the home of a vulnerable individual is taken over by a drug dealer in order to conduct illicit drug activity. Drug gangs may take over the homes of individuals with mental health difficulties, developmental disability or substance misuse problems, or rehoused homeless people.

This pattern of gang activity and drug trafficking has become known as 'county lines', which refers to the phone lines used by city-based dealers to sell drugs to individuals in rural areas. In addition to crack cocaine, there are concerns about the trade and use of novel psychoactive drugs such as 'spice', which are associated with violence because of their negative impact on mental health.

Child criminal exploitation (CCE) is common in county lines gangs, and occurs where an individual or group takes advantage of an imbalance of power to control, coerce, manipulate or deceive a child or young person; the victim may have been exploited even if the activity appears consensual. CCE is broader than illicit drug use and can include sexual exploitation and other scenarios whereby children are forced to commit crimes.

Gang membership and mental health problems

Gang membership is associated with a range of mental health conditions, including anxiety, psychosis, drug and alcohol dependence, conduct disorder, and antisocial personality disorder. The link operates in both directions: poor mental wellbeing can draw an individual to a gang, and gang involvement can negatively impact an individual's mental health.

Mental ill-health and gang affiliation share common risk factors, often relating to an individual's early ACEs (p.32) and the environments in which they grow up. Attachment to gangs may reflect a lack of attachment to family and the absence of role models or parental figures. Gangs may also provide both protection and employment for young men who are vulnerable and at risk of victimisation.

Long-term exposure to violence (whether as victim or perpetrator) is associated with psychological problems including PTSD (p.96) and depression (p.94). Girls involved in gangs can be particularly vulnerable to mental health problems resulting from sexual victimisation and intimate partner violence.

Gang-affiliated young people may also experience particular barriers and challenges to engaging with mental health and other services. The relationship between gang affiliation and poor mental health requires an interagency approach (p.272) that co-ordinates services across a wide range of organisations.

Ethnicity, crime, and psychiatry

Ethnicity in forensic psychiatry

Ethnicity is a vague concept that relies on self or social ascription to belonging to a group with common geographical origins, race, language, and religion. It can be erroneously used interchangeably with race (largely perceived by appearance and attributed to biological and genetic traits) and culture (shared system of concepts established by convention and reproduced by traditional transmission).

People who do not describe themselves as white British are over-represented amongst psychiatric service users in the UK, especially in secure services (p.258); with black and other minority ethnic groups being more likely to be diagnosed with schizophrenia, admitted to hospital compulsorily instead of voluntarily, secluded and restrained (p.196), or forcibly medicated. The over-representation is also evident in various stages of the criminal justice system, with nonwhite groups being more likely to be arrested, charged based upon weaker evidence, receive longer sentences, as well as being less likely to receive bail, so that there is marked over-representation in the prison population.

In RoI, there are very small numbers of nonwhite people (no more than 5% of the population) despite significant immigration since the 1970. However, Travellers[8] are substantially over-represented in secure units and prisons, and are said to have experienced widespread discrimination: they make up 0.5% of the population, but 15% of female prison inmates and 22% of male.

Concerns about racism

Over-representation of disadvantaged groups is potentially contributed to by racially influenced misdiagnosis, lack of culturally informed screening tests and assessments, misperception of behaviour and/or by racist attitudes and beliefs.

It is sometimes unclear how identity and values can be validly defined or appreciated in the individual, so as to be personally respectful and nondiscriminatory. For example, a young man born and raised in the UK may still define himself as African by heritage, but another young man with a similar background may define himself as British. Also, there is a danger that in validly perceiving difference, one may infer clinically irrelevant difference. In addition, some validly perceived differences may have practical significance (in terms of facilities required for religious observance, say) but have no moral or legal significance (for example, nobody is allowed to kill another person, no matter what their religious beliefs).

Taking difference seriously in forensic psychiatry

Forensic mental health care professionals must pay close attention to the identity and experience of individuals from groups different from their own during the process of assessment (p.149), formulation (p.146), and treatment (p.182). Cultural differences may also be a factor in engagement and

---

8 Irish people who adopted an insular nomadic lifestyle in the seventeenth century and became genetically distinct from the main Irish population. They are unrelated to Roma ('Gypsies').

alignment of agendas between the individual and the treatment team. It may be helpful, therefore, to talk to a wide variety of sources from within the same community, not just the family. Assessment must also consider the limitations and validity of using measures that have been normed on white Western, English-speaking populations (see psychological testing p.130). It is also important to consider whether a patient from a certain ethnic group may suffer increased distress and alienation from their community if facing criminal charges or incarceration.

It has been suggested (by the Bennett inquiry, p.780) that more staff in forensic units be recruited from nonwhite groups and from other countries. There is some danger, however, that this approach in isolation may lead to a focus on differences that should be irrelevant (such as skin colour), and to ignorance of differences that are highly relevant (such as who has power and control).

The concept of **empowerment** implies treating each person as an individual, without making assumptions about the person's identity and values. No patient should ever be excluded from accessing potential treatments or subject to more punitive or coercive risk-management measures (p.238) on the basis of judgments about ethnicity or culture that are irrelevant to valid clinical perception.

Clinicians need space to consider their own conscious and unconscious biases and to evaluate their own assumptions. Susceptibility to bias is normal; professionalism requires the ability to recognise and account for bias.

Extremism, terrorism, & radicalisation

Those who fundamentally reject a society's current consensus may be labelled 'extremist' or 'radical' in their views; those who also reject the social compact and advocate violent change, 'terrorist'. The terms are usually pejorative, but the moral status of extremists or terrorists can vary between observers and over time.[9] See Box 2.2 for definitions.

Box 2.2 Extremism, terrorism, and radicalisation

Extremism
Beliefs, attitudes, feelings, actions, and strategies far removed from the mainstream of a society and condemned by that mainstream

Terrorism[10]
The use of violence and intimidation, especially against civilians, in the furtherance of political aims

Radicalisation
The process of adopting an extremist belief system, including the willingness to use, support or facilitate violence in order to bring about social change

---

Terrorist acts cause an average of 21,000 deaths per year, 0.05% of all deaths, worldwide. The vast majority occur in Africa, the Middle East, and South Asia[11]; however, the small number that occur in Europe and North America attract most attention and media coverage. The risk of being directly affected by terrorism is small, but public fear of it disproportionate. Impacts are listed in Box 2.3.

Box 2.3 Impact of extremist and terrorist acts
Death of victims
PTSD and other mental disorders in witnesses
Anxiety-related mental disorders in the wider public
Social divisions, discrimination (e.g. against young, bearded Asian men)
Breaches of human rights (e.g. through internment, p.430)
Diversion of public resources into recovery and counter-terrorism (p.596)[12]

---

9   For example, as a co-founder of the African National Congress's armed wing *Umkhonto we Sizwe*, in the 1960s Nelson Mandela advocated violence against the apartheid government in South Africa: he was reviled there as a terrorist but lauded in the West as a 'freedom fighter'. By the time the ANC took power in 1994, after he had served twenty-seven years' imprisonment for treason (p.430), mainstream views had shifted, and he came to be seen as a national hero and icon.

10   This refers to terrorism as a social phenomenon. For its definition in criminal law, see p.430.

11   Particularly Nigeria and the Maghreb, Iraq and Syria and Bangladesh, Pakistan, and Afghanistan.

12   The estimated direct costs to the US economy of the 9/11 attacks on the World Trade Centre and the Pentagon on 11 September 2001 were over $20 billion.

Radicalisation

One model of radicalisation describes individuals as going through twelve stages, including feeling victimised, developing political grievances, rationalising successively more extreme political views, becoming isolated from family and friends in the mainstream and bonding with like-minded individuals, 'groupthink'[13] creating a consensus around the most extreme views, splits within the group leading to even more polarised factions, hatred of and prejudice towards the 'outgroup' (i.e. mainstream society), legitimation of the killing of outgroup members, and legitimation of martyrdom to achieve it.

A number of social variables are risk factors for radicalisation, including youth, personal experience of hardship or adversity, alienation and social exclusion, poverty,[14] and perception of widespread injustice (particularly towards the group one identifies with); also suggestibility and compliance (p.160) and mental disorders, particularly depression.[15] In contrast, factors protecting against radicalisation include recent bereavement and other major life events, and engagement in mainstream society (e.g. through volunteering, voting in elections, donating to charity or taking part in peaceful political protest).

Certain social institutions such as prisons and religious schools are particularly prone to facilitate radicalisation because they take in vulnerable individuals (e.g. the young, poor, and socially excluded) and promote the sense of cohesion against an external enemy that fosters radicalisation. Such organisations can reduce the risk of radicalisation by operating in a transparent, responsive, consistent, and respectful way (as opposed to punishing prisoners arbitrarily); showing concern for the humanity and individuality of members, despite their status; and creating opportunities for engagement with the mainstream (e.g. inviting police officers into the *madrassa* to allow different groups to learn about each other).

Deradicalisation

Just as extremist groups can facilitate individuals going through the stages of radicalisation (for instance, by exposing them to extremist material over the internet or isolating them from mainstream views or nonbelievers), the State can seek to reverse the process, although such interventions are controversial, and there is no agreement about how effective they are in reducing risk of terrorist violence.

Interventions include debates conducted with mutual respect; reconnecting people with family and friends who do not share extremist views; facilitating acquiring a stake in mainstream society, through education, employment, or peaceful political engagement and mediation. In addition, where a radicalised individual suffers from mental disorder, successful treatment of that disorder may reduce their risk of retaining or acting on extremist views.

---

13 'Groupthink' is a well-documented psychological process in which the desire for harmony or conformity within a group causes it to reach a consensus without critical evaluation. The consensus view will tend to the most extreme view because of 'confirmation bias' within a cohesive group (selectively attending to evidence favouring the group's view and suppressing contrary evidence).

14 This is disputed. Some studies have found the poor to be more vulnerable to radicalisation, having little stake in mainstream society to lose; whereas others (mainly on Western populations) have found well-off, well-educated individuals, with their greater degree of political engagement, to be more sympathetic to extremists' political aims and therefore more susceptible to radicalisation.

15 Up to 60% of individuals referred to the UK government's Channel programme (see p.596) have mental health issues such as depression, psychosis, dysregulated affect, or autistic traits.

Do mental disorders cause violence?

In the 1980s, the dominant view within forensic psychiatry was that those with mental disorders, other than antisocial personality disorder, were, overall, no more likely to be violent than any others in the population, and thus were unfairly stigmatised. From the mid-1990s onwards, there appeared to be a shift in the UK towards increased public and political fear of people with mental disorder resulting chiefly from several high-profile incidents of violence committed by patients.

The scientific evidence

From the mid-1980s onwards, evidence began to accumulate of a greater than average frequency of violence amongst people with mental disorder compared to the general population. However, an association between mental disorder and frequency of violence (compared to those without mental disorder) does not demonstrate that mental disorder *causes* that increased risk. Such an association may be due to:

- **Chance**—the lower the p value the less likely this is.
- **Confounding**—where another factor, such as poverty, increases violence rather than mental disorder, but greater poverty in the group with mental disorder creates the false impression that it is the mental disorder increasing the risk of violence.
- **Bias**—for example where those selected to be in the study are not typical of those with mental disorder in a significant way.
- **Measurement error**—for example where there are errors in identifying mental disorder or violence in the study.
- **Reverse causation**—for example the mental disorder emerging as a result of the violence.
- **Causation**—it is the mental disorder that is causing the increased risk of violence.

An association is more likely to represent causation where the association is strong amongst other factors (e.g. the association of violence with schizophrenia is as great as that between cigarette smoking and carcinoma of the lung), consistent across a variety of different studies (e.g. systematic reviews) and reversible (e.g. treatment of schizophrenia with medication decreases risk of violence).

A structured review in 2021 that examined the association between violence other than intimate partner violence and various mental disorders (schizophrenia, bipolar disorder, depression, ADHD, personality disorder, PTSD, and substance misuse disorders) suggested that the odds of violence in those with these mental disorders were two to four times greater than in those without. This was after adjusting for potential confounders, both statistically and by use of twin studies where one twin has the disorder, and the other does not. However, past criminality and substance misuse strongly predicted future violence in many of these disorders. An important finding to remember is that over a five-to-ten-year period, over 90% of those with the mental disorders studied were **not** violent.

Interpreting the evidence concerning your patient

The crucial point to bear in mind is that odds ratios, or risk ratios, arising from study findings relate to groups as a whole, not the individual. For example, a review finding that 5% of those with a diagnosis of depression commit violence over a five-to-ten-year period does not mean that your patient has a 5% risk of committing a violent act in this period. Think about your own car insurance, if you drive: your insurance company might allocate you to a group 5% of whom will have an accident this year, based upon your age, sex, and profession; but if you routinely drive whilst drunk your risk will be very much higher than that, whereas if you only ever use the car to drive to church on Sundays, it will be much lower. In the same way, your patient's risk depends upon their personal history, including, for instance, the circumstances of violence (the presence of active delusions, their engagement with your service, their insight, their recent substance use and their current levels of anger or hostility associated with past violent episodes). Hence you should make an individualised <u>formulation</u> (p.146) as part of their <u>risk assessment</u> (p.166) in order to develop a personal risk-management plan.

Homicide

Homicide is the killing of one human being by another. When it amounts to <u>murder</u> (p.414) it is conventionally regarded as the most heinous offence (although <u>genocide</u> and <u>crimes against humanity</u> (p.438) are arguably more heinous). Homicide can be legally permitted, for example in wartime or in <u>self-defence</u> (p.410).

Mental disorder and homicide

The nature of the association between mental disorder and homicide needs to be considered carefully (see also p.44). <u>Schizophrenia and other psychotic disorders</u> (p.72) are associated with an increased risk of serious assault or homicide, but personality disorder (particularly <u>ASPD</u>, p.82 and <u>psychopathy</u>, p.90) and <u>substance misuse</u> (p.76) are very much greater risk factors. Most homicides are committed by people with no mental disorder.

- Between 2006 and 2016 approximately 6% of homicides were committed by people with schizophrenia in England and Wales (approx. 1% of the population).
- The number of homicides by people with schizophrenia or other psychoses has generally declined over time in England and Wales. There were approximately 120 per year in 1980 and approximately 31 in 2016; numbers fell steadily during this period, apart from an increase in 1997–2006 thought to be due to illegal drug use.
- In a Swedish population study, 9% of homicide offenders had schizophrenia; 12% another psychotic disorder; and 54% a diagnosis of personality disorder.
- In a Canadian study of homicide suspects, 3.7% were mentally abnormal. No changes from 1987 to 2012 in the contribution of mental abnormality to homicides was found.
- Roughly 10% of people convicted of homicide have some form of abnormal mental state at the time of the offence, and of these two-thirds have psychosis.
- Approximately 11% of homicides are committed by people who have had contact with mental health services in the past year.

Victims

Victims of homicides by people with mental disorder are more likely to be acquaintances than strangers. Women with mental disorder who commit homicide are most likely to kill family members.

Infanticide and related behaviours

The intentional killing of an infant (a child aged up to twelve months) by its mother is regarded as separate from other homicides in many cultures because of the effects childbirth and the stresses of early child-rearing are believed to have on the mother's mind. There is a separate <u>infanticide offence</u> (p.414) in some jurisdictions.

- **Infanticide** is associated with:
  - A diagnosis of depression
  - Postpartum psychosis
  - Maternal childhood sexual abuse

- **Neonaticide** is the killing of a newborn child. It was historically suggested that neonaticide is typically unrelated to mental disorder. Recent studies contradict this and suggest a significant association. Pregnancies may be concealed, and the baby's body hidden.
- **Filicide** is the killing of a child (of any age) by a parent. Categorisations of filicide have been attempted:
  - Altruistic or mercy killing
  - Psychotic or other mental disorder (15% in one study in E&W, higher in other samples)
  - Accidental or angry and impulsive
  - Unwanted child
  - Spousal revenge

Up to 50% of women who kill their children will have some form of mental disorder. Categorisation oversimplifies, and most cases will be multifactorial.

Murder-suicide

Murder-suicide—the suicide of the perpetrator directly after the homicide—is uncommon but can create enhanced media attention. Most occur in intimate relationships, perpetrated by men. Substance misuse and previous criminal history is less significant than with other homicides. Depression is suggested as being commoner in perpetrators of murder-suicide when compared to other homicide (20%–60%). See Table 2.2.

Clinical issues

Many people charged with a homicide offence will have a psychiatric assessment. There are several specific clinical (pp.122–147) and legal and practical (pp.148–161) issues to take into account when assessing someone alleged to have killed, including the risk of suicide (p.176) by the perpetrator.

Table 2.2 Police recorded crime—rates per 100,000 citizens per year, 2016

Crime	E&W	Scotland	NI	RoI
Homicide	1.22	1.13	0.97	0.78
Murder-suicide	0.2–0.4	0.2–0.4	0.2–0.4	0.2–0.4

Rates derived from Eurostat homicide statistics. Intentional killing of a person, including murder, manslaughter, euthanasia and infanticide. Excluding attempted (uncompleted) homicide. Excluding causing death by dangerous driving, abortion, and help with suicide. These represent dramatic falls from the 2007 figures in the first edition of the handbook.

Nonfatal assaults

Attempts to compare statistics for nonfatal, nonsexual assaults are hampered by differing definitions of **assault**. In E&W over one million offences against the person are recorded each year, but this uses a very broad definition of **assault**, including some that result in no injury; where injury is sustained, the majority are minor (e.g. bruising, black eyes, and minor cuts). Proportions of offences against the person:

• Homicide <0.1%
• Death or serious injury caused by illegal driving <0.1%
• Violence with injury 39%
• Violence without injury 41%
• Stalking and harassment 20%

Jurisdictions vary (see <u>laws on assault,</u> p.416) but in general a person is guilty of assault if they intentionally or recklessly cause another person to apprehend the application of immediate unlawful force. Assaults therefore include being put in fear of violence, and can include psychological assaults. Some types of stalking behaviour fall within this definition. A person is guilty of **battery** if they intentionally or recklessly apply unlawful force to the body of another person. The distinction between assault and battery is often misunderstood, especially by nonlawyers.

Consent

Assault is defined by the presence or threat of unlawful force: that is, where there is no consent, and no <u>justification</u> (p.410) such as self-defence, defence of others or in some parts of the UK, the 'reasonable punishment' of a child.[16] People may consent to the use of force against them, though in a few cases the courts have ruled that assault has occurred nevertheless, on the grounds of public policy.[17] Similarly, gaining consent protects doctors from charges of battery; although in practice, failure to gain consent results in being sued for negligence rather than prosecution, because of the lack of malicious intent.

Offenders

The majority of nonfatal assault offenders (and victims) are young men between age sixteen and thirty years. The next largest group of victims are women who experience domestic violence.

Clinical issues

The majority of people treated in forensic psychiatric settings have committed nonfatal, nonsexual assaults. There is an established relationship between <u>mental disorder and committing assault</u> (p.44).

16 Under s58 Children Act 2004, which restricted the common-law defence of 'reasonable chastisement' to common assaults. Many consider this residual defence to breach art.19 UN Convention on the Rights of the Child (because it denies children equal legal protection to adults). It was abolished in RoI in 2015 and in Scotland in 2019, and in Wales with effect from 2022.

17 Such as in wartime cases in which soldiers consented to being shot, for example in the foot, to avoid further active service, and more controversially, in cases in E&W in 1990–93 in which people consented to sexual violence against them for masochistic pleasure (*R v Brown*, p.749).

Men who are repeatedly violent and who are imprisoned may be offered psycho-education groups in prison during their sentence.

In prison samples, 9% of people convicted of nonfatal violence have been found to have schizophrenia. Other studies have repeatedly found higher rates of mental disorder in people convicted of nonfatal assaults.

Many perpetrators of nonfatal assaults are under the influence of alcohol at the time; so substance misuse services may meet the needs of service users with histories of nonfatal assaults. Antisocial personality disorder is highly prevalent in populations of people convicted of nonfatal assault, but it is unusual for this group of people to be assessed or treated by forensic psychiatrists unless there is also an established history of mental illness, or some other psychological disorder (though some general psychiatric community services will treat ASPD). See Table 2.3.

Table 2.3 Crimes recorded by the police—rates per 100,000 citizens per year, 2016

Crime	E&W	Scotland	NI	RoI
Assault (violent crime)	799.53	73.47	59.78	76.03

Rates derived from Eurostat violent crime statistics, based on assaults. Dramatic differences are likely to reflect differences in legal definitions.

Fire-setting behaviours

There were over 3,900 deliberate fires in dwellings in Britain (excluding NI) in 2017-18. In England, this resulted in fifty-eight deaths and 131 severe injuries, and cost £2.5 billion. Almost half of attended fires are set deliberately.

Arson (p.422) is the crime of maliciously, voluntarily, and wilfully setting fire to a building or other property that is owned by another, or for an improper purpose, such as to collect insurance. Not all fire-setting behaviours result in a charge of arson, and not all fire-setting is pathological. Distinguishing pathological arson related to mental disorder is difficult. See Table 2.4.

- **Pathological fire-setting** in ICD11 is characterised by multiple acts of, or attempts at, setting fire to property or other objects, without apparent motive, and by a persistent preoccupation with subjects related to fire and burning. There may also be an abnormal interest in fire-fighting equipment, things associated with fires, and calling the fire service.
- **Pyromania** in DSM-5 is a pattern of deliberate, purposeful setting of fires. It is diagnosed if the individual experiences tension or affective arousal before setting the fire, and there is associated interest or fascination with fire, and pleasure or gratification when witnessing or setting fires.
- **Juvenile fire-setters** (e.g. aged ten to eighteen in E&W) are thought to start one in four fires. The majority are started by children aged five to ten, who may not understand the dangers of fire. Even though the majority of child-set fires are started out of curiosity, not malice, the damage caused, both in human and economic costs, is real and sometimes devastating. Factors informing the decision to prosecute include the fire-setter's age, the nature and extent of the individual's fire-setting history, and the intent.
- More **female** patients than males in high secure hospitals have an index offence of arson. There are also high prevalence rates of self-harm among this group. Women are more likely to set fire to property invested with emotional meaning (communicative act). Motives include revenge, hatred, and jealousy.

Clinical issues

There are various theoretical models of arson, including pyromania, abnormal fascination with fire, displaced sexual drive, displaced aggression or a communicative act. There is no definite association between sexual gratification and fire-setting. Fire-setting may be chronic or episodic; some may set fires frequently to relieve tension; others apparently do so during periods of unusual stress in their lives. Psychiatric disorders may be present in fire-setters: a study exploring the association of psychosis with arson found significantly higher rates of arson conviction amongst people with schizophrenia and other psychotic disorders. It was noted that the association was stronger than for other violent crimes.

- 14%–65% of arsonists fulfil criteria for personality disorder

- 8%–35% of arsonists fulfil criteria for a psychotic disorder
- 8%–48% of arsonists fulfil criteria for learning disability
- 35%–66% of offenders are intoxicated, and alcohol misuse is likely to be a significant factor

Assessment of fire-setters should include investigation of early experience of fire; personality assessment; a functional analysis; antecedent events, including the general setting and conditions, specific psycho-social stimuli and triggering events, and positive consequences that might reinforce future fire-setting (fire-setting might result in the perpetrator gaining a lot of attention) and the individual's current understanding of fire-setting and risk.

Additional clinical factors that should be considered are:

- parental violence and alcoholism
- history of attempted suicide
- psychotic or revenge motive
- social skills
- other family dysfunction
- evidence of sadistic traits or psychopathy (p.90)

Treatment, as well as of the underlying mental disorder, amounts to risk management (p.178) and might include fire-safety training, social and coping skills, anger and/or aggression management, self-esteem work, and relapse prevention. Specific cognitive-behavioural interventions for mentally disordered fire-setters have been evaluated with promising results.

Table 2.4 Crimes recorded by the police and fires recorded by the Fire Service—rates per 100,000 citizens per year, 2017–18

Crime	E&W	Scotland	NI	RoI*
Criminal damage	964	902	909	478
Arson	44	49	65	32
Fires in dwellings assessed as deliberate	580 England 420 Wales	1,030	495	

*different criteria to UK: criminal damage recorded as damage to property or environment; fires assessed as 'malicious'

Stalking behaviours

Definitions

The essence of the various definitions of stalking is that the behaviour involves repeated unwanted contacts and intrusions, in a way that would cause apprehension or fear in most people, for a period of over two weeks. Victims may perceive themselves as being stalked before (or sometimes only well after) this time period. Examples of stalking behaviours are shown in Box 2.4.

> **Box 2.4 Examples of stalking behaviours**
>
> Unwanted emails, telephone calls, letters, or social media contacts
> Following the victim or loitering near their home or workplace
> Giving unwanted gifts or ordering unwanted services (e.g. taxis, pizza)
> Monitoring the victim's use of the internet or telephone
> Issuing threats, including death threats
> Intimidating, slandering, libelling, or officially complaining about them
> Damaging the victim's property
> Assaulting the victim

Relevant crimes

The more serious behaviours associated with stalking are often crimes in their own right, such as <u>assault</u> (p.416), <u>sexual assault</u> or <u>rape</u> (p. 418), making <u>threats to kill</u> (p. 436), or <u>criminal damage</u> (p. 422). Most English-speaking jurisdictions have a form of antistalking legislation. Both the UK and RoI have specific <u>stalking or harassment offences</u> (p.432).

Epidemiology

A variety of community studies suggest that approximately 15% of Western populations are stalked within their lifetime. Stalking behaviours are more commonly perpetrated by men. Women are more likely to be victims of stalking. Psychiatrists and other mental health workers may be at particular risk.

Typology

There is no single agreed classification of stalkers. One widely adopted typology is that of Mullen, which comprises:

- **Intimacy seekers** – stalkers attempting to establish a close relationship with a desired person whom they are unreasonably convinced reciprocates their love. There is an association with loneliness in a person with a psychotic disorder.
- **Rejected** – responding to an unwelcome end to an intimate relationship (usually sexual) by actions intended for reconciliation or revenge. This type is associated with the greatest risk of violence.
- **Incompetent** – would-be suitors seeking friendship and/or sex by socially inappropriate methods without concern for the individual. They may pursue for brief periods and have more victims.

- **Resentful**—setting out to exact revenge or achieve validation for perceived wrong, often using legal means. They lack insight into the fear they cause and see themselves as victims.
- **Predatory**—pursuing a stranger for sexual gratification, or in preparation of a sexual assault. There is an association with paraphilias.

Clinical issues

Studies suggest 50% of stalkers have a mental disorder, the commonest being psychotic disorders, personality disorder, and substance misuse disorders. Specific psychiatric phenomena such as suicidal ideation, delusional misidentification, and psychopathy are associated with an increased risk of stalking-related violence.

Risks

Stalking behaviours may escalate, and include violent behaviours; stalking is therefore a risk factor for violence. Stalking with a sexual motive may be a risk factor for sexual violence. Tools (p.136) such as the SRP and SAM use structured professional judgement to assess stalking episode specific risks such as persistence, recurrence, and violence. Stalking involves a special relationship between the perpetrator and victim, meaning that conventional risk assessment may underestimate risk of violence.

Approximately 25% of stalking episodes result in violence in community samples, and serious violence in UK high-security samples.

Prognosis

One study suggests the median persistence of stalking behaviours (after the initial two weeks) is six months. Stalkers with psychosis are about three times more likely to stalk for over a year.

Management

Key principles of management include:
- supporting the victim in avoiding any contact whatsoever with the stalker (including confronting the behaviour) and seeking psychological support and legal advice;
- if the victim has a professional relationship with the stalker, transferring their care to another professional immediately; and
- if the stalker has a mental disorder, treating the underlying disorder if possible.

Specific treatment recommendations should follow logically from formulation and target the dynamic risk factors judged to be most relevant in persistence of stalking and stalking-related violence for the individual stalker. Restraining orders may be helpful, although risks to the victim may increase in the period immediately after one is issued.

Sexual offending and its social context

Sexual offences are overwhelmingly (but not exclusively) committed by men. The victims are overwhelmingly (but not exclusively) women, and to a lesser extent children.

Individual versus social causation

Psychology and psychiatry tend to account for sexual offending by way of individual psychopathology, implying that treatment or educational programmes are required, such as when <u>paraphilic disorders</u> (p.102) are diagnosed.

Other accounts emphasise social and cultural factors. This is supported by there being societies in which sexual offending is almost unknown; whilst rates of sex offending are highest in societies where derogatory attitudes to women or children are tolerated or supported (for example, with easy access to cheap pornography). Many sex offenders are also prolific criminal offenders, suggesting that their sexual offending is reflective of generally antisocial attitudes.

However, only a small proportion of men (let alone women) are sexual offenders; who come from across the social spectrum. Sex offenders appear to hold persistent and recognisable <u>distortions of beliefs and cognitions</u> (p.62) about their victims that drive offending behaviour and are not found in nonoffenders. There is considerable heterogeneity in motivation with some sexual offending best understood as being designed to control and humiliate. Supporters of the social deviance position counter that these distortions and beliefs are widespread in the community, and that detected sex offenders represent only those who are also highly antisocial or criminally incompetent—so that the overall rate of sex offending in the community would therefore be reduced if social attitudes towards the vulnerable (including women and children) were changed. Hence sexual offending is better understood as control and humiliation of the vulnerable, rather than as disorder of individual appetites.

Differences between sex offenders

There are real differences between

- the fetishist who collects sex toys,
- the viewer of illegal pornography,[18]
- the serial rapist,
- the recidivist paedophile and
- the parent who abuses their stepchild.

It is highly unlikely that one form of explanation can account for such heterogeneous behaviours, not all of which will be detected or result in prosecution. More likely is that different types of offender will variously better fit the social deviance and individual accounts. For example, individual deviance may provide a better theoretical understanding of a man who starts to

---

18 This varies from one jurisdiction to another. At present in the UK, it comprises child pornography, and 'extreme' pornography (realistically depicting scenes that are life-threatening or involve serious damage to the anus, breasts or genitals, or involve animals or corpses).

SEXUAL OFFENDING AND ITS SOCIAL CONTEXT 55

abuse his daughter in the context of his wife's illness or absence: but social deviance might better explain the same behaviour in a man who is also physically or emotionally abusive to his wife.

Personality disorder and sexual offending

The individual deviance/pathology model may extend to seeing sex offending as only one aspect of pervasive psychopathology, especially as part of diagnosed personality disorder. This has implications for the therapeutic response (p.246), if any, and perhaps legal compulsion (p.57).

Multiple perspectives

In assessing sex offenders (p.174), it is wise to address their social attitudes towards women and children, recognising the research that suggests that significant subgroups of nonoffending men share rape-supportive attitudes. However, it is also important to consider the individual psychological factors that may have facilitated the person's offending behaviour, not least because it is likely to be easier to intervene at the level of the individual. Only very rarely is serious mental illness or disability even partly explanatory of sexual offending.

Training

It is essential that all those working with sex offenders understand both social and individual deviance accounts of sexual offending. A sole focus on individual disorder or psychopathology is likely to mislead both clinician and offender.

Sexual offending against adults

Sexual offending refers to specific legally defined crimes such as <u>rape</u> and <u>sexual assault</u> (p.418), which differ between jurisdictions—as opposed to sexually inappropriate behaviour: inappropriate behaviour deemed to have a sexual motive (ranging from implicit sexualised suggestions that would not amount to an offence, to serious sexual violence).

Sexual offending as an aspect of mental disorder

DSM-5 and ICD11 include a number of <u>paraphilic disorders</u> (p.102), being sexual arousal patterns that focus on nonconsenting others or are associated with substantial distress or risk of injury to self or others. They include exhibitionism, frotteurism, voyeurism, fetishism, paedophilia, sexual masochism, sexual sadism, and other specified paraphilic disorder. They are *clinical* categories that do not automatically correspond to any criminal offence.

Epidemiology

<u>Surveys of victimisation</u> (p.23) give much higher estimates of sexual offending than those recorded by the police; for example the 2019 British Crime Survey (BCS) found that only 17% of rapes were reported, and 40% of those reported were dropped 'as victim does not support action' (often due to the intrusiveness and unpleasantness of the process), followed by other 'evidential difficulties'. Only 1.7% of reported rapes are prosecuted (58% of these resulting in conviction). Of rape victims, 90% know their attacker. See Table 2.5.

Table 2.5 Crimes recorded by the police—rates per 100,000 citizens per year, 2017-18

Crime	E&W	Scotland	NI	RoI
Rape	91.3	30.8	29.6	Publication
Sexual assault	133.1	96.9	In 'Other'	currently
Other	307.5	88.7	49.2	postponed

Rates include rape and sexual assault against men, as well as women, in most jurisdictions. Scottish and Northern Irish figures include attempted rapes. 'Other' varies between jurisdictions and includes offences such as grooming, soliciting for prostitution, incest, lewd acts, 'unlawful carnal knowledge', and assisting another in committing rape.

Association with mental disorder

The possibility of mental disorder being associated with sexual offending is not as well-researched as for violent offending, and is confounded by substance misuse and criminogenic factors. The great majority of sex offenders do not have a major mental illness (no more than 10%). One study has suggested that sex offenders were 4.8 times more likely to have schizophrenia and 3.4 times more likely to have bipolar disorder; other studies have found no such association.

<u>Functional psychotic disorders</u> (p.72) may be associated with some sexual offences through:

- disinhibition, arousal or irritability
- direct 'psychotic drive' (e.g. command auditory hallucinations)
- cognitive impairments or distortions secondary to psychosis
- poor social skills related to negative schizophrenic symptoms

The psychosexual profiles of mentally ill and non–mentally ill sex offenders are similar, and mental illness alone can provide only a partial explanation of sexual offending. There is strong familial aggregation of sexual crime.

Other mental disorders may be associated with sexual offending, including personality disorder (found in 30%–50% of sex offenders – especially ASPD and psychopathy, p.90), substance dependence, intellectual disability, Asperger's syndrome, and brain damage. Studies of personality in sex offenders show that some (though not, for example, rapists) tend to have more schizoid, avoidant, depressive, dependent, self-defeating, and schizotypal personality traits, compared to other offenders.

The importance of conviction

When people with major mental disorders commit sexual offences there is a strong tendency for them to be diverted (p.268) out of the criminal justice system to hospital. While this might enable them to receive initial treatment more rapidly than if they were to remain in the criminal justice system, it can complicate (or even render ineffective) any future psychological work on their sexual offending as lack of a conviction makes it easier for some patients to deny their commission of, or responsibility for, the offending behaviour.

Sexual offending against children

Child sexual abuse (CSA) can involve the commission of similar acts as sexual offences against adults, but they are usually separately classified.

Child sexual offending as an aspect of mental disorder

The paraphilic disorder most strongly identified with sexual offending against children is <u>paedophilia</u> (p.102), defined in DSM-5 as a paraphilic disorder in which a person has acted on[19] intense sexual urges towards prepubescent children or experiences recurrent sexual urges towards, and fantasies about, children that cause distress or interpersonal difficulty.

Defining paedophilia as a mental disorder carries no implication of lack of criminal responsibility; nevertheless, the term *paedophile* has been adopted in popular culture, particularly in the UK, to refer to anyone convicted of a sexual offence against a child, although such use of this term does not accurately reflect the heterogeneity of this group of offenders. See Box 2.5.

Box 2.5 Statistics on child sexual abuse

- About 11% of girls and 3% of boys suffer sexual abuse before the age of sixteen years.
- The incidence of sexual crimes perpetrated against children in the UK is 0.5–2 per 1000 children per year.
- About 70% of sexual abusers are someone the child knows; 33%–50% of abusers of girls, and 10%–20% of abusers of boys are family members.
- 37% of sexual abuse involving physical contact occurs in the child's own home.
- 2%–20% of sexual offences against children are committed by women (lower figures from crime reports, higher figures from victim studies).
- About 15% of sexual offences are committed by adolescent offenders.

Epidemiology

As with <u>sexual offending against adults</u> (p.56), CSA reported to the police provides a poor measure of the incidence of sexual offending against children, with reporting rates under 30% (to the police or any confidant). In 2018-19, only 4% of CSA offences reported to the police resulted in a charge; though 79% of charges led to a conviction. Even convicted offenders are seldom convicted again of similar offences: 20% in one estimate.

A greater proportion of female-perpetrated sexual offences are against children compared to male-perpetrated sexual offences.

Association with mental disorder

There is no known causal relationship between mental disorder and CSA. However, studies suggest that the following mental disorders are more common in child sexual offenders than in the general population: depression,

---

19 This may not mean molesting a child, but masturbating to a fantasy about children. DSM-5 has been criticised for not making plain that some people with paedophilic disorder resist the urge to abuse children.

bipolar disorder, social anxiety disorder, ADHD, learning disability, autistic spectrum disorder, and borderline, histrionic, and antisocial personality disorder.

In women convicted of sexual offences mental disorder may be more common than in men, although the relatively small numbers involved make comparison difficult.

Online-facilitated child sexual abuse

The range of behaviours in this category has grown considerably and now includes any engagement with online images of CSA, grooming, and sexting. The internet has either revealed an enormous previously unrecognised sexual interest in children or has produced an enormous increase in such interest. Research suggests that 4%–12% of men and 3% of women in the general population view images of CSA. Most do not have criminal records. Between a quarter and a third of online groomers are female.

Of people with convictions for image-related CSA, 0.5%–4% progress to abusive physical touching of children. Internet-based offenders with a previous conviction for any other offence are more likely to reoffend or escalate.

People charged with internet-based child sex offences often have difficulties with sexual self-regulation, plus have experienced a significant numbers of adverse life events prior to arrest.

Several typologies of internet-based offenders have been proposed. One distinguishes between **contact** and **fantasy** as the driving force (the former seeking to meet minors, the latter not); another is based on the degree of sophistication in using and hiding online activities; others are based on motive, such as:

• **emotional satisfaction**: reduction of emotional distress through seeking solace and comfort via the use of internet pornography.
• **intimacy deficit reduction**: satisfying some of the need for intimacy by using internet pornography.
• **hypersexuality**: high levels of sexual behaviour satisfied compulsively by use of internet pornography.

Other types of sexual offending

Indecent exposure

Legally this involves removing clothes to reveal genitals or (in some jurisdictions, p.419) other sexual body parts. DSM-5 includes <u>exhibitionistic disorder</u> (p.102) where there is distress and interference with life. There is no known association with any other mental disorder. See Box 2.6.

> **Box 2.6 Indecent exposure**
> - Indecent exposure is one of the commonest sexual offences. It also has the highest recidivism rate of all sexual offences.
> - Up to 4% of men and 2% of women report witnessing an exhibitionist act.
> - About a third of exhibitionists will also commit a contact sexual offence.

There is no established risk-assessment tool specifically for indecent exposure. The same risk factors as for other sexual offences are relevant. Exhibitionism is associated with decreased life satisfaction and higher scores on impulsivity and risk-taking tests.

DSM-5 divides exhibitionistic disorder by preferred victim: nonconsenting adults, prepubescent children or both. Another distinction, though not empirically validated, is between the inhibited, guilty exhibitionist (who, if male, typically displays a flaccid penis) and the angry, aggressive exhibitionist (who, if male, typically displays an erection).

Voyeurism

This involves spying on people undressing or engaging in sexual activity. Without consent, one form of it ('upskirting') is an <u>offence</u> throughout the UK (p.434), and voyeurism more generally is an offence in Scotland. About 11% of men and 4% of women self-report voyeurism. There is no known association between voyeuristic disorder[20] and other mental disorder.

Pornography offences

Use of extreme (sometimes illegal) pornography may be associated with coercive sexual behaviour and aggression. There is no known link with mental disorder.

Revenge porn

This involves disclosing private sexual photographs or films with intent to cause distress, and is an <u>offence</u> in the UK (p.434). Any association with mental disorder is yet to be investigated.

---

20 Voyeuristic disorder involves persistent and intense sexual arousal from deliberately observing an unsuspecting person who is naked, in the process of undressing or engaging in sexual activity, when this urge has been acted on with a nonconsenting person or causes significant distress or social impairment over six months.

Incest

There is no known association between mental disorder and sexual activity with siblings or other family members.

Being sexually abused as a child is associated with high levels of psychiatric morbidity.

Bestiality

One study suggested a 10% prevalence of bestiality amongst adolescent offenders. This group may have higher rates of mental disorder. There is limited evidence that bestiality is more common among psychiatric patients than general medical patients.

Necrophilia

Necrophilia (sexual activity with a corpse) is not proven to be associated with psychiatric disorder.

Abuse of position

Sexual offending may relate to perpetrators abusing positions of power against vulnerable victims (e.g. children). Doctors, teachers, staff at children's homes or learning disability hostels, and prison officers all have opportunities to abuse their position of trust in this way. There is no known association with mental disorder, but people with mental disorder are at increased risk of victimisation (p.179).

Motivations for sexual offending

Sexual behaviour is influenced by social and cultural values and stereotypes, sexual identity and gender role expectations, and physiological sexual appetites, fluctuating by age and stress level. In <u>formulating</u> (p.146) an offence, or <u>assessing sexual violence risk</u> (p.172), consider:

- **affective risk factors**: most sexual violence is driven by emotion (anger, hatred, and shame), often disinhibited by substance misuse.
- **criminogenic risk factors**: most sexual violence is committed by men with past convictions for violence, domestic or other family violence.
- **personality disorder**: including psychopathy, narcissism, and sadism, where sexual violence may be intended to intimidate or to kill.
- fantasies, and sexual arousal to images, of **harming or degrading victims**.
- **early childhood adversity** and **insecure attachment** are more common in sex offenders than in the general population, leading to problems making and maintaining intimate relationships.
- **self-soothing**: making the perpetrator feel (temporarily) better about themselves (common in online offending).[21]

Many sex offenders, however, report none of these risk factors.

Cognitive distortions and offence-supporting schemata

Cognitive distortions may facilitate offending, typically justifying harmful behaviour and excluding victims' perspectives. See Table 2.6.

Table 2.6 Cognitive distortions that facilitate sexual offending

Child sex offenders	Adult sex offenders
They were sexually mature	Women are devious, using sex to gain
Children enjoy sexual contact	She deserved it
No harm was done	Women never say what they mean
It helps child sexual development	Women want domination
Adults can do what they want to children	Men cannot control themselves

Cognitive schemata (value-laden beliefs about the world) are especially common drivers in sexual offenders. For example:

- **entitlement**—I am superior to victims, and entitled to take from inferiors.
- **dangerous world**—the world is hostile; I must control this by making others feel in danger.
- **unknowable women**—women cannot be understood; men are entitled to see women as devious; all encounters are adversarial.
- **women as sex objects**—women are always sexually available and cannot be hurt by sexual activity without physical harm.
- **uncontrollable male sex drive**—unfulfilled sexual desires harm men; once aroused, appetites must be fulfilled.

21 In other contexts 'self-soothing' can be an adaptive means of managing emotional distress.

Schemata specific to child sex offenders include:
- **children as sexual**—children are inherently sexual and can consent.
- **absence of harm**—there may be benefit to children; it is not real harm.
- **uncontrollable world**—events, emotions, and sexual feelings are out of my control.

Reality-distorting defences reduce shame and anxiety and are often driven by stereotypes about the role of the vulnerable in society (especially women) and distorted beliefs about masculinity.

Theories of sexual offending
All sex offending involves exploitation of the vulnerable and cognitive distortions that allow the offender to feel justified. Most sex offenders know their victims and use relationships to facilitate offending (which may be a key risk factor). Most victims experience the perpetrator as hostile, angry, and frightening, suggesting these affects are in the offender even if denied at assessment.

Models of sexual offending
The Ward and Siegert pathways model involves different routes to offending: deviant (impersonal, purely physical) sexual scripts, intimacy deficits (treating children as 'pseudo-partners'), emotional dysregulation (offending as a way of managing anger, low mood or low self-esteem), antisocial cognitions, and a combination of the four other pathways.

Against children
Finkelhor's 'four conditions model' describes:
- emotional congruence (claiming special connection with children, perceiving them as having emotional needs like theirs).
- sexual arousal to children.
- blockage of adult or peer relationships.
- willingness to overcome internal and external inhibitions.

Wolf's model complements Finkelhor's: adding childhood adversity leading to personality dysfunction; low-self-esteem, sexually deviant interests, and a cycle of fantasy, grooming and offending, cognitive distortions, and worsened self-image.

Against adults
- Hall and Hirschmann's 'quadripartite model of key vulnerabilities': sexual arousal, justifying cognitions, affective dyscontrol, and antisocial personality. Offending occurs when a 'critical threshold' is passed.
- Malamuth's 'confluence model': childhood experiences lead to individual differences in six key variables related to sexual promiscuity and hostile masculinity, shown to predict 'rape proclivity': sexual arousal to rape, dominance as a motive for sex, hostility towards women, attitudes facilitating aggression towards women, antisocial personality traits, and sexual experience.

Female sex offenders
These models should not be applied to female sex offenders, who constitute a small heterogenous subgroup, including sexual offenders with male co-defendants who they claim (truthfully or not) coerced them to sexual relationships with a minor. In assessment consider offence circumstances and relationship with the victim, criminogenic risk factors, personality dysfunction, and dysfunctional schemata.

Other types of offending

Criminal offences must be distinguished from behaviours that may indicate psychopathology. Psychiatrists assessing individuals charged with, or convicted of, nonviolent offences should ensure the criminal offence is not a social or behavioural manifestation of psychopathology that could be addressed therapeutically, or indicate increased risk of violence.

Property crime

Most nonviolent offences recorded by the police in E&W are offences involving theft of property: from homes, cars or commercial property. These offences make up about 40% of police recorded crime; this may be an underrepresentation of actual offences committed. Other types of property offence recorded are vandalism and criminal damage.

Perpetrators of theft are rarely mentally ill; social factors (p.28) are more relevant. They are likely to be socially disadvantaged and come from economically deprived urban areas.

Some offenders may steal to finance a drug or alcohol addiction. For some young offenders, repetitive property crime may be the start of an offending trajectory (p.36) that will escalate in severity. For other young offenders, property crime reflects temporary delinquency. Repetitive thefts of single items may reflect a mental disorder such as paraphilic disorder (p.102).

In terms of risk assessment, determine whether the pattern of acquisitive crime is combined with violent offending or other types of crime, which may suggest a more generally antisocial attitude.

Breaching legal sanction

A common form of other recordable offence is breaching of legal sanctions: violations of court orders, failures to pay fines, and breaches of probation or parole. The pattern of offending is important: repetitive breaches of legal sanctions may be indicative of impulsivity or antisocial attitudes. Repetitive breaches of sanctions regarding interpersonal contact with ex-partners or children may suggest stalking (p.52) or paranoid or hostile attachments in the context of domestic violence (p.26).

Fraud and crimes of deception

Fraud and other acts of deception cover a wide variety of criminal behaviours. There is no suggestion of a specific relationship between mental disorder and these offences, although repetitive fraud or deception may be associated with psychopathy (p.90) or factitious disorder (p.118). Fraud and computer misuse offences increased from 2017 to 2020. In about 60% of fraud incidents, there is no contact between the victim and the offender.

Drug offences

A conviction for a drug offence will not ordinarily indicate forensic psychiatric involvement, although drug misuse is common amongst mentally disordered offenders. Serious drug offences committed by people with mental disorder who require treatment may imply difficulties in assessing the risk of harm (supplying illegal drugs may be harmful in a societal sense but not in the direct and individual way that harm is usually addressed).

There are many hundreds of other specific offences and offence behaviours which have not been described here because they are relatively uncommon and/or are usually less relevant to forensic psychiatry.

Why divide violent & sexual offending?

Most criminal statutes identify offences as sexual rather than violent, regardless of physical harm done or the intention of the perpetrator. Why?

Social attitudes: patriarchal dominance

The division was probably originally based on societal attitudes towards women and children who were identified as victims (male victims did not figure). The earliest 'sexual' offences were largely confined to rape, sexual abuse of children, and anal sex (even if consensual), and reflected a view of women and children as the property of a man who was head of the family unit. Whilst medieval law recognised that there was an offence against the victim, the main wrong arose from the fact that the head of the household might now lose out financially since the woman or child was now 'spoiled' or damaged and would be unattractive in terms of a property-based marriage arrangement. Rape was therefore not only a criminal offence; it contained elements of a civil wrong or tort (p.548).

Consent versus assent

Social discourse continues to draw a distinction between sexual and violent offences, such that they are still recorded and considered as distinct. A possible basis for this may rest on issues of **consent**. Nonsexual offences against the person may involve the use or threat of unlawful force (p.48); whereas in some forms of sexual assault (e.g. unlawful sexual intercourse) the victim may have agreed to the act (i.e. assented), even if they have not legally consented.[22]

Is it a question of force?

In most jurisdictions, violent and nonviolent sexual offences are classified together in law, and separated from nonsexual violent offences. This classification obscures the intrinsically violent nature of sexual offences such as sexual assault, perhaps because defendants in these cases are keen to emphasise the 'sexual' nature because this suggests something consensual. For nonsexual offences, the mere threat of force causing fear of violence is sufficient to establish offences such as common assault (p.416) and affray (p.424).

Rape

The distinction between rape (p.418) and other violent offences may be due to concerns about false allegations. The prevalence of false allegations is unknown, but they are likely to be over-represented because they are frequently reported, whereas true allegations are known to be under-reported. There are also myths about rape (usually from a male perspective) which suggest that rape is just a bad sexual experience, especially if the victim and the alleged rapist have had a previous sexual relationship, and the victim has not suffered any other obvious physical injury.

These myths ignore the first-hand testimonies of both rape victims and rapists. Rape victims describe fear for their lives, and pain and shock at

22 Because, for example, they are too young to have the capacity to consent (see p.530).

the forcible intrusion into their bodies. Convicted rapists give accounts of enjoying terrorising and humiliating their victims, especially those who raped an ex-partner in response to being rejected, a common scenario. Risk factors for rape include previous convictions for violence or other criminality, substance misuse, high levels of <u>psychopathy</u> (p.90), and sexual arousal to violent material. Most convicted rapists have previous convictions for violence, and a small subgroup escalate from noncontact sexual offences such as indecent exposure to sexual assault and ultimately rape.

What questions are raised?

There are serious legal questions about the extent to which definitions of offences should be based upon the *victim's perception* of violence, as opposed to the *intent of the perpetrator*. It does not seem sensible to distinguish the use of force against one area of the body from other areas of the body. There may be a public interest in categorising those offences that are genital in nature and content, and which cause harm that does not involve direct physical force or contact: such as indecent exposure, offences involving pornography and those 'offences' committed by consenting adults, such as sadomasochistic practices.[23]

A proposal

The classification of sexual offences and violent offences separately potentially creates a mindset that illegal sexual acts are not violent. Reclassification in the following terms would partially address this issue.
- All violence, sexual or otherwise, classified together;
- Offences of breach of social taboos classified separately.

Statistics and measurement of crime would therefore correlate with the legal classification.

---

23 Sadomasochistic acts can be prosecuted as assault in E&W despite the consent of the 'victim', and despite the ECHR ruling that it was possible for the victim to consent to being assaulted in this way, because the ECHR also ruled that States could nevertheless criminalise such behaviour on the ground of its social unacceptability.

Mental disorders in forensic psychiatry*

* This chapter provides clinical information in a manner which emphasises the forensic aspects of the conditions described, focusing mainly on associated risks and mechanisms of harm, and their management. For comprehensive clinical information concerning each condition we recommend that you consult the *Oxford Handbook of Psychiatry* or another general psychiatry or specialist text.

Functional psychosis

Psychotic states of mind include:
• Altered *perception* of external reality
• Distorted *cognitions*
• Disordered *mood* (mania, depression, and fear)
• Hyperarousal secondary to the above

Box 3.1 Prevalence of functional psychosis
• General population: 0.4% (diagnosed; 10% symptom self-report)
• General psychiatric patients: at least 5%
• Prisoners: 10% male remand; 7% male sentenced; 14% female (both)
• Forensic psychiatric patients: 76%

Specific psychotic symptoms and violence

Paranoid symptoms involve abnormal, altered interpretation of relationships with others, especially imagining a relationship where none exists (e.g. believing that a news broadcast contains a special coded message for you). *Persecutory* delusions are paranoid delusions in which another person is perceived as intending harm.

Risk of acting violently increases if paranoid symptoms are present, regardless of diagnosis. Patients with paranoia have incorporated other people into their psychotic experiences, who may then be at risk of harm (e.g. from what the patient thinks is 'self-defence'). Delusions of persecution, being spied on and conspiracy are associated with violence. Violence may arise from resultant anger, confusion, fear, or panic.

Paranoid psychotic states can occur in:
• schizophrenia and bipolar disorder (p.92),
• a more circumscribed delusional disorder,

or

• transiently in borderline personality disorder (p.84) and
• during intoxication (e.g. with cocaine or amphetamines) or arising from alcohol dependence (p.76).

Encapsulated fixed paranoid beliefs may exist in the absence of other types of disordered reality testing, such as hallucinations. Paranoid delusional disorder, which can occur as an exacerbation of paranoid personality disorder, may be particularly resistant to treatment and may result in persistently high risk to others.

Threat/control override (TCO) symptoms occur most commonly in paranoid schizophrenia. TCO symptoms cause the patient to feel gravely threatened by someone and involve the perception of loss of control of self through the operation of external forces (e.g. command hallucinations or passivity phenomena). Unlike other psychotic symptoms, TCO symptoms have been shown in some research to be associated with violence[1] but this finding has not been universally replicated. More recent research has considered the relationship between threat symptoms (delusions) and anger as the mediating emotional state.

Schizophrenia and schizoaffective disorder

More than twenty primary studies have found an increased risk of violence in people with schizophrenia and schizoaffective disorders, even after factors such as substance misuse and sociodemographic status have been accounted for. The odds of violence with these disorders are three to eight times higher in men and four to fifteen times higher in women compared to the general population. People with schizophrenia had a rate of violence four times that of their siblings without the disorder, which suggests that factors in common (e.g. similar early childhoods, social factors) are not sufficient to explain the increased rates of violence observed in those with the disorder.

Although the odds of killing are about fourteen to twenty-five times higher than in the general population, this still only translates into a 0.3% lifetime probability of a person with these disorders committing homicide.[2] Lifetime risk of violence is about 24% (and 5%–10% after five to ten years of follow-up).

Other factors that further increase risk of violence in these disorders include substance abuse, poor impulse control, poor insight, not receiving medication, and other risk factors for offending (p.28).

Delusional symptoms or disorders

Delusional symptoms or disorders may be associated with violence. An increased risk of violence may occur in conjunction with the following types of delusions:

- Persecutory delusions (believing the victim means you harm).
- Misidentification delusions (e.g. believing the victim is another person whom you intend to harm).
- Delusions of jealousy (e.g. believing the victim is cheating on you).
- Delusions of love (believing the victim loves you, whereupon a sign of rejection may result in violence).
- Querulous delusions (beliefs giving ground for complaint against the victim).

Morbid jealousy (Othello syndrome) can occur in conjunction with many psychiatric diagnoses and is not necessarily psychotic. In 'delusional jealousy' there is an abnormal belief of partner infidelity.[3] This is often accompanied by intensive seeking of evidence to support the belief. It may be

---

1 This research finding refers to an association at the population level: that is, the group of patients with TCO symptoms are more often violent than those without such symptoms. See the discussion on considering population versus individual risks as part of risk assessment (p.166). The statements elsewhere in these pages about certain symptoms increasing risk of violence in patients are clinically observed correlations in *individual patients*, but not backed up by large-scale research studies.

2 Highlighting the importance of the distinction between relative risk (odds fourteen to twenty-five times higher) and absolute risk (0.3% lifetime prevalence).

3 The diagnosis is independent of whether the partner is, in fact, being unfaithful since it is based upon failure of reality testing.

difficult to distinguish from 'obsessional jealousy', paranoid personality disorder, or nonpathological extreme jealousy.

Erotomania (De Clerambault's syndrome) more often affects women. There is a belief that a person of importance is in love with the patient. It can occur in isolation as a delusional disorder or as a symptom of schizophrenia.

Induced delusional disorder is a delusional disorder experienced by an individual in prolonged, intimate contact with a person with psychosis, also known as 'folie à deux'—arguably wrongly, as the dominant partner is usually independently delusional. It is rare and sometimes associated with violent offending by both individuals (e.g. _R v Windle_, p.771).

Who is at risk?
Most victims of violent crime perpetrated by people with psychosis are not strangers but relatives, partners, or acquaintances. Approximately 60% of victims are family members, with less than 10% being strangers. People with psychosis are far more likely to be victims than perpetrators of violence or other crimes.

What is the risk?
* People diagnosed with psychosis are four to six times more likely to commit violent offences than members of the general population.
* The link between psychosis and nonviolent offending is not well established.
* Less than 10% of all violence is attributable to people with psychosis or other severe mental illness.
* In a year the probability of a person diagnosed with schizophrenia committing homicide is 1 in 3,000.
* Of homicides, 5%–10% are committed by people with schizophrenia (higher figures in Sweden; lower in the UK).

The increased risk of violence in people with psychosis is partly related to the following (in themselves, much more significant) comorbid risk factors:
* increased rates of substance misuse (eightfold increase in violence with this comorbidity).
* common comorbid personality disorder (twofold increase, and much higher for ASPD; see p.82).
* the same emotions (anger, panic) and desire to act that may be present if one were truly being persecuted.
* socioeconomic disadvantage.
* individual factors (gene/environment interaction studies suggest that 35% of the increased risk of violence in individuals with psychosis cannot be accounted for by factors shared with nonpsychotic siblings).

Alcohol & drug misuse and dependence

Misuse of alcohol or drugs is common in mentally disordered offenders. Having a mental disorder doubles risk of alcohol dependence and quadruples the risk of drug misuse; having comorbid mental illness and personality disorder increases risk further. Management of substance misuse is therefore an integral part of forensic psychiatry.

Box 3.2 Prevalence of substance misuse

- General population: harmful use of alcohol 16.6%; of drugs 35% (lifetime)
- General population: alcohol dependence 3.1%; drugs 4.3%
- General psychiatric patients: 20%–37%
- Sentenced prisoners: 50%–63% men; 33%–39% women
- Remand prisoners: 10%–61% men; 10%–69% women
- Forensic psychiatric patients: 51% drugs; 40% alcohol

The frequency of substance misuse in prison and secure psychiatric hospitals is an indicator of the failure of even intrusive security procedures to prevent <u>contraband</u> items being smuggled in (p.190). Patterns of drug use have changed with a surge in use of novel psychoactive substances such as 'spice'.[4] Amongst older drugs, cannabis, cocaine, amphetamines, and heroin are the most commonly used, in descending order.

Comorbidity with other mental disorders

Substance misuse in combination with mental illness and/or personality disorder is extremely common amongst forensic psychiatric patients. One study found that a fifth of male patients with schizophrenia were dependent on alcohol by age twenty-seven years.

Associations with offending behaviour

Alcohol and drug misuse are more strongly associated with violence and other offending than any other mental disorder (although there are many shared risk factors for drug use and interpersonal violence; see also Box 3.3). Including alcohol disorders, the odds of violence compared to the general population are increased sevenfold overall; excluding alcohol disorders, they are increased sixteen-fold for men and twenty-six-fold for women. Recent alcohol use is a risk factor for violent offending: half of those who commit assault are drunk at the time, as are two-thirds of those who kill. Illegal drug use may be a risk factor for acquisitive offending, to raise money to buy drugs.

---

4 A term for a group of synthetic cannabinoids, often sprayed onto shredded leaves and smoked.

- Alcohol use disorder roughly doubles risk of violent offending (and has a ten-year prevalence of violent offending of 8%).
- Cocaine is more strongly associated with domestic violence as compared with opioids or cannabis.
- Crack cocaine is more strongly associated with violence as compared with cocaine.
- Methamphetamine (and probably amphetamine) use is associated with violence.
- Novel psychoactive substances may be associated with violence.
- About 18% of those with a drug use disorder commit a violent offence over a ten-year follow-up.
- No definite association with violence: opiate intoxication or nicotine.

> **Box 3.3 Features of misuse and dependence that predispose to violence**
> - Acute intoxication—e.g. through disinhibition and disorganisation of behaviour (though cannabis and heroin intoxication *reduce* violence risk)
> - Withdrawal states—e.g. through agitation or paranoia
> - Dependence—e.g. through compulsion to obtain the substance
> - Neuropsychiatric sequelae of prolonged misuse
> - Associated personality traits—e.g. impulsivity and sensation-seeking
> - Social context—e.g. peer group, socioeconomic deprivation, childhood maltreatment and parental drug use

The combination of substance misuse and mental disorder increases the likelihood of violent offending further. One review revealed an eight- to tenfold increase in odds of violence in individuals with severe mental illness who abuse substances compared with the general population. In another study, violent offending increased by a factor of twenty-five for patients with schizophrenia who misused alcohol, compared with 3.6 for patients with schizophrenia who did not. A third study showed that 18% of patients with a major mental disorder will commit violence during the course of a year, rising to 31% for those with comorbid substance misuse, and 43% for those who also have personality disorder (p.78).

Other harms associated with misuse and dependence

- **Self-neglect**: chronically intoxicated or dependent users may fail to care for themselves.
- **Self-harm and suicide**: dysphoria is caused by withdrawal, and is much more likely to lead to self-harm in those disinhibited by earlier substance use.
- **Being a victim of violence**: one-third of assault victims are drunk at the time.

Personality disorder

Personality disorders (PDs) are pervasive disorders of affect, arousal and self-regulation, which result in personal or interpersonal distress or dysfunction. They usually emerge by early adulthood, can cause mild dysfunction or severe disability, and are exacerbated in their expression by stress and comorbid conditions, particularly mood disorders, psychosis and substance misuse.

Box 3.4 Prevalence of personality disorder*

- General population: 12%
- Primary care settings: 24%–30%
- General psychiatric patients: 50%
- Prisoners: 65% male; 50% female
- Forensic psychiatric patients: 60%–70%

*Studies tend to apply a low threshold for diagnosis.

There are three main clusters in DSM-5[5]: A (odd, eccentric), B (antagonistic, flamboyant), and C (anxious, fearful). See Table 3.1. ICD11 instead describes PD using severity levels (mild, medium, and severe) and specifying dominant traits.[6] The features of one PD may overlap with those of another in the same cluster,[7] so that a person may be diagnosed with more than one PD. People with PD may seek or avoid treatment.

Whereas all personality disorders are found in primary care and general psychiatry, forensic services deal primarily with cluster B PDs, particularly antisocial (p.82), borderline (p.84), and narcissistic (p.86). These are associated with rule-breaking and offending. PD is associated with increased risk of reoffending after discharge from secure units.

Table 3.1 Clusters of personality disorder traits

Cluster A	Cluster B	Cluster C
Paranoid	Antisocial	Avoidant
Schizoid	Borderline (emotionally unstable)	Dependent
Schizotypal	Histrionic	Obsessive-compulsive (anankastic)
	Narcissistic	

---

5 DSM-5 also includes a dimensional Alternative Model of Personality Disorder, based on severity of impairment amongst five trait domains (negative affectivity, detachment, antagonism, disinhibition, and psychoticism—maladaptive versions of the Five Factor Model traits of conscientiousness, neuroticism, agreeableness, extraversion, and openness to new experiences).

6 Similar to DSM-5's AMPD, these are negative affectivity, detachment, disinhibition, dissociality, and anankastia. A 'borderline pattern' qualifier can also be used. Categorical diagnoses are also possible.

7 As with a Venn diagram.

Comorbidity with other mental disorders

Comorbidity is the norm in forensic clinical populations; most patients meet criteria for multiple PD diagnoses (mostly ASPD, and BPD), often alongside a primary diagnosis such as schizophrenia. Depressive and substance misuse disorders are commonly comorbid with all PDs.

How do symptoms impact risk of offending or violence?

Most patients with PD only present a risk to themselves: self-harm, suicide and all-cause mortality are greatly increased in most personality disorders. Cluster B diagnoses are also associated with violence and offending, partly because of impaired ability to mentalise (p.208), as well as from symptoms such as hyperarousal, impulsivity, and dysregulated anger or fear. Violence risk is highest when individuals have comorbid conditions that also increase violence risk (e.g. paranoid psychosis, and substance misuse), and when there is a combination of the risk factors set out in Box 3.5.

Other clusters have less association with offending. Cluster A PDs involve poor reality testing and paranoid cognitions, but not dysregulated mood or impulsivity as in cluster B. Cluster C individuals may have dysregulated mood states, but not paranoia or impulsivity.

Box 3.5 Symptoms increasing risk of violence in PD

- Altered perception of reality—transient psychosis[8] or dissociation
- Paranoid cognitions and lowered threat perception threshold
- Dysregulated mood states, especially anger
- Hyperarousal secondary to the three causes above
- Lack of empathy
- Contempt of vulnerability in others (common in NPD)
- Impulsivity
- Lack of mentalising ability (capacity to reflect on actions)

Assessing risk associated with symptoms and signs in PD

Beyond general approaches to violence risk assessment (p.168), when assessing risk of violence in a patient with PD it is important to consider:
- history of violence to self or others, particularly convictions for violence.
- antisocial and unempathic attitudes to vulnerable people or carers.
- any insight or curiosity about their capacity for violence (as opposed to blaming others).
- comorbid mental disorder or substance misuse disorders (which may increase impulsivity, impair reality testing or cause disinhibition).

Who is at risk from violent offenders with PD?

As for mental illness, most victims of violent crime perpetrated by people with personality disorders are family members, partners, or otherwise known to the offender. Health care professionals may also be at increased

---

8 Transient periods of psychosis are common in both BPD and ASPD when under stress, and often associated with pseudohallucinations of a 'voice' instructing self-harm and/or harm to others.

risk from offender patients with personality disorder. Children may be at particular risk from parents with personality disorders.

Personality disorder and psychiatric injury

Personality disorder can also be relevant to claims for <u>compensation after injury</u> (p.640) because it may increase the plaintiff's vulnerability to injury and damage caused by the defendant (the so-called <u>eggshell skull rule</u>, p.641). For example, in one case the claimant's pre-existing histrionic PD was held to have exacerbated the damage caused by the defendant.

Antisocial personality disorder

Antisocial personality disorder (ASPD) is associated with offending and rule-breaking behaviour. It involves significant **impairment** in:
- identity (e.g. self-esteem derived from personal gain).
- self-direction (e.g. failure to conform to lawful or moral behaviour).
- empathy.
- interpersonal intimacy (being manipulative, deceitful, callous, or hostile).
- inhibition (irresponsibility, impulsivity, and risk-taking).

<u>Conduct disorder</u> (p.108) and <u>ADHD</u> (p.106) frequently precede the development of ASPD.[9] Conduct disorder is more likely in children with genetic vulnerabilities in serotonin regulation[10] who experience maltreatment.

ASPD is distinct from <u>psychopathy</u> (p.90). Almost all patients with psychopathy also meet the diagnostic criteria for ASPD, but few patients with ASPD display signs of psychopathy.

Box 3.6 Prevalence of ASPD
- General population: 1%–4% (6% male; 2% female)
- General psychiatric patients: 1%–18% (70% in substance use disorders)
- Prisoners: 63% male remand; 49% male sentenced; 21%–31% female
- Forensic psychiatric patients: 40%–70%

Individuals with ASPD rarely seek help, including primary care. ASPD is seen commonly in substance misuse services, and forensic psychiatric and prison populations. It is more commonly diagnosed in males. However, as for BPD, in more severe manifestations the gender gap is reduced, and in forensic psychiatric populations it is often comorbid with BPD. ASPD symptoms decline with increasing age.

How do symptoms impact risk of offending or violence?

Most criminal rule-breaking by patients with ASPD involves theft and fraud, especially in the context of comorbid drug use. A minority are violent to others. Specific symptoms that increase the risk of violence in ASPD include:
- Drug induced disturbances of perceived reality.
- Paranoid attitudes and cognitions; especially likely if drugs are misused.
- Hyperarousal.
- Lack of empathy, especially if there is evidence of contempt for distress in others.
- Impulsivity and lack of mentalising ability (capacity to reflect).
- Grandiosity (which contributes to contempt for others, especially if there are also narcissistic traits).

---

9 A childhood history of 'conduct disorder' is required to diagnose ASPD under DSM5.
10 Particularly the low-activity allele of the gene for monoamine oxidase A.

People with ASPD experience others as having agency and control, and often see themselves as being victimised, minimising their responsibility for violence they perceive as self-protection or retribution.

Assessing risk associated with symptoms and signs in ASPD

ASPD is associated with a tenfold increased risk of violence (p.44): eightfold in women, thirteen-fold in men. Reoffending risk is also increased. Beyond general approaches to risk assessment (p.168), other warning signs include escalating forms of violence (including violence to self in the form of severe self-harm) and evidence that the patient believes that other people are belittling or shaming them. Comorbid BPD may increase risk in the context of hostile attachments to others[11] and dissociation (p.100). Paranoid states make individuals with ASPD more likely to misperceive or overestimate threat and to carry weapons. Impulsivity means they are more likely to use them. Risk of violence is increased with comorbid conditions that are also associated with violence, such as severe mental illness and substance misuse.

ASPD is also associated with increased likelihood of:
- substance misuse disorders (three to five times higher rates).
- homelessness.
- physical health conditions.
- death by suicide or misadventure.

Who is at risk from violent offenders with ASPD?

Any person may be at risk from an individual in their environment with ASPD (particularly when they are in gangs, 38). Those who form attachments to them (e.g. partners) are at greatest risk.

---

11 Relevant to stalking and harassment.

Borderline personality disorder

Borderline, or emotionally unstable, personality disorder (BPD or EUPD) results in **impairment** of:
- identity (e.g. emptiness, unstable self-esteem).
- self-direction.
- empathy (difficulty recognising others' needs, hypersensitivity to insult).
- intimacy (intense unstable relationships, preoccupation with abandonment).
- affect regulation.
- inhibition (e.g. impulsivity, risk-taking).
- reality testing (transient psychotic states and dissociation).

A major symptom of BPD is *intense attachment*: to children, partners, professionals, and animals. These attachments tend to oscillate, with intense idealisation followed by hatred, especially if the relationship is threatened. BPD often involves physical attacks on the body in self-harming behaviours and impulsive suicidal behaviour. Intrusive thoughts of harming self or others may be experienced as pseudohallucinatory 'voices'.

Of those with BPD, 70% report childhood mistreatment. Genetics, dysfunction of the limbic system and endogenous opioid receptors and hyperresponsivity of the hypothalamic-pituitary-adrenal axis may be important in aetiology. A 2016 study estimated prevalence of BPD to be equal across genders. People with BPD are care-seekers and are thus prevalent in psychiatric services, particularly psychotherapy, eating disorders, crisis and forensic services.

Box 3.7 Prevalence of BPD
- General population: 1%–6%
- General psychiatric patients: 11%–20%
- Prisoners: 23% male remand; 14% male sentenced; 20% female
- Forensic psychiatric patients: 24%–60%

BPD patients are less able to 'self-soothe' or tolerate uncertainty, and therefore often act out their feelings rather than acknowledging and managing them. Acting out feelings such as anger may involve self-harm or violence. People with BPD may 'split' experiences into very good or very bad. This splitting (p.312) can be projected into others, including staff teams who may find that some members strongly like and others dislike the patient.

How do symptoms impact risk of offending or violence?

BPD is prevalent in perpetrators of all kinds of family violence. Perpetrators may be male or female. In one study 36% of people with BPD reported carrying out an act of violence, usually towards someone with whom they were in an intimate relationship of need or dependence. Instability of relationships is a risk factor for violence in people with BPD.

A population study of 14,753 British adults concluded that the association between BPD and violence was mostly explained by comorbid ASPD, psychopathy, and substance misuse. The exception was serious intimate partner violence (IPV), for which the BPD itself was a relevant risk factor. Violence risk factors specific to BPD include:
• Attempts to avoid feared abandonment.
• Intense anger and hostility.
• Impulsivity.
• Any history of stalking, especially where there has been a previous relationship or IPV.
• Severe and repetitive self-harm.

Assessing risk associated with symptoms and signs in BPD

As perceived abandonment is an identified risk factor for violence, history taking and assessment should focus on loss of relationships, both actual and threatened, whether recent or not. Perceived abandonment is likely to increase arousal and perceived threat, potentially increasing risk of violence and self-harm. Special attention should be paid to abrupt changes in routine or physical or psychological security (e.g. bereavements, new accommodation, and carer change).

Those with BPD tend to become dependent upon care, and may perceive attempts to withdraw elements of a care package, or to discharge them, as rejection and abandonment, resulting in acting out through self-harm or violence. Thus there is a particular risk that patients remain inappropriately detained in secure conditions.

Who is at risk from violent offenders with BPD?

Anyone who is in a caring relationship with someone with BPD is at risk, including parents, partners, and children. Ex-partners may be especially at risk, and the risk may persist after the relationship ends. Healthcare professionals may be at risk of angry outbursts and sometimes violence if they are perceived as uncaring or abandoning.

Treatment

Five psychological treatments have an epidemiological evidence base in BPD: dialectical behavioural therapy (DBT, p.208), mentalisation-based therapy (MBT, p.208), schema-focused therapy (SFT, p.209), transference-focused dynamic psychotherapy (p.212), and systems training for emotional predictability and problem solving (STEPPS, p.218). Training staff is of particular relevance when treating BPD in secure settings because patients/prisoners may form intense attachments to staff, which increase the risk of boundary violations (p.302).

Narcissistic personality disorder

Like other cluster B PDs, NPD causes impairment in self-identity, self-direction, and interpersonal functioning, with a range of severity. Comorbidity with other PDs is common. Early descriptions were based on psychoanalytical theory[12]; later accounts attend to cognitive and interpersonal psychology.

NPD is most easily understood as an elaborated psychological defence against feeling vulnerable. Its symptoms include a pervasive pattern of grandiosity (in fantasy or behaviour), sense of entitlement and lack of empathy. Two aspects of the same psychopathology are described: an overtly *grandiose* and arrogant form, and a *vulnerable* anxious form. Both presentations feature excessive focus on self, preoccupation with a belief in one's special status, exquisite sensitivity to status, and competition and envy to the point of paranoia. A sense of entitlement may be seen as justifying exploitation and bullying.

Box 3.8 Prevalence of NPD

- General population: 1% (0.1%–6.2%)
- General psychiatric patients: 2%–16%
- Prisoners: 8% male remand; 7% male sentenced; 6% female
- Forensic psychiatric patients: 26%

Aetiology is unknown but it is likely that exposure to emotional neglect or abuse and attachment insecurity in childhood increases risk. Temperamental factors exacerbated by parental overindulgence and/or having a parent with NPD traits may also have some influence.

How do symptoms impact risk of offending or violence?

Studies of incarcerated offenders find that NPD is a robust predictor of conviction for violence, especially in females.

- Comorbid NPD, ASPD, and BPD carries significantly increased risk of violence to others, especially if other violence risk factors are present. Approximately 40% of those with NPD have a comorbid substance abuse or anxiety disorder; 30% have comorbid depression.
- Grandiosity and sense of entitlement are risk factors for violence by people with NPD. Violence is usually manifested in intimate partner violence.
- NPD is common in <u>stalkers</u> (p.52) and may contribute to the association between stalking and violence.

---

12 Particularly the psychoanalyst Otto Kernberg, who introduced the concept of narcissistic personality structure, based on libidinal investment in an infantile representation of the self.

- NPD traits such as grandiosity may contribute to the risk of other kinds of unusual violence such as acts of terrorism, spree killings, serial killings, and sexual violence to strangers. The perpetrators with NPD may see the violence as justified because of their unique abilities or as a response to unacceptable rejection and humiliation by the victim.

Assessing risk associated with symptoms and signs in NPD

Risk assessment utilises the same principles as for any other mental disorder. The presence of pro-social factors (e.g. education, employment) may be protective or make an offender more dangerous and resourceful.

Forensic psychiatrists may be asked to assess risk in people whose NPD traits give rise to fantasies of extreme violence. In such cases, it is important to assess the usual violence risk factors and assess how anxious the individual is about what might happen, any mood component to the fantasies, and what defence mechanisms (p.212) are used to manage self-esteem.

Suicide risk is increased in people with NPD but may be hard to assess accurately because of grandiosity and 'apparent good self-esteem'.

Staff may need particular warning and support to prevent boundary violations (p.302), as offenders with NPD may be skilled at manipulation.

Who is at risk from those with NPD?

Any individual who challenges the defences of the individual with NPD may be at risk. Similarly, any individual in a position where they may be exploited may be at risk of becoming the victim of offending.

Paranoid personality disorder

Paranoid personality disorder (PPD) is principally characterised by a pervasive pattern of suspiciousness and distrust of others and rigid misperception of others' intentions as hostile.

Signs of PPD include persistent beliefs that others are deceiving, harming or exploiting them, or that partners are unfaithful to them, and preoccupation with feelings of betrayal, anger, and hurt. Rigidity of thought is common, resulting in grudge-holding and revenge fantasies. Controlling behaviours are common; as in NPD, people with PPD may be exquisitely sensitive to slights; the two diagnoses may be comorbid. There is clearly a spectrum of cognitive rigidity between PPD and paranoid psychosis (p.72), and distinguishing them may be difficult.

> **Box 3.9 Prevalence of paranoid personality disorder**
> - General population: 0.5%–7% (12% male; 3% female)
> - General psychiatric patients: 7%–10%
> - Prisoners: 29% male remand; 20% male sentenced; 16% female
> - Forensic psychiatric patients: 18%

Aetiology is unknown; there is evidence of increased rates of PPD amongst close relatives of those with schizophrenia or delusional disorder, hinting at a genetic or shared environmental association. As with other PDs, it is likely that early childhood adversity and insecurity of attachment play a part in the development of PPD.

How do symptoms impact risk of offending or violence?

A 2016 meta-analysis of 23,444 members of the UK general population showed an association between paranoid ideation and a doubling of the odds of violence (not explained by psychosis or comorbidities). Although not a study of PPD, it highlights the importance of paranoia in violence. People with PPD rarely seek help, so studies are often based on legally identified samples.

It is likely that comorbid mood disorders may increase the risk of suicide (especially in high-risk groups such as middle-aged males), which is accentuated because of the profound social isolation experienced by individuals with PPD.

Most people with PPD do not appear to get into trouble with the law, despite profound suspicion and mistrust of others. Violent offending risk is likely to increase if there is co-morbidity with NPD and ASPD. Offending may take the form of stalking or harassment offences, often against a professional or official that the perpetrator believes has failed or harmed them in some way. Relational violence is rare because people with PPD are less likely to make intimate attachments.

Violence in PPD is often reactive and extreme; its execution may be carefully planned. Individuals with PPD have been identified as perpetrators of spree killings and terrorist offences.

Assessing risk associated with symptoms and signs in PPD

The general risk factors for violence should be explored and assessed as above. As for NPD, much depends on the context of the concern, and whether there has been a recent change in relational status or a loss event. Specific issues in risk assessment in PPD relate to the reluctance of people with PPD to reveal their mental state or inner thoughts, and the ease with which new people may be incorporated into their paranoid world view. Comorbid mood dysregulation may lead to increased levels of paranoia without warning.

The risk from PPD lies in its irrationality and associated unpredictability. Making a therapeutic alliance may be difficult and unsuccessful even in the long term. Changes to a containing environment or imposed social interaction with others may increase risk.

Staff need training about the unpredictability of violence by people with PPD and the futility of attempting to persuade patients out of their beliefs using rational argument.

Psychopathy

Psychopathy is a particular expression of severe personality disorder, characterised by *callous unemotional traits* and *extremely antisocial attitudes*. Its features overlap with those of ASPD (p.82) and NPD (p.86); it is conceptually distinct from both.[13]

Psychopathy is the result of a complex interaction of genetic vulnerability, limbic system abnormality, and early childhood adversity.

> **Box 3.10 Prevalence and comorbidity of psychopathy**
> - General population: 0.1%–1.2%
> - General psychiatric patients: no data
> - Prisoners: 15%–25%
> - Forensic psychiatric patients: 15%–30%

Community prevalence studies use self-report measures in students which do not include criminality as a criterion, emphasising arrogance, and cruelty. Prison studies usually use the Hare Psychopathy Checklist (PCL-R, p.170) which is observer-rated, uses multiple information sources and is commonly part of violence risk assessment (p.168) for serious offenders. The mean PCL-R score across all forensic psychiatric patients is 18–20.

PCL-R psychopathy has two factors[14]:
- Factor 1 (Callous unemotional): arrogant interpersonal style, grandiose, glib, and deceitful; lacks empathy, lacks remorse, and has shallow and labile emotions and deficient affective experience.
- Factor 2 (Antisocial): impulsive behavioural style, sensation-seeking, and lack of planning; irresponsible, parasitic lifestyle.

A score of 30 or over (25 in Europe) indicates psychopathy. Male and female psychopaths are similar, but prevalence in female offenders is lower.

How do symptoms impact risk of offending or violence?

Psychopathy substantially increases risk of violence, especially in released prisoners with PCL-R scores above 25–30. One study estimated that over half of offences involving severe violence were related to psychopathy.

Features of psychopathy that increase risk of harm to others include:
- Predatory attitudes towards others.
- Grandiosity and paranoia.
- Contempt for others' distress.
- Intelligence, deceitfulness and planning capacity.

---

13 The current concept of psychopathy is derived from Pritchard's concept of 'moral insanity' and Cleckley's work *The Mask of Sanity*, whereas the broader concept of ASPD has separate roots in Henderson's 1939 classification, *Psychopathic States*, and NPD is derived from Kernberg's theories.

14 Robert Hare, the author of the PCL-R, divides each of these into two 'facets'.

- Remorselessness.
- Impulsivity and lack of capacity to reflect on actions.

Psychopathy may manifest in repeated offending behaviour, including crimes of deception, theft, and violence, and as interpersonal dysfunction, which may or may not involve interpersonal violence. There is some debate about whether criminality is essential to psychopathy.

Risks associated with symptoms and signs in psychopathy

In prisons and forensic psychiatric settings, most psychopaths are known high-risk offenders, and risk is augmented by other violence risk factors. When assessing risk in this group, it is important to consider:

- Is the level of violence escalating?
- Are there any other risk factors present, such as other mental disorders or substance misuse?
- Is there an identifiable victim?
- Is there a lack of anxiety or remorse for past offences?

Risk assessment should involve different disciplines and sources of information, and should not be based on one clinician's single view or self-report.

Who is at risk from violent offenders with psychopathy?

Any person is potentially at risk from individuals with psychopathy. Strangers may be harmed, usually in the context of robbery or exploitation. Some predatory psychopaths specifically target women or children for harm, and may groom their victims beforehand. Men with mild to moderate degrees of psychopathy may be perpetrators of domestic violence and cruelty to children within the home. Higher-functioning psychopaths may prefer to use deceit and emotional manipulation rather than violence to achieve their purposes, and they may not have criminal records.[15]

Staff need training in the potential for deception by patients with psychopathy. Supervision and reflective practice (p.308) are essential to prevent inappropriate relationships. Many inpatient secure services will not admit offenders with high levels of psychopathy, who are more likely to be found in prison or high-security hospitals.

15 One study found the rate of psychopathy amongst corporate executives was around 20%.

Bipolar disorder

Bipolar disorder involves discrete episodes of mania (or hypomania) and depression. Mania involves extreme, elevated mood, often with grandiosity, sleeplessness, and recklessness; hypomania is less extreme and does not include psychosis. Functioning must be disturbed for over a week, with symptoms unexplained by drugs or physical illness.

- Bipolar I disorder diagnosis requires at least one episode of mania, and a roughly equal ratio of manic (or hypomanic) and depressive episodes.
- Bipolar II involves only hypomania, and a higher ratio of depressive episodes.

> ### Box 3.11 Prevalence of bipolar disorder
> - General population: 0.7%
> - General psychiatric patients: 4%
> - Prisoners: 1% whether male or female, sentenced or remand
> - Forensic psychiatric patients: approximately 5%

Comorbidity with other mental disorders

Between 65% and 90% of all people with bipolar disorder have one or more comorbid mental disorder, typically anxiety-related disorders (pp.96,98) or impulse-control disorders (e.g. ADHD, p.106); commonly under-diagnosed. In offenders, 50% have alcohol or drug dependence (p.76). If present, alcohol and substance misuse generally increase during manic phases, and to a lesser extent during depressive phases.

Manic features that may predispose to violence & offending

- Elation
- Hyperarousal
- Impaired judgement
- Impulsivity
- Irritability
- Intolerance of frustration
- Hypersexuality
- Psychosis (p.72), especially intrusive hallucinations or grandiose or persecutory delusions

Associations with offending behaviour

The odds of violence in those with bipolar disorder are about five times greater than in the general population; the rate of violence is highest when there is comorbid substance misuse disorder. Risk of violent crime is also somewhat higher in siblings of those with bipolar disorder. Lifetime prevalence of violence conviction is about 11% in men with bipolar disorder and 2% in women (<5% over ten years of follow-up). Of violence convictions, 70% are in those who are over five years postdiagnosis.

The offences most commonly committed are minor and include: <u>common assaults</u> (p.416), offences related to intoxication with alcohol or drugs; threats of violence, <u>damage to property</u> (p.422), <u>theft</u> (p.426), forging cheques, or failure to pay, or <u>sexual indecency</u> (p.419). The victims in most cases are strangers.

Serious offences are less common but include: <u>GBH</u> (p.416), <u>arson</u> (p.422), sexual assaults including <u>rape</u> (p.418), causing death by dangerous driving, and (very rarely) <u>homicide</u> (p.414). A small number of <u>stalkers</u> (p.52) suffer from bipolar disorder.

Other harms associated with manic states
- **Self-neglect** : overactivity preventing self-care
- **Reputational or financial damage** due to poor judgement
- **Vulnerability to sexual or financial exploitation** due to grandiosity and poor judgement

Those in manic states not uncommonly enter into contracts unwisely. A psychiatrist may be called upon to report on whether the patient had the <u>mental capacity</u> (p.540) at the time to understand the nature and the implications of the contract they made, which may determine whether or not the contract can be enforced.

Depression & other affective disorders

The main cause of depression is major depressive disorder. Depressive episodes can also occur in bipolar disorder (p.92), dysthymia, cyclothymia, schizophrenia (p.73), substance misuse (p.76), personality disorder (p.78), stroke, and other conditions.

Box 3.12 Prevalence of major depression
- General population: 6.9%–22.3% (lifetime)
- General psychiatric patients: 15%
- Prisoners: 14.9%–29% (7.8% severe)
- Forensic psychiatric patients: approximately 5%

In a meta-analysis of 33,588 prisoners worldwide no significant difference was observed in depression prevalence between male and female adult prisoners. A large cohort study showed a gender difference for depression prevalence in adolescent prisoners (29% females; 11% males).

Comorbidity with other mental disorders

Of people with major depression, 9.2%–82.5% have one or more comorbid mental disorders, most commonly substance misuse or dependence (p.76), anxiety-related disorders (pp.96,98), and impulse-control disorders (e.g. ADHD, p.106). Major depression may follow traumatic brain injury (p.112).

Associations with offending behaviour

Recent evidence suggests that depression may be a risk factor for violence. A cohort study found that adolescents with depression have about twice the odds of conviction for violence compared to community controls (after adjustment for previous violence and socioeconomic status). Two other adolescent cohort studies suggested that the odds of violence may increase as depressive symptoms worsen.

Depressed adults have about three times higher odds of committing violent crimes than community controls. Comorbidity with other known risk factors for violence (particularly substance abuse) leads to the highest risk of violence to others.

However, the rates of violent crime committed by those with depression are far lower than for mental illnesses such as schizophrenia (p.73). The vast majority of people with depression do not pose a risk to others; ten years after diagnosis, fewer than 5% have committed violent crime. They are a far greater risk to themselves, far more likely to be victims of crime (compared to the general population), at risk of self-neglect, lacking in motivation to care for themselves, and likely to exhibit self-harm or suicide. Irritability and lack of a normal perspective on the future may contribute to violence (e.g. in domestic homicide).

Distinguishing between psychotic and nonpsychotic depression is important. Women with psychotic depression can be at risk of killing their loved ones (especially children), as well as themselves; in the belief that the future for themselves and their loved ones is hopeless, the most loving response being <u>mercy killing</u> (p.413). A similar phenomenon may occur for men (particularly older men) who kill their spouse when suffering from severe depression.

Other harms associated with depression

• **Self-neglect**: lack of motivation to care for oneself, or others
• **Self-harm or suicide:** see p.176

Depression is also relevant to forensic psychiatrists as a frequent consequence of <u>victimisation</u> (p.179) and of punishments such as <u>imprisonment</u> (p.448), and may form the basis of a claim for <u>compensation</u> (p.640) in certain circumstances. Psychiatrists can be asked to assess the risk that imprisonment (or <u>deportation</u> or <u>extradition</u>, p.558) will lead to a deterioration in mental state, or other harm.

Posttraumatic stress disorder

In this context, 'trauma' means an exceptionally severe, life-threatening, and distressing event, or a series of events that cumulatively are exceptionally severe and distressing. The relationship between such trauma and crime is complex. Posttraumatic stress disorder (PTSD) is one possible sequel of trauma.

Box 3.13 Prevalence of PTSD
- General population: 3%–5%
- General psychiatric patients: 14%–43%
- Prisoners: 0.1%–27% men; 12%–38% women (approximately 1:3)
- Forensic psychiatric patients: 36%–58%

Diagnostic controversy

A PTSD diagnosis requires, in essence, severe psychological disturbance following trauma, involving *involuntary re-experiencing* of the trauma, *hyperarousal*, *avoidance* of stimuli associated with the trauma, and *emotional numbing*.[16] Amnesia (p.636) for the traumatic event is common, and usually dissociative in nature.

The diagnostic requirement of an objectively traumatic event generates a risk of circular thinking: that is, of regarding an event as objectively traumatic because a person repeatedly and involuntarily re-experiences it. This is an issue in compensation claims (p.640), especially given the familiarity of the concept of PTSD amongst the lay population.

Comorbidity with other mental disorders

Imprisoned people with PTSD have double the odds of substance misuse and triple the odds of anxiety, depression, and suicidality, compared to those without PTSD. Its prevalence in people with schizophrenia in forensic settings is higher than in general psychiatric samples. People with psychosis and PTSD tend to have more positive psychotic symptoms, heightened paranoia, and more violent thoughts, feelings, and behaviour. The relationship between psychosis, PTSD, and violence is not fully understood.

Associations with offending behaviour

There is no definite causal link established between PTSD and offending behaviour. However, PTSD is associated with violence in prison, community reoffending, and military combat. Comparing deployed British soldiers with PTSD to those without PTSD, risk of violent offending is about two to three

---

16 It is distinct from the concept of complex PTSD (p.669), which is far less widely accepted. This condition, closely related to the competing concept of borderline personality disorder (p.84), is often associated with the kind of prolonged physical, sexual, or emotional abuse that forensic patients often suffered as children.

times higher, with about 9% of those with PTSD violently offending in the seven years after deployment, compared to 3% without PTSD.

There are a number of factors which are important to understanding offending behaviour seen in people with PTSD:

• **Hyperarousal**, resulting in a heightened emotional and physiological state may predispose to impulsive and reactive violence.
• Psychological preparedness or **hypervigilance**, where the person with PTSD may be 'on the lookout' for threat or danger and correspondingly respond inappropriately to a stimulus as if it were a threat.
• **Impulsivity** and **anger** are commonly seen in PTSD and may provide a mechanism through which violence is perpetrated.
• **Flashbacks** may precipitate a violent response as a direct result of experiencing a threatening event.
• The violent response may occur in a state of **dissociation**. Dissociation is a common feature of PTSD, and violence may occur more frequently in this semiconscious state.
• **Nightmares** may result in violent actions during sleep or immediately on waking.

Combat veterans with a diagnosis of PTSD have been shown to be more likely to show reactive violence (as opposed to instrumental violence, p.26) than those without PTSD.

PTSD as a consequence of offending

The traumatic trigger for development of PTSD in forensic psychiatric in-patients may be their index offence in up to 70% of cases. PTSD is more likely to be a consequence if the offence was unplanned and if the offender has no significant criminal history.

Treatment of PTSD caused by offending may have to be pursued along-side treatment of mental conditions that were (possibly causally) associated with the offending.

Relevance to forensic psychiatrists

PTSD, whatever its origins, may also be relevant to forensic psychiatrists when their patients face imprisonment or deportation (p.558), as it may form the basis of a claim that, in exceptional circumstances, the imprison-ment or deportation would breach the patient's human rights (p.516) be-cause of its impact on their PTSD and consequent risk of suicide or other self-harm.

In forensic services that treat victims of offending (p.234), PTSD is the most common diagnosis.

Suffering PTSD after an injury or other major incident is one of the com-monest reasons for claiming compensation for psychiatric injury (p.640), which requires psychiatric evidence.

Anxiety disorders

These include generalised anxiety disorder (GAD), obsessive-compulsive disorder (OCD), social anxiety disorder, panic disorder, phobias, and more broadly, adjustment disorders, including grief reactions. They are the most common class of mental disorder, affecting approximately one in five adults. Anxiety is also a prominent symptom in depression (p.94) and PTSD (p.96).

> **Box 3.14 Prevalence of anxiety disorders**
> • General population: GAD 3%; SAD 5%; OCD 1%; panic 3%;
>   phobias 10%
> • General psychiatric patients: no data
> • Prisoners: GAD 10%–15%; OCD 2.5%–4%; panic 9%; phobias 1%–3%
> • Forensic psychiatric patients: no data

Studies focusing on the prevalence of neurotic illness as a single group have found rates of approximately 10%–45% in prisoners, well in excess of the general population. This excess has not been seen in all studies.

Associations with offending behaviour

Although community research suggests that anxiety disorders are more common in men who self-report violent behaviours compared to those who do not, there is no evidence that anxiety disorder per se affects an individual's risk of violence or other offending behaviour. Anxiety disorders are commonly comorbid with other mental disorders and substance misuse. One in three men and one in six women with an anxiety disorder abuse alcohol, and 70% of adults with cannabis dependence have an anxiety disorder.

Severe anxiety may predispose to dissociation (p.100), which itself may disinhibit the patient, allowing them to do things they would not otherwise do.

Other associations

Severe forms of anxiety disorder arising after injury or a major incident, particularly severe adjustment disorders, may form the basis of a claim for compensation for psychiatric injury (p.640), in the same way as PTSD.

Dissociative and conversion disorders

Concepts of 'conversion' (of psychological conflict into the experience of physical symptoms) and 'dissociation' (from psychological conflict) evolved from psychoanalysis, but are now defined pragmatically by their symptoms. Whether their aetiology involves trauma, emotional conflict, or manifestations of underlying neurophysiological disturbance is debated.

Box 3.15 Prevalence of dissociative and conversion disorders

- General population: around 10%
- General medical patients: 5% conversion (M:F 1:2–10), 10% dissociative
- General psychiatric patients: around 10%
- Prisoners: no data
- Forensic psychiatric patients: no data

The prevalence of these disorders has steadily declined since the late-nineteenth century (when they were known as 'hysteria' and might affect a third to a half of some sections of the population at some stage in life); at the same time, personality disorders have become more commonly diagnosed.

DSM-5 describes dissociative and conversion (or 'functional neurological symptom') disorders as broadly involving impairments in mental integration: of consciousness, memory, identity, emotion, perception, body sense, motor control, and behaviour. Box 3.16 below shows the subtypes recognised in DSM-5 and ICD11.

Box 3.16 Dissociative and conversion disorders

- Dissociative amnesia with/without fugue
- Trance and possession trance disorders (ICD11 only)
- Dissociative identity ('multiple personality') disorder
- Depersonalisation-derealisation disorder
- Secondary dissociative syndrome (ICD11 only)
- Ganser's syndrome (ICD11 only)
- Dissociative neurological symptom disorder (sensory, motor)

Comorbidity with other mental disorders

Dissociative states are more common in patients with other mental disorders, specifically PTSD (p.96), anxiety disorders (p.98), depression (p.94), and organic syndromes (e.g. after traumatic brain injury, p.112). In one study, nearly half the subjects with conversion disorder also experienced dissociation.

The dissociative symptoms of 'depersonalisation' (a sense of oneself as altered or unreal) or 'derealisation' (a sense of the world as altered or unreal) are reported in normal individuals subjected to high stress, such as soldiers in battle.

Associations with violence

- A substantial proportion of individuals with dissociative symptoms have experienced or witnessed severe violence (as victim or perpetrator).
- Individuals in a dissociative state are said to be released from acting as they might ordinarily do, and act 'out of character'. However, it is unwise to assume that violence is related to dissociation without very clear other evidence to suggest it. Full dissociation requires amnesia for the event.
- There is some limited evidence to suggest that having trait dissociation (i.e. a 'dissociative disorder' rather than transient dissociative state) makes future violence more likely.

Dissociative amnesia

Genuine amnesia for commission of a violent offence arises most commonly from **dissociative amnesia** (subsequent dissociation from the memory of events that occurred during normal consciousness, also known as 'psychogenic amnesia'). By contrast, a **dissociative state** at the time of the offence, with consequent dense amnesia, is very rare (and difficult to confirm).

Of people alleged to have offended violently, 20%–30% claim amnesia (p.636) for key events, including 10%–70% of murder suspects. This may be malingered (p.118), the result of psychosis (p.72), or a sleep disorder (p.115), but in many cases arises from dissociative amnesia (often without a past history of a dissociative disorder).

Dissociative amnesia for offences is associated with offences committed in a state of high emotional arousal, where the victim is known intimately to the offender and where the offender has drunk alcohol (the greater the degree of violence involved, the greater the likelihood of dissociative amnesia). Often the amnesia is patchy, with 'islands' of memory, usually beginning with absence of memory of events close in time to the violence or other cause of emotional arousal. Very commonly, it is complicated by intoxication at the time, raising the possibility of alcohol blackout (p.637).

Somatoform disorders and chronic fatigue

These disorders, which are related to but distinct from the dissociative and conversion disorders, have no known association with violence or other offending behaviour. However, they may very occasionally be of relevance to forensic psychiatrists, such as when they form the basis for a claim for compensation after injury (p.640).

Paraphilias

These are a heterogeneous group of conditions in which the individual exhibits culturally atypical sexual behaviours (p.54) that are longstanding (present for at least six months), cause them or those around them marked distress, and interfere with normal daily life. They tend to involve an inappropriate sexual target (e.g. prepubescent[17] children in paedophilia, animals in bestiality, or inanimate objects in fetishism) or inappropriate means of obtaining sexual gratification, as in exhibitionism, sadomasochism, frotteurism,[18] or voyeurism. Some, but not all, paraphilic behaviours are also sexual offences (p.418).

Sex addiction is not currently a recognised mental disorder, although paraphilic disorders often involve an out-of-control quality whereby sexual activities dominate daily life. Paraphilias may develop as psychological defences to unprocessed emotions.

> **Box 3.17 Prevalence of paraphilic disorder**
> - General population: 3% exhibitionism; 8% voyeurism; 3%–5% paedophilia
> - General psychiatric inpatients: 13%
> - Prisoners: no data
> - Forensic psychiatric patients: no data
> - Convicted sex offenders: 25%–75%

Existing data are from Western countries. Self-reporting bias is a limitation. The sexual behaviours which are considered abnormal vary between cultures. The internet has made paraphilic pornography vastly more available: it is unclear to what extent this has normalised atypical sexual behaviours, or simply demonstrates that paraphilias are more common than previously acknowledged.

Paraphilias are more common in men (with woman exhibiting perhaps 10% of the male prevalence). Females and males are similar in demographic, clinical, and offence-related characteristics. The most common paraphilias amongst women are paedophilic (36% of the male prevalence in one study), sexually sadistic (29%), and exhibitionistic (29%).

It is important in diagnosing paraphilias to adhere to a proper medical concept of mental disorder (p.54) and respect the diversity of human sexual expression not leading to distress, harm, or violation of the rights of others. Not all atypical or criminal sexual behaviours are paraphilic disorders.

---

17 The DSM-5 and ICD11 definitions of paedophilia specify prepubertal children (i.e. younger than elven years old). 'Hebephilia' refers to sexual attraction to pubertal children. Paedophilia may relate to sexual abuse experienced as a child, but most children who are sexually abused do not develop paedophilia.

18 Nonconsensual rubbing against another person in a sexual manner (e.g. on public transport).

Comorbidity with other mental disorders

High rates of comorbid mental illness and personality disorder have been reported in those with paraphilia—for example 93% of patients with paedophilia in one study had comorbid mental disorders, most commonly mood disorder and/or substance misuse. Comorbid psychotic illness is rare. Approximately 75% of individuals with paraphilias who commit sexual offences suffer from personality disorder, and one-fifth from psychopathy (p.90). Paraphilias have been suggested by some authors to be more common in patients who also suffer from autistic spectrum disorders (p.104) or ADHD (p.106). Most research concerns paraphilic sex offenders only.

Associations with offending behaviour

In most jurisdictions, behaviours associated with certain paraphilias are in themselves illegal (e.g. bestiality, paedophilia, or frotteurism, the latter of which amounts to assault, p.416, and consensual sadomasochistic practices in some jurisdictions, including the UK). Some paraphilias (e.g. fetishism) may contribute to other crimes (e.g. theft, p.426, of underwear from a washing line).

Other harms associated with paraphilias

Self-harm or **accidental death**[19] (e.g. from extreme sadomasochism) One study suggested that psychiatric inpatients with paraphilic disorder were more likely to have attempted suicide than those without.

---

19 Claims of 'accident' given by defendants charged with murder of a sexual partner may be viewed skeptically.

Autistic spectrum disorders

People with autism spectrum disorders (ASDs)[20] are over-represented in forensic mental health populations. Intellectual disability, which may occur in more severe forms of ASD, is considered separately (p.110).

Box 3.18 Prevalence of autistic spectrum disorders

• General population: 1.1% (2.0% men; 0.3% women)
• General psychiatric patients: no data
• Prisoners: no data
• Forensic psychiatric patients (high security): 1.5%–5%

ASDs may be under-recognised in forensic psychiatric settings, with many patients diagnosed having previously been diagnosed with schizophrenia (p.73) and/or schizoid personality disorder (p.78). See Box 3.19.

Box 3.19 Autistic spectrum disorders

Persistent multicontext deficits in social communication and interaction [21]
  • in social-emotional reciprocity and
  • in nonverbal communicative behaviours and
  • in developing, maintaining, and understanding relationships
Restricted, repetitive patterns of behaviour, interests, or activities
  • stereotyped or repetitive movements, object use, or speech and/or
  • inflexible adherence to routines, sameness, or rituals and/or
  • intense/focused, highly restricted, fixated interests and/or
  • hyper- or hypo-reactivity to (or interest in) sensory input
Present from early developmental period, causing clinically significant impairment in social/occupational function, unexplained by other condition
... with/without disorder of intellectual development
... with/without absence/impairment of functional language
... with/without loss of previously acquired skills
... associated (or not) with another medical, genetic, or other condition

---

There is a wide range of cognitive abilities associated with autism; with some being high-functioning, whilst others have significant cognitive disability. The level of functioning appears to have an effect upon the characteristics of the offences they may commit. Some studies suggest that people

---

20 The term *autistic spectrum* has both entered common parlance and probably become overused, including in clinico-legal contexts.

21 Simplified version of DSM-5 and ICD11 criteria. Older terms are still often in use, including *pervasive developmental disorders* as a group term, and syndromes including classical autism, atypical autism, Asperger syndrome and childhood disintegrative disorder (Heller's syndrome).

on 'the autistic spectrum' commit more violent offences and criminal damage (as well as stalking, noncontact sexual offences, arson, and cyber-crime). However, rates of offending overall may be the same as in the general population, and most individuals with ASD do not offend.

Features of ASDs that may predispose to violence

- Lack of concern for outcome
- Social naivety
- Lack of awareness of outcome
- Lack of empathy
- Misinterpretation of others' behaviour (e.g. as hostile)
- Social or sexual rejection, bullying, or family conflict
- Comorbid drug and alcohol use
- Comorbid personality disorder
- Comorbid ADHD

Formulation of offending behaviour in ASDs

- **Theory of mind** deficits, including a tendency to egocentricity, resulting in lack of awareness of their impact upon victims and of what is 'wrong' in social and emotional terms, including being less able to recognise fear in a victim.
- Deficits in **social reciprocity**, which may predispose to sexual offences in particular (e.g. in an individual who wants sexual contact, without appreciating the complex reciprocal interactions that must occur between two potential partners in order for it to be consensual).
- **Restricted, repetitive interests** that may, for example, include fire-setting, or may lead to the commission of bizarre and sometimes persistent crimes without apparent ordinarily understandable motive (e.g. where the 'motive' is merely repetition of the act).[22]
- Other determinants of offending may be **revenge** for persistent bullying; **explosive responses** to particular stimuli or changes in routine (which can be extremely violent) and **susceptibility to exploitation**, with coerced involvement in criminal activity.[23]

---

22 Nevertheless, despite the lack of an understandable motive for crime, patients with autism spectrum disorder often still have the legal <u>intent</u> (p.402) to commit the crime and may therefore still be convicted.

23 See for example offences of <u>encouraging and assisting</u> (joint enterprise, p.408).

ADHD

Attention deficit hyperactivity disorder (ADHD), attention deficit disorder and hyperkinetic disorder (a narrower definition) are terms used for a syndrome characterised by persistent overactivity, impulsivity and difficulties in sustaining attention. The occurrence of the symptoms both within and outside the home, the presence of both inattention and overactivity, plus the presence of conduct disorder (CD, p.108) are all associated with a more serious condition that is less responsive to treatment, and which has poorer outcome. Its relevance to adult forensic psychiatry lies partly in its association with developing adult antisocial personality disorder (p.82).

Evidence suggests that inattentive and overactive/impulsive subtypes of ADHD have distinct profiles. Those with the hyperactive-impulsive subtype are characterised by extreme overactivity, with oppositional and aggressive behaviours. Conduct problems are their most prevalent school-based difficulties, and they have high rates of school suspension and special educational placement. Children with the hyperactive-impulsive profile are at increased risk of long-term antisocial behaviour problems and poor school adjustment.

Children with ADHD are also more likely than those without to have intellectual disability (p.110).

Box 3.20 Prevalence of ADHD
- General population: 5%–10% during school age; 2%–4% during adulthood
- General psychiatric patients: 17%
- Prisoners: over 30% of young offenders (p.580); 26% adults
- Forensic psychiatric patients: no data
- The prevalence rate is four times higher amongst males than females

How do symptoms impact risk of offending or violence?
- Impulsivity, hyperactivity, and inattention in school can result in poor attainment at school, which is itself a risk factor for adult offending.
- Impulsiveness may reflect deficits in frontal lobe executive functions (p.134), with a tendency to commit offences through having poor control over behaviour, poor ability to consider the consequences of actions, and a tendency to focus on immediate gratification.
- ADHD symptoms may also lead to more opportunistic patterns of offending.
- Children with ADHD display a greater degree of difficulty with resisting aggression; with oppositional and defiant behaviour, and conduct problems (most commonly lying, stealing, truancy, and physical aggression).

What is the risk?

- Hyperactivity at age eleven to thirteen significantly predicts arrests for violence up to age twenty-two years, especially amongst boys who have experienced delivery complications.
- Odds of arrest for violence are three to four times higher in ADHD than the general population.
- After four years of follow-up, about 15% of men with ADHD and 4% of women have a conviction for violence.
- Each comorbid condition further increases the risk of delinquency or offending.

Conduct disorder and ODD

DSM-5 defines conduct disorder (CD) as 'a repetitive and persistent pattern of behaviour in which the basic rights of others or major age-appropriate societal norms or rules are violated'. This must manifest in at least three of: aggression to people and animals, destruction of property, deceitfulness or theft, and serious violations of rules.

Oppositional defiant disorder (ODD) refers to a pattern of conduct problems characterised mainly by angry/irritable mood, argumentative/defiant behaviour, or vindictiveness (and typically occurs in pre-school years). ODD is distinct from CD, and is less pervasive, but may be a developmental precursor of CD. The behaviours of ODD are typically of a less severe nature than those of CD and do not include aggression towards people or animals, destruction of property, or a pattern of theft or deceit. ADHD (p.106) is often comorbid with ODD and CD.

Box 3.21 Prevalence of CD and ODD

- General population aged fifteen through nineteen: ODD 2.9%; CD 5.8% boys; 3.4% girls
- CAMHS patients: no data, but one of the commonest referral reasons
- Youth detention: CD 90% of young people in the secure estate
- Forensic psychiatric patients: no data

CDs constitute a third to half of all clinical referrals to CAMHS, and chronic CDs are the single most costly disorder of adolescence.

Risk factors for CD

- Low parental supervision
- Parental conflict
- Inconsistent, harsh disciplining
- Soft neurological signs
- Impulsivity
- ADHD

Genetic vulnerability to impulsivity interacts with abusive environments to cause an increased risk of CD in adolescence.

Childhood onset CD requires the presence of symptoms before the age of ten years, with poor peer and family relationships present, and problems tending to persist into adulthood (p.36). Adolescent-onset conduct disorder requires the absence of symptoms before the age of ten years. These individuals tend to be less aggressive and have more normative peer relationships. They often display conduct behaviours in the company of a peer group engaged in these behaviours, such as a gang (p.38). Their prognosis is much better than the early onset group.

How do symptoms impact risk of offending or violence?

By definition, the antisocial behaviours indicative of CD increase the risk of offending. Of children with CD, 40% will go on to become young offenders (and 90% of young offenders had CD in childhood); whereas ODD is not particularly associated with offending behaviour.

Aggressive children are unpopular because they have low levels of pro-social skills. This not only leads to social isolation (a risk factor for offending) but makes it more difficult for them to establish supportive relationships with nondeviant peers (a protective factor).

Cognitively, individuals with CD exhibit hostile attributional bias, so that they interpret ambiguous social situations as threatening. Affectively, anger and irritability are the main states. Where there is a history of childhood maltreatment, this may lead to exhibition of similar symptoms, such as hypervigilance, aggression in response to any fear stimulus, and fearful interpretations of others.

Other harms associated with ODD and conduct disorder

ODD can cause family disruption and school exclusion. It is also a risk factor for CD, which is associated with delinquency and noncriminal rule-breaking. Many conduct-disordered young people are never considered to be young offenders because their illegal behaviours escape detection or may be below the threshold for being criminal.

What is the risk from CD?

There are different developmental trajectories (p.36) for antisocial behaviour, and the development of CD is a significant marker for the development of so-called life course–persistent antisocial behaviour.

A subgroup of individuals with CD will go on to develop ASPD (p.82). Risk factors include early onset, a wide range of symptoms, greater severity and frequency, symptoms ranging across situations (home, school), and hyperactivity.

In adolescence, the emergence of paranoid symptoms, and narcissistic or passive–aggressive personality traits, are most associated with later antisocial behaviour and violence.

Intellectual disability

Intellectual disability (ID) refers to significant intellectual functional impairment (usually an IQ below 70), plus significant impairments in social functioning or adaptive behaviours associated with everyday skills, both present before age eighteen years. People with ID are at increased risk of other developmental disorders and mental illness, as well as victimisation.

The term 'learning difficulties' is often used for specific or generalised intellectual impairment that does not meet all of these criteria.

Box 3.22 Prevalence of intellectual disability

- General population: 1.5%–3%
- General psychiatric patients: no data
- Prisoners: 0.5%–10% (up to 60% of male prisoners have learning difficulties)
- Forensic psychiatric patients: no data

Frequency of offending in patients with ID is higher than in the general population, ranging internationally from 2% to 10%, depending on study methodology. People with ID, and to an even greater extent learning difficulties, are over-represented in prison settings, and probably also in secure hospital settings. Reviews of high security indicate ID patients have the longest duration of stay, possibly from lack of community resources to facilitate discharge. Prisoners with ID also have higher rates of psychotic and other common mental disorders, as well as cannabis use, suicidality, and self-harm compared to the general prison population.

How do ID symptoms impact offending or violence?

Lower intellectual function, rather than the syndrome of ID, is a risk factor for offending. Low-average IQ or borderline intellectual functioning is the level of disability most strongly associated with offending (an IQ below 70 is actually associated with a *reduced* risk of offending). However, ID may represent a proxy for other risk factors for offending: lack of employment or daytime activity or significant personal relationships (social exclusion, more generally, may also serve to explain the observed association between ID and offending).

Low intelligence at age three years significantly predicts officially recorded offending up to age thirty years. Poor school attainment, common in people with ID, is also linked to offending. People with ID are at higher risk for conduct disorder (p.108) and ADHD (p.106) in childhood, and are more likely to be rejected by their peer group. Deficits in verbal skills, memory, and visuo-motor integration are also related to offending behaviour, independent of low social class and family adversity.

It is also likely that any increased prevalence of offending observed in ID is due to a greater likelihood of detection of crimes committed. People with ID are <u>vulnerable suspects</u> (p.574), often lacking appropriate support and legal representation from early stages in the criminal justice process, with particular vulnerability to being <u>suggestible</u> and/or <u>compliant</u> (p.160).

ID and sexual offending

Many people with ID have low social competence: they have not learnt the rules that define acceptable and unacceptable behaviour, resulting in friendly acts being misperceived as sexually inappropriate or even aggressive. Sexual offences may result from inappropriate, impulsive expression of emotion, rather than premeditated acts (see also pp.56–69).

Sex offenders with ID have low specificity for age and sex of their victim, but with a greater tendency to offend against younger people and male children. Offences may not be carefully planned.

The traditional view that sexual offending is more common amongst people with ID is difficult to substantiate. However, there is stronger evidence for increased recidivism amongst sexual offenders with ID compared to people without.

Associations with other offending

There is no significant difference in the frequency of **property offences** between individuals with ID and those without. Of people convicted of **fire-setting**, 10% have ID.

Acquired brain injury

Brain injuries acquired after birth include traumatic brain injury (TBI). Impact to the head can lead to loss of consciousness, posttraumatic amnesia, confusion, and neurological deficits. Glasgow coma scale (GCS) score after injury, duration of unconsciousness, and the period of memories lost to posttraumatic amnesia determine whether TBI is mild (concussion), moderate or severe.

Neurocognitive sequelae may be permanent or transient (from weeks to months). Psychological trauma associated with injury may also impact presentation. Transient postconcussion symptoms occur in 30%–80% of TBI independently of any permanent brain injury and can predispose to violence. Transient symptoms may involve:

- Physical symptoms: headache, dizziness, photosensitivity, tinnitus, double vision, and insomnia.
- Psychological symptoms: irritability, anxiety, depression, restlessness, aggression, mood lability, impulsivity, and loss of alcohol or drug tolerance.
- Cognitive symptoms: poor concentration, confusion, impaired judgment, amnesia (p.636), and other memory deficits.

Box 3.23 Prevalence of traumatic brain injury

- General population: 0.3%–2% (TBI-associated disability)
- General psychiatric patients: 17%–43% (inpatients, including minor TBI)
- Prisoners: 36%
- Forensic psychiatric patients: 22% in high security (60%–70% have neurological impairment); 23%–50% in other services

---

Several studies and reports have suggested a link between TBI and criminal behaviour. Large population data suggest that 9% of TBI patients go on to commit violent offences, with double the odds of the general population (after adjustment for confounders such as class, substance misuse and comparison to unaffected siblings).

Features of TBI that predispose to violence

Particular focal brain lesions are associated with the highest risk of violence. Lesions in the frontal lobes can produce personality changes and disrupt planning and organisation of behaviour (executive function, p.134). This can result in disinhibition, which can be linked to violence. There is some evidence to indicate that damage to the temporal lobes, particularly the amygdala and hippocampus, is also associated with aggressive behaviour.

Certain factors that predispose to TBI also predispose to violence: poor premorbid social functioning (p.135, antisocial behaviour, and history of alcohol/substance abuse (p.76).

TBI is also associated with self-directed violence, including suicide. In one study 5.5% of suicide victims had acquired brain injuries within the previous three years.

Associations with offending behaviour

There are a number of hypotheses about why traumatic brain injury may increase the risk of violent behaviour (discounting the specific effects related to the site of a localised brain injury, see above):

- Cognitive impairment affecting recognition of legal boundaries and motivation to adhere to laws.
- Impulse-control deficits.
- Personality changes (disinhibition, suspiciousness).
- Disturbances in emotional functioning (irritability, affective lability).
- Poor social judgement.
- Increased vulnerability to involvement in criminal activity.
- Comorbid antisocial personality disorder/psychopathy.

Epilepsy and sleep disorders

Epilepsy and sleep disorders are rarely associated with violence. Both are occasionally raised within defences (p.412) to criminal acts. Interest in epilepsy and parasomnias in forensic psychiatry began with cases involving automatism (p.612). Malingering (p.118) and dissociative disorders (p.100) should also be considered when epilepsy, or a sleep disorder, is proposed as explanatory to an (alleged) offence.

Box 3.24 Prevalence of epilepsy

- General population: 0.5%–1% (point prevalence)
- General psychiatric patients: no data
- Prisoners: 1%–6%
- Forensic psychiatric patients: 5% (special hospital)

Prevalence of parasomnias

- General population: 2%–25%

Comorbidity with psychiatric disorders

- Prevalence of any mental disorder in patients with epilepsy: 20%–60%
- Psychosis: 2%–9%
- Depressive disorders: 20%–60%
- Substance abuse: 20%–50%
- Autistic spectrum disorders: 5%–46%

Some neurologists suggest that comorbid psychiatric symptoms form part of seizure disorder. However, there is growing evidence of a complex bidirectional relationship where psychiatric comorbidity may predate epilepsy.

Sleep disorders are not associated with mental disorders.

Violence and epilepsy

There is no general association between violent acts and epilepsy. Epilepsy may be associated with complex behaviours outside ordinary conscious control, rarely resulting in violence.

Ictal violence (violence committed during a seizure) is rare and generally not goal-directed. Violence is more likely in complex partial seizures than generalised tonic-clonic seizures. Most offending probably occurs in the postictal or interictal period, sometimes in the presence of an external influence (e.g. suggestion from another person).

A potential confounding factor is that brain abnormalities of the temporal or frontal lobes that may cause complex partial seizures may also independently influence violent behaviour. Such abnormalities may have a role in the controversial diagnosis of intermittent explosive disorder (p.669); there is an apparent lack of memory for explosive episodes of sudden uncontrolled violence.

Assessment of link between epilepsy and violence

Assessment of a person with epilepsy alleged to have committed a violent offence should involve consideration of:

- Diagnosis of epilepsy by at least one neurologist (with expertise in epilepsy).
- Epileptic automatism established by clinical history and closed-circuit TV-EEG monitoring capturing violence.
- The violent act should be within behaviour characteristic of the patient's usual seizures.
- Whether the offence is senseless or out of character.
- Whether there is any obvious motive, planning, premeditation or concealment of the offence.
- Clinical judgement by a neurologist or neuropsychiatrist regarding the likelihood of the violence being a result of a seizure.

Sleep disorders (parasomnias)

Sleep disturbance is a common component of many psychiatric disorders. This is distinct from parasomnias which involve partial arousal from sleep, such as sleep walking or sleep terrors (NREM sleep arousal disorders) and REM sleep behaviour disorder.

Sleep disorders and violence

Where violence occurs in adults with sleep disorder, it is more common in males with childhood history of parasomnias, including nocturnal enuresis. Sleep terror disorder and sleepwalking overlap and may be present in the same episode. Sleep deprivation, alcohol, marijuana, and caffeine may provoke sleepwalking.

Victims of crimes associated with sleep are usually known to the perpetrator. The sleepwalker may not appear to hear cries from or recognise their victim.

Whether the episode occurred in REM or non-REM sleep may be significant, but not necessarily crucial. The notion that an individual in REM sleep is paralysed and therefore cannot be violent is no longer accepted. Speech and actions in REM sleep may therefore involve dream enactment.

The possibility of nocturnal epilepsy can further confuse assessment. It may need to be considered as an alternative diagnosis.

Assessment of link between sleep disorders and violence

The following should be considered at assessment.

- Is there a previous history of parasomnias in childhood or adulthood?
- Was violence preceded by a period of stress for the perpetrator?
- Did arousal from sleep occur soon after sleep onset?
- Is there evidence of complex, goal-directed behaviour?
- Was the victim well known and loved?
- Was there evidence of recognition or seeking out of the victim?
- Was there a period of confusion following the attack?
- Is there amnesia for the event?
- Was there any obvious motive, planning or premeditation?
- Was there any concealment of the offence?
- Was the offence senseless or out of character?
- Was the violence preceded by a period of poor sleep?

Organic disorders: dementia & delirium

Dementia is a syndrome characterised by global cognitive decline. Dementias can be subdivided into cortical (Alzheimer's disease, Pick's disease), subcortical (Parkinson's disease, Huntington's disease, and Wilson's disease), cortical-subcortical (Lewy body dementia), and multifocal (CJD).

Delirium is a transient acute disturbance of brain function, physically caused, which is more likely to occur in individuals with some underlying degree of brain deterioration.

Box 3.25 Prevalence of dementia
- General population: 7% (over 65 years); 33% (over lifetime)
- General psychiatric patients: no data
- Forensic psychiatric patients: 19%–33% (over 60 years)
- Prisoners: 7% (increased from 1% in 2011)

Prevalence of delirium
- General population: no data

Comorbidity of dementia with other mental disorders
- Delusions (paranoid) and hallucinations with dementia: 20%–40%
- Anxiety and/or depression: 50%
- Cognitive deficits vary with dementia type

Association between dementia and offending behaviour

Dementia is primarily a disorder of old age. People older than sixty-five years old account for less 0.5% of all violent offenders. Behavioural and psychological symptoms of dementia (BPSD) and neuropsychiatric symptoms include agitation and aggression. This may include shouting, verbal insults, hitting, biting, and other physical violence. These behavioural symptoms may occur with other psychiatric and physical disorders.

People with Alzheimer's disease have five-fold increased odds of aggressive behaviours over healthy individuals, not differing by dementia subtype. There is no increase in those with mild cognitive impairment (a dementia precursor).

No specific offence is clearly associated with dementia. However, sexual offences may be more common in elderly people with dementia compared to those with other psychiatric disorders. Minor offences are more common.

Assessment

Anyone presenting with aggressive or offending behaviour for the first time in older age should be assessed carefully to exclude dementia, especially if the offence is serious.

Likewise, in those with a history of <u>alcohol abuse</u> (p.76), the possibility of alcoholic dementia or delirium should be considered, especially if such a defendant claims <u>amnesia</u> (p.636) for an offence. Other problems that may be mistaken for dementia include <u>depression</u> (p.94), <u>head injury</u> (p.112), <u>intellectual disability</u> (p.110), and sensory impairment.

Management of offending behaviour in dementia

Nonpharmacological methods should be first line. If agitation, delusions or hallucinations are causing extreme distress or creating a risk to self or others, antipsychotics can be considered at minimal dose for minimal time, alongside psychological and environmental interventions (long-term treatment is associated with serious adverse events—including stroke and death). In moderate to severe Alzheimer's disease, when memantine is indicated, this is the preferred treatment for agitation. Carbamazepine may also have a role in some cases of agitation in dementia. Review treatment every six weeks, with attempt at discontinuation.

Delirium

Delirium can be associated with a wide range of medical conditions including dementias, alcohol or drug intoxication or withdrawal, medical or surgical conditions such as urinary retention. It can be associated with aggressive behaviour. The management of aggression in delirium will usually be by management of the underlying cause. Sedation should be avoided, unless necessary to manage any immediate risk of harm to self or others. If pharmacological management is required, then ordinary principles of <u>rapid tranquilisation</u> (p.200) should be observed.

Other organic disorders

Some organic disorders (e.g. traumatic brain injury) may result in organic personality change and violence. Alcohol intoxication may be enhanced in its effect in causing violence in an individual with underling brain damage or degeneration. Organic psychosis may be associated with increased criminality.

Malingering and factitious disorder

Malingering and factitious disorders involve intentional dishonesty in reporting symptoms of physical or mental illness. In **malingering** this is pursued for external, tangible gain, such as avoiding prison, military service, moving from a prison to a hospital or financial compensation. It is not a mental illness, so is 'detected' rather than diagnosed.

Factitious disorders involve lying for psychological gain: the most familiar form is *Munchausen syndrome*, where individuals seek medical investigations. *Factitious disorder by proxy* is rare but has involved high profile incidents of parents harming and killing their children, and healthcare staff their patients.

Prevalence of malingering

It is inherently difficult to obtain good data on fraudulent behaviour. Rates are typically higher in milder than severe forms of 'illness', and in civil than in criminal cases; this is believed to be due to the relative burdens of proof.

Box 3.26 Prevalence of malingering and factitious disorder
- General population: less than 1%
- General psychiatric patients: 0.4%–0.8%
- Prisoners: no data
- Forensic psychiatric patients: no data
  US data from medicolegal reports malingering in up to:
- 30% of personal injury and disability cases
- 20% of criminal cases
- 40% of mild traumatic brain injuries
- 8% of general medical cases

Types of malingering

Malingering involves a continuum of deceptional intent and gain, and four types have been defined:
- **Invention** of symptoms where none exist.
- **Perseveration** of symptoms that once existed.
- **Exaggeration** of genuine symptoms: considered the most common type.
- **Transference**, or attributing genuine symptoms to a false cause.

Assessment of malingering

A nonaccusatory empathic approach has been shown to encourage disclosure of malingering where it is present. Malingerers can be less interested in secondary loss (e.g. unemployment) and remedial supports (e.g. occupational therapy) than secondary gain (e.g. compensation). Collateral interviews can help but be aware others can be colluding or unintentionally manipulated. No symptom or sign is pathognomonic but be mindful of:

- Temporal anomalies in symptom onset and delayed request for help.
- Significant discrepancies between medical reports or assessments.
- Significant variation between self-reported and objectively measured pathology.

Psychometric testing

Psychometric tests can support an opinion, but even malingering-specific tests cannot 'prove' malingering. There are four major types:
- **Biomarkers**: physiological markers such as heart rate—the basis of the polygraph.
- **General psychometric tests**: looking for implausible patterns across a general battery.
- **Malingering-specific tests**: designed to detect feigned symptoms.
- **Symptom validity tests**: designed to detect feigned cognitive deficits.

Presenting findings

False clinical optimism, confirmatory bias and over-reliance on psychometric testing without understanding its limitations have all been shown to limit correct detection of malingering. Even experienced clinicians have found it difficult to identify actors simulating illness.

As malingering is not a psychiatric illness, but a state of lying, clinicians should be very cautious about trying to 'prove' its presence. It is usually optimal to describe how well, or atypically, a presentation fits with a proposed illness, which is the clinician's area of expertise.

Malingerers have been shown to have higher rates of personality disorder, substance use, unemployment, past litigation, and financial problems. However, these are common issues more generally, and attempts to link such factors and any external incentives—even if clear and confirmed—to an individual is liable to draw censure about impartiality.

If psychometric testing is used, expert witnesses might face cross-examination about these, based on the <u>Daubert questions</u> (p.659):
- Has the technique been tested in field conditions and subjected to scientific review?
- What is the known or potential rate of error?
- Do standards exist for the control of the technique's operation?
- Has the technique been generally accepted within the relevant scientific community?

An individual may be exaggerating or lying *and* have a genuine illness; and no malingering tests or assessment can determine motivation for this. It is usually best left to a court, or trier of facts, to determine whether inconsistencies are best explained by malingering. Distinguishing between malingering and factitious disorder based upon the presence or absence of external gain can be difficult. There can be cases where there appears to be no evident external gain, and yet the behaviour persists, so that the presumption must be that there is some form of internal psychological gain. Clinically what may matter is formulating and understanding the behaviour so as to attempt to modify it (e.g. within prison health care).

Assessment in forensic psychiatry

The forensic psychiatric assessment

There are important ethical and legal distinctions to draw between assessing a patient in a health context and a defendant or litigant in a legal context. However, whatever the context, and whoever is doing the assessment (an individual forensic psychiatrist, or a psychologist and psychiatrist or a psychiatric team), the clinical process should be essentially similar, albeit sometimes somewhat modified, or added to, in light of any legal questions known to be in play. (See also the advice on assessment specifically with a view to providing reports (pp.678–710), including the ethical requirement (p.773) to explain the context and purpose of the assessment, and the fact that there may be no therapeutic relationship or doctor-patient confidentiality.)

Process

A forensic psychiatric assessment may involve some or all of the following:

- Understanding the context in which the assessment takes place, and adjusting as necessary by making special considerations (pp.148–161).
- Obtaining information from an appropriate range of sources (p.142), including the history as reported by the patient/defendant/litigant, relevant family members and others[1]; medical and other records such as education and social services files and your own mental state and physical examinations.
- Performing or requesting specialised psychological tests (pp.130–139), the nature of which will depend upon the clinical issues at hand but might include tests of personality (p.124), attitudes (p.128), intelligence (p.134) or other aspects of psychological or neurological functioning.
- Ordering biological or other investigations (p.140), if necessary, including, for example, brain imaging and EEG investigations and investigations to relevant general medical conditions.
- Reaching a diagnosis or differential diagnosis (p.144) and an individualised formulation (p.146).
- Assessing the risks of various possible harms (pp.166–179).
- Constructing treatment (pp.182–234) and risk-management (pp.238–253) plans.

Contemporaneous clinical notes should be made that clearly record whether information from the interviewee is paraphrased or literally their words, and whether it was elicited from open or closed (leading) questions—which may be important legally as well as medically. Occasionally, it may be appropriate to make an audit or video recording of part of an interview, with consent.

Always be aware that your clinical notes can become part of legal proceedings, including subsequent unpredicted proceedings such as an action in negligence (p.550) or a tribunal. Your notes may also be made available to the interviewee or be disclosed during legal proceedings to others you might not expect, as the normal rules of confidentiality (p.320) do not always apply. Clinical notes should therefore be constructed with precision and care.

---

1 In a legal context, you may need permission to speak to informants who are also witnesses.

Assessment of personality

What is personality?

Personality, from the Greek *persona* (mask), has no single definition, but there are several theories of its nature and function.

- Some theories emphasise the **social aspect** of personality: how individuals perceive the world and interact with others.
- Other theories emphasise the **individual nature** of personality: the psychological structures and capacities of the individual, such as affective traits, psychological defences, affective and arousal regulatory systems, plus cognitive biases and attributions.

Personality is enduring and influences how an individual appraises and interprets the world and therefore affects how they tend to behave in given social situations. This can be psychiatrically significant, whether or not the individual's personality is 'disordered', since personality traits can affect the way that symptoms of mental illness are expressed, and/or how well an individual with mental disorder functions.

What is personality disorder?

Personality disorder (p.78) is a disorder of the psychological constructs above. It can be defined as an **enduring** disturbance of **characteristic** aspects of the self, usually present since adolescence that:

- manifests in **dysfunctional patterns** of thinking, feeling, behaving, and relating to others;
- is present across **most** personal and social **situations**;
- is developmentally or culturally **inappropriate**; and
- causes substantial **distress** or **functional impairment**.

Assessment of personality and PD

Personality and PD can be assessed by clinical interview, combined with a wide range of sources of information, and by psychometric tests validated on large populations.

Clinical psychological assessment tends to suggest the presence of PD (or its absence) on the basis of personality structure as measured psychometrically, in terms of statistical variance from the mean, often without reference to functional consequences. As function can depend upon context, an individual with a psychological vulnerability to PD may appear non-disordered for many years until their PD is exposed by a change of circumstance. Psychiatric diagnosis, however, requires evidence of dysfunction.

Assessment for PD may be indicated where there is persistent behavioural and/or interpersonal disturbance in the absence of obvious cognitive impairment or mental illness. More broadly, a personality assessment will inform understanding of any patient, and assist with risk assessment, treatment planning, and risk management.

Selection and use of personality assessment tools

There is a wide variety of personality assessment tools (p.137), each with its own orientation, strengths, and weaknesses. They vary by the conceptualisation of personality that underpins them. For example, the Eysenck

Personality Questionnaire and the NEO-PI-R[2] are based on **trait theories**; whereas the Millon assessment tools view personality in terms of the degrees of various **dimensions of pathology** present.

Validity of PD assessment tools

There is considerable debate about the validity of self-report tools for underpinning the diagnosis of PD, since many individuals exhibiting PD have inaccurate ideas of how others see them, and will complete self-report instruments according to their own distorted perspective. There may also be motivation to look 'good' or 'bad', such as where the measure is to be used in a court report or to inform risk assessment. Other informants may be more reliable, but can also be biased—and have no access to the subjective experience of the person assessed. It is therefore important to incorporate both self-report and informant data. Paper or computer-based instruments can be helpful in reducing interviewer bias, particularly with individuals who may have antisocial or borderline PD, who may be antagonistic or hostile, and who may thereby distort the interviewer's perception of the individual.

Single versus multiple assessments

One-off assessments for PD are notoriously unreliable, particularly at a time of crisis; ideally a single assessment should be regarded as only a screening assessment, and lead to a more detailed examination. If only a single interview is possible, this emphasises the importance of collateral source data. Assessment using different approaches, more than one assessment test and paradigms, for example those of psychiatry and psychology, can also aid validity and reliability.

Measuring severity

There are no standardised assessments for the severity of PD. However, aside from high psychometric scores, more severe PD will probably result in greater impairment of function, and sometimes satisfaction of criteria for more than one PD diagnosis or <u>cluster</u> (p.78). More severe PD is also more likely to be associated with comorbid mental illness.

Personality disorder and risk assessment

Most people with PD do not present a risk to anyone. However, there are subtypes of PD (pp.82–91) which are associated with significant risk of violence to others, and these are over-represented in forensic populations.

Psychopathy

Probably the most meaningful risk feature in PD is the degree to which the individual demonstrates <u>psychopathic</u> (p.90) traits, such as callous and unemotional, or unempathic, attitudes to others.[3] The Psychopathy Checklist Revised (<u>PCL-R</u>, p.170) provides a measure of these traits.[4]

---

2 This refers to the first three factors the test measures: Neuroticism, Extraversion and Openness to new experiences. The others in the **Five Factor Model** are agreeableness and conscientiousness.

3 Psychopathy is not a diagnosis per se; it represents a subset of <u>antisocial PD</u> (p.82).

4 Strictly, the PCL-R is a diagnostic tool and not a risk assessment instrument, but it is frequently used as a component of <u>violence risk assessment</u> (p.168) because of the strong correlation between psychopathy and risk of violence.

Normative scores

Personality tests can be normed on either the general population, as is the EPQ, or on a clinical population, as is the MCMI-III. However, most personality assessment tools have not been standardised on forensic populations. This may not necessarily be a problem since deviance from nonforensic norms may be of importance in formulation (p.146) (though it limits the opportunity to study treatment outcomes).

Cultural factors

PD occurs in every culture, but it may have different presenting features, and different social ramifications, in different ethnic/cultural groups.

Most personality assessment tools were devised and developed in the context of Western cultural values. They may therefore miss cultural values and attitudes that are of psychological salience to individuals from other backgrounds. Hence, it is not recommended that such assessment tools be used with individuals from non-Western cultures. Individuals, and informants, should be clinically interviewed by professionals conversant with the relevant cultural values and beliefs. There are also limitations of conducting many tests with deaf people.

Sexual attitudes and behaviour

Assessing attitudes

Assessing behaviour

Sexual attitudes and behaviour

The assessment of sexual attitudes and behaviour, coupled with assessments of mental state and personality (p.124), will usually be undertaken in order to give an opinion on the risk of sexual offending (p.172), treatment (p.221), or on whether any legal defence applies (p.412). Reported deviant sexual fantasies, or abnormally high levels of sexual arousal, may prompt a request for specialist assessment; although deviant fantasies are also present in the nonoffending population. Some sex offenders develop depression, either in conjunction with their offending or in response to treatment, which must also be assessed for.

Most sexual behaviour services will not assess or treat prior to conviction since response to treatment is often poor, because the acceptance of disorder required to succeed is inconsistent with seeking to deny or minimise an offence at trial.

Assessing attitudes

The concept of 'attitudes' may be flawed because of its imprecision, but it has long been the basis of most clinical assessment and research, and there is no currently available alternative concept. The relationship of attitudes to personality traits (p.124) is complex. One view is that attitudes are more amenable to change than personality traits. Attitudes supportive of sexual offending have been shown to have a small, yet reasonably consistent, relationship with sexual recidivism.

Assessment of sexual attitudes requires a clinical interview and collateral history; supplemented by standardised assessments such as the RSAS, EWT, and ACS (see p.137 for the names and definitions of these tests). The aim is to understand the patient's cognitive distortions and relevant schema.

Cognitive distortions

Cognitive distortions (p.62) amount to patterns of thinking that tend to allow the individual to ignore others' perspectives (especially the victim's) and to justify their offending behaviour. It may be difficult to assess such distortions in a way that is free from desirability bias: that is, not endorsing items that are obviously socially unacceptable. An analysis based solely on cognitive distortions is an oversimplification, and underlying core beliefs, and possibly other motivations for sexual offending (p.62), should be taken into account.

Schema

Schema (or schemata), derived from cognitive therapy (p.62), have been described as implicit theories that people hold to explain the world around them. They may be considered to be underlying modes of thinking of which cognitive distortions are the superficial representations. Schema that have been described as motivating sexual offenders are described on p.62.

Assessing behaviour

Behaviour is assessed using a combination of clinical interview, collateral history, official records, including police and social services records, and direct observation.

Clinical interview

An interview directed at assessing sexual attitudes and behaviour should cover:

- Sexual development and early sexual experiences.
- Masturbation—frequency, fantasy, and public/private.
- Sexual partners—number, gender, and age.
- Consideration of paraphilia (p.102) and deviant sexual interests.
- Sexual preoccupations.
- Strength of sexual arousal.
- Violence in sexual relationships (fantasised and actual).
- Use of pornography.

Pornography

Use of pornography in general has not been shown to cause sexual offending. However, pornography depicting sexual violence has been shown to affect self-reported likelihood of rape or other sexual offending. More generally, the content of pornography preferred by an individual is an important guide to their sexual attitudes. Viewing child pornography is a form of sexual offending against children (p.58). The causal impact of use of child pornography on child sexual offending is not clear (see p.59).

Psychological testing

Aside from its role in personality assessment (p.124), psychological assessment can assist in case formulation (p.146), risk assessment (p.166), assessing treatment need, potential treatability, and likely treatment outcome. Psychometric tests, scales or instruments may be used as part of that wider clinical assessment, including to help formulate more precisely the relationships between the characteristics of an individual and their risk profile or criminogenic 'needs'.

Selection and use

There is a large number of tests available (see specific psychological tests p.136). However, for a test to be useful it should be **reliable** and **valid** (see below). It should be documented and reviewed in the scientific literature and be accompanied by a manual describing the test's development, psychometric properties and procedure. The standard administration recommended in the manual should be followed, whether it is directed solely at clinical issues or ultimately at clinico-legal questions.

There is a range of different kinds of psychological tests in use. The most common types are self-report tests, structured clinical judgement tools, and risk assessments. When tests become outdated (e.g. due to change in the general population) they are usually revised and updated.

Note that some tests require the administrator to be trained in a relevant profession (e.g. a clinical psychologist, or a mental health professional more generally: for example, the PAS, p.137) and/or in that specific test (e.g. the MCMI, p.137). The manual will state who should use and interpret the test, and what qualifications are needed (see also Box 4.1).

Box 4.1 Cultural considerations

Many psychological tests are standardised on Western populations and would not be appropriate for use with individuals from other cultures. Some tests are more culturally dependent than others, especially those with a significant verbal component. When conducting tests via an interpreter, the interpreter may need careful briefing.

Reliability

This is the repeatability or reproducibility of results from a test or measure. It should give consistent results:
• Each time it is applied to an individual (**test-retest reliability**), and
• When applied by different clinicians (**inter-rater reliability**).

There are several different statistical methods of measuring reliability, including correlation coefficients for test-retest reliability, Cronbach's alpha for internal consistency and Kappa for inter-rater reliability. Such reliability coefficients range from 0 (no reliability) to 1 (perfect reliability), and a test with a reliability coefficient of below 0.7 should not be used clinically or in legal proceedings (if it is, then it should be reported with warnings).

Reliability varies across samples and populations, and the test manual should be able to provide further details, together with normative scale information and details of test validity.

Validity

The validity of a test refers to whether it measures what it is designed to measure (and purports to measure). There are three main types of validity:

- **Content validity** refers to the item content, and how well it represents the behavioural domain to be measured.
- **Criterion validity** refers to the effectiveness of the test, as compared with results from a 'gold standard' test (the criterion), and it can be further subdivided to **concurrent** validity, which refers to how well the results compare with the criterion measured at the same time, and **predictive** validity, which refers to how well the results predict the criterion measured in the future (for example, how well the test predicts the individual's future behaviour).
- **Construct validity** refers to how well the test measures a relevant theoretical construct or trait (e.g. how well the items in an IQ test each correspond to related known properties of intelligence).

Normative scores

Standardisation, an essential part of psychometric test construction and development, involves the test being administered to a representative sample of people for whom the test was developed. Standardised tests provide norms for several different populations.

Interpretation of results

Test scores should be interpreted with an appropriate comparative sample: that is, the scores obtained by the individual should be interpreted by comparison with those of an appropriate population (e.g. all forensic patients or all violent criminals). For example, saying that Mr X has a PCL-R score of 15 carries little meaning; saying that this is well below the conventional cut-off score of 25 (or 30) for a diagnosis of <u>psychopathy</u> (p.90) is helpful, but saying that this places him in the twenty-sixth percentile of forensic inpatients, and that this means that 74% of forensic inpatients have a greater degree of psychopathy, is more useful still.

The score for a test should not be applied for a purpose for which the test was not developed. For example, a test designed to measure risk of violence after discharge from a forensic psychiatric hospital, such as the <u>VRAG</u> (p.171), will not give meaningful results if applied to young offenders in a <u>YOI</u> (p.580).

Test data should be integrated and interpreted in relation to other sources of data. Scores should not be over-generalised or used in isolation. That is to say, the test results should be placed by the assessor in the context of the assessment as a whole. For example, a diagnosis of ID, or an explanation of that patient's behaviour, should not be based on an IQ score alone, but on that IQ score interpreted in the context of other assessment findings.

Disclosure of tests or test scores

Detailed descriptions of subtle psychological tests may undermine the validity of the test, as potential future test subjects may then be more likely to be able deliberately to distort their responses. That said, it is difficult for another expert to evaluate the test findings (e.g. for the purposes of cross-examination, p.714) if a certain amount of detail is not provided; and that this justifies accepting the risk of the disclosed information becoming publicly available. Experts should be aware of the implications and ethical issues involved in disclosure or nondisclosure.

Problems in presenting test results in legal fora

Psychological tests are constructed by scientists, and then used and interpreted by professional clinicians. Each understands the strengths and limitations of any given test, including the limits of its interpretation and the importance of validating results by placing them in the context of a full clinical assessment.

However, when a test is used to come to clinical conclusions that are then applied to a legal question, and the clinician is subject to examination and cross-examination (p.714)—especially in front of a jury—there is much scope for deliberate lawyerly 'misunderstanding' of the test method, results, and interpretation. For example, a barrister might take individual questions within an instrument and question the expert witness on those questions, attempting to belittle the test by a process of disaggregation, deliberately not understanding that the items in the test are only valid as a whole. Resisting such techniques of deliberate misunderstanding can require much skill, and calmness, again especially in front of a jury, as well as preliminary discussion with the barrister on the same side, to advise what questions would enable a proper and balanced understanding of the test to be communicated by the expert.

Psychological test domains

Anger and violence

Attitudes towards violence, and levels of anger, are relevant to both risk assessment and general attitudes to offending. Measures can also be useful in evaluating the outcomes of anger management groups and other therapies.

Competency or capacity

Individuals may be competent to carry out different sets of tasks. Fitness to give legal instructions, <u>fitness to plead</u> (p.602) or competence to make medical decisions are most commonly relevant issues. There are a number of instruments that assess <u>mental capacity</u> (p.522) in the context of treatment, but most are derived from US populations and have not been standardised in the UK.

Executive function

This consists of higher-order cognitive skills associated with the ability to engage in independent, goal-directed behaviour. It can be broken down into different domains of functioning (e.g. verbal/visual productivity, cognitive flexibility, inhibition, organisation and planning), and different tests tap into different domains. Impairments in EF have been linked to dysfunction in the frontal lobes.

Intellectual/cognitive function

An individual's intelligence refers to a variety of different domains, including the ability to solve problems, reason, apply previous knowledge to new situations, learn new skills, and conduct abstract thinking. An Intelligence Quotient (IQ) can be used to measure general intelligence, being a unitary measure with a mean of 100 and a normal distribution. There are various tests that assess specific aspects of cognitive function, such as executive function, verbal performance, processing speed, and memory.

Feigning and malingering

Feigning refers to exaggerating or fabricating symptoms, regardless of intent. <u>*Malingering*</u> (p.118), which is more difficult to ascertain, refers to conscious fabrication or gross exaggeration of symptoms, in relation to cognitive deficits, amnesia, and psychiatric symptoms. The SIRS/SIMS (Structured Inventory of Reported/Malingered Symptoms) and the TOMM (Test of Memory Malingering) may be used.

Memory

There are three stages of memory:
- **Encoding** (laying down new memories),
- **Storage** (creating a permanent record) and
- **Retrieval** (recalling the stored information).

And three types of memory:
- Working memory (temporary holding and manipulating information in consciousness),
- Long-term memory (storing information for a long time), and
- Sensory memory (storing sense impressions).

Various cognitive tests are designed to measure different types and stages of memory processing.

Mood and anxiety

There are various tests that measure mood and anxiety.

Personality profiles

Personality Profiles should not be used in isolation, particularly not in relation to risk assessment (p.166), which can be an issue in assessing psychopathy (p.90). There are a number of instruments available for assessing personality, as listed on p.137. (See assessment of personality (p.124) for more details.)

Premorbid functioning

Various tests estimate the level of intellectual or cognitive functioning before an illness or head injury. Most are based on vocabulary or reading ability. Any discrepancy between current and premorbid estimates will be highly significant in that it will provide an indication of the degree of deterioration. However, any difference does not equate with clinical significance.

Response distortion

Scales such as the Paulhus Deception Scale (PDS) are specifically designed to identify individuals who deliberately distort their responses and present themselves in a positive light when asked to complete psychological assessments and rating scales. The PDS assesses two forms of distortion, Self-Deceptive Enhancement (SDE) and Impression Management (IM). SDE aims to examine the tendency to give honest but inflated self-descriptions, reflecting a tendency to unconsciously portray oneself as more favourable and socially acceptable. IM is designed to measure a deliberate tendency to present oneself in a positive light and is associated with faking or lying.

Sexual deviance

This may be appropriate to assess in the context of risk assessment (p.166), particularly risk of behaviour such as rape or child abuse. Sexual deviancy (p.62) is usually assessed in terms of deviant erotic object choice or the association of sexual arousal with anger or hostility for victims.

Suggestibility and compliance

See p.160 for a discussion of interrogative suggestibility and compliance, which may be relevant for retracted confessions (p.608). The tests, GSS1, GSS2, and GCS (p.137), were designed for use in relation to police interviews, but are applicable to any interview situation.

Traumatic experience

There are various measures available that assess post trauma symptoms. However, in the forensic population it is common for individuals to have experienced multiple traumatic events and not all tools are good at accounting for complex trauma. Psychometric tests do not always distinguish between trauma as a consequence of earlier events and trauma as a consequence of offending.

Specific psychological tests

Instruments for risk assessment are listed on pp.170–175. This list is not exhaustive: only those instruments more commonly encountered in forensic settings have been included.

Table 4.1 Specific psychological tests

Key	
A	Test is specifically for children and adolescents
F	Test has a prominent functional/performance element
IS	Based on structured or semistructured interview
QS	Questionnaire based on self-report
QI	Questionnaire administered by interviewer
P	Test has a prominent visual/pictorial element
R	Includes information from medical & other records
TP	Includes information from third-party informants
V	Test has a prominent verbal (word-based) element
*	Training in the specific test required

Cognitive: intellectual functioning		
WAIS-IV	Wechsler Adult Intelligence Scales—4th edition*	**QI,V,F,P**
WISC-V	Wechsler Intelligence Scale for Children—5th edition *	**QI,V,F,P, A**
WASI	Wechsler Abbreviated Scale of Intelligence*	**QI,V,F**
MMSE	Mini Mental Status Examination	**QI,V,F**
ACE-III	Addenbrooke's Cognitive Examination	**QI,V,F**
QT	Ammons Quick Test	**QI,P**
Raven's	Raven's Progressive Matrices	**QI,P**
Cognitive: premorbid functioning		
NART	National Adult Reading Test	**QI,V**
SGWRT	Schonell Graded Word Reading Test	**QI,V**
TOPF	Test of Premorbid Functioning*	**QI,V**
Cognitive: memory		
WMS-IV	Wechsler Memory Scales—4th edition*	**QI,V**
CMS	Camden Memory Scales	**QI,F,P**
RBMT	Rivermead Behavioural Memory Test	**QI,V,F,P**

Cognitive: executive/frontal lobe functioning		
BADS	Behavioural Assessment of Dysexecutive Syndrome	**QI,F**
DKEFS	Delis-Kaplan Executive Function System	**QI,V,F**
H-B	Hayling-Brixton Test	**QI,V,F**
Trails	Trails A&B	**QI,F**
Stroop	The Stroop Test	**QI,F**
WCST	Wisconsin Card-Sorting Test	**QI,F**
CAMCOG	Cambridge Cognitive Examination	**QI,V,F**
FAB	Frontal Assessment Battery	**QI,V,F**

Personality: dimensional		
MMPI-2	Minnesota Multiphasic Personality Inventory-2*	**QS,V**
MCMI-IV	Millon Clinical Multiaxial Inventory-IV *	**QS,V**
MACI-II	Millon Adolescent Clinical Inventory-II *	**QS,V, A**

Personality: diagnostic		
IPDE	International Personality Disorder Examination *	**IS,V**
MSI-BPD	McLean Screening Instrument for BPD	**IS, V**
PAI	Personality Assessment Inventory	**QS,V**
PAS	Personality Assessment Schedule	**IS,V,R,TP**
PCL-R	Psychopathy Checklist Revised *	**IS,V,R,TP**
PDQ-IV	Personality Diagnostic Questionnaire—4th edition	**QS,V**
SCID-5-PD	Structured Clinical Interview for DSM-V*	**IS,V**

Suggestibility and compliance		
GSS1,2	Gudjonsson Suggestibility Scale 1 or 2	**IS,V**
GCS	Gudjonsson Compliance Scale	**QS,V**

Sexual offending		
MSI-II	Multiphasic Sex Inventory - II	**QI,V**
RSAS	Rape Supportive Attitude Scale	**QI,V**
RMS	Rape Myth Scale	**QI,V**
EWT-V2a	Empathy for Women Test, version 2a	**QS,V**
SAQ	Sex Attitudes Questionnaire	**QI,V**

ACS	Abel Cognitions Scale	**QI,V**
QACSI	Questionnaire on Attitudes Consistent with Sex Offending	**QI,V**
Anger and violence		
STAXI-II	State-Trait Anger Expression Inventory	**QI,V**
PI	Provocation Inventory	**QI,V**
NAS	Novaco Anger Scales	**QI,V**
WARS	Ward Anger Rating Scale	**QI,V**
MVQ	Maudsley Violence Questionnaire	**QI, V**
Competency		
CST	Competency Screening Test	**QI,V**
CAI	Competency Assessment Instrument	**QI,V**
FTPA	Fitness to Plead Assessment	**QI,P,V**
IFI	Interdisciplinary Fitness Interview	**IS,V**
MacCAT-T	Macarthur Competence Assessment Tool for Treatment	**IS,VF**
Posttraumatic stress disorder		
CAPS	Clinician Administered PTSD Scale	**QI, V**
TSI	Trauma Symptom Inventory	**QS, V**
PDS	Post Traumatic Stress Diagnostic Scales	**QS, V**
IES-R	Impact of Events Scale	**QS, V**
Blame attribution		
BAI	Blame Attribution Inventory	**QI,V**
Fire-setting		
FSAS	Fire-Setting Assessment Schedule	**QI,V**
FIRS	Fire Interest Rating Scale	**QI,V**
SDS	Severity of Dependence Scale	**QI,V**
Mood		
BDI-II	Beck Depression Inventory—Second Edition	**QI,V**
BAI	Beck Anxiety Inventory	**QI,V**
GHQ	General Health Questionnaire	**QI, V**
Suicidal intention		
SSI	Scale for Suicide Ideation	**QI, V**
BHS	Beck Hopelessness Scale	**QI,V**

| SISQ | Suicidal Ideation Screening Questionnaire | **QI, V** |
| SADPERSONS | Screening questionnaire for suicidal ideation | **QI,V** |

Trauma

DAPS	Detailed Assessment of Posttraumatic Stress	**QI, V**
TSI	Trauma Symptom Inventory	**QI, V**
CAPS	Clinician Administered Posttraumatic Stress Disorder Scale	**IS**
CTQ	Childhood Trauma Questionnaire	**QI, V**
IES	Impact of Events Scale	**QI, V**
PDS	Posttraumatic Stress Diagnostic Scale	**IS**

General psychopathology

PANSS	Positive and Negative Symptoms in Schizophrenia	**QI, R**
PSE	Present Status Examination	**IS**
SCAN	Schedules for Clinical Assessment in Neuropsychiatry	**IS**

Malingering

| SIRS/SIMS | Structured Inventory of Reported/ Malingered Symptoms | **QI,V** |
| TOMM | Test of Memory Malingering | **QI,V** |

Many of the cognitive function tests listed above can also be used for malingering.

Use of biological investigations

One purpose of conducting biological investigations in psychiatry is to identify any medical condition that may be affecting brain function. These include brain imaging and electroencephalography (EEG), plus potentially a
wide range of blood and urine tests, and very occasionally karyotyping and
other genetic tests. Another purpose is to monitor the impact of psychiatric
medications on various organs.

Biological investigations are rarely specific to forensic psychiatric evaluation and the principles of such investigations are the same as for patients
receiving general psychiatric care.

Indications for investigations

Forensic psychiatric inpatients may be investigated using biological techniques more frequently than in general psychiatry. This can occur because:
• There are higher rates of head injury in people convicted of violent acts
  necessitating brain imaging and EEG investigation.
• There are higher rates of physical ill-health amongst forensic psychiatric
  patients, including sexually transmitted infection and diabetes.
• Forensic patients often have comorbid drug and alcohol misuse
  disorders requiring urine drug testing and/or breath analysis to test
  for drug or alcohol use, as well as investigation for possible effects of
  chronic substance misuse.
• Patients in forensic psychiatric services are more likely to be prescribed
  high-dose antipsychotic medication, resulting in the need for more
  frequent blood and ECG monitoring.
• Forensic psychiatric patients are more likely to be prescribed clozapine,
  necessitating frequent blood test monitoring.
• Forensic psychiatric patients are more likely to be required to undergo
  plasma monitoring of antipsychotic blood levels in order to test
  compliance with oral medication.

Where a patient in hospital or a prisoner is facing a serious charge, the
threshold for ruling out an organic cause of their condition should be low.
The criminal justice stakes are high. This can mean that no stone is left un-
turned when otherwise a 'wait and see' approach might be clinically appropriate. Also, even subtle abnormalities of brain function can lay the
foundation for a <u>mental condition defence</u> (p.412), most commonly that of
<u>diminished responsibility</u> (p.624) in relation to a charge of murder.

Given the current poor state of knowledge about the biological basis of
mental disorders and the paucity of specific tests available, there is no place
at present for routine biological investigation in the diagnosis of mental disorder or in assessing the cause or risk of violent behaviour.

Biological investigations should not be performed without a specific indication, such as suspicion of a condition that is diagnosable through the use
of the test in question, checking medication compliance by testing the blood
level of a drug, or monitoring for side effects of medication.

Presentation of the results of investigations

Caution should be exercised in reporting abnormalities of, or affecting, the brain to courts in relation to possible mental condition defences. This is because brain function does not directly map on to legal questions relating to criminal responsibility: largely the law asks questions that science cannot directly answer; and science answers questions that the law does not ask (i.e. they have different paradigms and <u>constructs</u>, p.354). For instance, a brain CT scan showing frontal damage, even combined with neuropsychometric tests suggesting impaired <u>executive function</u> (p.134), may imply a disability in medical terms, but this might have little or no relevance for criminal responsibility when <u>translated into the particular legal context</u> (p.358).

Information-gathering and liaison

A comprehensive psychiatric assessment takes account of not only information arising from the patient/defendant/litigant but also information from third parties. This includes obtaining all relevant medical and other (including legal) records wherever possible. Although perhaps often impractical in general psychiatry, this level of information-gathering is the standard required in forensic psychiatry, and is essential for risk assessment (p.166).

The following sources should all be considered. In terms of information governance, it is important to consider the use to which information will be put, how long the information will be held, and whether consent is needed for third-party discussions. Some information may be too time-consuming to obtain.

From the patient, defendant, or litigant

- History
- Mental state examination
- Physical examination
- Results of tests, investigations and psychometric assessments
- Letters, diaries and other documents written by the patient (usually used only with their consent)

From informants

- Family members
- Friends and colleagues
- Teachers, employers
- Other professionals who have known the patient for a considerable length of time (e.g. former doctors and social workers)

From records

- GPs
- Other psychiatric and general hospitals
- Previous psychiatrists
- Social workers from adult and child & family social services
- School reports and academic assessments
- Police criminal record and police intelligence reports, including records held under Multi-Agency Public Protection Arrangements (p.592)
- Housing and hostels
- Employers
- Reports from independent sector agencies (e.g. volunteering schemes)

From current and past legal papers

- Prosecution case summaries
- Witness statements
- So-called unused material for court cases (e.g. witness statements not placed in the prosecution bundle)
- Statements collected by the defence
- Court records, including previous judges' comments on sentencing
- Probation presentence and other reports
- Court reports written by other experts

Potential ethical problems

Where defendants are admitted to hospital before trial, they may forget they are not simply a patient, and disclose legally relevant information that might be harmful to their defence. Patients should be informed that clinical records may be subject to legal disclosure during the trial, and that the prosecution may see information that might undermine the defence case. This is another example of how forensic patients need to be reminded that absolute confidentiality cannot be guaranteed (p.320).

Potential legal problems

Witness statements (both prosecution and defence) may be important sources of information in assessments of defendants. They may recount acts or statements made by the defendant that might, for example, indicate their mental state at the time of an alleged offence. Such statements will have been collected within a legal model (p.355) for legal purposes, and so the clinician may wish to interview the witness directly, to ask more specifically about their mental state or behaviour within a medical model. There might be legal restrictions on interviewing, however, and this should not be pursued without first seeking the permission of the prosecution or defence (the side who has not instructed you), or the court, on the advice of the instructing solicitor.

A further problem arises when some of the information on which a clinical opinion is, or should properly be based is legally privileged, or otherwise inadmissible in court (p.382) for example because it lists previous offences. If the clinician needs to take this information into account in order to reach their opinion (e.g. as part of a risk assessment) they may need to include it in a section of their court report (p.694), but should be careful to avoid disclosing the information whilst giving evidence in court (p.712), unless directly instructed to.

Diagnosis

The purpose of diagnosis is to categorise symptoms and signs, and to express them in internationally accepted standardised terms that enable accurate, succinct communication. A diagnosis may also indicate the prognosis, and the likely response to treatments. Wherever possible, diagnoses are based upon knowledge of the aetiology and pathology of the condition, but such knowledge is often lacking in psychiatry. As a result, most psychiatric diagnoses represent syndromes rather than diseases, including possible overlap between syndromes (especially with different personality disorders within one cluster (p.78)).

The lack of objective biological criteria for many psychiatric diagnoses, particularly the 'functional' conditions with no identified neuropathology, means that value judgments (p.674), and other subjective factors, may affect the diagnostic process, something that must be guarded against, including through the adoption of values-based practice (p.288).

Diagnosis in forensic psychiatry

Diagnosis has particular ethical importance in forensic psychiatry because it may be crucial to legal processes that have major non-health-related implications for the subject: such as determination of culpability or detention in prison versus hospital (the law's wish to 'categorise' therefore often creates clinico-legal incongruence). Legal (especially criminal) processes may require forensic experts to go beyond diagnosis and offer a narrative formulation (p.146): an understanding of how the diagnosis relates to the behaviour of concern in the individual.

Diagnostic classificatory systems

There are two main diagnostic classifications: the World Health Organisation's International Classification of Diseases, Eleventh edition, psychiatric section (ICD11 Chapter 6) and the American Psychiatric Association's Diagnostic and Statistical Manual, Fifth edition (DSM-5). Some prefer the DSM-5 because it sets out the number of criteria to be met for diagnosis; others prefer ICD11 because of its international basis and its clearer system of numerical codes. Both ICD11 and DSM-5 made major revisions to several diagnostic areas, particularly personality disorder, where degrees of severity are now recognised in terms of affect regulation and impairment of interpersonal function.

Forensic psychiatrists should exercise caution in the use of DSM and ICD in legal settings. The use of defined criteria can be useful when it allows others to see how an expert came to their diagnosis. However, such criteria are an aid to, and not a substitute for, the exercise of clinical judgment. Lawyers may focus 'forensically' on the criteria, and (sometimes deliberately) seek to undermine the expert's view, based solely upon the presence or absence of specified numbers of criteria (in DSM). The more 'narrative' approach of ICD can lay the expert open to 'getting lost' in the wordage. Experts should resist cross-examination that treats DSM or ICD like a 'cookbook', and emphasise the importance of describing the full clinical picture across time.

Diagnosis, symptoms, behaviour and offence

There is rarely a direct or simple <u>relationship</u> between mental disorder and complex behaviour (p.44). It is important not to confuse diagnosis with behaviour, or with a criminal offence (or to attempt to <u>treat the behaviour or offence</u>, p.338): a woman with depression (*a diagnosis*) sets a fire (*a behaviour*) as a result of suicidal feelings (*a symptom*). She may then be charged with arson (*a criminal offence*).

Diagnosis cannot be inferred solely from behaviour, and people can behave 'abnormally' or antisocially in the absence of any psychiatric disorder. Inferring diagnosis from behaviour can lead to circular reasoning if the diagnosis is then used to 'explain' the behaviour. This is a particular risk in cases of unusual behaviour which is also criminal (such as <u>stalking</u> (p.52) or child homicide).

Diagnostic tools

Like other doctors, psychiatrists usually make diagnoses based upon clinical assessment of signs and symptoms. However, structured diagnostic interviews (e.g. the <u>SCAN</u> or <u>SCID-5-PD</u>; pp.137, 139), devised for research purposes, can also be used to aid diagnose psychotic disorders and personality disorders. Clinicians require training for such interviews to be reliable or valid, and they should be used with caution in complex legal disputes.

Formulation

Formulation offers a narrative hypothesis about the <u>underlying causes, precipitants and maintaining factors</u> (see pp.28–43) of a person's psychological, interpersonal and behavioural dysfunction. It is distinguished from diagnosis by being individualised, theoretically driven and focused upon *understanding* rather than *categorisation* (in terms of known clusters of symptoms and signs, and/or underlying pathology, as they occur in populations of individuals).

Formulation is of particular importance in forensic psychiatry because of its role in both offering an understanding, sometimes narrative, of criminal offending, and evaluating and helping to manage and reduce patients' risk to others. Formulations must do justice to the treatment need, to patients' individuality, and to the risk of harm they may pose. They should include both 'risk' and 'resilience' (protective) factors. Essential elements to consider in constructing a formulation include:

- **Salient developmental features**: here particular attention is paid to both genetic vulnerability and exposure to fear/loss experiences in early years. A history of disrupted attachments and chronic fear experience is associated with an increased risk of developing mental disorders, especially PD, and is also associated with unempathic attitudes towards the self and others.
- **Any indication of early (preteen) antisocial values and attitudes**: this is a bad prognostic sign, as is any antisocial behaviour before the age of ten years, or callous and unemotional attitudes in preteens (which are resistant to repair or reparation). Any indicators of positive responses to care and attention, or enduring attachments, should be noted as resilience factors.
- **Later attachment history and adult relationship patterns** should be included. Are adult relationships intense, unstable, conflicted and short-lived (as in BPD) or distant, cruel, or exploitative (as in ASPD)? Are any of these features causally relevant to any index offence?
- **Elements of impaired reality testing at the time of an index offence**: distinguish cognitive distortions from delusional belief. How much is the impairment a feature of the person's everyday world view, and how much was it situational? Did drugs and alcohol misuse play a part?
- **What the individual themselves makes of the offence**: are they shocked, baffled, or in denial? What <u>psychological defences</u> (p.212) are they now using, and which might have facilitated commission of the offence?
- **Risk factors for violence in this individual's case**: might they be relevant in in-patient settings and therapeutic relationships?

Common theoretical formulation models

Formulation is a core competency of mental health practice; however, there is no agreement on one model, and different models may be either complementary or conflicting.

Biopsychosocial: the classic psychiatric formulation, a two-dimensional table comprising biological, psychological, and social factors that are deemed to *predispose* to the current or anticipated problems, *precipitate* them, perpetuate (*maintain*) them or *protect* against them.

Cognitive-behavioural: a formulation based upon the CBT model (p.206) of interrelated thoughts, emotions, sensations, and actions, triggered by negative automatic thoughts and underlain by core beliefs. Like the biopsychosocial model it considers *predisposing*, *precipitating*, *maintaining* and *protective* factors.

Narrative: an individualised, largely unstructured formulation, although it may isolate and classify individual factors. It represents an individual's story from one perspective, is specific to the formulator and often seeks to explain a particular outcome, such as why patients became ill or why they offended. The scenarios found in the HCR20 (p.170), and other risk-assessment instruments, are examples of narrative formulations (for an example see Box 4.2).

Psychodynamic: a formulation founded in psychodynamic or psychoanalytic theory, incorporating elements such as defences, drives, and internal objects.

Legal (e.g. criminal): narrative formulation (often contested) constructed from evidence for use during trial (p.566) and sentencing (p.442), comprising elements such as means, motive, intention (p.402), and opportunity.

Box 4.2 Example case summary and narrative formulation

Mr Jones is a twenty-three-year-old man charged with the murder of his stepfather. He was admitted to hospital from prison because of concerns about depression and suicide risk. In his early childhood, he was exposed to neglect and physical harm and taken into care between the ages of four and six years. He was returned to his mother's care but was exposed to further repeated physical violence from stepfather from the age of eight years. He was antisocial at school from age ten and was permanently excluded at fourteen for violence. His first conviction was at age fifteen for criminal damage, and he has multiple convictions for theft and criminal damage. Last year he assaulted his mother, breaking her arm, but she did not press charges. He has had no intimate relationships but does have one friend from school whom he still sees. He is also in touch with his foster mother.

Resilience factors include intelligence and an absence of substance abuse history. *Risk factors* include early loss and fear experiences, mental illness, preteen antisocial attitudes and a complex and angry relationship with his mother. Therefore his mother may still be at risk from him, and therapeutic relationships with females should be carefully monitored. He is likely to be paranoid with male authority figures, and male staff will need to respond to him carefully and not rise to provocative behaviour.

Special issues in forensic assessments

Forensic assessments need attention to context and purpose, especially if the assessment is to be the basis of a medico-legal report or potentially give rise to enhanced or extended detention.

- The persons being assessed should be informed fully at the outset about the nature and purpose of the assessment; for example, if it is for a move to a more secure placement, they should be advised of this. If it is for a court report then they should be advised that the usual clinical limits on confidentiality will not apply, and the report will be disclosed (p.320) to individuals who are parties in the court proceedings (unless the defence have control of the report). If they refuse to be assessed, they should also be informed that a report may still be produced containing opinions based solely on other sources of information.
- If they agree to assessment, then their consent (p.660) to the assessment and the associated report must be recorded. This is so even where a court has ordered that a report must be submitted: if the person refuses consent, a report should be submitted that includes stating this. It might also include information from other sources, if appropriate (but see pp.322, 334, and 342 on the ethics of doing so).
- You should consider the potential conflict in role between assessing a person for potential treatment only and having to present a report to a court or tribunal. There are advantages and disadvantages to treating mental health professionals giving expert testimony. They may be the person in the best position to offer a clinical opinion; however, they may be biased (p.674) in regard to its legal application, or the assessment may adversely affect the subsequent therapeutic relationship.
- In criminal cases, it is vital to consider the stage of the legal process the person is at when conducting the assessment as this will have implications for what the person might want to disclose, particularly pre-trial (p.398); see also the caution on information-gathering during admission to hospital before trial (p.143).
- Although caution should be exercised in gaining and interpreting information from the person being assessed, given that he or she may be involved in legal proceedings, this should not result in distortion of ordinary clinical procedure. It is inevitable that doctors ask patients direct questions which, to the lawyer, amount to leading questions (p.160). As a result vigilance should include attempts to check and confirm information, both within the interview and through access to other sources of information. You may also need to focus on some clinical aspects more than others e.g. the mental state at the time of the offence.
- The quality of a report to court depends upon both the clinical assessment and proper consideration of records and legal papers (e.g. the case summary and witness statements, p.142). Although a report may appear adequate at face value, any inadequacy is likely to be displayed clearly through the process of cross-examination (p.714). Length is no indicator of quality.
- Starting the interview by asking about family and personal history often puts people at their ease, enhances the reliability of information gained, and provides initial hypotheses about diagnosis (p.144) and

formulation (p.146). This may make it easier when asking about more sensitive matters directly relevant to the legal issues, especially in criminal cases, p.694) when defendants may feel ashamed or frightened.

- Take into account any cultural or ethnic (p.40) differences between you and the person being assessed. Try to avoid biased assumptions based upon such factors, especially in regard to interpreting potential psychopathology. Such factors may also have significance in terms of experience of vulnerability and perceptions of power disparities. Supervision (p.308) by an appropriately experienced colleague, or retrospective peer review, can be of great assistance in avoiding bias.

- Do not forget that individuals caught up in the criminal justice system, especially children and young people (p.154) and those with intellectual disability (p.110), can be highly vulnerable—whatever they are alleged to have done. Particular issues to watch out for include suggestibility and compliance (p.160) within police interviews. It is also not unusual for alleged offenders to be defensive and wary with strangers; this may not be evidence of paranoia!

Special issues in prison settings

There is evidence from UK and international prevalence studies that mental health problems are very common in prisoners and those held in correctional facilities[5] (Box 4.3).

Box 4.3 Prevalence of psychiatric disorders in prison population

- Psychosis—10% men; 7% women
- Mood and anxiety disorders—39% men; 75% women
- Personality disorder—75% men on remand; 50%–60% all sentenced
- Illicit substance use—85% men; 69% women

Psychiatric assessments are therefore often needed to address risk management and consideration of transfer to hospital for treatment. Some forensic psychiatrists work directly in prison in-reach psychiatric services (p.270); this page focuses on visiting psychiatrists.

Both forensic and general psychiatrists may be asked to see prisoners: to assess for a <u>court report</u> (pp.678–709); in response to a prison request for <u>transfer to hospital</u> (p.271), or for a statutory assessment, such as preparing a <u>Parole Board Report</u> (p.696).

Prior to a prison visit

- Check whether there are any day or time restrictions on visits, and whether the prison imposes a notice period (e.g. at least forty-eight hours). Also check what ID you need to bring, and restrictions on items you can take in (rules vary by security category and individual institution).
- Contact the mental health in-reach service or prison healthcare department to arrange the visit. Ideally such assessments will be in the health care unit; if there is no health care unit, then the assessment may have to take place in the legal visits suite. This is problematic because such suites may be noisy and not conducive to a mental health assessment; in addition, the legal visits department may not have access to the patient's medical records.
- Be aware that prisoners will only be available to be seen at certain times: usually two hours in the morning or afternoon. Time your visit accordingly, and phone before you travel.
- Review all the case papers and other relevant documents in advance.
- Prepare your plan of assessment, including specific questions you wish to ask of the prisoner and records you wish to see.

On arrival

- Arrive early, as it may take thirty to sixty minutes to pass security checks. Remember to take approved photographic ID, often a passport, driving licence, and/or employment ID (some prisons require more than one).

5 During and after the Covid-19 pandemic many assessments of prisoners were carried out remotely, which method gives rise to different issues.

- Certain items are restricted (e.g. mobile phones, Dictaphones, and memory sticks). You may be allowed to leave these in lockers, but it is worth checking prior to your visit.
- Expect a personal search (usually a rub-down or pat-down search, as well as one involving an electromagnetic 'wand'); as well as searches and/or x-ray screening of your coat and bag, and being sniffed by a drug-search dog.

During the visit

- If appropriate, obtain information from the sources listed below as well as from the patient/prisoner.
- Ask the prisoner to sign a consent form for access to their medical records. If you are given access to these records, you will not be able to remove them, so all notes need to be made in full and in situ (defence lawyers can gain them and send them to you).
- Remember that, with the exception sometimes of healthcare staff, it will usually be inappropriate to share confidential medical information with prison staff.
- Ensure that the prisoner is aware of the nature and purpose of the assessment, the limits on the usual doctor-patient confidentiality, and their right to refuse. Bear in mind that prisoners will often soon forget this and begin confiding in an empathic doctor, so you may need to remind them of the limits on confidentiality, and how and why this information is going to be used or disclosed.

Sources of information

- Inmate Medical Records (IMRs) held by NHS or prison healthcare staff, including all electronic records
- Healthcare staff who know the patient/prisoner
- Prison officers who know the patient/prisoner
- Disciplinary and wing records (often a useful record of behaviour)
- If in use, consider Assessment, Care in Custody, and Treatment (ACCT) forms and Form 2052 SH: these are suicide and self-harm care planning documents

After the assessment

- Write in the medical record that you have completed an assessment, whatever your role; include your contact details and, if appropriate, a summary of the clinical outcome of your assessment. You may have to ask a colleague to make this note for you if you do not have access.
- If the assessment is solely for a legal report, the notes made should usually refer only to the fact of the assessment and not your clinical findings, or its legal implications.
- If you think that the prisoner's mental health is at risk and/or suspect the risk of harm to themselves or others is sufficient to breach confidence, then under the _Egdell_ principle (p.754), you should liaise with the prison mental health team and document this in the relevant records.

Special issues with women

Women are a minority of offenders, especially violent offenders. In 2017 only 26% of those prosecuted and 5% of prisoners in the UK were female; only 2% of convicted women received immediate custodial sentences; and the average duration for women was 10 months compared to 17.6 months for men. Convicted women are less likely to reoffend, and they are often responsible for dependent children, 91% of whom are then forced to leave their homes in order to be cared for (this is rarely noted in pre-sentence reports). The commonest offences for which women are convicted are TV licence evasion, shoplifting, theft, and fraud.

Differences between male and female offenders

Although there are far fewer female offenders than male, there are both similarities and differences. They differ from men in that they are numerically far fewer, less likely to have histories of violence, and tend to be older at their first offence. They are more likely to have sought mental health treatment prior to imprisonment, they tend to report more drug and alcohol problems, and self-harm more in prison. All female offenders in prison are more likely than males to self-harm, although rates of completed suicide are lower.

Female violence perpetrators

A comparatively small number of women commit acts of violence: between 2015 and 2017, fifty-three women received a life sentence for murder in the UK, compared to 752 men. However, the proportion of prisoners serving a sentence for violence is similar in male and female prisons (29% and 26%, respectively). Only 2%–4% of women prisoners are serving a sentence for sexual offence. Female violence perpetrators have more histories of domestic violence, but similar experiences of childhood adversity.

Some women commit acts of violence in partnership with a violent man or fail to protect vulnerable children from them. In 2017, 1,000 women were cautioned or prosecuted for cruelty or neglect of children in the UK, compared to 600 men.

Like males, female violence perpetrators usually victimise those who are dependent upon them, or related to them in close relationships, and violence to strangers is rare; unlike men, they are unlikely to be members of gangs or to use weapons. Female stalkers, however, may target strangers or professional contacts. In rare cases, women may kill partners in the context of severe domestic violence; arguably this can present particular problems for courts in applying the defences of <u>diminished responsibility</u> (p.624) and <u>provocation</u> or <u>loss of control</u> (p.630) fairly.

Risk factors for violence in women

- In both sexes, previous violence or <u>criminality</u> (p.20), <u>antisocial personality disorder</u> (ASPD, p.82), and <u>substance misuse</u> (p.76) increase the risk of violence. ASPD is comparatively less common in females, but in females the risk is further increased where there is comorbid <u>BPD</u> (p.84) and unmet <u>social needs</u> (p.28).

- In both sexes, paranoid <u>psychotic disorders</u> (p.72) increase violence risk, but this is especially true of women with postnatal psychoses who may present a significant risk to their newborn babies. Paranoid thoughts about any child (not just newborns) should always be taken very seriously in terms of risk, especially if combined with other unexplained fears and suicidal thoughts. The risk period for postnatal psychosis may extend into the first postnatal year.
- Violence by women tends to occur in the context of relationships. This includes terrorism-based offences; a small number of women are radicalised online and invited to marry into terrorist groups. These alliances give rise to high risk and unpredictable violence.

Mental disorder in female offenders

Prevalence studies of mental disorder in prisons have found similar rates of mental disorders in both sexes for most disorders, with the exception of ASPD, which is twice as common in men. BPD is particularly common in female prisoners (Box 4.4).

> ### Box 4.4 Prevalence of mental disorder amongst female prisoners
>
> - Psychosis: 14%
> - Depression 15%–21%
> - Personality disorder 50% (ASPD 21%; BPD 20%)

A subgroup of female prisoners require treatment in secure psychiatric settings: usually because they are psychotic, suicidal, self-harming, or are otherwise difficult to manage in prison. Most can be safely treated in <u>medium secure</u> (p.258) <u>services for women</u> (p.260), and only a tiny minority will require treatment in <u>enhanced medium security</u> (p.258) or <u>high security</u> (p.258). This latter group resemble their male counterparts in terms of their antisocial personality traits.

Risk assessment in female offenders

Most risk-assessment tools have been standardised in relation to male offenders, and their generalisation to female offenders is of doubtful validity. The base rate for violence in females is so low that predictive risk factors are much harder to establish. Some studies suggest that there are risk factors like prostitution and multiple pregnancies which affect only women, although these are unlikely to predict violence.

The victims most at risk of violence from women are their children. Studies of child homicide show that mothers and fathers are equally at risk, and that the majority of mothers had a mental disorder at the time of killing. Therefore when assessing the risk of violence in female offenders, it is crucial to consider whether she has children in her care. It should also be remembered that women who have been violent to others still have a higher risk of <u>suicide or self-harm</u> (p.176) than of being violent to others again.

Special issues with children & youths

Forensic and child & adolescent psychiatrists may be asked to assess children and young people aged ten (the lowest age of criminal responsibility, p.406) to seventeen years, who present a risk to others and appear to suffer from mental disorder.[6] Young people may pose a risk of harm to others or themselves (especially other young people) through violence, sexually inappropriate behaviour, fire-setting, or property damage. Only a minority persistently commit offences into adulthood (p.36), or commit serious offences. As with adult offenders, only a small proportion come into contact with psychiatric services.

Young people who end up in the youth justice system (YJS) often have multiple vulnerabilities. Challenges include the nebulous nature of emerging mental ill-health in comparison to adult presentations, and the reluctance of young people to engage with services due to stigma.

Approaches to assessment

When assessing children and adolescents, one difference from an adult psychiatric assessment is the need to recognise that individuals are still developing, and that future maturation may impact the treatment and prognosis of any identified conditions or problematic behaviours.

Various measures are used by mental health professionals to assess both criminogenic and mental health needs that link with desistance in this population. A number of mental health screening tools have been developed for YJS use in the UK. Some screening tools focus on broader needs which have the capacity to undermine mental health and emotional wellbeing.

- The Salford Needs Assessment Schedule for Adolescents (SNASA) can be used to identify psychosocial and mental health needs by Youth Offending Teams (YOT, p.585) in E&W.
- The SQIFA (Screening Questionnaire Interview for Adolescents) is a universal screening tool administered to all young people on initial contact. Those identified as having a need are then referred for the second stage, the SIFA (Screening Interview for Adolescents). This is administered by YOT health workers.
- A more in-depth clinical assessment may need to be undertaken by a psychiatrist or psychologist. The SAVRY may also be used which is the best structured risk assessment.
- The ASSETT Plus assessment tool is used by YOTs in the UK, focussing on criminogenic risks and needs. This has an increased emphasis on better assessing speech and communication needs and learning difficulties which were not addressed well by the ASSET.
- The Comprehensive Health Assessment Tool (CHAT) was developed for young offenders in custody across E&W. It is a semistructured assessment developed to provide a standardised approach to health screening and consists of five parts that are administered at various time points following admission to the secure estate.

6 No psychiatrist lacking substantial higher training in child and adolescent psychiatry should undertake assessment of those less than 18 years of age; in regard to alleged serious offending the assessor should ideally be dually trained in both child and adolescent *and* forensic psychiatry

Table 4.2 Rates of mental disorders in the general population and in young people in custody

Disorder	General population	Young people in custody
Any clinically recognisable	14.4% (11–16 year olds) 16.9% (17–19 year olds)	90%
Conduct disorder	6.2% (all 11–16 year olds) (7.4% male; 5.0% female)	90% (males)
Emotional disorders (c.f. anxiety, depression)	9% (all 11–16 year olds) (7.1% male; 10.9% female) 14.9% (17–19 year olds)	13%–21%
Suicide	8 per 100,000 (males) 3 per 100,000 (females)	2 to 9 deaths per year in E&W from 2012 to 2018
Drug dependency	25% (cannabis only) 16–19 years	52% males 58% females
ADHD	1.7%–9%	12%
Autistic spectrum disorders	0.6%–1.2%	15%
Communication disorders	5%–7%	60%–90%
Intellectual disability	2%–4%	23%–32%
Foetal alcohol syndrome	0.1%–5%	10.9%–11.7%
Traumatic brain injury	24%–31.6%	65.1%–72.1%

A review of the inquests and investigations into deaths of young people in custody found that many had had significant interaction with community agencies before entering prison, yet there were failures in communication between these agencies and the prison. There is likely a failure of some vulnerable young people being diverted out of the CJS at an early stage, being exposed to unsafe cells, segregation, restraint, and bullying, with limited access to needed therapeutic services.

A long-standing concern in youth justice is the over-representation of nonwhite groups, and this is high on the YJB agenda.

Children as witnesses

Children often require special measures when giving evidence (p.157).

Special issues with witnesses

Occasionally, a forensic psychiatrist may be asked to assess a witness who is thought to have a mental disorder that might affect their legal competence to give evidence, or impair their credibility or reliability[7] as a witness. This is distinct from considering the same issues in a defendant, as part of addressing their <u>fitness during police interview</u> (p.573), <u>fitness to plead</u> (p.602), and <u>fitness to give evidence</u> (p.606).

Note that only impairments of credibility or reliability as a witness *because of mental disorder* are relevant; an expert should never attempt to bolster a witness's credibility (sometimes known as 'oath-helping'[8]).

Assessment can be hampered by inability within legal process to secure the medical records of a witness.

Competence of witnesses

Within criminal proceedings, to be <u>fit to give evidence</u> (p.606) a witness must be able to:

• understand questions put to them as a witness, and
• give answers which can be understood.

Psychiatric evidence might be relevant to deciding whether a witness meets these two tests, but it is for the court to decide whether they are competent or not, and if so, how much weight to give their evidence (see also <u>addressing the ultimate issue</u>, p.664). One suggestion for the psychiatric assessment is to consider two questions:

• Is the witness's ability to understand the oath impaired by mental or other disorder, and if so, how?
• Is the witness's ability to recall and recount what he or she has witnessed impaired by mental or other disorder, and if so, how?

Answering these questions may also require psychological assessment, including of cognitive function, <u>suggestibility,</u> and/or <u>compliance</u> (p.160)[9]. Conditions that might impair competence to give evidence include dementia, psychosis, and intellectual disability.

The court will determine the competence of witnesses during a <u>voir dire</u> (p.719), based upon a comprehensive psychiatric assessment addressing these legal questions.

Reliability of witnesses

Even if a witness is considered competent to give evidence (or determined to be competent by the court), there may still be issues of reliability: relevant to the weight that a jury might properly place on their evidence. If instructed to assess witness reliability, this should involve a full psychiatric assessment. This will form the basis for considering whether there is any

---

7 Credibility refers to whether a witness is thought by the court to be telling what they believe to be the truth; reliability refers to whether their evidence is accurate.

8 Medieval courts treated statements by witnesses as proven fact if a fixed number of 'oath-helpers', often twelve, stated before the court that they believed the witness to be telling the truth.

9 Suggestibility and compliance have not yet been accepted as relevant to the competence of a witness (as opposed to a defendant) in the UK or RoI. However, this may not always be the case, and assessments of the reliability of the witness or a police interviews with them may be requested.

reason why the witness, as a result of mental disorder, might be at risk of not giving a reliable account to a jury. For example, fluctuating delusions might change the account the witness would give at different times.

Specific issues of reliability that are sometimes put to psychiatrists include the reliability of childhood memories (especially memories of sexual abuse recovered after psychotherapy, p.668, that are subsequently alleged to be false), and the reliability of a witness or victim (such as a victim of rape or sexual assault) who gives inconsistent accounts of the alleged offence or act in apparently inconsistent ways. Such inconsistencies should not be taken as evidence of unreliability even if the witness in question has a mental disorder that potentially bears upon this issue. Unless you have special expertise in these areas, it may be more appropriate for the issue to be considered by a forensic psychologist or psychotherapist (p.11).

Fitness to attend court

Mentally disordered witnesses and defendants may not be able to attend court to give evidence because of their mental condition. The court will usually expect evidence from a treating psychiatrist before adjourning (p.607) or allowing the case to proceed in the absence of the witness or defendant.

Vulnerable witnesses

Vulnerable witnesses include witnesses under the age of seventeen, witnesses suffering from an intellectual disability or other mental disorder, the elderly, or a witness whose quality of evidence, in the opinion of the court, is likely to be diminished by reason of fear or distress in testifying. The witness may well be competent to give evidence, and not considered unreliable in doing so, but require special measures to be applied when attending court. These may include:

• allowing supporters to sit with them;
• using screens or video links to separate them from the defendant(s);
• restricting public and media access while they give evidence;
• making proceedings feel less formal, for instance by removal of wigs;
• using communication aids such as computers or interpreters; and
• granting anonymity, especially if there is a serious risk of intimidation.

Advice may be sought from The Advocates Gateway, which provides free advice about working with vulnerable witnesses and defendants.

Ethical pitfalls

Assessing the competence and reliability of witnesses is an area of practice where there are particular dangers not only of addressing the ultimate issue (as above), but also of exceeding one's area of expertise (pp.295, 304, 655) and allowing one's own values to affect one's opinion (pp.330, 674).

Special issues with victims

Victim issues are common in forensic psychiatry. Most commonly, the victim(s) of patients under forensic psychiatric care may be family members who are also involved in the patient's rehabilitation. They may also have some rights to information about the patient's discharge pathway and may exert some influence over the patient's progress. Victims' views can sometimes have a significant effect upon to where a patient is rehabilitated and how. Forensic teams have to address risk to identified victims in their risk-management plans.

Forensic psychiatrists may have duties to prevent their patients causing further harm to their victims, and to warn identifiable future victims (see p.296), but the extent of these remains unclear with the law still evolving.

Forensic patients may well have been a victim of crime themselves, as a child or an adult or both, and may report posttraumatic symptoms, meeting criteria for PTSD and complex PTSD (p.669). Other psychological effects of victimisation include depression, anxiety, substance misuse, paranoia, intense anger, and shame. These feelings can contribute to the risk of victims becoming perpetrators themselves.

Victims and the criminal justice system

Victim surveys (p.22) data show that the lifetime likelihood of being a victim is high for minor offences but low for serious ones. Men and boys are more likely to be victims of violence generally, but women and girls are at much higher risk of sexual violence and violence by partners. Males are at more risk than females overall of violence by strangers. There are differences in whether victims report a crime, including their relationship to the perpetrator, age, and socio-demographic status.

Assessment of victims

It is uncommon for forensic psychiatrists to be directly involved in the assessment of victims. However, the following includes situations where a victim assessment might be performed:

- A forensic psychiatrist, not involved in assessing or treating the defendant, may (rarely) assess the psychological needs of a victim in relation to risk assessment (p.166).
- In civil litigation, the victim might be assessed when damages needs to be assessed in cases of negligence (p.548) by another health professional, or concerning compensation (p.640) for trauma in a claim for personal injury.
- As with other witnesses (p.156) there may be concerns about a victim's reliability in providing evidence in court, perhaps because of their suggestibility or compliance (p.160) or unreliability of posttraumatic memory. Victims as witnesses may suffer further trauma and exacerbation of their posttraumatic symptoms as a result of giving evidence.
- In family proceedings (p.554), an expert might be required to carry out a competence or needs assessment on a child whose parents are undergoing divorce or other relevant proceedings.

It is invalid to assess an alleged victim as part of an attempt to determine whether an offence was or was not committed against them. For example, it may be argued that if a victim has signs or symptoms of PTSD they 'must' have been a victim of the alleged offence. There is no evidence for drawing such inferences.

Vulnerable victims and special measures in court

Some victims may be especially vulnerable due to their age or intellectual disability or other comorbid condition. Specialist assessment may be needed; for example, assessment of children's experience of victimisation is best carried out by a child psychiatrist.

The courts may take <u>special measures</u> (p.157) to reduce the stress of testifying for victims, and to maximise their reliability as witnesses. Measures include: the removal of gowns and wigs for child witnesses, use of video live-link systems that allow people to testify via closed circuit television, or screening witnesses from defendants; and prerecorded videotaped evidence. Other measures include the protection of certain witnesses from cross-examination by the accused and restricting the <u>cross-examination</u> (p.714) of alleged rape victims about their sexual history. Court appointed intermediaries can also provide support for witnesses who are victims.

Suggestibility and compliance

Suggestibility

Interrogative suggestibility refers to the tendency of individuals to accept information communicated to them during formal questioning within a closed social interaction (for example, a police interview or a clinical interview[10]). The two main components are susceptibility to accept leading questions ('yield'); and susceptibility to critical feedback from the interrogator leading to a change in answer ('shift'). Research has indicated that it is difficult to fake suggestibility.

Associations with suggestibility
- Poor memory recall
- Low intelligence
- High emotionality and anxiety
- High social desirability
- Fear of negative evaluation
- Low assertiveness and self-esteem
- Negative life experiences and trauma

Suggestibility is typically associated with underlined and compliant confessions (p.608) and can be more likely if the suspect is unsure of what they have, or have not, done.

Compliance

This refers to the tendency to go along with propositions, requests or instructions for some immediate instrumental gain,[11] in full knowledge of doing so. It can result in a coerced-compliant confession (p.608), when suspects confesses to something they know that they have not done, possibly due to external pressure.

Relevance to legal proceedings

A person's degree of suggestibility and/or compliance may be relevant in a psychological assessment in relation to the reliability of their testimony, whether they are the defendant, the victim, or a witness. The courts are most concerned with retracted confessions (p.608), which may or may not have been false. The relevant expert is usually a psychologist, except where the person suffers from a diagnosable mental disorder, in which case psychiatrists and psychologists usually work together.

Evidence of unreliability may render the confession inadmissible, or admissible but with expert evidence to suggest that less weight should be given

---

10 It could also in principle relate to giving oral evidence in court as a witness (p.156), including defendant witness, but there does not appear to be any specific literature on this.

11 This should not be confused with the related psychological concept of **acquiescence**, which is the tendency during psychological testing to respond to questionnaire items with the answer 'yes' or 'true', whatever the content of the question.

to it. The 'Guildford Four' and 'Birmingham Six'[12] cases are two notorious examples of psychological evidence being used to assist in overturning convictions based upon confessions that were subsequently recognised to be unreliable.

Assessment of suggestibility and compliance

There are specific psychological tests to assess an individual's degree of suggestibility (Gudjonsson Suggestibility Scale, versions one, GSS1, and two, GSS2, p.137) and compliance (Gudjonsson Compliance Scale, GCS, p.137).

However, demonstrating either does not suggest, of itself, that the interviews were unreliable. It is also necessary to examine in detail the police interview transcripts and tapes, including addressing the manner of the questioning, interviewer bias, confirmation bias, and misleading questions, as well as the evident individual traits of the interviewee, in order to determine whether such traits operated within the interviews. Here attention should be paid to leading or closed questions, the subject appearing to take on information originating in things said by the interviewer, and undue pressure by the interrogator. In the case of a defendant, the absence of a solicitor during questioning, or of an appropriate adult (p.574) if needed, may also be relevant.

Suggestibility and compliance in oral evidence

- If a vulnerable defendant or witness is to give evidence then the assessment findings, and potential relevance to questioning, especially in cross-examination, should be described to the court.
- Vulnerable individuals may well still be able to testify under the right conditions, with additional support as necessary (such as the special measures described for vulnerable witnesses and victims giving evidence, pp.156–159).
- Through an application by a solicitor to the judge, the jury may potentially be informed of the psychological factors that might make the individual's testimony less than normally reliable.

---

12 Both cases concerned explosions in the UK caused by the Irish Republican Army, as part of a campaign designed to force the British to leave Northern Ireland. There was huge public pressure for convictions of those responsible; in the absence of safeguards such as those later enacted in the Police and Criminal Evidence Act 1984 (p.739), the police were able to pressurise suspects they believed to be guilty to give confessions that turned out to be false. The distinguished forensic psychiatrist to whom this handbook is dedicated, the late Dr James MacKeith, was, with Professor Gisli Gudjonsson, an important expert witness in the Irish bomb case appeals.

Risk assessment*

---

* This chapter should be read in conjunction with p.332.

Risk assessment: techniques & values

What risk assessment is not

In medicine, harms (e.g. death during surgery, or the side-effects of a drug) may arise as a 'cost' of attempting to benefit the patient. Risk-benefit ratios reflect this risk of doing harm. In psychiatry, this might mean, for example, the risk of causing persistent orofacial dyskinesia by treating psychosis with an antipsychotic drug.

However, risk assessment in psychiatry also relates to harm arising from the patient's own (mentally disordered) behaviour: harm to themselves through suicide or self-harm, or harm to another, such as rape or assault or murder. The universal desire to prevent such harm creates an expectation, fuelled by a lack of societal understanding of the nature of mental disorder and its potential consequences, that it must be possible to predict it. However, detailed prediction of something as complex and multifactorial as human behaviour is impossible, and likely to remain so.

Prediction versus prevention

The major unrecognised distinction in public discourse about risk is that between predicting behaviour or harm and preventing it, as if the former were essential to achieving the latter. However, to take an extreme example, all community homicides by patients with schizophrenia could be prevented by detaining them indefinitely in hospital. The majority of homicide inquiries have concluded that although the killing could not have been predicted often it could have been prevented through such measures: not through better risk assessment, but by having a lower threshold for detention, greater numbers of hospital beds, and/or better community services (albeit by diminishing patients' liberty and quality of life).

What risk assessment is[1]

Statements about risk in psychiatry are usually couched in terms such as 'the probability of this man, with his current symptoms and in his current circumstances, killing his wife, is unacceptably high'.[2] Implicit within this is a values-based (p.288) trade-off between preventing the patient harming his wife, and restricting his liberty. Because harms cannot be predicted accurately, there will always be **false positives** (where the State restricts the liberty of a patient who would not have caused harm on that occasion) as well as **false negatives** (in which action is not taken and harm occurs).

This is not to say that there are no data at all, and that risk assessment consists solely of value judgments; merely that our best estimates of the data (the probability of killing his wife on Tuesday) are very poor estimates, and that we must use some element of value judgment to set these poor estimates against each other (the cumulative estimate of the probability of him killing his wife, and the estimate of the harm done to him by restricting his liberty by only allowing escorted leave, p.191, say).

---

1 For worked examples of risk assessment see the *Oxford Casebook of Forensic Psychiatry*.

2 Other factors, such as the availability of appropriate treatment for his mental disorder, would still be necessary to justify detention under mental health legislation (see p.466).

Risk assessment, therefore:
- is imprecise and subject to great uncertainty,
- involves value judgments, and
- does not relate to specific events or times.

It relates to conditions, circumstances, and situations, plus exacerbating and protective factors (e.g. 'in the presence of untreated command auditory hallucinations, if disinhibited by alcohol or drugs, with access to a suitable weapon, and if unsupervised by a trusted relative or professional, he would be at high risk of assaulting or killing the subject of those hallucinations, e.g. his wife').

Should psychiatrists assess risk at all?

There is a great social, political, and legal demand for risk assessment (as well as for impossible harm prediction), and for risk management (p.238): that is, acting to reduce the risk through the understanding of it garnered via risk assessment. Moreover, some techniques of risk assessment, such as some actuarial measures (p.166), are right more often than by chance, and a few, used properly, do better still, such as the HCR20 (p.170).

Psychiatrists may be tempted to eschew risk assessment altogether—it is time-consuming, controversial, can feel ethically dubious in certain circumstances, and is often proved 'wrong' (when someone assessed as low risk causes harm, and vice versa, but by definition, some low-risk patients will still cause harm, just a smaller proportion than of high-risk ones[3]).

However, what is the alternative? Psychiatrists must decide whether or not to act in one way or another with each patient they see. Are such decisions to be guided without consideration of possible harms at all (e.g. prescribing drugs without considering the risk and severity of side-effects for this patient)? If not, how are such harms to be brought into consideration without some form of risk assessment procedure? For all the justified criticisms of the risk assessment techniques described in the following pages, risk assessment is inherent not only to medicine in general but to psychiatry in particular. It is unavoidable. Indeed, you do it even when you do not intend to do it. What matters is knowing not only the technical but also the ethical basis (p.322) of what you do.

---

3 This is one of the conundrums of risk assessment: even when the probability of a particular harm at the level of the population or group is well-known (e.g. it is well-established that around 10% of patients with schizophrenia will commit assault at some point in their life), the probability of the harm at the level of the individual is very rarely well-known (i.e. there is currently no way of telling whether *this* patient with schizophrenia is one of that 10%).

Approaches to risk assessment

Human behaviour is determined by multiple internal and environmental factors: assessing the risk of any given behaviour occurring is complex and difficult. Moreover, the research evidence informing practical risk assessment is weakened by major methodological limitations. Psychiatrists must therefore be cautious in attempting to assess such risks (including on <u>ethical grounds</u>, p.322), particularly where there is no intended or likely therapeutic benefit, as with some reports for criminal courts (p.694). They must be more careful to eschew <u>harm prediction</u> (p.164). They must be able to demonstrate (for example, to a future <u>homicide inquiry</u>, p.598, or court in a <u>negligence</u> case, p.548) that they performed their risk assessment carefully and in accordance with recognised good practice.

How well can risks be assessed?

The empirical evidence on risk assessment is undermined by biases and confounding variables:

- Studies in clinical settings tend to over-estimate risk: inpatients are at greater risk (because the risk was usually a reason for the admission).
- The diagnostic criteria for some disorders include harmful behaviours.
- The population prevalence of most harms (e.g. violence, suicide) is low.

For all these reasons, the prospective accuracy (positive predictive value) of psychiatric risk assessments is poor: of those labelled as 'high risk', particularly high risk of violence, several will not cause the harm in question for each that does.

Actuarial approaches

These are based upon statistical estimates of risk in groups of people. They perform better in some controlled studies than clinical judgment alone.[4] However, they have several flaws:

- They have a low positive predictive value, as explained above.
- They are limited by their reliance on **static factors** (e.g. a record of previous violence) and limited use of **dynamic factors** (such as the presence of active psychotic symptoms), and therefore cannot adequately measure changes in risk.
- They mostly ignore **protective factors** that reduce risk.

Group membership versus individual risk

Actuarial risk assessments inform you only about the aggregate risk of the group to which the individual belongs; not about the individual themselves. For example, studies that demonstrate that most eight-year-old boys presenting with acute abdominal pain have appendicitis, whereas most eighty year olds with the same presentation have intestinal obstruction (due to bowel cancer, say), provide information about the aggregate risks of the two conditions in eight and eighty year olds presenting with acute abdominal pain. This is useful, but insufficient: to decide what to do, you must

---

4 That is, they have better 'receiver operating characteristics', and offer greater improvements in risk estimation over chance than does unstructured clinical judgment.

also consider factors that show your patient is typical of the group, or in some way atypical. Such individual factors (for example, pyrexia in the child, or weight loss in the geriatric) must be added to the results of psychiatric actuarial risk assessments—which is exactly what structured professional judgment (see below) seeks to do.

Professional judgment approaches

These are based upon the judgment of an individual clinician or a team of clinicians, preferably from different disciplines; and can be **unstructured** or **structured**. In the latter case, the structure can act merely as an aide memoire (as in the case of the SDRS, p. 171) or can incorporate some actuarial elements (e.g. the HCR20, p.170).

When used alongside individual knowledge of patients and their environment, structured clinical risk assessments like the HCR20 have been shown to improve the outcomes of clinical decision-making.

Structured professional judgment in practice

All medicine involves assessment of the individual on a background of aggregate epidemiological data. Risk assessment judgments must take into account individual factors (sometimes based upon understanding of pathology, and including protective factors); the individual's history of symptoms associated with past behaviour[5]; as well as their membership of a group known to carry a given risk.

Although risk assessment instruments focus almost exclusively on the risks of violence, sexually inappropriate behaviour, self-harm, and suicide, the forensic psychiatrist must address a much broader array of behavioural risks, including:

- absconding or escape,
- drug use,
- medication noncompliance,
- self-neglect,
- exploitation,
- harm from others,
- relapse, and
- others, such as property damage.

Hence risk management (p.237) requires more specific information than just a single number, or even a restricted range of numbers: it requires knowledge of patients, within an individual formulation (p.146) of their condition and past behaviour.

---

5 Although there may not be epidemiological evidence that a particular symptom is associated with violence, a clinician may have good historical evidence that it is associated for their specific patient, within their own 'biography of behaviour'.

Risk of violence

The law defines <u>dangerousness</u> (p.672) as if it were a largely stable and consistent aspect of a person. Clinically, however, the *risk of harm*[6] is dynamic, and it depends at any given time on the interaction between the individuals, their mental disorder (if any), and their circumstances. The aim of a risk assessment for violence is to identify risk factors that arise within individuals, any disorder, and their circumstances, so as to develop a <u>management plan</u> (p.238) to minimise that risk.

Assessment of risk of violence

Specific <u>prediction</u> of violent acts is not realistic (p.164). Risk estimates are inexact: no method is adequately sensitive and specific. The integration of validated <u>structured assessment tools</u> (p.170) into routine clinical practice is widely accepted. Because risk is dynamic, risk assessments are more reliable in the short term.

Relevant individual and group factors

Most of these combine elements of group factors that are assessed by <u>actuarial measures</u> (p.166), such as being an active substance misuser, with individual factors assessed by clinical judgment, such as only misusing the substance when in the company of a particular friend. Note also protective factors.

Most important risk factor
- History of previous violent acts, including violence to people, animals, and property, with as much detail as possible on the nature and circumstances of each act (e.g. whether weapons were used, the relationship with the victim)

Biological factors
- Psychiatric disorders, especially schizophrenia and personality disorder[7]
- Neuropsychiatric disorders such as dysexecutive syndrome
- Specific psychiatric symptoms such as thought insertion, passivity phenomena, paranoia, persecutory delusions, and command hallucinations[8]
- Any symptom historically associated with violence in this individual
- Intoxication, withdrawal, or dependence (substance misuse)
- Response to psychiatric treatment

Psychological factors
- Personality traits and other persistent psychological patterns affecting behaviour, such as sadism, callousness, suspiciousness, affective instability, and impulsivity, and especially <u>psychopathy</u> (p.90)
- Personal resources such as planning, stress tolerance and problem-solving skills, and ability to use tactics other than violence (protective)

6 It is important to emphasise the distinction in giving expert evidence, since judges commonly fail to appreciate the technical and ethical distinctions between the two.

7 Known in the aggregate to be epidemiologically associated with violence (this only applies to a very small proportion of disorders and symptoms).

8 Collectively known as <u>threat/control override symptoms</u> (p.72).

- Personal and cultural attitudes towards violence
- Concordance with treatment (protective)
- Insight into mental disorder and into the risk of violence (protective)
- Specific intent or plans to act violently, or motivation to do so (grievances, resentments)

Social factors

- Developmental factors including experiences of childhood abuse or maltreatment, and age when significant violence was first used
- Social resources such as friends, relatives or employment, and especially intimate partners (protective)
- Opportunity to act violently (e.g. access to weapons and potential victims)
- Availability of destabilising factors such as drugs and antisocial peers
- Monitoring or supervision by family, friends, psychiatric services, police, probation, or other agencies (protective)

Assessment instruments

Violence risk assessment instruments (p.170) tend to consider a range of static and dynamic risk factors, the precise use of the factors depending upon the development of the instrument, and often on the population upon which it was normed, or for whom it was intended. Many of the risk prediction instruments overlap, for example the HCR20, SORAG, and VRAG all include the PCL-R. Care must be taken to ensure that the instrument is appropriate for use on members of the group to which the individual belongs. Most of the tools require specific training.

Structured risk assessments are more useful when risk is high and the behaviour relatively common; they are less accurate in relation to acts with low population prevalence, such as homicide. They are better predictors of violence in those with some personality disorders than psychoses (probably because the former are defined in part by violence), and less reliable when used for assessing change in risk (as when deciding on discharge, for example).

Violence risk assessment instruments

Structured professional judgment

HCR20 version 3[9] (Historical, Clinical and Risk management twenty-item scale):
- Twenty items in three domains (Historical, e.g. 'early maladjustment'; Clinical e.g. 'negative attitudes'; and Risk e.g. 'plans lack feasibility').
- Includes emphasis on 'scenario based' planning originating in individual risk scenarios.

SAPROF (Structured Assessment of Protective Factors for Violence):
- It is good practice to use this as an adjunct to the HCR20, for an overall view of the balance of risk and protective factors.
- Also comes in a youth version (SAPROF-YV).

SARA (Spousal Assault Risk Assessment):
- Twenty-item tool assessing risk of future violence in men for spousal assault.

SAVRY (Structured Assessment of Violent Risk in Youth):
- The most commonly used risk assessment for adolescents.
- Twenty-four items in four domains (historical, social/contextual, individualised clinical, and protective factors).

Purely actuarial tools

PCL-R (Psychopathy Checklist—Revised):
- Twenty-item scale measuring 'psychopathy' rather than risk assessment, but has been shown to have reasonable predictive power.

PCL-SV is a screening version with predictive validity in institutional and community patients

PCL-YV (Youth Version):
- Is a modified version for use in adolescents.
- ●*There are ethical controversies (p.322) about its use.

OGRS (Offender Group Reconviction Score):
- A statistical reconviction scale used by probation officers in presentence reports.

Probation services use the actuarial **OASys** (Offender Assessment System) for adults, and **Asset-Plus & Onset** for adolescents, but these are not strictly comparable to clinical risk assessment tools.

The table on the following page lists less-frequently used tools. Tools for assessing sexual violence are shown on p.174.

9 See the *Oxford Casebook of Forensic Psychiatry* for worked examples of using the HCR20.

Table 5.1 Less-frequently used violence risk assessment instruments

Instrument	Name	Type
SDRS	Short Dynamic Risk Scale	SPJ
EPS	Emotional Problems Scale	SPJ
RAMAS	Risk Assessment Management & Audit System	SPJ
VRAG	Violence Risk Appraisal Guide	Actuarial
EARL-20B/21G	Early Assessment Risk List (Boys/Girls)	Actuarial
YLS/CMI	Youth Level of Service/Case Management Inventory	Actuarial
START	Short-Term Assessment of Risk & Treatability	SPJ

Risk of sexual offending

Most sexual offenders have no mental illness, and only some have personality disorder or intellectual disability. Forensic psychologists and probation officers carry out most assessments of sexual offenders; psychiatrists and clinical psychologists are only involved when mental illness is suspected.

Risk assessment should be a prelude to <u>risk management</u> (p.246), and so should include <u>formulation</u> (p.146) and help to identify treatment needs. Risk factors for reoffending are not necessarily the same as for the index offence. Aggregate risk factors come from literature on (predominantly) convicted male sex offenders; use caution in generalising to other groups, including unconvicted men with concerning behaviours or fantasies.

Clinical assessment

Probably the most widely used approach to psychiatrists' assessment of risk of sexual offending is <u>clinical judgment</u> (see p.167). A full history and mental state examination should be supplemented by a detailed psychosexual history including: childhood victimisation, violent sexual fantasies, sexual behaviour, and attitudes towards women to sex with children. Comorbid mental disorders should also be considered, particularly alcohol and drug misuse, psychosis, mania,[10] learning disability, and personality disorder. Consider in particular the nature of the relationship between the symptoms of the disorder and the behaviour in the individual.

Actuarial tools

Actuarial tools predict recidivism more accurately than unstructured clinical judgment. They address static factors and produce a broad statistical probability of recidivism (i.e. the probability in a group of offenders similar to the patient). They do not address the cause of the risk, or its management. While they have been found to be good at identifying people at low risk, they tend to over-estimate 'high-risk' cases. They are also poor predictors of risk in first-time offenders, young people, and women.

The psychopathy checklist (<u>PCL-R</u>, p.137) is not specific to sexual offences but is one of the most reliable predictors of sexual reoffending.

Psychological evaluation

Dynamic factors have been the major focus of sex offender treatment programmes, particularly cognitive distortions, fantasies and deviant sexual arousal, sexual preoccupation, interpersonal relationships and intimacy deficits, anger, impulsivity, and emotional dysregulation. These are considered at clinical interview and in psychometric evaluation.

Penile plethysmography (PPG)

Penile plethysmography is a technique for assessing sexual arousal, heart rate and galvanic skin response in males, in response to various audio[11] and visual stimuli. It assesses sexual arousal by measuring penile tumescence. It is

---

10 Disinhibition in mania and psychosis enables a patient to act on pre-existing fantasies.

11 Audio rather than visual stimuli are preferred, especially in the USA, because they can be simulated, whereas visual images of child sexual abuse cannot (apart from manga or computer images).

part of clinical assessment of some sex offenders and is occasionally used to measure treatment response. Its validity is open to question, at least when used in isolation, partly because some offenders can use their own thoughts and images in order to avoid responding to the stimuli.

Polygraphy

There is ongoing debate about the accuracy of the polygraph ('lie detector') in the assessment of sex offenders—although there is general consensus that it does afford better assessment of deceitfulness than other approaches. It may therefore be helpful in increasing the rate of offence-related disclosures. It is used on a trial basis with some offenders in the UK.

Other issues in risk of sexual offending

- Internet pornography offences (p.59) do not necessarily confer an increased risk of contact sexual offences. Assessment should concentrate on examining all other risk factors (as above).
- Indecent exposure or exhibitionism (pp.60, 102) is considered to be more predictive of contact sexual offending if the perpetrator exhibits in multiple places, pursues or touches the victim, displays an erect penis, or masturbates during exposure.

Structured clinical judgment

As in the other areas of risk assessment, the best approach is to use clinical judgment structured by the use of an appropriate tool (p.174), and taking into account all the elements set out in the preceding paragraphs.

Comparing assessment tools

Tools tend to consider a range of static and dynamic risk factors, the precise combination often depending on the population on which it was normed or for whom it was intended. Most of the tools require specific training. It is vital to be aware of the limitations of the instrument across different groups, including by culture, ethnicity, gender, and age.

Sexual behaviour risk assessment instruments

Structured professional judgment

RSVP (Risk of Sexual Violence Protocol):
- Twenty-two item risk assessment for sexual violence in offenders older than eighteen years. Based on structured professional judgment using formulation and scenario planning.

ARMIDILO-S (Assessment of Risk and Manageability of Individuals with Developmental and Intellectual Limitations):
- A structured risk and management guideline instrument developed by the Scottish <u>Risk Management Authority</u> (p.594).

Purely actuarial tools

Static-99/Static 2002:
- Actuarial assessment of static, unchanging factors validated to predict risk of sexual and violent reoffences in male adult sex offenders only. Contains all four items from RRASOR plus items concerning relationship history, violent offences, and stranger victims.

RM2000 (Risk Matrix 2000):
- Uses static factors to predict risk (up to fifteen years later) in men older than eighteen years with at least one conviction for a sexual offence. It is mainly used by the Probation and Prison Service.
- It consists of three scales (S, sexual reconviction; V, violent reconviction; and C, a combination of both).

SORAG (Sexual Offending Risk Appraisal Guide):
- Fourteen items designed to predict violent reoffending among sex offenders. It is a better predictor of general violence than other sexual offender risk measures.

J-SOAP-II (Juvenile Sex Offender Assessment Protocol, version 2):
- A checklist to aid in the systematic review of risk factors associated with sexual and criminal offending. Designed to be used with boys aged twelve through eighteen years convicted of sexual offences or with a history of sexually coercive behaviour.

ERASOR (Estimate of Risk of Adolescent Sexual Offence Recidivism):
- Uses both static and dynamic factors assessing risk of sexual offending in adolescents (historical sexual assaults, sexual interests, attitudes and behaviours, psychosocial functioning, and treatment).

HM Prison Service also uses the **SARN-TNA** (Structured Assessment of Risk and Need—Treatment Needs Analysis) as part of its national sex offender treatment programme.

Table 5.2 lists less-frequently used tools.

Table 5.2 Less-frequently used sexual behaviour risk assessment instruments

Instrument	Name	Type
RRASOR	Rapid Risk Assessment of Sex Offender	Actuarial
Stable-2000/7	Stable Risk Factors (c.f. Static-2002)	Actuarial
VPS-SO	Violence Prediction Scheme—Sex Offender	Actuarial
SONAR	Sex Offender Needs Assessment Rating	Actuarial
SVR-20	Sexual Violence Risk Twenty-Item Scale	SPJ

Risk of suicide and self-harm

Although frequently assessed together, deliberate self-harm and completed suicide are epidemiologically and phenomenologically distinct, and tend to be associated with different mental disorders.

Prevalence

In the UK, suicide accounts for the greatest loss of years of life after coronary heart disease and cancer (Box 5.1).

> ### Box 5.1 Suicide rates in England & Wales
> - General population[12]: 11.2 per 100,000 per year (ratio 3:1 male: female)
> - General psychiatric patients: 15% (attempts)
> - Prisoners and police custody detainees: 80 to 90 per 100,000 per year
> - Forensic psychiatric patients: no data

In prisons, the rate of self-inflicted deaths and self-harm has risen significantly since 2012. Suicide accounts for 30% of deaths in custody. Half the suicides of English prisoners are amongst those <u>on remand</u> (p.398). In custody 5%–6% of men and of women 20%–24% self-harm. Suicide is a much greater risk than violence amongst psychiatric patients.

Risk factors for completed suicide

Research on completed suicide has identified the following risk factors, although many have low specificity and sensitivity, and immediate versus long-term risk cannot be distinguished:
- Previous self-harm is the most important factor—completed suicide is fifty times more likely compared to someone who has never self-harmed.
- Mental disorder—especially mood disorders (major depression, bipolar disorder), alcohol or drug dependence, schizophrenia, and cluster B PD.
- Cognitive factors—hopelessness, impulsivity, aggression, dichotomous thinking, cognitive constriction, problem-solving deficits, over-generalised autobiographical memory, and suicidal thoughts.
- Reasons for hopelessness such as terminal illness, prospect of prolonged imprisonment, and loss of a key relationship.
- Social isolation—being single, separated, or widowed.
- Losses—personal (bereavement and divorce), financial, and status.
- Conflicts with others.
- Being male.
- Stated intent—two-thirds of those completing suicide have informed someone of their intentions.
- Older age (except in schizophrenia and drug abuse, where younger age at diagnosis increases the risk of completed suicide).

12 This figure is for the UK; the rate is considerably higher in Scotland (16.1 per 100,000).

- Physical ill health, especially chronic or painful illnesses.
- Economic factors—unemployment or poverty.
- Criminal history—including early delinquent or assaultive behaviour and arrests for intoxication (6% completed suicides had outstanding charges).
- Incarceration—with increased risk for those on remand, those with a long, or life sentence, those convicted of murder/manslaughter, and those with alcohol use problems.[13]

Assessment of stated suicide intent

- Conduct an unhurried, sympathetic interview
- Provide space for patient to reveal thoughts and self-destructive intent
- Explore historical risk factors and ongoing difficulties, including mood swings, impulsivity, and aggressive tendencies
- Discuss potential precipitants (e.g. stressful life problems): particularly interpersonal, separation, illness of family member, court appearance, and recent personal physical illness
- Mental state examination for psychiatric disorder
- Specific questioning on current suicidal intent
- Direct questions concerning thoughts of suicide, specific plans, and preparatory acts (e.g. stockpiling tablets, gaining access to means)
- Homicidal thoughts as part of act (e.g. thinking of killing a spouse or child to spare them from (perceived) intolerable suffering)
- Consider whether the patient's self description is coloured by illness or their situation, by obtaining a history from an informant
- Consider use of Beck Suicide Index (helpful in measuring changes in risk, but not absolute risk)
- Explore protective factors (e.g. family, relationships, pets, and religious beliefs) and discuss how the individual might be kept safe

Although assessment is particularly difficult if statements of suicidal intent are made repeatedly and/or interpreted as threats, it is important to take them seriously as the risk of completed suicide in those who have threatened suicide is high.

Factors in an attempt suggesting higher risk of future suicide

- Lethality of method
- Act carried out in isolation
- Timed so intervention is unlikely
- Taking precautions to avoid discovery
- Preparations anticipating death
- Preparation for the act
- Communicating intent to others beforehand
- Extensive premeditation
- Leaving a note
- Not alerting helpers after the act
- Anger at failure of earlier attempt
- Admission of ongoing suicidal intent

13 Though a lower risk for black or black British prisoners.

Other specific risks

The <u>general principles</u> (pp.164–138) are the same as in the assessment of all risks. Consider risk factors and their relationship with mental disorder, assign an overall level of risk, consider scenarios in which the harm is particularly likely to occur, and then move on to consider <u>risk management</u> interventions (p.238).

Fire-setting

Only a small proportion of acts of <u>fire-setting</u> (p.50) result in any conviction for <u>arson</u> (p.422) so the risk of fire-setting should therefore be considered routinely. There are no specific assessment tools, and very few demographic and clinical variables have been identified that distinguish the most dangerous fire-setters.

In young people, fire-setting has been shown to be associated with:
• Previous fire-setting.
• Aggression, frustration, and boredom.
• More school-related difficulties, including truancy.
• Peer rejection.
• Parental mental ill health or inter-parental conflict.
• Poor social skills.
• Binge drinking.
• Low levels of parental supervision.
• Maltreatment or abuse.

Fire-setting by adults is associated with:
• Early age onset of fire-setting.
• Alcohol/substance abuse.
• Antisocial personality disorder.
• Long-lasting enuresis in childhood.
• Psychosis.
• Learning disability.
• Interest in or excitement from fire.
• Evidence of planning.
• Previous arson endangering life.

However, many individuals with such features will not set fires.

The **meaning of the fire-setting** to the individual is almost certainly the most important aspect of assessing and managing its risk. Common meanings include a source of revenge, an opportunity for self-harm or suicide, a way of controlling others, a source of sexual gratification, and a way of reducing internal tension. Assessments should also address fire-setters' emotional state and any cognitive distortions before, during, and after setting the fire, and their reaction to having set it.

Hostage-taking

The taking of a hostage may be a component of an offence or may occur after detention in prison or hospital in response to frustration or in an attempt to manipulate others. Assessment of the risk of hostage-taking should incorporate a detailed functional analysis of any previous incidents. There is no empirical basis for addressing the risk of hostage-taking, but a structured clinical judgment approach allows for formulation of different scenarios, with implications for risk management (p.244).

Absconding and escape[14]

The risks of these behaviours occurring, and what might then occur if the patient did abscond or escape (including suicide and violence), require constant consideration in secure hospitals, taking up a large amount of a clinical team's time. The consequences of absconding or (especially) escape frequently include adverse media coverage, no matter how carefully the risks were assessed.

Factors found to be associated with **absconding** include:
• Young, male detained patients.
• Transferred prisoner.
• Previous absconding.
• Diagnosis of schizophrenia.
• Multiple previous admissions.
• Longer total hospital admission.
• Previous history of violence.
• Season (more incidents in spring and summer).
• Recent verbal aggression or substance misuse.

So many patients exhibit these various factors that individual formulation of past episodes, and current evidence relevant to them, are essential in making decisions about leave (p.486) or observations (p.190).

Escape is, fortunately, sufficiently rare that no clear specific risk factors have been identified.

Victimisation and exploitation

People with serious mental illness are at increased risk of being a victim of violent crime compared to the general population. People with mental disorder in prison are more likely to be victims of violence compared to prisoners without mental disorder. Both groups are also more likely to be exploited financially, sexually, or criminally, particularly by gangs (p.38). However, vulnerability must be considered individually, based on investigation of past experiences and circumstances of victimisation.

Other risks

Other risks not specific to patients in forensic psychiatric services include:
• Self-neglect.
• Risks associated with driving or operating machinery.
• Physical health complications.
• Iatrogenic risks relating to treatment.
• Risks of drug or alcohol use.
• Risk of relapse.
• Risk of committing nonviolent crime.

---

14 Escape involves a breach of security, such as climbing a wall or cutting a hole in a fence, whereas absconding merely involves leaving without permission, or failing to return on time.

Risk assessment in nonclinical settings

Subjects who are not patients

Risk assessment, as performed by psychiatrists, is a procedure designed for use with patients, and clinicians' professional judgments are derived from their experience with patients. The actuarial instruments (p.166) sometimes used in risk assessment are normed on patient populations: that is, they identify the group of patients, with one or more relevant factors, that a patient most resembles. Both professional judgment and actuarial instruments are therefore **invalid** when conducted on people who do not have mental disorder. This may be particularly relevant to clinicians asked to assess the risk of offenders reoffending when they do not suffer from any diagnosable mental disorder, and psychiatrists should decline such requests. In Scotland, conducting work on behalf of the Risk Management Authority (p.594) may present this issue.

Assessments outside clinical settings

It is frequently necessary for a clinician to make an assessment of risk in prison, or some other nonclinical setting. However, care must be taken to ensure that the setting does not influence the process of information gathering (for example, by giving the patient an incentive to conceal relevant information lest it result in further punishment), nor distort the clinician's judgment (for example, by regarding the patient not as a person with a mental disorder but purely as an offender who deserves punishment rather than assistance).

Assessments by nonclinicians

The risk assessment procedures used in psychiatry presuppose a professional background on the part of the assessor. For example, consider item H9 on the HCR20 (p.170), the presence of personality disorder. The assessor not only needs specific training in the HCR20, in order to know the criteria for determining whether a particular diagnosis and level of severity are sufficient to score positively on the item. They also need the clinical skills to be able to obtain the information from the patient, or other sources, necessary for making a diagnosis of personality disorder; plus the professional judgment and knowledge required to decide which specific diagnosis, if any, is appropriate.

Clinical risk assessment instruments should therefore not be used by nonclinicians. However, there are other risk assessment instruments designed for nonclinical settings, such as OASys (p.170), used by the probation (p.584) and prison services (p.578); and the Asset and Onset (p.170), used in the Youth Justice System.

Chapter 6

Treatment

Aims of treatment

The aims of treatment of mentally disordered offenders are both similar to those of other psychiatric patients and different because criminogenic needs (those associated with offending) must also be addressed.[1] As well as an additional focus of treatment, this introduces an ethical dimension which is not present in the treatment of nonoffender patients.

Clinical aims

Forensic psychiatry aims, like the rest of medicine:
• to preserve life and postpone death by the successful treatment of disease and
• to improve quality of life by ameliorating symptoms and/or rehabilitation (p.264).

Many forensic patients struggle with persistent symptoms and behaviours such as assaults on others or self-harm. The only amelioration offered may be involuntary medication, detention in a locked ward, and restraint (p.196). Although long-term containment and seclusion may be therapeutic interventions, from the patient's perspective they resemble indefinite detention, which is difficult to justify if the patient has committed no serious crime. Even where legal (see p.482), not all such medical treatments (p.337) are ethically justified, especially when appropriate psychological treatments are not offered.

Criminogenic risk reduction

Forensic psychiatric services also aim to reduce the risk the patient poses to others (see p.352). To the forensic psychiatrist, this aim, and the risk management (p.237) techniques it involves, presuppose a link between mental disorder and violence (p.44) or other harms, which will sometimes be present (e.g. if a person attacks in response to command auditory hallucinations), but may well not be (e.g. if an offender has previously suffered from mania but is currently well).

In theory treatment for risk is secondary to the clinical aims above; that is, if there is a link between symptoms of the disorder and offending, treatment of the former will also address the latter. However, where there is no treatment that will effectively meet the clinical aims, but there is one that will reduce risk of harm to others, giving or withholding treatment may pose an ethical dilemma (p.337)—such as deciding whether to give an antilibidinal drug (p.201) to a sex offender with a personality disorder that has not responded to psychological or social therapies.

For the forensic psychiatrist working in a multidisciplinary team (p.312), the risk reduction aim may lead to tensions with other professionals with differing understanding of their duties. For example, nurses may consider the patient's wellbeing their only focus, and may not accept a duty to assist in reducing risk to others. Conversely, forensic psychologists sometimes use their professional expertise to address criminogenic needs in the absence

---

1 This does not contradict our advice that risk assessment should not be conducted by clinicians on nonmentally disordered offenders (see p.180), but recognises that, in assessing mentally disordered offenders, there are often relevant factors which go beyond their mental disorder.

of mental disorder (p.329), with the aim of reducing risk to others and minimising reoffending. To what extent, if any, is it appropriate for a forensic psychiatrist to be involved with such clients?

Principles of treatment

The principles of the Reed Report (p.781) state that forensic psychiatric services are expected to work together with other agencies in order to provide care that is:

• based upon the individual needs of the patient,
• provided in the community wherever possible,
• provided as close as possible to the patient's home,
• provided in the least restrictive or secure environment possible; and
• aimed at maximising rehabilitation and prospects of independent living.

Balancing benefits and harms

A further principle concerning decisions about treatment is that a decision to treat (or not) must take into account the severity and likelihood of the harms that the treatment might itself cause, including loss of liberty or agency, and balance these against the magnitude and likelihood of the desired benefits. An example is the prescription of long-acting depot antipsychotic medication (p.201): this may cause serious side-effects such as obesity and tardive dyskinesia which may be irreversible. Prescribing a treatment, no matter how well-intentioned, that foreseeably causes more harm than good may be ethically unjustifiable (p.302) and result in disciplinary (p.557) or even negligence (p.550) proceedings—especially if the aim was solely risk reduction.

Treatment settings in forensic psychiatry

Forensic psychiatry is practised in secure hospitals, community services, prisons, and law courts. Different treatment options will be available in each setting, in terms of legal coercion (p.186).[2] For instance, in a secure hospital it may be appropriate to order antipsychotic treatment under mental health law[3] for an acutely psychotic patient who capacitously (p.482) refuses treatment. In prison, treatment cannot usually be given without consent,[4] so the antipsychotic could only be given voluntarily. In courts and police stations, giving an antipsychotic even with consent may be inappropriate in practice, because of the lack of trained staff or facilities to deal with side-effects.

Treatment interventions in forensic psychiatry are nearly always[5] delivered in environments that could be considered coercive, because the subjects of treatment or intervention are legally restrained or detained. Forensic professionals must take into account the setting in which the treatment is to be delivered, and the impact this may have on consent, the effectiveness of any treatment, and any adverse effects. The legal context associated with a particular setting may also have an effect on how treatment is administered.

Impact of the setting

Forensic psychiatry is often practiced in settings which are nontherapeutic, and where public safety and discipline are the primary values of the culture. Even prison health care centres are subject to prison rules. The prisoner-patient may find the institution highly coercive, and when combined with anxiety about ongoing criminal proceedings, may find it difficult to trust the doctor. The coercion may be strong enough to affect the prisoner's capacity to consent to treatment or information sharing. Even if their consent is legally valid,[6] ethically the context alters the nature of the interaction, which is one reason that it is normal medical practice in prisons not to compel patients lacking capacity to accept treatment under mental capacity law (p.522), unless serious harm would result.

This coercive environment needs to be considered when recommending treatments to prisoners awaiting trial on remand, who may think that the treatment will affect the outcome of their trial and their sentence: for instance, offering a place in a sex offender treatment group (p.221) to someone awaiting trial on charges of sexual assault (p.419) might create an

---

2 And occasionally because the security of the setting can itself be therapeutic: for example a patient with borderline personality disorder (p.84) may feel 'contained' in a secure hospital, lessening the manifestations of their disorder and enabling them to commence psychological work (see p.204). This is different from legally describing security as treatment in its own right (p.340).

3 Where this allows treatment without consent (p.482) for capacitous patients (broadly speaking, E&W, and Scotland).

4 The exceptions are the treatment of a patient under the common law rule in *Munjaz* (p.763) to prevent an immediate risk of significant harm, or of incapacitous patients under mental capacity legislation (p.522).

5 Other than those delivered in the community—which meta-analytic reviews have shown to be the most effective for reducing offending behaviours.

6 *Freemen v Home Office* (p.756).

incentive to participate insincerely in order to hope to reduce the sentence if convicted. For this reason, good practice is often not to offer offence-related therapies until after conviction.

Even in secure psychiatric settings, patients may experience coercion that affects their consent. All secure services restrict autonomy and choice in the name of risk reduction, and patients are aware that many treatment decisions may be taken without them and in discussion with third parties (like the Ministry of Justice) without their express consent. Forensic patients are also aware that to some extent they have to agree with the team's formulation of their problems and that gaining increased liberty depends on their compliance and cooperation, whether sincere or not. There are particular problems associated with the **treatment of substance misuse**, which is generally mandatory for all forensic patients; however, the mandate conflicts with treatment models that emphasise an individual's readiness, voluntariness, and willingness to change. Nevertheless, such mandatory interventions can be effective even in prison settings.

Coercion and treatment

Definition: objective and perceived coercion

There are ethical and philosophical problems in <u>defining coercion</u> (p.324). Research on coercion in psychiatry has addressed two forms:

- **objective coercion**, measures such as detention in prison or under mental health law, seclusion, forced medication, restrictions on the use of the telephone, contact with friends, and leave from the unit, and
- **perceived coercion**, the patient's own experience of lacking control or influence over what happens to them (cf. <u>agency</u>, p.324).

The latter is ethically and practically likely to be of greater significance.

Research has also demonstrated that clinical concepts are too narrow, in seeking to reduce coercion to a single measurable concept. A social science perspective involves seeing coercion as the product of the beliefs and expectations of, and interactions between, patients, staff, and society—though this concept is much more difficult to study.

Measuring coercion

Scales have been devised to attempt to measure the experience of perceived coercion, based upon patients' self-reports, and objective coercion, which includes readily recorded restrictive practices.

The most commonly used measure of perceived coercion is the MacArthur Perceived Coercion Scale (**MPCS**), which contains five true-or-false items. These items do not address coercion or perceived coercion directly but instead focus on control, decision making, choice, freedom, and initiation of treatment, with the implication that perceived coercion emerges from these constructs. The Forensic Restrictiveness Questionnaire (**FRQ**) is directed at forensic psychiatric care and patients.

Instruments such as the MPCS show that measured perceived coercion is not well correlated with legal status. This suggests that either the measure is too inaccurate, or that patients cognitively reconstruct their experience from that of 'being coerced', into (for example) 'being cared for'. A recent Indian study suggests that patients' perceptions of coercion decrease as symptoms lessen and global functioning improves.

Prevalence of coercion

Studies show that patients report significant levels of perceived coercion, but find no consistent association with objective coercion. Even voluntary patients can perceive coercion; in one US study, 10% of voluntary patients felt coerced, while 35% of involuntary patients did not. A British study found one-third of voluntary patients felt coerced; a Nordic study of different centres and countries reported similarly. This study also found that 74% of involuntary patients experienced high levels of perceived coercion.

Recent reviews suggest that perceptions of coercion are affected by a range of variables, especially the context of admission, the therapeutic alliance with the psychiatrist, and the experience of being treated respectfully. This may explain why there is little correspondence between legal status and perceived or reported experiences of coercion and legal status. For example, power relationships between staff and patients may be expressed differently depending on whether the ward is open (unlocked) or locked; in secure services and on locked wards, the staff may feel more confident and relaxed about safety and may therefore use less controlling language, whereas on open wards, staff may feel they need to be more verbally controlling and then come across to patients as arrogant or dismissive. This may then make patients (whether voluntary or involuntary) feel unable to speak up for themselves.

Domains of coercion

Coercion is located within many domains of the lives of those with mental disorder, and arises from multiple sources.

Patients report experiencing coercion within psychiatric institutions during their care and treatment, not only at admission. One study involving a narrative analysis of patient interviews identified coercion through:

* not being allowed to go home or out,
* the use of mechanical or personal restraint,
* being coerced to take medication,
* being threatened with sanctions, and
* not being allowed to make decisions.

In another study between 24% and 40% of voluntary patients reported restrictions on leaving the ward, whilst up to 73% of involuntary patients reported such restrictions. Almost half of all involuntary patients experienced forced medication, compared with up to 28% of voluntary patients. There is also evidence of increasing experience of coercion, and use of leverage, in the community: coercion may be an everyday aspect of community mental health work.

Clinical importance of perceived coercion

Aside from the ethical implications of coercing patients (p.324), it is important to consider the effect on treatment outcomes (p.232). If perceived coercion has negative therapeutic effects, it is important for clinicians to understand how to minimise that perception. Even if coercion has therapeutic effects that are neutral or positive, it is important to consider when it is ethically appropriate to use coercion. If the effect of perceived coercion is to worsen treatment outcomes, this reduces the ethical justification for coercion and loss of liberty.

Factors associated with perceived coercion

* **Demographics**: The evidence is mixed. Several studies have failed to find an association between perceived coercion and age, gender, ethnicity, and social class; whilst others have found high levels of coercion correlated with older age and nonwhite ethnicity, white ethnicity and female gender, higher levels of education, and single marital status.
* **Psychopathology**: Studies of the relationship between diagnosis or psychopathology and perceived coercion also present an unresolved picture. However, it is important to identify whether patients' reports of coercion have their basis in illness-related symptoms, and perceptual biases, or are derived from real events or circumstances.

- **Procedural justice**: This has been found to be negatively associated with perceived coercion. Patients who feel unfairly treated or not listened to tend to report higher levels of perceived coercion on admission.
- **Information**: Patients are often ill-informed about their legal rights, and in one ethnographic study there was a finding that information was often deliberately withheld from patients by staff. The provision of sufficient good-quality information has been found to reduce perceived coercion.
- **Pressure**: Perceived coercion is strongly correlated with *negative pressure* (threats and force designed either to press a patient into hospital admission or to persuade them of the negative consequences should they refuse), but not with *positive pressure* (persuasion and inducements brought to bear to convince the patient of a likely positive outcome). The involvement of police increases perceived coercion; the same pressure from a family member or friend reduces it. Clinical pressure, whether positive or negative (i.e. inducements or threats by staff) increases patients' perception of coercion on admission to hospital.

All such research highlights the importance of relationships and context.

Attitudes to treatment
Perceived coercion is associated with patients adopting more negative attitudes towards treatment, independently of whether it affects therapeutic outcome. Patients who feel coerced into admission are:
- less accepting of medical accounts of their conditions,
- less satisfied with treatment, and
- more likely to hold negative views of their experiences.

Even when objectively coerced patients retrospectively acknowledge their need for hospitalisation, they retain their negative opinions.

Future treatment
Patients' experiences of coercion make them less likely to seek treatment in the future. One study in California reported that 47% of respondents admitted to avoiding traditional mental health services for fear of being committed, and a recent study of individuals with schizophrenia spectrum conditions found that 36% reported fear of coerced treatment as a barrier to seeking help for a mental health problem.

It is unclear, however, whether perceived coercion affects patients' compliance with future treatment once it has begun.

Clinical outcome
The relationship between patients' attitudes and clinical outcome is difficult to assess, and evidence for associations between perceived coercion and therapeutic improvement is scarce and inconsistent.

Two independent studies have found that patients with high perceived coercion are more likely to report little therapeutic gain, and to show less symptomatic improvement on the Brief Psychiatric Rating Scale and Global Assessment Scale, but others have reported that patients who viewed their admission as coercive had higher levels of functioning at discharge.

Therapeutic use of security

In mental health services, security level is justified by a patient's risk to self or others.

What defines different levels of security?

- **Environmental** or **physical security**: perimeter and internal features of a service such as fences, locked doors, key chains, and soft cutlery.
- **Relational security**: sufficient trained staff, good communication, meaningful activities, and well-understood ward dynamics, relationships, and patient histories.
- **Procedural security**: practices such as searches, inspections, investigating and learning from incidents, and staff pre-employment checks.

The contributions of the types of security differs between facilities and contexts. In some psychiatric settings (e.g. the community), relational security is the most important, and the others have little or no role.

What determines a patient's security level need?

Security level should be the least restrictive[7] option possible to contain risk to self and others. This requires detailed risk assessment (p.163), including multidisciplinary perspectives (p.312) and, in more complex cases, the use of a toolkit such as the DUNDRUM (p.194).

Determining security need within risk management plans should be rational and objective, based upon the *gravity* and *immediacy* of the risk of harm, and the local availability of resources, with acknowledgement of the ethical balance to be struck between safety and coercion.

Patients subject to restriction orders (p.510) undergo security need assessment by the relevant Ministry (p.586) using its own criteria, which may ignore clinical advice; courts may request security information for defendants subject to court proceedings; tribunals (p.373) can recommend changes in security level—and in Scotland, order the patient to be transferred.[8]

Transition between levels of security

Security need should be reassessed regularly. This may involve changing procedural security (such as frequency of observations), relational security (e.g. appointing someone who knows the patient well as primary nurse), and/or physical security (e.g. moving to another ward or unit). Typically, such measures, which are external to the patient, can be relaxed as patients recover and become more able to contain their own behaviour.

Observation and engagement

Observation is important procedurally and relationally for monitoring a patient's mental state and behaviour, and for engaging them in therapeutic dialogue. It is solely clinically determined. Common 'levels' of observation are:

---

7 A principle set out in the Reed Report (p.781) and E&W's Mental Health Act Code of Practice.

8 By deeming the patient 'detained in conditions of excessive security' under ss264–273 MHCTA.

- **General**—keeping the patient in mind, being aware of their location.
- **Intermittent**—unobtrusively checking on and/or speaking to the patient frequently (typically twice or four times per hour; e.g. for patients at high risk of disturbed or violent behaviour or suicide).
- **Continuous**—keeping the patient within eyesight at all times, including at night (e.g. for patients at imminent risk of harming themselves or others).
- **Enhanced**—as above, but with observing staff within arm's reach at all times (e.g. for patients likely to act very quickly if the opportunity arises).

Leave outside the secure environment

Within secure rehabilitation patients should be offered opportunities to demonstrate that they can safely exercise choice when under decreasing supervision and control. Leave to have more freedom is a gradual process: beginning within detaining units, then within secure perimeters, and then (in less than high security) outside secure perimeters, first escorted then unescorted. Leave decisions should be based on risk assessment, including risk of <u>absconding</u> (p.250), taking into consideration:

- mental state stability,
- insight and engagement,
- rapport with staff,
- motivation to abstain from risk behaviours,
- past behaviour on leave, and
- potential impact on victims.[9]

The relevant Ministry authorises (or refuses) leave for <u>restricted patients</u> (p.510), including transferred prisoners (whose parole status is not relevant to leave). Leave (or <u>suspension of measures</u> in Scotland, p.486) can be granted by the <u>RC/RMO</u> (p.468) for unrestricted patients. Leave should always be described by its therapeutic purpose, destination, escorting arrangements, transport arrangements, plus other conditions (e.g. agreeing to urine drug testing on return).

Can increases in security be therapeutic?

Many patients experience security measures as <u>coercive</u> (p.186). Increased security increases a patient's <u>deprivation of liberty</u> (p.532), sometimes posing <u>ethical dilemmas</u> (p.322) if justified only for their own wellbeing. However, increased security may allow a sense of containment (e.g. for hypervigilant patients), reduced use of sedating medication, and, as a result, more psychological and social therapies. For nonoffender patients exhibiting risky behaviours, increased security may help them feel safer from abandonment. There is a danger that such patients can become dependent on secure care (which is not recommended for chronically suicidal patients).

---

9 This is more likely to determine detailed leave arrangements (including communication with the victim) rather than whether leave occurs or not.

Problems in the use of security

- Ethical tension between security (focusing on risk reduction) and therapy[10] (focusing on patient welfare).
- Disputes between services (p.272) or teams, about required security levels, during which patient's treatment needs may be neglected.
- Public perception may prevent some high-profile patients moving to lower security, no matter how well they do in treatment.[11]
- Facilities and policies of units at the same security levels may not match.
- Need may fall between different security levels (e.g. a patient's behaviour may be unmanageable in a low secure unit, but their risk may not meet the threshold for the medium secure unit, leading to concerning long-term seclusion; p.196).
- Units may apply blanket restrictions applying to all patients regardless of needs, creating injustice and leading to complaints.
- MDT staff may become polarised when balancing secure and therapeutic needs, becoming either highly 'risk averse' (giving no leave) or excessively focused on the therapeutic value of leave.

---

10 Mental health legislation (though not human rights law, p.516) defines *treatment* widely so as to authorise the use of security measures, including seclusion (p.196). However, this does not mean that security on its own amounts to treatment.

11 Substantial and/or prolonged use of community leave may indicate an unmet need for lower security.

The DUNDRUM toolkit

The DUNDRUM[12] quartet is a validated set of structured professional judgment instruments (p.167) that aim to assess a patient's objective need for security (p.190). It comprises:
- D1 Triage Security (level of security required),
- D2 Triage Urgency (urgency with which it is required),
- D3 Programme completion (readiness for reduced security), and
- D4 Recovery (evidence of change in readiness).

Each of the four scales is made up of several items, rated on their own four-point scale (e.g. for TS1 Seriousness of violence: 0 none, 1 minimal, 2 repeated assaults, 3 use of weapons, and 4 homicide). They are intended to supplement, not replace, professional judgment.

Table 6.1 Factors in each DUNDRUM measure

TS1 Most serious violence	P1 Physical health
TS2 Most serious self-harm	P2 Mental health
TS3,4 Immediacy of risk	P3 Drugs and alcohol
TS5 Special factors (e.g. sadism, PCL-R)	P4 Problem behaviours
TS6 Absconding	P5 Self-care and activities of daily living
TS7 Ability to obtain weapons	P6 Education, occupation and creativity
TS8 Victim sensitivity	P7 Family and social networks
TS9 Complex needs	
TS10 Institutional behaviour	
TS11 Legally required security	
TU1 Safety of current setting	R1 Stability of mental disorder
TU2 Mental health	R2 Insight
TU3 Suicide prevention	R3 Therapeutic rapport
TU4 Humanitarian need	R4 Use of leave
TU5 Systemic issues	R5 HCR20 dynamic risk items
TU6 Legal urgency	

Strengths
- Aide memoire to professional risk assessment.
- Validity—considerable research evidence for its discriminative power.
- International applicability—not limited to any specific jurisdiction.
- Transparency—patients can see what they need to achieve to move to a lower security setting (from the D3 and D4 tools), and can complete self-rated version of these to highlight differences in perception.
- Aggregation—security needs for a group of patients can be summated, to facilitate decisions on resources and commissioning.

12 Dangerousness, UNDerstanding, Recovery, and Urgency Manual.

Limitations

- Scoring options may not cover all possible scenarios.
- Local resources may not include the security level recommended (e.g. too few high secure beds).
- Recommended programmes may not be available, preventing higher P1–7 scores.

Seclusion and restraint

Seclusion and restraint may be required during an acute phase of illness, or behavioural disturbance arising from severe personality disorder, as part of a risk management plan (p.238). Seclusion can be therapeutic, making a distressed patient feel safer, but this is controversial. Similar clinical settings use seclusion variously. Seclusion and restraint are contentious, and regulated under mental health law[13] and codes of practice, though both are legal forms of treatment (p.482).

Prevention and de-escalation

Prevention of violent incidents (p.240) is better than responding to them. Reducing incidents by well-designed physical and relational security (p.190), including sufficient staff, space and privacy, predictable routines, meaningful activities, and a sense of being respected and having a voice (which reduces perceived coercion, p.186). Observation (p.190) of patients, and de-escalation techniques (using body language and speech, and helping them to find a nonviolent solution to their distress or anger) are also preferable to restraint or seclusion.

Restraint

Restraint involves the physical holding of a patient to inhibit their behaviour. In the UK, this is always achieved by staff (not mechanical restraints). Restraint may manage an immediately dangerous situation (to the patient or others), and/or allow giving medication (p.200) if it is essential and cannot otherwise be given.

Restraint should be a last resort. There should be a plan for ending it quickly; for example, by giving the patient PRN medication whilst restrained. Restraint should be:
• for the minimum period necessary,
• carried out by trained staff using approved techniques that do not cause pain,
• proportionate to the situation,
• carried out with no more than reasonable force,
• accompanied by monitoring of physical health,
• accompanied by a request for a doctor to attend urgently, and
• used only when resuscitation equipment is available.

Restraint can be **fatal** for the patient, particularly if they are prone (facedown) and pressure is applied to the back, such as by a staff member sitting on them. This position should not be used. Patients' airway and breathing should be continuously monitored during restraint.

Seclusion

Seclusion (usually supervised, compulsory solitary confinement in a bare, locked room) can reduce harm to patients or others in hospital settings, but

---

13 For example, in RoI s69 MHA makes it an offence to restrain or seclude a patient unless it is necessary to prevent injury and complies with the MHC's rules.

may be harmful and traumatic.[14] Attempts to reduce its use have produced mixed results; few specialist forensic secure services have eliminated it altogether. It is used rarely or not at all in many European countries.

Seclusion may be considered:

• when there is a need to contain severely disturbed behaviour and other methods have failed;
• only if absolutely necessary;
• not as a punishment or threat, or because of staff shortage;
• only when satisfactory resources are available; and
• only when there is a seclusion policy.

During seclusion, there must be continuous observation of the patient's physical condition, mental state, and behaviour, with regular reviews of their condition and of the need for continued seclusion: usually at least two-hour reviews by nursing staff, four hourly by a junior doctor, and twice daily by a senior doctor (see Box 6.1). Automated electronic monitoring systems are available.

Box 6.1 Factors to consider in seclusion reviews

• Physical health, including injuries from the original incident
• Food and water intake
• Mental state
• Interaction with staff
• Attitudes and beliefs, especially relating to staff and any victims
• Hostility, threat, or violent behaviour

Longer term seclusion

Persistent severe violence can occasionally be managed only by repeated periods of brief seclusion, or even longer term seclusion. In these exceptional circumstances, legislation, codes of practice, and local policies may allow for this, subject to safeguards.

Reducing restrictive practices

There are coordinated projects in the UK and elsewhere aimed at reducing restrictive practices like seclusion and restraint, motivated by evidence of their adverse effects. Reduction programmes include leadership, training, debriefs with the patient, prevention tools, and therapeutic environmental guidelines. These, and QI initiatives, have reduced use in some settings. The use of medication may reduce the need for prolonged restraint and/or seclusion, but requires careful balancing of its risks and benefits.

Legislation in E&W[15] requires mental health organisations to have policies on, train staff in, monitor the use of, and investigate incidents associated with, physical, mechanical, and chemical restraint and isolation.

---

14 Distinguished from 'time out', where there is a voluntary agreement between the patient and staff to spend time alone—usually in their room—as a method of de-escalation.
15 Mental Health Units (Use of Force) Act 2018.

Physical treatments

Physical treatments other than medication play a very small role in forensic psychiatry.

Electro-convulsive therapy (ECT)

ECT may be used as part of the treatment of mental illness within forensic psychiatry as it is within general psychiatry. It is only recommended for severe treatment-resistant (or acutely life-threatening) depression, mania, or catatonia.

Legal rules and ethical guidance for the general use of ECT apply to patients in forensic psychiatric settings, although the complex nature of the presentation of many forensic psychiatric patients means that ECT is comparatively more commonly used for conditions other than depression, especially in <u>high secure</u> (p.258) hospitals, because other treatments have been tried and have failed.

Transcranial stimulation

Transcranial direct current stimulation using much lower voltages than ECT, and repetitive transcranial magnetic stimulation (rTMS) using localised magnetically induced currents, are intended to produce similar therapeutic effects to ECT without side-effects such as memory impairment. There is some evidence to support the effectiveness of rTMS for depression.

Neurosurgery

Neurosurgery for mental disorder (**psychosurgery**) is exceedingly rarely used.[16] Severe treatment-resistant mood disorders and very severe treatment-resistant obsessive-compulsive disorder are the only remaining indications, and only if the patient has <u>capacity to consent</u> (p.522) and actively requests it after all other treatments have failed.

Deep brain stimulation (DBS)

DBS is used most commonly in neurological disorders such as Parkinson's disease. There are no specific indications in forensic psychiatry, but there is ongoing research into its effect in psychiatric disorder, most frequently in OCD, Tourette's syndrome, and severe depression. The legal status of DBS (as a form of neurosurgery, or otherwise) is uncertain in some jurisdictions.

---

16 In part because of the controversial history of prefrontal leucotomy. Introduced in 1935, when most patients with schizophrenia would have lifelong debilitating symptoms and be detained indefinitely in hospital, it seemed a valid alternative to dangerous treatments such as cardiazol shock therapy, insulin-induced coma, or barbiturate-induced 'deep sleep'. Moniz, who developed the technique, received a Nobel Prize in 1949. However, from the mid-1940s onwards it became clear that it deprived patients of their personality and a degree of humanity. It died out gradually as antipsychotic drugs became available in the late 1950s and 1960s.

Pharmacology

Most patients in forensic psychiatric services are treated with medication, either for their primary mental disorder or for symptoms and manifestations of their mental disorder.

Acutely disturbed or violent behaviour

Medication is considered when psychological and behavioural approaches are insufficient to manage such behaviour. **Rapid tranquilisation** should then be used to assist in managing the risk of harm to self or others, and to help reduce the patient's distress. To avoid polypharmacy, wherever possible antipsychotics and other drugs used in rapid tranquilisation should be the same as those regularly prescribed to the patient. For an example protocol see Box 6.2.

Box 6.2 Example rapid tranquillisation protocol after de-escalation has failed

1. Oral treatment
   • Lorazepam 1–2mg or promethazine 25–50mg
   • *or* if **not** on regular antipsychotic, olanzapine 10mg *or* quetiapine 100–200mg *or* risperidone 1–2mg *or* haloperidol 5mg
   • *or* buccal midazolam 10–20mg
   • Repeat once after 45–60 minutes
2. Intramuscular treatment
   • Consult senior colleague and consider patient's legal status
   • Lorazepam 1–2mg (have flumazenil to hand)
   • *or* promethazine 50mg
   • *or* olanzapine 10mg (do **not** combine with im benzodiazepine)
   • *or* aripiprazole 9.75mg
   • *or* haloperidol 5mg (high risk of dystonia, ideally only after ECG)
3. Intravenous treatment
   • Diazepam 10mg over at least 5 minutes (have flumazenil to hand)
   • Repeat after 5–10 minutes up to three times
4. After any im or iv drug, monitor temperature, pulse, BP, and respiration every 5–10 minutes for an hour and then every 30 minutes

FOR EXAMPLE ONLY: DO NOT USE IN PLACE OF LOCAL POLICY

Local guidelines, or authoritative published guidelines such as those from NICE or the Maudsley Hospital, should be consulted. Individualised pharmacological strategies are recommended.

Zuclopenthixol acetate ('Acuphase') may be used for patients with psychosis who have not responded to repeated short-acting drugs. It has effects that last for up to seventy-two hours. It should **not** be used for rapid tranquilisation because it takes at least two hours to have a significant effect. It should not be used in people who have never taken antipsychotics.

Violence and psychosis

Antipsychotic medication can have an indirect impact on violence by ameliorating symptoms that might predispose to violence, such as command auditory hallucinations or perplexity. Second-generation antipsychotics, particularly clozapine and olanzapine, may have more impact on violence and aggression than first-generation ones in inpatients.

Long-acting injectable (depot) formulations are used more frequently in forensic psychiatry, due to poor adherence to oral medication by many patients, and because the harms associated with relapse (e.g. renewed violence or offending) are often more severe.

Personality disorder

No medication is recommended as primary therapy in personality disorder, but it can be used to treat or prevent comorbid mental illnesses or as adjunctive treatment for certain symptom domains:
- Cognitive-perceptual—consider low-dose antipsychotic.
- Affective—consider mood stabiliser or antidepressant.
- Impulse-behavioural—consider SSRI.
- Anxious-fearful—consider anxiolytic or SSRI.

Disturbed or violent behaviour in intellectual disability

Intellectual disability does not itself respond to any currently available pharmacological treatment. Medication may be indicated for comorbid disorders such as psychosis, depression, or epilepsy. Antipsychotic medication to manage challenging behaviour is overused and lacks supporting evidence. Discontinuation should be gradual to minimise unpredictable behavioural deterioration.

Antilibidinal medication

Pharmacological treatments are an option for some patients with paraphilias (p.102), or those who commit sexual offences (p.418) or show inappropriate sexual behaviour (p.246), though evidence of benefit is limited.
- **SSRIs** are used for treatment of paraphilic disorders, particularly when there is comorbid depression or OCD. They can impair libido and delay ejaculation. They may reduce urges, fantasies, and compulsive behaviour.
- **Medroxyprogesterone acetate** (a progesterone derivative) and **cyproterone acetate** (a synthetic steroid similar to progesterone) are antiandrogen drugs that reduce testosterone, luteinising hormone, and follicle-stimulating hormone levels. They reduce the intensity and frequency of sexual fantasies and urges but have significant side-effects, including depression, feminisation, gynaecomastia, and weight gain. They should only be considered in conjunction with psychological treatment.
- **Gonadotrophin-releasing hormone** (GnRH) analogues are used to manage sexual deviance and hypersexuality. They are more potent than MPA and cyproterone but appear to have fewer side-effects.

Antipsychotics should not be used as antilibidinal medication. Phosphodiesterase inhibitors (e.g. sildenafil) increase libido, but have not been shown to increase the risk of sexual offending.

Physical health in secure settings

People with enduring mental disorders experience poorer physical health. The average life expectancy of people with schizophrenia in the UK is fifteen years less[17] than that of the general population. Over half of this excess mortality is from disease. Personality disorders are also associated with greater rates of physical ill-health.

Reasons for lower life expectancy in forensic psychiatry

Many forensic patients were exposed to high levels of childhood adversity, which is associated with extreme stress and, amongst other findings, a potential for reduced immune response. Patients often have unhealthy ways of managing distress (e.g. substance misuse, over-eating, and smoking[18]) which contribute to poor health. Iatrogenic harm occurs from <u>pharmacological treatment</u> (p.200), including obesity, diabetes, and cardiovascular disease. One study found that many forensic inpatients gained most of their weight during their inpatient stay.

Additional factors include:

• poor health awareness,
• fewer opportunities for healthy living,
• low detection rates for medical illness, and
• poor compliance (e.g. because of persecutory ideation).

Interventions

Health promotion should include information, advice and resources on:

• **Smoking**—smoking cessation programmes are effective for some, and many secure services are now smoke-free.
• **Nutritional (dietetic) advice**—focusing on healthy eating and reducing drinks and foods with high sugar and fat content. There is conflict between allowing patients choice in what they eat (even when they lack capacity) and encouraging healthy eating. Takeaways are often part of the culture in secure units. Some propose starting treatment for the consequences of poor nutrition (e.g. metformin for diabetes) at the earliest opportunity.
• **Exercise**—forensic patients need access to exercise, including organised gym sessions and sports therapy. Facilities at forensic units vary.
• **Weight loss** requires both practical and psychological interventions, as low self-esteem may reduce the motivation to lose weight.

Infection control

Infection outbreaks such as in the 2020 SARS-Cov-2 pandemic present complex challenges for those in prison, hospitals, and courts (including staff). Avoiding close contact and restricting movement involve difficult dilemmas. Important measures include space planning, monitoring of

---

17 Though, hearteningly, when the first edition of this book was published it was twenty-five years less.
18 Nicotine in cigarettes may decrease some side-effects and may ameliorate some of the neurological deficits of schizophrenia.

symptoms, and case numbers using best available guidelines and data (on transmission modes and duration, social distancing, and personal protective equipment), plus frequent testing and vaccination.

Monitoring physical healthcare

Forensic psychiatric patients and prisoners are entitled to the same quality of physical healthcare as others. Legal restrictions on liberty should not prevent proper monitoring of physical health; some services have General Practitioners or Physician Associates who assist with this. NICE and other guidelines on the physical healthcare of patients on psychotropics known to have associated physical health risks should be followed. See Box 6.3.

Box 6.3 Typical recommended physical health monitoring during antipsychotic treatment

At baseline (e.g. at admission), and every six to twelve months thereafter:
Calculate BMI, and enquire about diet and exercise
Enquire about EPSEs, akathisia, TD, and other possible side-effects
Perform a systems enquiry and physical examination
Measure fasting glucose and lipid levels, U&E, LFTs, and TFTs
Perform an ECG and calculate QTc

Psychotherapies in forensic psychiatry

Psychological therapies can promote recovery from mental disorder, reduce distress, and aid psychological growth and resilience. There is an extensive range of therapies with these objectives, some supported by evidence-based guidelines such as those from NICE. Many therapy techniques can be effective if the therapist and patient establish a therapeutic alliance and the technique is matched to the problem. Mild to moderate disorders may respond to psychotherapies alone; more severe disorders usually need adjuvant medication.

Psychological treatment planning is complex, particularly in forensic psychiatry. Most patients have severe and multiple comorbidities, and there is a lack of good evidence about what order of treatments is most effective. Most studies focus on reoffending as an <u>outcome measure</u> (p.275) and leave unclear what psychological needs were addressed. Recovery can be influenced by factors outside the therapy, such as the prison regime or authorities' refusal to accept evidence of progress.

Psychological formulation

Psychological treatment of offenders begins with a <u>formulation</u> (p.146) of how the mental disorder relates to risk of offending, which can lead to an agreement with the patient about treatment aims. Therapeutic interventions should address dynamic risk factors for violence, including substance misuse and long-term effects of adverse childhood experience.

Prison and probation interventions

In prisons, forensic psychologists offer offence-related work only; clinical psychologists—if present—address mental disorder. Prisoners have available psycho-education and <u>cognitive skills programmes</u> (p.220). Some programmes address particular offending types; some address generic cognitive skills. Substance misuse programmes are offered by community third sector services. Probation services offer psychoeducational interventions, mainly addressing substance misuse and family relationships.

The national UK programme for offenders with personality disorder (<u>OPD</u>, p.260) screens all offenders for personality disorder and offers formulations for those above the threshold. These help in planning interventions during the sentence, and in allowing Integrated Risk Management Services in the community to manage offenders with PD after release. The programme also aims to make all prison environments 'psychologically informed' (**PIPEs**), and employs psychologists, psychiatrists, and psychotherapists to deliver a Therapeutic Community model (<u>TCs</u>, p.216) for suitable prisoners in several prisons in E&W.

Therapeutic techniques in secure services

- <u>Cognitive-behavioural therapy (CBT)</u> (p.206) addresses conscious cognitive distortions. CBT-based psychoeducational groups may initiate patients into psychological therapy. They are unlikely to be sufficient alone to address most forensic patients' needs.
- <u>Dialectical Behaviour Therapy (DBT)</u> (p.208) impacts affect dysregulation and impulsivity; it is useful for preparation before offence-based work that may be distressing.

- <u>Mentalisation-Based Treatment (MBT)</u> (p.208) and <u>psychodynamic therapies</u> (p.212) work to improve reflective skills and awareness of dysfunctional defences. NICE recommends MBT for <u>borderline</u> and <u>antisocial</u> PD (pp.84, 82).
- Schema-focused therapy (<u>SFT</u>, p.209) focuses on attitudes and beliefs.
- Arts therapies (p.210) are especially useful for those struggling to articulate their thoughts and feelings; NICE guidelines recommend them for people with thought disorder.
- <u>Eye Movement Desensitisation Reprogramming (EMDR)</u> (p.222) targets persistent posttraumatic stress disorder (<u>PTSD</u>) (p.96) symptoms.

<u>Group therapies</u> (p.214) offer pro-social experiences and perspective-taking practice. Initial group programmes address anxiety and mood regulation (a DBT feature). Later groups may offer manualised violence reduction, or sex offender groups may use cognitive theory to help offenders understand their risk. These groups are best followed by participation in either MBT and/or structured reflective groups that offer space to consider offence meanings and related affects.

Therapy planning

Planned therapy sequences should ideally address diagnosis, psychopathology, index offences, risk reduction, and rehabilitation in an integrated way. Therapies should not be terminated abruptly: this may increase violence risk.

Encouragement is often needed to attend therapy, which may be disparaged by patients (as may medication). Teams should not collude with resistance, but, instead, empathise with how difficult it can be, emphasising its purpose. Most patients will understand that whether discharge (including by tribunals) is likely will be affected by the level of cooperation with therapy. For many, this will be the first time they have taken their minds seriously, which may well be difficult at first.

There is currently no evidence for claims that patients can have 'too much therapy', or that they must not have different therapies concurrently. Each case must be assessed according to clinical need, and treatments in any complex therapy plan must be integrated. All should be delivered and supervised by trained staff. UK secure unit quality standards recommend access to a range of therapists: arts, psychodynamic and occupational therapists, psychologists, and forensic medical psychotherapists.

Cognitive-behavioural therapy

CBT, first developed by Aaron Beck in the 1960s, is based upon the idea that disorder is not caused by events themselves but by the perspective the patient takes on them. Its origins lie in classical learning theory, with its focus on observable behaviours and the assumption that irrational thinking processes are influential and maintained through reinforcement. CBT is a relatively short-term, collaborative therapy that addresses this by focusing on current problems, where the goals are symptom relief and the development of new skills. It is comparatively well evaluated.

Rationale

Behaviours and emotions are determined by the person's cognitions and core beliefs (ingrained views about oneself, others, and the world). Some pathological emotions are the result of cognitive distortions (such as those in Box 6.4), and these are more easily influenced than underlying emotions. CBT aims to 'change the way you feel by changing the way you think'.

Regarding offenders, the assumption is that the foundations of criminal activity are dysfunctional patterns of thinking. By changing routine misinterpretation of events, offenders can modify antisocial aspects of their personality and consequent behaviour.

Box 6.4 Examples of cognitive distortions amenable to CBT

- Polarisation: things are either wholly good, or wholly bad
- Filtering: selectively attending to the bad, dismissing the good
- Overgeneralisation: this happened once, therefore it will always happen
- Catastrophisation: focusing on the worst, no matter how unlikely
- Assuming conclusions: not checking evidence for or against your view
- Personalisation: thinking things relate to you when they don't

---

Techniques

The therapist aims to assist the patient to monitor cognitions, identify cognitive errors, understand maladaptive schema, explore strategies to challenge and change these, and examine the resultant effects on behaviour. CBT makes use of behavioural, cognitive, and experimental techniques.

- Behavioural techniques include activity scheduling, graded assignments, exposure, response prevention, distraction, relaxation training, and assertiveness/social skills training.
- Cognitive techniques include education, reading assignments, identifying automatic thoughts; Socratic questioning, a thoughts diary; and role play, thought rehearsal, cognitive restructuring, and examining the evidence.

There is a wide range of therapeutic techniques that fall under the CBT umbrella. These include rational and emotive therapies (REBT), mindfulness-based CT (MBCT), cognitive analytic therapy, SFT, (p.209), and systems training for emotional predictability and problem solving.

CBT in forensic services

CBT remains the commonest psychological treatment modality for offenders in hospitals, prisons, and the community. It targets symptoms (e.g. emotional dysregulation or psychosis) and offending behaviours, including the thoughts, choices, attitudes, and meaning systems that are associated with antisocial behaviour and lifestyles.

Initially, CBT was mainly used in prisons, primarily in group programmes addressing offending behaviour, particularly anger management, sexual offending, and addictions. Many of the accredited Offending Behaviour Programmes have a strong CBT emphasis, such as Enhanced Thinking Skills, Reasoning and Rehabilitation, and Sex Offender Treatment Programmes. A main focus of the latter is the sex-related <u>cognitive distortions</u> (p.128) that promote offending. CBT can also help an individual to develop skills necessary to function well outside forensic settings.

It has been argued that CBT approaches are not universally applicable to all groups of offenders (also see Box 6.5). Manualised programmes developed for the mainstream male prison population need to be adapted for other groups, including women, people from other cultures, and offenders with mental disorder, intellectual disabilities, or traumatic brain injury. The manual may be more appropriately labelled 'a guide for treatment' (some are highly prescriptive, others less so). Meta-analyses show that CBT is effective in affective disorders, including in offenders, but that its efficacy in psychotic disorders is less certain.

Box 6.5 Principles for successful CBT treatment with offenders

- Interventions should use the cognitive-behavioural and social learning techniques described in this section.
- Patients should have some ability and willingness to think about their thoughts and feelings.
- Reinforcements should be mainly positive, not negative.
- Treatment interventions should be used primarily with high-risk offenders, targeting criminogenic need.
- Where appropriate, community interventions are more effective than those in institutional settings.

DBT, MBT, and SFT

These therapies all invite the patient to think about how early childhood adversity led them to develop dysfunctional ways of managing negative affects like sadness and anger, and how these dysfunctions have impacted their personality development and interpersonal functioning. They then offer different strategies for improving psychological function. Technically, they share an emphasis on the here-and-now of the therapeutic process, and encourage patients to be consciously aware of their thoughts and feelings as they happen. The interventions described on this page are not mutually exclusive, and individuals could be offered various interventions at different stages of rehabilitation within their therapy plan (p.205).

Dialectical Behavioural Therapy

DBT emphasises the development of mindfulness skills, which can reduce affective dysregulation and impulsivity. These help patients gain enhanced awareness of feelings and thoughts, which allows for the implementation of skills in managing stress and improving relationships with others. The manualised DBT treatment programme begins with mindfulness, and revises this in between the other skills modules:

• emotion regulation,
• distress tolerance, and
• interpersonal effectiveness.

The programme involves group work on the skills modules, with simultaneous individual therapy, and homework to practise skills. The individual sessions are where the dialectical process of synthesising apparently opposed ideas (e.g. learning to accept some things through meditative techniques, and change others through cognitive exercises) takes place. DBT therapists are required to undertake formal training and attend regular supervision.

Evidence for DBT's effectiveness in treating borderline PD (p.84) is now strong, and NICE guidelines recommend its use. It has also been shown to be effective for mood disorders, self-harm and suicidal ideation, and substance misuse. Full DBT is offered in some forensic services, and more limited DBT skills groups are widely available for patients with emotional dysregulation. The educational component may be especially useful before other therapies commence; some services now train all ward staff in basic DBT skills to ensure support is available between sessions.

Mentalisation-Based Treatment

MBT is a NICE recommended treatment for personality disorder, based on attachment theory,[19] psychodynamic insights, and systemic therapy (p.218). It is effective for borderline and antisocial PD, and more broadly for the treatment of impulsivity and self-harm.

It comprises both group and individual sessions over about eight-teen months, and focuses on social **perspective-taking** and **reflective skills**. Therapists must be trained, accredited, and supervised to prevent splitting

---

19 Bowlby's theory that all emotional development springs from care-giving relationships in infancy.

(p.312). MBT psycho-education programmes are widely used in the prison <u>OPD programme</u> (p.260); teaching staff basic MBT skills improves their competence in working with people with PD.

Schema-Focussed Therapy

Like DBT and MBT, SFT is an integrative psychotherapy, developed for the treatment of personality disorders. It combines cognitive therapy with Gestalt[20] therapy, object relations theory,[21] and attachment theory. It invites patients to become aware of negative **schemas** (i.e. dysfunctional belief patterns about the world that developed in their childhood) and change them using cognitive therapy and reflective psychodynamic techniques. SFT has been successfully used with offenders with PD in forensic services in Holland and Canada.

Arts psychotherapies

Arts psychotherapies use creative arts, image, body, and sound as platforms for psychological change. They are based on theories of mind and show how despite symbolic function impairment in mental illness, participants can develop imaginative methods to aid recovery and sense of self. Arts therapies do not require any artistic talent in order to be effective.

The principal types of arts therapies are:
• drama therapy,
• art therapy,
• music therapy, and
• movement and dance therapy.

Arts therapies can be valuable for those who find it difficult to verbalise experiences, and can bypass defences to access hidden meanings without the participant feeling exposed. They can be especially useful for paranoid patients, and those who struggle with the stigma of diagnosis and offending, allowing the processing of trauma safely from a distance through metaphor.

Although their efficacy is not well researched in adults (and there are practical difficulties in doing so), case studies provide some evidence of positive responses, particularly with difficult-to-engage or 'stuck' patients with negative symptoms.

Arts therapies with forensic patients

There is a long history of the effective use of all arts therapies in forensic services. There can be both group or individual sessions, and elements of arts therapies can be used alongside other psychology programmes. They are particularly suitable for:
• patients who have suffered significant childhood abuse and neglect and who struggle to speak about this;
• patients who cannot name and describe emotions (alexithymia) or verbalise their thoughts; and
• patients who may be articulate but are affectless in their accounts of themselves and others (e.g. those with ASPD, and some other sex offenders).

Arts therapies can also be a useful for introducing patients who lack social skills to pro-social relationships. In being part of an arts therapy group patients have the opportunity to create, individually or together, and sharing work offers the chance to be a valued member of a group.

The same risks apply to the arts therapies as to any psychological therapy in forensic practice; that is, concerns about professional boundary violations (p.302), attempted manipulation of the therapist, or lack of facilitation support.

Arts psychotherapists are trained to master's or doctorate level, and use in depth clinical supervision with other experienced arts psychotherapists to process work. As they are often single practitioners, working part time in a service, it is important that they are protected against isolation from clinical teams and from being the target of projections.

Psychodynamic psychotherapy

Psychodynamic psychotherapy

Individual psychodynamic therapy works to enhance the ability to think about difficult feelings rather than act them out in dysfunctional ways. Its structure focuses on the predictability of the therapeutic frame (the time, duration, and location of sessions), while allowing the patient freedom to select the material for discussion. The additional technical aspect is close attention to the therapeutic relationship and the therapist's experienced feelings about the patient. This is based on evidence that interpersonal attachment patterns from the patient's childhood are unconsciously repeated in relationships that involve closeness and vulnerability, including therapeutic relationships (where the unconscious repetition is known as **transference**). Where the patterns arise from adverse childhood experiences (p.32), behaviours and relationships in adulthood will be dysfunctional, and associated with poor affect regulation and ability to mentalise (p.208).

Sessions explore the psychological strategies (**defences**, see Box 6.6) the patient uses to cope with feelings, that worsen matters long-term and distort reality, and how dysfunctional relationship patterns are repeated in present day experience—including in offending and in the relationship with the therapist. Sessions usually last fifty minutes, and may take place weekly (in dynamic psychotherapy) or up to four times per week (in more intense psychoanalysis).

> **Box 6.6 Examples of psychodynamic defence mechanisms (from most to least mature)**
>
> - Sublimation: using negative affect healthily, e.g. channelling aggression in sport
> - Humour: overtly expressing negative affect in a safe, pro-social form
> - Suppression: recognising but consciously delaying attending to negative thoughts
> - Intellectualisation: focusing on abstractions, ignoring emotional aspects of a topic
> - Displacement: directing negative affect to an unthreatening target, e.g. bullying
> - Dissociation: emotional numbing, cutting off emotional reaction to stimuli
> - Repression: keeping a desire unconscious, resulting in memory lapse or naïveté
> - Acting out: directly acting on an unconscious desire without awareness of it
> - Projection: attributing negative affect to other people, then reacting to it in them
> - Denial: flatly refusing to accept aspects of reality or grossly distorting them
> - Delusional projection: attributing negative affect to nonexistent objects

Psychodynamic therapy in forensic settings

There is no clear evidence associating psychodynamic interventions and reduced offending. Systematic reviews have linked psychodynamic psychotherapy to improvements in complex psychopathology relevant to offending, including affect regulation, maintaining supportive relationships, and improvement in personality and affective disorders.

Forensic patients who experienced extensive abuse at the hands of caregivers may find individual psychodynamic therapy stressful, especially those who struggle to verbalise feelings. Education, DBT, (p.208), or small-group therapy may be indicated beforehand. Unprepared forensic patients may become highly aroused and agitated in individual work, or behave seductively with therapists. Careful attention to the history and index offence may elicit warning factors.

Contraindications

This therapy is rarely recommended for those who are acutely psychotic[22] or have high PCL-R (p.137) scores. Such work is technically difficult, and should not be attempted by junior staff. Evidence for group therapy (p.214) and therapeutic communities (p.216) is stronger for these patients.

Early in therapy, patients often become more aware of painful feelings (e.g. distress, anger) they had previously avoided. It is crucial that therapies are not stopped as this awareness develops. Patients and their teams should be made aware that they may feel worse before they begin to understand and manage their feelings better, and plan accordingly. No therapy should be abruptly terminated; there should be at least one meeting between therapist and patient to end the work.

Confidentiality

All therapists need to work closely with forensic clinical teams. Some psychodynamic therapists assert that complete confidentiality (including from the patient's team) is a technical requirement. Usually a compromise is reached whereby limited confidentiality is offered and the patient knows that information relevant to risk will be shared. If therapists fail to share their views with clinical teams, this limits the therapy's value, invites splitting (p.312), and increases the risk of therapists colluding with patients in hiding aspects of their mind, which may replicate the index offence, increasing risk.

22 In the psychiatric sense of exhibiting delusions, hallucinations, or similar symptoms, not in the (related, but much broader) psychodynamic sense of disrupted relationships with internal objects.

Group therapy

Group therapies are widely used in forensic work in prisons and secure services with staff and patients.

Benefits of groups

- Promotion of pro-social behaviours and attitudes (e.g. rule-keeping)
- Promotion of interpersonal skills and turn-taking
- Decreased shame and social isolation (both criminogenic risk factors)
- Education about offending and its effects
- Promotion of hope and reduced hopelessness (a potent risk factor for suicide)
- An economically efficient way of providing interventions to individuals with similar problems

A working knowledge of group dynamics is essential for the assessment of relational risk in inpatient settings, and for managing forensic institutions.

Disadvantages of groups

- Patients are usually anxious about groups so resist joining them.
- Poorly run groups may allow offenders to support each other's antisocial attitudes and beliefs: a concern with ASPD and young offenders.
- Groups can be difficult to engage with for offenders who are paranoid, avoidant, or who struggle with shame.
- Very anxious or antisocial offender patients may be destructive of the group process.

Group interventions in prisons

All offence-related interventions in prisons are delivered in groups. Group therapy forms the basis of therapeutic communities (p.216) in prisons and in some PIPEs (p.204). There is some limited evidence that inmates who complete treatment in prison therapeutic communities show reduced recidivism rates.

Group interventions in the community

For offenders with community penalties or those on licence (p.448), the Probation Service (p.584) in E&W offers a range of group interventions related to the OPD programme for those who have assaulted others. There is some limited evidence that these programmes reduce recidivism. The Portman Clinic in London provides out-patient group and individual psychodynamic psychotherapy to offenders, including child and internet sex offenders.

Group therapy in secure psychiatric units

Group therapy may be targeted at an offence-related issue, symptoms of a disorder, or the distress associated with current experience. As many forensic patients have poor affect and arousal management skills, and deal with anxiety in antisocial ways, it is important for groups to be highly structured in terms of time, place, and content. Some groups have a set focus (e.g. CBT for psychosis); in others, group members are responsible for the session content (i.e. the patients set the agenda). This is important technically in order to promote responsibility and agency. Therapists need to be active and confident.

There is good-quality evidence that both cognitive and psychotherapy groups are effective in both reducing distress and increasing social functioning in patients with PD and other complex disorders. Group therapeutic factors, such as learning from each other, may be effective in reducing criminogenic risk in terms of increasing pro-social skills and reducing social isolation.

There is increasing evidence that group work (e.g. within DBT, p.208) is optimal for patients with moderately severe PDs of all types. There is less evidence about the effectiveness of group therapy for individuals with severe ASPD or high levels of psychopathy. Group programmes that only focus on cognitions and manual completion may overlook other kinds of psychopathology, especially hostility, deceptiveness, and cruelty to others.

Staff groups

All staff working in secure care with complex patients should have access to reflective practice (p.308), which provides time to review their work with patients. Working with such disturbed patients has an emotional impact on staff, and emotional reactions to patients are clinically relevant to understanding patients and avoiding inappropriate responses. Reflective practice should be delivered in groups, ideally involving all the members of a clinical multidisciplinary team. Group meetings are essential as a reminder to staff that reflection on the work is a professional necessity, and they can also be used to apply values based practice (p.288).

Therapeutic communities

Therapeutic communities (TCs) in the 1960s offered alternatives to traditional disease treatment models in psychiatry. Today, TCs are specialist, highly structured residential communities for patients with particular needs, where all aspects of the environment form part of an intense psychosocial treatment shared by staff and patients. They feature:

• **Democratisation**, sharing decisions where possible;
• **Permissiveness** of feelings, curiosity, and identity rather than behaviour;
• **Communalism**, sharing everything within the community; and
• **Reality confrontation**, not colluding in avoidance of what is distressing.

TCs for personality disorder

Systematic reviews suggest that TCs effectively reduce distress and improve social functioning in patients with mild to moderate PD, especially borderline PD (p.84). The therapeutic benefit is not fully realised until about twelve months after completion, with less effect if the patient left the TC early. Programmes generally last one to three years.

It is likely that such TCs' benefits arise from:

• offering education about mental states, social rules, and rule-keeping;
• promote mentalising (p.208) and cognitive skills in the self-regulation of negative affects, and a culture of curiosity about mental states;
• reinforcing pro-social behaviours and increasing anxiety about antisocial behaviours (most TCs quickly respond to rule-breaking, and require rule-breakers to take responsibility for their behaviour);
• decreasing social isolation and allowing residents to make secure attachments to the programme and the community (of particular value to those with highly adverse childhood experiences resulting in insecure attachment patterns); and
• decreasing shame about distress and increasing affective regulation skills.

TCs for prisoners and forensic psychiatric patients

Given the high prevalence of personality disorder amongst prisoners, there has been considerable interest in providing TCs in prisons. In theory, the TC approach should have particular benefits for prisoners with ASPD and BPD, but, by nature, antisocial people may be antagonistic to pro-social structures or seek to attack them. Prisoners cannot be coerced into a TC programme; also many TCs will not take prisoners who are on psychotropic medication, which is a problem for those with comorbid psychosis and mood disorder.

Modified TCs have been set up in several prisons in the UK (e.g. HMP Grendon); there are three TCs in medium secure psychiatric services as part of the OPD network (p.260). There is some evidence that they reduce future violence risk. Varying effectiveness of different TCs may relate to their particular structure and style.

TCs work best when staff are well-trained and 'buy in' to the model. Running a prison TC requires close attention to therapeutic boundaries, relationships between staff and prisoners, and between the prisoners. Staff need supervision and reflective spaces to help them stay with the primary task of helping the residents take more responsibility for their own behaviour and mental wellbeing.

Systemic and family therapy

Systemic and family therapy

Systems theory asserts that interactions, relations, and context are of primary importance in understanding the behaviour of an individual. The systemic therapist considers the individual in terms of their significant life contexts, especially interpersonal relationships.

In a forensic context, systemic therapists are informed by ideas of 'pattern' and 'process' in relationships; systemic formulation includes consideration of the intergenerational transmission of attitudes and beliefs concerning violence, and life-cycle experiences, as well as the context of the referral.

Systemic therapy can be used with different types of offenders in different contexts. Systemic work can also aid risk assessment, provide psycho-education to family members, facilitate reparation, deal with any specific factors within the family system that contributed to offending, and provide an opportunity for victims (including victimised offenders) to come to terms with their traumatic experiences.

Domestic/intimate partner violence

A significant number of couples presenting for couple or family therapy report violence within their relationship. However, therapy should not be attempted where there is still a high risk of further violence, and there should be an agreement that both partners are committed to finding a way to live together safely.

There are a number of interventions available for perpetrators of child physical abuse. These include parenting programmes, parent support programmes, and family preservation models, relying on crisis intervention and case management.

Mentally disordered offenders

Many patients in medium secure units suffer from schizophrenia, with or without personality disorder, and their victims are most commonly family members.[23] Family interventions have been shown to improve outcome and the management of schizophrenia. Therapeutic change that occurs in collaboration with the wider systems, especially the family, around the individual is more likely to be sustained. Family therapy, and less technical family interventions, are not always available in secure settings, mainly due to a lack of appropriately trained therapists and resources.

Young offenders

Family-based systemic interventions have been shown to be effective for a proportion of childhood behaviour problems.

Multisystemic Therapy (MST) is an intervention used to treat young people at risk of care or custody in the age range of eleven through seventeen years. It is an intensive, family- and community-based, individualised programme that targets systems around the young person. There are a

---

23 The nature of the relationship with family members in family therapy can be legally important in terms of whether the therapist has a duty of care to them and whether they effectively become 'patients' (*ABC v St George's Healthcare NHST & others* [2020] EWHC 455).

few adaptations of MST suited to young offenders: Multisystemic Therapy–Problem Sexual Behaviour, Multisystemic Therapy–Substance Abuse, and Multisystemic Therapy–Family Integrated Transitions. The latter adaptation aims at transitioning young people from residential or secure settings back into the community.

Treatment Foster Care Oregon is an intervention for young people who are 'looked after'. For young people referred by youth justice services, the intervention is targeted at serious and persistent young offenders for whom the alternative to fostering would be custody or (in E&W) an Intensive Supervision and Surveillance Programme.

Functional Family Therapy (FFT) is another manualised systemic, cognitive-behavioural model of therapy that targets eleven to eighteen year olds with antisocial and violent behaviour.

In 2020, the Youth Endowment Fund awarded funding to pilot adapted versions of MST and FFT for ten to fifteen years olds at risk of criminal exploitation.

Offender treatment programmes

Risk, needs, and responsivity

Interventions directly offence related are based on the Risk-Needs model, which states that interventions should adhere to three principles:

- The **risk** principle—higher risk offenders should receive more intervention.
- The **needs** principle—treatment targets should focus on criminogenic need.
- The **responsivity** principle—the intervention should be one to which the offender is receptive.

For general offenders, this approach appears to reduce recidivism.

Good Lives model

This is a more holistic intervention, developed in response to critique of the Risk-Needs model. It uses a strengths-based approach, similar to the mental health recovery model (p.264). In RoI, the programme is called Better Lives. It starts from the position that offenders must respect others' rights to wellbeing and freedom, and deserve the same respect in return. The programme aims to improve individuals' ability to formulate and select goals, construct plans and implement them freely, in eleven areas of 'primary goods', ranging from healthy living, to work, to inner peace, and to creativity.

Both the Good Lives model and the Risk-Needs model can be complemented by formulations (p.146) based on assessment of adverse childhood experience and psychological defence mechanisms. Both models also assume the use of pharmacological and psychological treatment for symptoms of mental disorder. Interventions may be offered individually or in groups.

Delivering psychological treatment to offenders

Interventions for violent offenders

Psychological interventions are structured and manualised for delivery in prisons. They typically address **antisocial attitudes** and **cognitive beliefs** that support offending. Some are brief and target a single factor (e.g. anger management); others are longer multifactorial programmes focusing on cognitions, anger management, skills training, and relapse prevention. Evidence for their effectiveness is limited.

There are specific forms for young offenders (e.g. Aggression Replacement Training (ART), Equipping Peers to Help One Another (EQUIP), and MST, p.218). These are not aimed at the most violent young offenders.

Interventions for domestic violence may be offered by prison, probation or specialist centres. They may be based on a variety of theories and generally utilise cognitive-behavioural techniques. They may be offered to individual, couples, or groups.

However, for violent offenders, a purely cognitive model does not address relational factors with the victim (affecting 70% of offenders) nor unconscious unresolved distress from early attachment insecurity (a known risk factor for violence). Violence perpetrators (in hospital or prison) may benefit from long-term therapies which address relational risk factors, past and present (e.g. with staff). Violence perpetrators may also need therapies that help them to come to terms with the consequences of their offences, and the implications for their future life. They may need a portfolio of different therapies integrated with each other.

Interventions for sexual offenders

Sexual offending one of the first areas in which standardised programmes were developed, including the Sex Offender Treatment Programme (p.247). This and other interventions based on cognitive models of sex offending are now seen as less effective and may even increase the risk of reoffending in some cases.[24] Other models that examine insecure attachment and negative affect management now appear more effective.

Accredited Offending Behaviour Programmes

Offending Behaviour Programmes are an integral part of work carried out by UK prison and probation services (see p.586). They are accredited by an MoJ panel (CSAAP). There are currently more than forty accredited programmes in E&W.[25]

---

24 An RCT published by the MoJ in 2017 showed that after eight years, there was an increased risk of sexual and child image offences in SOTP completers, compared to matched controls. A later meta-analysis showed that there were benefits from some aspects of SOTP treatment.

25 Scotland has no national programme, though there are local initiatives. Northern Ireland's Probation Board runs substance misuse and violence reduction programmes only. Prisons in RoI run some programmes, including sex offender treatments as above, but do not have an accreditation system.

Other psychological therapies

Eye Movement Desensitisation Reprogramming

Having built a therapeutic relationship, the EMDR therapist encourages the patient to recall traumatic images, thoughts, emotions, and bodily sensations, while undertaking bilateral stimulation, most commonly repeated eye movements. It has been shown to be effective in patients with PTSD (p.96) with intrusive traumatic memories, including from their own offences.

Psychological treatments for substance misuse

These are often group-based and usually utilise a model of recovery, abstention, or harm reduction and relapse prevention. Most treatment for substance misuse is provided by primary care or third sector programmes like Turning Point and Addaction in the UK. Alcoholics Anonymous and Narcotics Anonymous have been shown to be effective for those who engage. Few of these interventions have been tested in secure forensic services, mainly because patients are involuntarily abstinent.

Psychoeducational interventions may be of value when patients are leaving secure conditions. Interventions in secure settings tend to focus on increasing motivation to address substance use, increasing awareness/management of high-risk situations (both external and internal to the patient) where substances will be tempting and supportive exposure/management of triggers and cravings for substances. There is a focus on developing a balanced lifestyle and identifying occupations as an alternative to substance use.

Motivational interviewing (MI)

MI is a psychoeducational approach to help people with substance misuse, and other problems, engage with recovery. It is based on the Stages of Change model, which recognises that people go through different phases of motivation before they are able to give up a dysfunctional behaviour:
• Precontemplative—not open to considering change.
• Contemplative—ready to consider change.
• Preparation—intending to change, planning change.
• Action—changing behaviour.
• Maintenance—sustaining changes in behaviour.
• Termination (no longer any risk of the old behaviour) or Relapse (returning to the dysfunctional behaviour).

It involves an interviewing style that emphasises 'rolling with resistance', 'avoiding argumentation', and 'developing discrepancy', aiming to explore and resolve ambivalence: promoting patients to see themselves as capable of making changes. MI may be the starting point to move an offender towards engaging in other psychological interventions.

Nursing, relational security, and milieu

Nurses and health care assistants (HCAs) have a crucial role in establishing relational security (p.190) in teams, on wards, and in community settings. Their work establishes the therapeutic atmosphere or 'milieu' that influences recovery through the medium of team dynamics.

Inpatient care

Long-term residential secure care is a specific intervention in its own right, and the framework for recovery in forensic care. Patients are admitted to ready-made communities where they will have to make relationships with staff and patients as part of their care. Relationships with staff (especially ward nurses and HCAs) are crucial to individual recovery.

The ward team will influence the ward milieu, which has an important influence on recovery. Most patients arrive in agitated and antisocial states of mind, and have to take a risk in trusting staff to help them recover and give up their old behaviours. Ward staff need to feel confident in talking to patients; de-escalating distress; modelling pro-social behaviour, and managing their emotional responses to patients. Staff need an adequate understanding of mental disorder, how it affects risk of violence, and how it may impact on staff. Reflective practice (p.308) is crucial in supporting this work.

Because nurses and HCAs spend so much time with patients, they need additional support to make and maintain professional boundaries (p.302). This is especially true in those services that offer treatment to patients with ASPD and BPD (pp.82, 84). Staff have to maintain a boundary between being personally supportive and encouraging, yet not compliant or vulnerable to collusion with rule-breaking. This is difficult to do well for long periods of time; other staff have a role in supporting nursing colleagues in maintaining boundaries and reflective understanding of feelings provoked by the work.

Other skills include the ability to maintain continuing attention to changes in risk, combining therapy with security, and understanding the ethical and practice aspects of working in what can be highly coercive environments.

Community settings

Where forensic nurses and HCAs work in community settings the same principles of relational security apply, even though the work may be significantly less intense.

Challenges to relational security

There are challenges in maintaining relational security and a therapeutic atmosphere:
- Nursing staff are usually responsible for the imposition of rules and day to day security measures (to some extent, even where there are separate security staff), which may involve conflict with patients.
- Rules may infantilise patients and anger those who feel that they are being patronised or belittled.
- Nurses are responsible for the immediate management of violence and aggression, to a greater extent than other staff groups, and are therefore more often victims of assaults.

- Inpatient nursing staff experience high levels of stress as a result of the constant fear of violence associated with managing people with a history of violence.
- Nurses may over-identify with patients, and collude with them in boundary-breaking; a particular problem in services that treat personality disorder.
- Nurses may also avoid patients that they fear or dislike, and fail to enforce boundaries with them as a result.
- Although nursing teams spend the most time with patients, these issues apply to other professionals also, and it is important that they are not projected only onto nursing teams, causing splitting (p.312).

When things go wrong

An antitherapeutic culture in secure settings is one where bullying, coercion, deceit, and denial flourish. This may involve staff bullying patients, staff colluding with patients, or both. All these behaviours have been reported in secure psychiatric settings (e.g. the Blom-Cooper and Fallon inquiries, p.780). Such antisocial environments do not help patients become more pro-social, and increase the risk of inpatient violence towards staff.

A forensic psychiatric milieu is more likely to become antisocial if:
- Nursing staff are expected to deliver care that they do not perceive as therapeutic, resulting in a perception that their skills are under-utilised or under-valued.
- Nursing staff do not feel supported by other members of the MDT, or are in dispute with them.
- There is no attention to team dynamics, and staff cannot access reflective practice groups and supervision (p.308).

Other settings

There can be very different roles and issues for forensic nurses in:
- prisons where there may be opposition to a compassionate approach to prisoners;
- community settings where the role may be coordinating care; and
- court e.g. diversion schemes (p.268) where nurses and others may be expected to regard those they assess as defendants first and patients second.

Social work

Forensic social workers operate in a range of contexts, in secure inpatient settings, and in community teams, supporting and sometimes supervising mentally disordered offenders. In the social care context, social workers are often employed as Criminal Justice or Youth Justice social workers. They are involved in gatekeeping and ensuring that service users are managed with the least restrictive level of <u>security</u> (p.190). They often work within multi-disciplinary teams and bring a social and family perspective to treatment.

Some social workers take up additional training to become accredited under mental health law, as an Approved Social Worker[26] (<u>ASW</u>, p.468). In the UK, the DHSC Forensic Mental Health Social Work Capabilities Framework sets out the knowledge and skills required of forensic social workers, usually including a minimum three years' experience postqualification.

Roles of the forensic social worker

These include:

- statutory duties under mental health law, such as applications for detention, consultation with relatives and carers, discharge, and supervision;
- writing social circumstances reports (including for tribunals);
- planning community care;
- liaising with (and making applications to) local authorities and other bodies, particular in relation to accommodation and social care;
- consideration of the needs of past or potential victims;
- <u>safeguarding</u> of children and vulnerable adults (p.590); and
- assessing and managing risk from the perspectives above.

Carers, children, and families

Forensic social workers lead on safeguarding of children and adults. For inpatient or detained patients, they maintain links to the wider family and community where the patient will likely return and are central in risk assessment and planning towards balancing the needs of the wider system as well as the individual service user. They take the lead in gathering social histories and keeping family members informed about a patient's treatment; as well as liaising with the relevant local authority to arrange carers' assessments when necessary. If a patient has children and it is the role of the social worker to liaise with Local Authority child protection services to ensure that any ongoing contact with the patient is in the child's best interest and is safely managed.

Some social workers have expertise in assessing the safety needs of children, and their carers' capacity to protect them. They may have experience of working with young people in the care system ('looked-after children') who may also be in contact with the CJS. They have a role in completing a family assessment, including advising whether there is any domestic or

---

26 Known as a Mental Health Officer in Scotland and an Approved Mental Health Professional (AMHP) in E&W. Nurses, OTs, and psychologists can also become AMHPs but not ASWs.

spousal abuse, and in identifying potential concerns regarding child protection such as abuse or neglect. In most cases, however, this work would be performed by a social worker from the local children and family social services department, who would liaise with the forensic social worker.

Young offenders

Social workers have a number of special duties with respect to young offenders. These are often undertaken by specific social work Youth Offending/Justice Teams in E&W but usually by Local Authority social work teams elsewhere, particularly when the youth is already known to social services or is a 'looked-after child'. Social workers specifically assigned to work with young offenders will often be required to meet with them and their families prior to court or in Scotland a <u>Children's Hearing</u> (p.386), and liaise with other agencies to identify the most appropriate intervention and <u>placement.</u> (p.218). They may write and make recommendations to court (or a Children's Hearing in Scotland) and undertake a range of noncustodial activities which are intended to rehabilitate young offenders but also to divert them from more severe custodial sentences including restorative practice.

Occupational therapy

Occupational therapists (OTs) are specialist therapists: where 'occupation' refers to practical, purposeful activities that allow people to live independently with a sense of identity and purpose. Occupations include categories of self-care, productivity, and leisure. OTs aim to realise potential and overcome barriers preventing meaningful occupation; they work holistically to assess, maintain, or develop skills needed to flourish, promoting recovery (p.264) and social inclusion, and preventing relapse. They clarify and acknowledge patients' aspirations and strengths, conveying hope and helping patients make their own choices about their interests and needs.

Forensic occupational therapy

There is increasing recognition of the links between poor occupational performance, poor mental health, and offending. More OTs now work with mentally disordered offenders. Forensic OT is a recognised sub-profession. In secure hospital settings, OT adapts to security restrictions that contribute to occupational deprivation. Forensic OT interventions include developing satisfying, balanced routines within inpatient and community settings, learning and maintaining skills for personal and domestic activities of daily living (e.g. budgeting, cleaning, cooking, transport, IT), improving self-management of health conditions, health promotion (e.g. exercise, sleep, and nutrition), and facilitating access to work, education, and leisure activities, which contribute to pro-social networks. Interventions are provided one-to-one or in groups.

The role of the occupational therapist

- OTs complete assessments on how a patient's mental state impacts their ability to carry out independent living. Detailed histories of patients' roles and routines and help to build a picture of the individual's life.
- Assessments highlight strengths and weaknesses informing collaborative goals.
- OTs help motivate individuals in working towards these goals and increasing interest in developing life skills and purposeful occupation, including within the confines of an inpatient unit.
- Risk assessment impacts opportunities open to patients, and the OT must, in conjunction with the MDT, carry out risk assessments when planning appropriate interventions (e.g. access to tools).
- Interventions focus on increasing responsibility and autonomy.
- OTs have a role in supporting an individual to access the employment and educational opportunities which are offered within forensic inpatient settings and in the community, so these are set up before discharge to act as protective factors during transition to community life.
- In community teams, forensic OTs support patients to engage in employment/education/leisure activities, maintain life skills, and enhance social networks to support ongoing recovery.
- OTs evaluate interventions regularly, making adaptations where necessary and reviewing goals with patients.

Model of human occupation (MoHO)

Forensic OTs use self-rating scales, structured and semistructured observations, interviews, standardised assessments, and outcome measures. The majority of standardised tools are based on the MoHO or others such as the Model of Creative Ability, which seeks to:

• prioritise a patient's holistic needs;
• explore how an individual's view of their own performance capacity impacts their choices (often people with offending histories have difficulty identifying things to be proud of, or are unrealistic in goal setting);
• explore values which support pro-social choices and identities; and
• give a rationale for intervention.

It is recommended that OTs routinely use standardised outcome measures to assess and demonstrate patients' progress. MoHO assessments form part of the <u>DUNDRUM quartet</u> (p.194) for assessing forensic patient' readiness to move to a less secure setting.

Vocational rehabilitation

What is it?

Vocational rehabilitation has been described as a process enabling people with functional, psychological, developmental, cognitive, and emotional impairments or health conditions to overcome barriers to accessing, maintaining, or returning to employment or other meaningful occupation.

There are different methods of helping people access work:

- Pre-vocational Training—preparatory work prior to employment.
- Supported Employment—employment in a standard environment with on the job support.
- Work schemes within secure units.

Barriers to employment in forensic psychiatry

Forensic patients are faced with a number of barriers to employment: institutionalisation, stigma, discrimination, poor support, concern over benefits, disempowerment, poor education, absence of recent employment, restricted freedom and choice, low expectations of self and society to engage in and succeed in pro-social activities like employment, poor motivation, and the co-existence of an offending history.

Why is it necessary?

- Of offenders with mental illness, 75% are unemployed and lack structure or a daily routine. Rates are even higher for people discharged from secure hospital care (up to 90%).
- Meaningful activity alleviates boredom, which is often associated with acting out, addiction, and reoffending.
- Employment instability is associated with offending and increased risk of all-cause mortality.
- Employment can have a beneficial impact on many other factors related to quality of life, including:
  • increased income;
  • achievement of valued social responsibility;
  • greater socialisation (practicing social skills and developing tolerance to co-operate with others);
  • increased self-esteem;
  • improved physical health;
  • improved mental health, including preventing relapse and readmission;
  • opportunities to use skills;
  • opportunities to give something back to the community; and
  • provision of an indicator of progress in recovery.
- Reoffending rates can be reduced.

What exists?

- Individual schemes within secure hospitals
- Arrangements directly with employers
- Partnerships with charities
- Vocational rehabilitation provided by people from clinical and nonclinical backgrounds

- Various models are used by services; the Individual placement and support (IPS) model is the most structured and well-defined form of supported employment. It is based on the philosophy that anyone is capable of gaining competitive employment, provided the right job, with appropriate support, is identified

---

Example

First Step Trust is a charity providing training and employment for people excluded from work because of mental health problems or other disadvantages. They run work projects within secure hospitals as well as other settings.

Does it work?

As with any intervention, there is a need to define its aim. Vocational rehabilitation as an intervention is difficult to evaluate as a large majority of people with severe mental disorder will remain unemployed:

- For people with severe mental illness supported employment (including IPS) is the most effective intervention for employment.
- There is limited evidence on impact on symptoms, quality of life, or social functioning (a conclusion limited by under-powered studies).
- The majority of evidence is from the USA, not the UK or RoI.
- Research is needed to generate an evidence base for patients in forensic psychiatric settings.

Evaluation of treatment

Forensic psychiatric care combines mental health care and offender rehabilitation. Its evaluation focuses on such <u>outcome measures</u> (p.275) as:

- reduction in mental symptoms and distress,
- improvement in social and/or psychological functioning,
- reduced relapse or readmission rates, and
- reduction in offending or risk of offending.

These mirror measures developed by researchers in the field of offender rehabilitation. There have been periods of therapeutic optimism and pessimism over the last fifty years; since the 1980s the emphasis has been on 'what works', based on meta-analytic studies of interventions and an evidence-based approach to assessment, management and treatment. High costs of secure care have also driven attention towards efficacy and efficiency.

Reduction in offending

<u>Reconviction rates</u> (p.22) are a principal measure, partly because they are easy to measure, and partly because of social anxiety. Reconviction within two years is the standard across studies in E&W, but studies that continue beyond two years offer more information. Evaluation studies typically compare the reconviction rate of a group of offenders who have participated in an intervention/treatment and others who have not.

Metanalytic reviews suggest that offender treatment and rehabilitation have a small impact upon recidivism. That there is not a larger effect may be because many other factors are involved. For example, patients may relapse into substance misuse because of external stress, which increases their risk for recidivism, but which is unrelated to the effectiveness of the treatment they received.

Violent offender interventions

These include short programmes targeted at a single factor (e.g. anger management) and longer group programmes addressing multiple factors (e.g. cognitive skills, victim empathy, risk factors for violence, and relapse prevention). The most effective interventions target negative affect/anger, antisocial attitudes, and relapse prevention. Their effectiveness with forensic psychiatric patients is unclear.

Sex offender treatment

There have been recent doubts about the effectiveness of CBT programmes for sex offenders, and concerns that the prison programmes may increase, not reduce recidivism. However, these programmes continue to be offered in prisons. It is not clear if they can/should be used with all types of sex offender, nor what impact mental illness may have on their effectiveness. It is possible that medication may be useful in reducing sexual arousal.

Intimate Partner Violence (IPV) interventions

These are usually offered by probation services or prisons. There is little or no evidence for their effectiveness in reducing IPV, and treatment for substance misuse may be more helpful. Since many IPV perpetrators have mild-moderate degrees of BPD, NICE recommended interventions may be helpful for these offenders.

Young offenders

Reduced youth reoffending is associated with a focus on criminogenic, rather than clinical, needs. Effective interventions are structured and multimodal. Individual programmes should have a cognitive component that addresses attitudes, values, and beliefs supportive of antisocial behaviour. There is some evidence for the effectiveness of early prevention, parenting programmes and systemic interventions, such as <u>MST</u> (p.218), that address family, community, and wider risk factors. There is also some evidence that such interventions reduce costs long-term.

Effective programmes

The literature suggests that, in order for an offender programme to be effective, it needs:

- a theoretical framework supported by empirical research;
- to involve assessment to determine risk of future offending;
- to target the criminogenic need;
- to be structured, clear and directive;
- high treatment integrity (i.e. the delivery of the programme is carefully planned and model-based);
- to be multimodal, cognitive-behavioural, and skills-oriented; and
- to be community based rather than in institutions.

Mentally disordered offenders (MDOs)

Most Offending Behaviour Programmes have been tested in white, adult, male offenders without significant mental health or learning difficulties. There are few data for offenders with mental disorders such as paranoid schizophrenia or personality disorder. It is not clear as yet how to integrate attention to both criminogenic and psychopathological risk factors for different offender groups.

The following interventions for mentally disordered offenders are assumed to produce better outcomes, but lack a sound empirical base:

- use of <u>restriction orders</u> (p.510) (although uncontrolled studies do suggest association with reduced reconviction rate),
- depot as opposed to oral antipsychotics, and
- higher level supervision of offenders in the community.

Difficulties evaluating the effectiveness of forensic care arise from:

- some outcomes (like severe violence) having a low community prevalence,
- difficulty in constructing RCTs,
- the intervention itself potentially affecting how the outcome is measured (e.g. it is easier to track offenders on restriction orders),
- interventions that are multiple and complex,
- lack of clarity concerning what aspects of mental change are important,
- lack of clarity in how to measure them, and
- difficulty defining and measuring meaningful outcomes (outcomes that are easy to measure may not be important to the treatment and those that are important to the treatment are hard to measure).

Treatment of victims

Who should treat victims?

Clinicians involved in treating offenders should know about, and be capable of assessing, trauma reactions, and should also understand the rights and needs of victims from the perspective of their role with the perpetrator. Also, many perpetrators have also been victims. Understanding 'victimology' offers to those treating offenders depth of understanding about the impact of their patients' offending, and valuing of the importance of the victim perspective. It is crucial, however, that, in individual cases, clinicians do not treat perpetrators and victims of the same crimes.

Victims' needs

The psychological effects of being a victim of a crime include <u>PTSD</u> (p.96) and other traumatic stress reactions, substance/alcohol abuse, personality disorder (where the offending occurred during the victim's childhood), depression, and anxiety disorders. There are both short-term reactions and long-term effects.

Help-seeking is influenced by a victim's cultural background, expectations, and knowledge of what services are available, as well as by the severity of posttraumatic symptoms. Apart from help with their psychological and emotional needs, victims may need practical help, information, and financial support. In E&W, the charity Victim Support offers this kind of assistance, without charge. There are similar organisations in Scotland, Northern Ireland, and the Republic of Ireland, all of which offer:

• someone to talk to in confidence,
• information on police and court procedures,
• help dealing with organisations,
• information about compensation and insurance, and
• links to other sources of help including practical and physical support during trial.

There are other voluntary sector organisations that offer support to victims, and in addition, mental health services offer traumatic stress services.

Considerations in secure health settings and prisons

Victims of offences may still be linked with the perpetrator, particularly if they are a family member. However, victims have no rights to attend care planning meetings unless they are also a carer, when it is in their role as carer that they attend. By contrast, <u>Parole Boards</u> (p.582) are required to consider victim statements and wishes when considering release of prisoners, and victims are entitled to attend hearings. In tribunals victims' needs and wishes must be ascertained both by the treatment team and the Victim Liaison Teams in the relevant Ministry.

Working with perpetrators generally means a high likelihood of having contact with victims of their offences, as a large proportion are family members. So victims may well attend care planning meetings or be involved in interventions with the offender (e.g. systemic therapy, or restorative justice processes, which bring those harmed by crime and those responsible for the harm into communication, in an attempt to repair harm and finding positive ways forward). Careful consideration of the needs of the victims should be made in conjunction with the multidisciplinary team, including social workers, particularly when children are involved. Victims of mentally disordered offenders have rights to inquire about discharge planning through the Probation Service and treating teams have duties to <u>disclose information to victims</u> in certain circumstances (p.544).

Perpetrators as victims

Many perpetrators will have been <u>victimised</u> (p.179) themselves and experience high levels of posttraumatic symptoms. A substantial number of offenders have been victims of crime, in adulthood and childhood. Childhood abuse is associated with increased risk of developing personality and mood disorders in adulthood (see p.32). Psychological interventions should consider the relationship between traumas experienced and the index offence. The commission of the index offence may itself be traumatic, providing the trigger event for many forensic psychiatric inpatients with PTSD, especially family homicide. Suicide risk after family homicide remains high for perpetrators indefinitely.

Offender discharge/release into the community

Victim issues may sometimes determine that an offender is not permitted to return to their area upon discharge from hospital or prison, or there may be special restrictions put in place to protect the victim from contact.

Risk management

Risk management: general principles

Risk management is intimately related to risk assessment, and flows from it, even if some risk factors cannot be easily reduced or managed. These pages should therefore be read in close conjunction with those on risk assessment (p.163).

Treatment versus risk management as primary goals

There are important ethical differences between the primary goals and methods of treatment in psychiatry, and risk management; albeit one can serve the other. The primary aims of treatment (p.182) are to benefit the patient by improving mental health or reducing psychopathology and suffering; whereas the primary aim of risk management is to minimise the risk of harm to the patient or to others.

There is therefore unavoidable ethical tension (pp.322, 337, 339) within risk management because of the potential for conflict between the interests of the patient and of others. Risk management must therefore include ethical reflection, including upon the costs of measures proposed, such as perceived coercion (p.186), and their benefits, for the patient, and upon how any conflicting impacts upon the patient can be justified not only in terms of the patient's own benefit but also in terms of the benefits to others. Psychiatrists must show that they have conducted this ethical balance, and have explicitly discussed it with the patient (especially if the patient does not agree).

Principles of risk management

The following list is for guidance only. Some principles may conflict, and trade-offs may be necessary.

- Separate out the various **potential harms to the patient**, from **harms to others** and consider the risk (and the patient's perception) of each.
- Base the risk management plan on a careful risk assessment (p.163). Even in an emergency, you can carry out a basic risk assessment in your own mind within a few seconds, perhaps while walking to the scene.
- Apply the risk assessment, and particularly its actuarial (p.166) elements, in the context of your own understanding (e.g. your narrative formulation, p.147) of the patient.
- Take into account the setting in which the risk management plan is to be carried out (e.g. inpatient ward, prison, hostel, or patient's home).
- If the only risk assessment that can be carried out in the circumstances and time available is incomplete, make gathering further information part of the risk management plan, and update your assessment later; in the meantime, err on the side of caution (e.g. emphasising safety and security).
- Focus on both avoiding and preventing potential harms, and on a plan for dealing with them if they do occur.
- Treat underlying causes (especially mental disorder) whenever these can be identified, not just the problem symptoms or behaviours.
- Where there is a choice of actions to reduce risk, begin with those having the most positive, or least negative, impact upon the patient (e.g. in a plan for managing the risk of violence, prioritise problem-solving counselling sessions above seclusion; p.196).

- Only include actions that compromise the patient's freedom or that run contrary to their expressed wishes if they are **proportionate** and **justifiable** responses to the harms the plan aims to prevent, both technically and ethically.
- Bear in mind the legal context in which the plan will be carried out, and in particular whether any elements with which the patient does not agree are justified by a relevant legal power to act (e.g. under mental health (p.466) or mental capacity (p.522) legislation) and fall within local policies and codes of practice.
- Ensure that the whole team and the patient know and understand the plan, not just the individuals who compiled it. If there is conflict within the team, ensure that it is expressed and addressed, so that at least all members feel consulted.
- Work collaboratively with other agencies in managing risk (see p.252).
- Review the plan, and the underlying assessment, whenever the situation changes materially, and in any event at appropriate intervals (e.g. at ward rounds or CPA meetings), and more often if the plan involves significant additional restrictions on the patient's liberty.

Specific risks relevant to forensic psychiatry

See other specific risks addressed elsewhere:
- Risk of violence (p.240), including specific scenarios such as hostage-taking (p.244).
- Risk of sexually inappropriate behaviour (p.246).
- Risk of suicide and self-harm (p.248).
- Risk of absconding or escaping (p.250).
- Other specific risks (e.g. fire-setting, terrorism, stalking, or exploitation; pp. 42, 52, 178).

Management of violence

The following recommendations are drawn from NICE guidelines and the findings of homicide inquiries (p.598).

Risk assessment

A structured risk assessment (p.166) should form the basis of the risk management plan, including a formulation (p.146) of both disorder and violence. Then **keep the risk assessment continuously in mind:** think about how and when risk factors might change.

Mental illness and violence

- **Symptom control** can often directly reduce the risk of violence (see also p.44).
- Do not accept **noncompliance** with medication, or with other key aspects of the care plan—keep encouraging and/or enforcing compliance every day.
- Make use of the legal powers (pp.474, 510) available to ensure compliance with relevant aspects of the care plan.
- **Intervene early** when relapse is reasonably foreseeable. The law does not require relapse to have occurred before the patient can be recalled (p.589) or readmitted, as long as there is clear evidence that relapse, or other cause of enhanced risk related to mental disorder, is imminent if no action is taken.[1]
- Recognise that treatment and rehabilitation will often need to be **long-term.** For some patients, a series of brief admissions is of much less value than a prolonged admission, and can even be counter-productive.

Substance misuse and violence

Substance misuse alone can be a sole, or additional, reason justifying re-admission or recall; it can legally be the sole basis for recall if there is a clear history of illness relapse associated with the substance use. Whenever legal powers allow (e.g. under a restriction order (p.510) in E&W, or a community Compulsory Treatment Order (p.488) in Scotland), consider setting explicit **conditions** of abstinence and drug testing, with an explicit expectation that breach of the condition will lead to recall for inpatient reassessment.

Inpatients and violence

- On hospital wards, violence can be made less likely by well-designed physical environments; sufficient staff, space, and privacy; predictable routines; meaningful activities; and a sense of being respected and having a voice (see also p.289).

1 The definitions of 'mental disorder of a nature ... which warrants ... detention ... in hospital for assessment [for] the protection of other persons' in the E&W MHA, and in very similar terms in the MHNIO, and of 'mental disorder [causing] a serious likelihood of ... immediate and serious harm' in the RoI MHA, allow such early intervention. The Scottish requirement in the MHCTSA to demonstrate that it is likely that the mental disorder significantly impairs the patient's judgment makes early intervention slightly more difficult, as does the capacity test in the MCANI. See p.474.

- <u>Observation</u> of patients (p. 190), and **de-escalation** techniques (using body language and speech to calm a patient, then helping them to find a nonviolent solution to their problems) can reduce the chances of the patient becoming violent.

General advice

- Set **clear, operationalised criteria** for intervention and readmission/recall into the care plan. Make sure the patient knows those criteria; and stick to them.
- **Early intervention** when a patient with a history of violence behaves in a risky fashion, even if the mental state seems unchanged, is crucial. Do not rely solely on past clinical presentations; they may be falsely reassuring.
- Do not obsess about the 'correct diagnosis' with complex patients. Instead, focus on the treatment plan, risk assessment, and risk management plan, taking into account all the differential diagnoses.
- Take **carers' concerns** about risk, especially changes in risk, seriously; investigate and respond to them.
- General services should, when their risk assessment indicates a high risk of serious violence, make routine use of **forensic services** for advice.
- **Share assessments** of risk openly and honestly with the patient, carers and relevant services, within proper bounds of <u>confidentiality</u> (p.320).
- Remember that **risk of violence cannot be eliminated** (or even <u>predicted</u>, p.164), only minimised.

The management of specific violent incidents is described on p.242.

Managing acute behavioural disturbance

Sudden changes in behaviour may pose an immediate management problem, especially if they increase the risk of violence. Work collaboratively with other staff and seek help from senior or other colleagues and/or the police, unless you (and the colleagues with you) are sure you can manage the situation safely. Do not expose yourself, other staff or patients, to unnecessary risks.

On arriving at an incident

- Establish the nature of the incident before intervening (e.g. by telephone before arrival if time permits, or by speaking to other staff on arrival).
- If time allows, gather as much detailed information as possible, particularly if the patient or patients involved are previously unknown to you.
- If no colleagues are available to help, summon other assistance before intervening (e.g. by pressing an emergency call button on a hospital unit, or by shouting if others are nearby, or by mobile phone).
- Clear the area of other patients and inessential staff.

Speaking to the patient

- Make clear who you are, why you are there, and how you can help.
- Be calm, clear, honest, and respectful.
- Listen to what patients say, and observe their body language—try to understand how they feel as well as what they think.
- Empathise with their emotional state (this does not include agreeing with unreasonable things they might say or believe).
- Repeat information back to show you have understood.
- Allow patients to express themselves to you, and to see that you understand, before moving on to how to resolve the situation.
- Be clear about what cannot be avoided or negotiated away (e.g. giving up a weapon, accepting PRN medication), and focus instead on aspects over which the patient can safely be allowed to exercise choice (e.g. whether to take medication orally or intramuscularly, whether to acquiesce quietly or to be restrained by staff).
- Show that you are focused on solving the problems the patient presents, in an appropriate way (e.g. acknowledging their distress over the refusal of another patient to let them use their mobile phone, helping them to think through whether and when they might be able to use another phone, promising to assist with requesting leave if appropriate to use a payphone elsewhere once the patient is calm and the situation is under control).
- If the situation cannot be made safe by such de-escalation techniques, consider <u>restraining</u> the patient (p.196) to prevent further harm.

Once the incident is under control

- In the immediate aftermath of an incident on the ward, consider an increase in the <u>security level</u> (p.190) and the use of <u>seclusion</u> (p.196) or enhanced <u>observations</u> (p.190), if necessary.
- Treat any acute aspect of mental or physical disorder that may have impacted the situation (e.g. give food or fruit juice if hypoglycaemic; offer PRN medication for acute psychosis).

- Even if the patient is calm, consider asking them to have a period of 'time out' away from other patients if there is a risk of the situation re-escalating.
- Consider calling the police (if not already called), particularly if serious harm has been caused, or if there is an ongoing risk of further violence that cannot safely be dealt with.
- Consider facilitating the prosecution[2] of the patient (p.346) if their behaviour amounted to a criminal offence.
- Review the patient's **care plan**, if there is evidence of a link between the violent incident and their mental or physical disorder, their treatment, or the context of treatment.
- Document the incident, your actions, and colleagues', and the reasons for your actions, carefully in the patient's clinical record: this will encourage clarity of thought and provide a proper record available for future scrutiny.

After the incident

The experience of dealing with acute incidents can often be traumatic for staff, the patient, and other patients who witnessed it, especially if serious injury or harm was caused.

- Before staff leave after the incident, ensure that they obtain medical treatment for any injuries, and check whether they feel distressed in any way by the incident.
- Ensure that an appropriate person (e.g. the relevant manager if they were not involved in the incident, or a more senior manager) offers staff the opportunity to leave work if they are too distressed to continue working safely, arranges cover, and arranges counselling if needed.
- Apply the same principles to yourself—consider asking to go home if you are not fit to continue working, and consider requesting counselling through your Occupational Health department.
- Ensure that you or someone else completes an incident report according to local policies (this is in addition to documenting the incident in the patient's notes).
- Request, and take part in, a debriefing and/or critical incident review after the incident, if one is necessary.

---

2 This will usually require the victim to be willing to make a statement to police, but the police can accept evidence from others, and in exceptional circumstances (particularly cases of domestic violence) the CPS in E&W, the Procurator Fiscal in Scotland, and the NI Public Prosecution Service can prosecute without the agreement of the victim or chief witness. The RoI DPP does not appear to have a policy allowing prosecutions without the victim's consent, however.

Hostage situations

A hostage situation occurs where one or more persons are held against their will, without legal authority, in a location that is known to others; often the aim is to use hostages as 'bargaining chips' to coerce others to meet certain demands. Hostage situations may cause significant psychological and physical harm to the hostages and any witnesses. Forensic professionals may be asked to assess an individual who has previously taken a hostage during an index offence or a period of detention. They (rarely) may be asked to advise the police during a hostage event.

Assessment of risk

The assessment of the risk of hostage-taking should form part of every new admission to a secure mental health setting. If there is a previous history of hostage-taking, risk assessment should incorporate a detailed functional analysis of any such incidents. There is no empirical basis for specific risk prediction. However, the <u>HCR-20</u> (p.170) allows formulation and management of different relevant scenarios. Poor affect regulation (especially anger and hopelessness) may be risk factors for hostage-taking.

Hostage negotiation

This should be undertaken by trained negotiators, usually combined with police involvement and command. Negotiation with hostage-takers requires skill and training. It is essential for the role of the negotiator (who communicates directly with the hostage-taker) to be separate from the role of the incident commander (who has authority over the entire scene and personnel). The **longer the negotiations last**, the more likely a peaceful outcome.

The following factors are important considerations during the negotiation:
- **Motivation**. The hostage-taker will want to obtain something, usually something material, or an action by the authorities. However, hostage-taking may also reflect an attempt to influence an important person in the hostage-taker's life, like a partner or parent, or to intimidate or punish the hostage themselves. The motivation for the hostage-taking may not always be obviously rational and may be driven by high levels of emotion, especially if impulsive.
- **Risk**. If the hostage is a direct target (as in some prison or family hostage incidents), this may increase the risk to the hostage. Risk may also increase if the hostage-taker is suicidal or has recently had a relational loss of some kind. In mental health settings, negotiators will need information from clinicians to understand the hostage-taker's motivation and risk.
- **Planning and resources**. Hostage situations which are planned may differ from those which are impulsive in terms of demands, risk, and the resources held by the hostage-takers. Negotiators may need information from clinicians about the capacity of the hostage-taker to plan and carry out threats, their access to weapons, and so on.
- Ideally, both parties in the negotiation will show a **willingness to discuss the issues**. However, this cannot be assumed with all hostage-takers. The negotiator should not make dishonest or undeliverable offers.

Hostage responses to capture

Since the 1970s, there have been case reports of hostages forming positive attachments to their captors, as a defence against fear and vulnerability, especially if their captivity is prolonged. The evidence for a specific syndrome (such as the so-called Stockholm syndrome) is limited; reports of this are confounded by the reality of the need for hostages to try and make personal relationships with their captors in order to survive. It is much more common for hostages to experience extreme and persistent terror which results in PTSD and associated disorders (p.96).

Role of the psychiatrist in hostage negotiation

- In a mental health setting, the hostage-taker's psychiatrist may not always be the best person to negotiate with the hostage-taker; the primary nurse or someone altogether independent may be better.
- A forensic psychiatrist may act as a consultant to a negotiating team (as in the Lindt Café siege in Sydney in 2014), but there is a risk of exceeding one's competence unless one has been trained to undertake this task.
- If the hostage-taker is a known patient, the hostage-taker's treating psychiatrist may breach confidentiality to provide the negotiator with relevant information about the patient's mental state and personal circumstances if it is considered that the disclosure will bring about an early end to the incident and save the lives of the hostages.

The termination phase

This is brief and can have three outcomes:
- the hostage-taker surrenders peacefully (the usual outcome in secure mental health care);
- the hostage-taker is captured, harmed, or killed; or
- the hostage-taker's demands are met and the hostage-taker escapes, usually to be pursued by police.

Postincident support and advice

All those involved (including the perpetrator) are at risk of developing stress reactions, and some kind of immediate postincident support is helpful. Further support may be needed during critical incident reviews, and any associated external or internal inquiries. For perpetrators, failed hostage situations may intensify shame and hopelessness and increase suicide risk.

Managing problematic sexual behaviour

Exactly what amounts to such behaviour is socially defined and contextual: for example commenting on a person's sexual attractiveness might be problematic on wards but acceptable at home amongst friends. In addition to legally defined sexual offences, problematic sexual behaviour in psychiatric contexts often includes:

• Exposure (not necessarily of genitals).
• Inquiries about other people's sexual behaviour.
• Requests for sex.
• Remarks on sexual desire.
• Inappropriately sexualised language.
• Comments on the appearance of others.
• Pornography.
• Prostitution.
• Inappropriate sexual relationships (e.g. between a patient and staff member, or a prisoner and prison officer).
• Sexual contact with other vulnerable patients who lack capacity to consent to it.

Diagnostic associations

• Sexual offending arising from <u>sexual attitudes and behaviour</u> (p.128) combined with a comorbid mental disorder
• Disinhibition secondary to mania, psychosis, or neurological disorder
• Socially inappropriate behaviours associated with intellectual disability
• Hypersexuality in dementia

Approach to management

Management should be based on <u>formulation</u> (p.146) of potential problematic sexual behaviour and its <u>motivation</u> (p.62). For instance, offenders with 'avoidance goals' (who recognise offending is wrong but use inappropriate coping tactics in high-risk situations) require a different approach from those with 'approach goals' (who deliberately set out to commit sexual offences).

• Take a multidisciplinary (and multiagency) approach.
• Identify the problematic behaviours and related factors such as mental state, substance use, environment, and cognition.
• Gather detailed background information from multiple agencies.
• Analyse the nature, frequency, and circumstances of behaviours (e.g. within the antecedents, behaviours, consequences, the ABC) model).
• Target interventions based on the formulation, with measurement of the intervention's likely impact on nature, frequency, and severity.

Interventions

Many of these are only appropriate for convicted sex offenders.

Pharmacological

• Treatment of underlying mental disorder.
• Hormonal drugs that <u>suppress libido</u> (p.201) may be helpful as an adjunct to psychological treatment if the person has high levels of sexual arousal, masturbation, and preoccupation with sexual fantasies interfering with daily life—but evidence of effectiveness is extremely weak.

- Other medications that affect libido such as SSRIs may occasionally assist treatment of offenders with <u>paraphilic disorder</u> (p.102).
- A stepwise approach is recommended when considering antilibidinal drugs, beginning with drugs with the fewest side-effects.

Psychological treatment programmes
- The risk, need, responsivity theory for managing sex offenders matches treatment to the offenders' risk of reoffending and their strengths, and identifies criminogenic needs.
- Relapse prevention models focus on identifying high-risk situations that could lead to reoffending, and on eliminating dynamic risk factors including cognitive distortions.
- The <u>Good Lives Model</u> (p.220) of sexual offending is a strengths-based approach. The focus is on enabling the offenders to lead a different kind of life ('the new me'): achieving their goods without recourse to offending.
- The Sex Offender Treatment Programme (SOTP) is a group cognitive-behavioural programme usually delivered in prison, by prison staff and psychologists. SOTP in prisons and the community has now been replaced in E&W by a strengths-based programme called Horizon.
- <u>Multisystemic therapy</u> (MST-PSB, p.218) has the strongest evidence for managing problematic sexual behaviour in adolescent sex offenders.

Other
- Legal <u>sanctions</u> (p.442) can be used to manage risk of sexual offending.
- Local volunteer projects for supporting sex offenders in the community have developed since the 1990s. They focus on social isolation and loneliness as risk factors for reoffending. These projects also offer social support and reintegration with the goal of reducing reoffending.
- Compulsory polygraph ('lie detector') tests have been piloted in the UK since 2014 after research demonstrated their role in facilitating information disclosure by serious sex offenders who are managed by probation in the community, alerting offender managers to possible deception, and focusing risk management work. They are currently used for high-risk sex offenders released from prison on licence.

Managing the risk of suicide & self-harm

General psychiatrists tend to possess particular expertise in managing the risk of suicide and self-harm, and may be consulted if necessary.[3] However, forensic psychiatrists also need to be familiar with its management. Forensic psychiatrists may also be asked to advice on suicide in the context of deaths in custody (p.598).

Working with patients who want to harm or kill themselves

• Treat the underlying mental disorder.
• Include safety plans and other risk-reduction measures in the care plan.
• Allow twenty-four-hour access to staff (e.g. via a crisis phone number).
• Offer crisis resolution, such as problem-solving counselling.
• Consider admission to hospital, movement to an observation cell if in the police station, or transfer to the healthcare wing if in prison.
• If the risk is acute, consider enhanced observation (p.190).

Safety measures in hospitals and prisons

• Consider the use of multiagency partnerships for suicide prevention.
• Minimise availability of means of suicide or self-harm so far as is appropriate and possible in the setting.
• Use special ligature-free cells or rooms where available.
• Ensure provision of services for employment and support with debt and social isolation.
• Refer high-risk prisoners to a peer-support scheme (e.g. Listeners) and/or request that they be placed on a prison observation system (e.g. ACCT, Assessment, Care in Custody and Treatment in E&W).
• Observe medication being taken to prevent stockpiling for overdose.
• In secure mental health units, search visitors, patients after leave, and rooms as necessary to prevent acquisition or fashioning of means of suicide or self-harm.

Managing suicide attempts and self-harm

• Take immediate life-saving measures as necessary.
• Assess the situation rapidly and determine what has taken place (in particular, if an overdose is suspected, establish what has been taken and how much, including by asking the person if conscious, and searching the immediate area for bottles and packs).
• Transfer people who have swallowed objects or inserted them into their anus, vagina, or other orifices to A&E for investigation, and specialist removal, which may involve surgery.
• If transferring to A&E, send a summary of diagnosis, current mental state, legal status, risks, and management plan, with a suitable trained escort.
• If not transferring to A&E, ensure frequent appropriate monitoring of the patient and consider investigations as needed (e.g. U&E, LFTs, or specific drug levels after overdose).

---

3 Useful information may also be found in the *Oxford Handbook of Psychiatry*, or a general psychiatry textbook.

- Only suture wounds or treat other injuries if you are confident that your skills are sufficiently good and up-to-date; a cosmetically sensitive area is not involved; and no deep structures (nerves, tendons, or blood vessels) might be affected.
- Consider the nature of <u>post-incident interventions</u> (p.245) for staff and other patients/prisoners after the situation has been made safe.

Absconding, escape and other risks

Detained patients may not leave the secure perimeter without permission. Unauthorised departures include **absconding** (being outside the perimeter without permission) and **escape** (leaving by breaching security, e.g. climbing over a wall). If patients are deemed to be at high risk of escape or absconding, they may need to be managed in a higher security level (p.190).

Managing absconding or escape risks begins with a risk assessment for absconding or escape (p.179). This should include attention to **peak occasions** for escape or absconding (e.g. after conviction; when opportunity arises, such as when attending court or hospital for medical treatment); and **history** of escape or absconding. Risk assessment should also attend to **personal risk factors** such as family breakup, issues pertaining to children, or illness in relatives. Lastly, the assessment should consider potential **harms after absconding**, including suicide and harm to identifiable victims which might justify breach of confidentiality (p.320).

Risk management interventions

The key risk management intervention is granting or withholding leave (p.191), or setting terms of leave (e.g. number of escorts, duration, or destination). Escape risk is reduced using the appropriate level of security (p.190) and observations (p.190). Risk management plans incorporating such measures reduced absconding rates by 25% in one group of hospitals.

- Two studies of absconding suggested that the peak time is early afternoon, when nursing shifts change. Increased vigilance during handovers may reduce risk of absconding.
- The first few days and weeks after admission, after renewal of detention or receiving other bad news, or after transfer from another ward or unit are periods of increased risk of absconding or escape.
- Leave should be planned in advance considering staff numbers available.
- Every period of leave should be logged when planned, when the patient leaves, and when they return.
- A description of patients and their clothing on the day, and any contraband items signed out to them (e.g. mobile phones), should be made before they leave.
- Escorting staff should have a means of summoning assistance while out on leave (e.g. a mobile phone with relevant numbers pre-set).
- Leave terms should be relaxed gradually (e.g. increasing duration, or reductions in escort number).
- Staff should have a method of contacting patients on unescorted leave (e.g. a mobile phone given to the patient for the period of leave).
- Staff on the ward should be actively aware of when the patient is due to return, and should have a predetermined protocol to follow if they do not return on time. The sooner absconding is detected, the greater the chance of locating the patient quickly.
- Wards should have up-to-date photographs of patient and information about next-of-kin and contact information of any known associates or locations they are likely to visit.

After a patient has absconded or escaped

Without delay, the staff member detecting the incident should:
- Notify the police, giving them the description of the patients and their clothing, a brief risk assessment and information on their mental state, their legal status, the time and location where they were last known to be, and any other relevant information (e.g. addresses where they might have gone).
- Inform senior colleagues, who will:
  - Consider sending appropriately trained staff to a location where the patient is thought to be—if it is safe.
  - Consider informing potential victims.
  - Make plans for managing the patient upon return (e.g. admitting the patient to a more secure ward, if appropriate).
  - Request a postincident debriefing.
  - Managing other specific risks.

The general principles of risk management (p.238) apply to a range of behaviours associated with risk.

Fire-setting

When a patient is assessed as at significant risk of fire-setting (p.178):
- A functional analysis of previous incidents of fire-setting should be undertaken to understand the motivation, risk factors, as well as any relationship with mental disorder or mental state. A summary of this analysis should be recorded in the risk management plans.
- There should be regular room searches to ensure there are no materials in patients' rooms that could be used to set fires (e.g. newspaper; the absence of matches or a lighter should not be too reassuring as they might be acquired, or an electric socket used).
- Smoking and lighter use should be supervised.

Following an incident of fire-setting on a ward, depending on the damage, other patients may need to be moved increasing distress and other risks, such as escape (p.250). Both staff and patients will need to be debriefed.

The Firesetting Intervention Programme for Prisoners and Firesetting Intervention Programme for Mentally Disordered Offenders (FIP-MO) are two UK psychological treatment programmes for adults who have committed arson. However, it is not clear how effective they are or what factors predict future risk of fire-setting. There is some evidence that arsonists may have poorer social and relational skills than other offenders, implying that work on self-esteem and assertiveness may reduce the risk of future fire-setting.

Exploitation or victimisation

Where an incident of apparent abuse (physical, sexual, material, financial, or emotional abuse; neglect; discrimination; or institutional mistreatment) indicates that a vulnerable adult (e.g. a psychiatric patient) is at risk of exploitation or victimisation, the care team in the UK have a duty to follow the Safeguarding of Vulnerable Adults (SoVA, p.590) policy in force in their local area.

In Scotland, there are also legal powers (p.542) to remove a vulnerable adult to a hospital or other place of safety, and to ban people who may be endangering them from having contact with them.

Working with police & other non-health agencies

Forensic mental health systems commonly have to pursue multiagency working; the collaboration of individuals from different professional backgrounds, organisations, and services, usually having varying primary purposes but with the shared aim of improving public safety. Hence, they often need to work with the police and other non-health agencies as part of a risk management plan, particularly where the patient is, or is planned to be, in the community. This raises technical, legal and ethical issues (p.314).

General principles

Whatever the legal or administrative structure, if any, under which you are working with other agencies, the same general principles apply:

- Although you may be co-operating on a specific issue, health services and criminal justice agencies explicitly adopt different, potentially conflicting, primary goals (p.352). For example, when working with the probation service (p.584), your aim will be to promote the patient's welfare, whereas the probation service's will be to protect the public, which may lead them to use more coercive methods than you would sanction.
- The primary legal and ethical duties that apply in your normal clinical work continue to apply when working jointly with other agencies.
- Most notably, you continue to owe your patient a duty of confidentiality (p.320), and you cannot disclose confidential information about them to partner agencies unless you have their consent, or permissible grounds for disclosure exist. The basis for breach of confidence is not 'need to know' (a health-related concept) but 'significant risk of serious harm to the public' (*Egdell*, p.754).
- Other agencies are not subject to the same duties as you, and may use your information or assistance for purposes that would amount to breaches of your duties to your patient.
- In preparing documents for inter-agency working, always do so in accordance your duty of confidentiality. Never disclose whole clinical reports, only selected information directly relevant to public protection.
- Always satisfy yourself as to what will be done with your information, or assistance, before disclosing it.

Public protection meetings

MAPPA (p.592) arrangements in the UK provide a mechanism for agencies to work together in the management of the risk of harm to others posed by certain offenders, including certain MDOs. However, joint working with other agencies with offenders not covered by MAPPA is still possible under informal or ad hoc co-operation arrangements, guided by the principles set out above.

Multi-Agency Risk Assessment Conferences (MARAC)

In a fashion similar to the MAPPA, inter-agency working to protect vulnerable individuals, particularly victims of domestic violence, is now commonplace, and most areas of the UK now have a standing MARAC for discussing and co-ordinating agencies' safeguarding (p.590) and other plans.

Multi-Agency Sexual Exploitation meeting (MASE)

A MASE meeting is held when a child/young person is deemed medium or high risk of sexual exploitation. Professionals will work together to assess the risk and develop strategies needed to reduce risk, which may include disruption tactics to suspected perpetrators.

Working with voluntary agencies

Many voluntary organisations are created out of a desire to work with the most excluded members of society. The relationship between these and mentally disordered offenders may be complex and can present ethical and ideological dilemmas for the volunteers working for these organisations.

Public health approach to violence

The public health approach provides a framework for understanding and preventing violence. Central to this is the implementation of interventions that successfully address risk and protective factors in individuals, families, communities, and populations, aimed towards reducing violence at a community and/or population level. Hence the World Health Organisation has proposed that violence should be addressed by pursuing a strategic, coordinated approach involving a range of agencies, including partnerships between statutory and voluntary organisations.

Forensic
psychiatric services

The structure of forensic services

Forensic psychiatric services in the UK and RoI include services that inreach into the criminal justice system (CJS, p.566), and specialist services for high-risk patients with mental disorder who need secure inpatient care and/or community supervision.

Inreach into the CJS

Each of the services in Table 8.1 has access to different kinds of forensic psychiatric service, which vary between (and within) jurisdictions. Some 'forensic' services are provided by general adult psychiatric services.

Table 8.1 CJS institutions and their forensic psychiatric services

Police stations	Police liaison CPNs (p.269)
Courts	Court diversion teams (p.268)
Prisons & YOIs	Prison inreach & inpatient service (p.270)
Probation services	Various, see below

A range of forensic services liaise with probation services (p.584). Probation services often run behavioural group programmes for offenders; some forensic psychiatric services offer similar groups, particularly psychology-led behavioural programmes for sex offenders, and these may be organised jointly with the probation service and/or accept referrals from it. Other services, such as Offenders with PD Pathfinder teams in E&W, offer liaison and advice to probation officers.

Secure psychiatric services

In parallel with general psychiatric services, forensic services comprise the following main components:
• Secure hospital wards: low, medium and high (p.258);
• Outpatient clinics, particularly for forensic psychology; and
• Community forensic services (p.266).

Forensic services accept patients from general adult services, prisons, courts, and (rarely) the community. A significant proportion of patients at each level of security (and in the community) will have 'stepped up' or 'stepped down' from another level. In addition, there are highly specialised services, often in the independent sector, such as for patients with autistic spectrum disorders (p.104) or who have suffered traumatic brain injury (p.112).

Parallel or integrated services?

Regional and local secure forensic services were not established until the late 1980s.[1] Forensic services are low-volume, high-cost services which only manage high-risk patients. They gatekeep secure beds, which can lead to disputes with other parts of the mental health service. Conversely, general

1 Following the recommendations of the Glancy and Butler reports (pp.780, 781) in 1974.

services are often reluctant to take patients directly from secure care because of concerns about persisting risk. This is particularly true of patients with both psychosis and personality disorder.

The existence of separate general and forensic services has led to the following questions, which have been answered in different ways in different parts of the UK and RoI:
• Should general inpatient wards expect to receive patients from forensic services before discharge, or should forensic services manage them until they are ready for discharge to the community?
• Should forensic inpatient services discharge their patients to the care of general community teams, or should Community Forensic Teams (p.266) be established?
• Should low secure wards be within general services or forensic services, or within both?

In some parts of E&W there are Trusts that offer a full range of forensic services, including community teams; in Scotland and RoI, by contrast, forensic services are largely confined to central secure hospitals.

Overall, secure services attract a disproportionate proportion of national mental health budgets; in E&W, some 20% of the budget is spent on the fewer than 10,000 patients who occupy secure beds.

Secure hospital settings

A secure hospital or unit is one with the capacity to detain patients who pose a significant risk of harm to others, restrict their movement and activities, and prevent escape. Security level (p.256) is a function of physical architecture, procedures, and relational factors such as numbers of staff, and is defined in most cases by government specifications. There are three main levels of security: high, medium, and low.

High-security hospitals

The number of high secure beds has fallen as those at other levels have risen, and there are now approximately 1,000 in the UK and RoI. They now admit only those whose mental state and behaviour pose a **grave and immediate** risk of serious harm to the public (including healthcare professionals) that cannot safely be managed at a lower level of security. There are five high-security hospitals:

• Ashworth Hospital in Merseyside (228 beds, men);
• Broadmoor Hospital in Berkshire (212 beds, men);
• Central Mental Hospital in Dundrum,[2] County Dublin (102 beds, mixed);
• Rampton Hospital in Nottinghamshire (322 beds, mixed); and
• State Hospital in Carstairs, Lanarkshire (144 beds, men).

Some wards at the State Hospital specialise in patients with intellectual disability (p.110), as do some units at Rampton Hospital, which also has a specialist unit for deaf patients.

Average length of stay at high-security hospitals has increased in recent years, partly because lower-risk patients who need shorter admissions are no longer admitted there, and partly because better physical healthcare means that persistently high-risk patients who cannot be discharged are living longer (25% of the high secure population have been detained for over ten years).

Medium security (Regional Secure Units)

There are approximately 3,500 medium secure beds in the UK & RoI, with around 50% provided in the independent sector. The largest number of medium secure beds are for men; there are also beds for women, for adolescents, and for men or women with intellectual disability.

The average length of stay in MSUs is rising; with 19% remaining for more than five years. Medium secure services admit from general services, low and high secure services, and prisons. Reduction in general community and inpatient services may contribute to increasing length of stay, as well as the increasing number of prison transfers who require higher security.

Women's Enhanced Medium Secure Services (WEMSS)

WEMSS exist to replace physical security with enhanced procedural and relational security measures to the maximum extent possible. There are forty-six beds in three WEMSS units across E&W, in London, Manchester, and Leicester. They were developed in response to two observations:

2 Due to be replaced in 2022 by a larger hospital in nearby Portrane, with 170 beds (of which fewer than half will be high secure in all aspects).

- many women in high secure hospitals had not committed offences warranting detention in high security, but
- their behaviour was too disruptive to the environment of standard women's medium secure wards for them to be transferred there.

Low security

Services that amount to more than a general psychiatric ward with a locked door, but that do not meet the specifications for medium security, are loosely described as 'low secure'. In 2013, there were estimated to be around 2,500 such beds in the UK.

Diagnoses of borderline and antisocial personality disorder, in addition to severe psychotic or mood disorders, are common amongst patients admitted to low secure ward. Some services offer beds to support PICU services; others offer them as stepdown rehabilitation from medium secure services. Many low secure units are indistinguishable from locked rehabilitation wards. Some low secure units are part of specialist forensic services (so that patients must be at risk of harming others, even if also themselves), with staff having specialist forensic skills; others sit within general services.

Special provision in secure settings

Personality disorder and the Offender Personality Disorder (OPD) pathway

Secure hospital services in the UK[3] specifically for people with personality disorder form part of the OPD pathway.[4] The OPD strategy was commissioned to improve identification and assessment of offenders with PD, providing psychologically informed services for the most high-risk and complex cases. One of its main aims is to ensure many more offenders with PD are treated in prison settings, with transfer to hospital only for those unable to benefit from the prison service.

Women's services

Even the highest-risk women very rarely pose a grave and immediate risk of serious harm to the public (as opposed to being difficult to care for in general women's secure services), and there has therefore been a general move to avoid admitting them to <u>high-security</u> (p.258) units. Instead, they are cared for in specialist medium secure units (e.g. <u>WEMSS</u> in E&W, p.258), and specialist prison units.

Intellectual disability (ID) services

There is one high secure hospital, Rampton Hospital, and several medium secure units for this population across the UK plus at the Central Mental Hospital in RoI. Some specialist community services are now being developed. There is also little provision for those in the 'borderline' range of intellectual functioning who have deficits in social skills; this group tends to be overlooked by both general and forensic psychiatric services.

Autism spectrum disorders (ASD) services

Offenders with ASDs often find themselves in generic forensic secure settings, where they can be difficult to manage, or in intellectual disability services if this is also diagnosed. There are a few providers in E&W that cater specifically for patients with ASDs, both with and without intellectual disability, mainly in the independent sector.

Acquired brain injury (ABI) services

As with individuals with ID and ASDs, individuals with ABI may be treated in mainstream forensic services or nonforensic ABI units. There are a limited number of forensic specialist services for people with complex physical, cognitive, and functional difficulties that typically follow brain injury, who demonstrate socially inappropriate behaviour and need medium or low security; they are mainly in the independent sector in E&W.

---

3 RoI, with lower patient numbers, does not have diagnosis-specific secure services (except for patients with intellectual disability).

4 This replaced the discredited former Dangerous and Severely Personality Disordered (<u>DSPD</u>, p.15) programme.

Deaf services

Deaf and hard-of-hearing patients suffer a greater lifetime prevalence of mental disorder (40% as against 25% by one estimate), but can struggle in mainstream psychiatric service because of the oral nature of many therapies, and because the vast majority of staff are unable to communicate using sign language, and lack awareness of aspects of deaf psychology and culture. Three specialist general psychiatric services for deaf patients cover the UK between them. In addition, at least three independent sector hospitals provide specialist secure units for deaf people, alongside Rampton Hospital.

Older prisoners

An ageing prison population has created a range of policy and practice issues for prisons and secure mental health services. Older prisoners' physical, social, and psychological needs are complex. Prisons designed for fit, healthy adults have to adjust to the unplanned and unexpected roles of care home and even hospice. Increasingly, prison staff are having to manage not just ageing prisoners, but end of life issues. Secure services may struggle to provide care for prisoners who suffer dementias, and there may be insufficient secure beds for those prisoners/patients who cannot be rehabilitated into the community.

Adolescent forensic services

In E&W, which has extensive facilities for the <u>detention of children</u> (p.580), a small number of specialist secure psychiatric units have been developed for adolescents. These aim to divert some adolescent mentally disordered offenders from custody. They often face difficulty in transferring patients to appropriate facilities, particularly community services, when they reach eighteen years of age.

Scotland,[5] NI, and RoI[6] currently have no secure inpatient units specifically for adolescents, who must therefore be treated in secure children's homes or adult psychiatric units.

5 Until a new twelve-bed adolescent secure unit opened at Woodland View, Ayrshire in 2021.
6 Until a new unit in Portrane, County Dublin, opens in 2022.

Gender identity issues in secure care

The sex difference in relation to violent offending is stark: 80% of violent offenders are male. Some have argued that genes on the Y chromosome confer some extra risk for violence (in interaction with other factors such as poverty and substance misuse). However, it is also argued that gender role stereotypes about masculinity confer increased risk; especially the 'toxic masculinity' which is associated with denigration of vulnerability and a strong sense of entitlement. There is no evidence that transgender status alone is a risk factor for violence or criminality, though it may interact with other risk factors; nor any evidence that changing gender alters risk.

Transgender people in secure inpatient care

Like being homosexual, being transgender is not a mental disorder. Transgender people are at higher risk for some mental disorders, including gender dysphoria: that is, psychological distress arising from incongruence between the gender they identify with and their sex assigned at birth. There is no evidence that gender dysphoria is associated with any increased risk of criminality and violence.

Teams may need to distinguish those people who feel uncomfortable with the gender in which they were raised, and seek psychological help for this, from those who seek to transition into a new identity. Not everyone with concerns about their gender identity will wish to transition surgically or hormonally, but those who seek to do so should be supported with access to the services with appropriate expertise. A Gender Recognition Certificate (GRC) allows a person to change their legal gender by self-determination in RoI, or after a medical assessment and living consistently with their gender for two years in the UK (regardless of whether they decide to change their body).

In secure services, some patients will seek to transition as part of their recovery and care pathway. This is a complex area, with little research to guide clinicians. Although the desire to transition is not itself evidence of mental disorder, any associated risks can be hard to assess in the context of severe mental illness and personality dysfunction. It is also known that trans-individuals are at increased risk of being bulled and abused, and services need to be alert to <u>safeguarding</u> (p.590).

Transgender people in prison

Forensic psychiatrists may occasionally be asked to assess prisoners who either have transitioned before admission to prison or who seek to do so while in prison. The numbers of identified trans-prisoners has greatly increased in the last decade, with a much greater increase in numbers of transwomen than transmen. In E&W, HMPPS updated its policy framework and guidance about the management of trans-prisoners and the importance of respect for their legal rights in 2020, and closed a special prison unit for transwomen in favour of an integrated system. Transgender Case Boards review the needs of trans-prisoners, and consider transfers based on rights and risk. They can determine the location of a transgender prisoner lacking a GRC (those with GRCs are located based on their identified gender). In Scotland, guidelines state that transgender patients without a GRC should be housed with the gender with which they identify.

There are well-publicised cases of transwomen who have completed suicide after admission to male prisons. There are also well-publicised cases of transwomen prisoners who have sexually assaulted other prisoners in female prisons, and a relatively high proportion of transwomen have been convicted of sexual offences,[7] although they nevertheless pose a low risk of violence to others. A multidisciplinary approach to assessment and management in partnership with prison authorities is recommended, to minimise the risk of stigma.

7 According to the UK Centre for Crime and Justice Studies, 48% compared to 19% of the general male prisoner population and 2% of the ciswomen prisoner population.

Rehabilitation & recovery

Earlier models of work with forensic patients and offenders were socially excluding and stigmatising. Recovery and rehabilitation emphasise personal responsibility and social inclusion.

The **recovery model** is based on a model in addiction services. It assumes that people with mental illnesses can be rehabilitated back into society even if they still have symptoms and problems. The recovery model emphasises individuality and personal values; it encourages professionals to understand the patients' experience in terms of their personal narrative, as opposed to defining them by their diagnosis or offence.

Rehabilitation in offender care involves attention to both risk reduction and managing offender identity. Models such as the Good Lives Model (p.220) and the Desistance Model resemble recovery models in that they emphasise attention to personal agency and values and focus on pro-social activities with others.

Core principles

- Recovery is an essential part of the rehabilitation of mentally disordered offenders.
- All individuals have the capacity to learn and grow.
- Wherever possible, forensic patients should be helped to re-establish pro-social community roles that promote reintegration, including education and work.
- Personal support networks are vital to both recovery and rehabilitation.
- Attention to the individual's personal goals and values is key.
- Whenever possible, forensic patients should be helped to exercise autonomy and agency in relation to their mental illness and risk to others.
- All individuals should be treated with respect and dignity.
- Diagnoses are used only to inform treatment and not to discriminate against service users.
- Culture and ethnicity play an important role in recovery as sources of strength and enrichment for the individual and services.
- Interventions should be person-centred, and focus on strengths and resilience.

Barriers to implementation in forensic psychiatry

The core principles may be particularly difficult to achieve with forensic patients who continue to hold antisocial values. Recovery and rehabilitation may be compromised by concerns about security and risk, which may also lead to perceived coercion (p.186); with a risk of staff exhibiting 'double speak'. Also:

- The court or the Ministry of Justice may impose mandatory requirements on the individual to receive treatment or complete intervention programmes, which challenge the duty to respect patient autonomy wherever possible.
- Similarly, legal restrictions may interfere with optimal recovery and rehabilitation programmes.

- Attention to risk management often conflicts with patient autonomy and may mandate interventions that increase social exclusion.
- Stigma surrounding patients' offences may mar their social identity, so that they are excluded from their communities (e.g. murder, rape).
- Justice agencies and mental health tribunals may not understand recovery and rehabilitation, but focus only on medication as 'treatment'.
- Secure services may lack trained staff who can deliver psychosocial rehabilitation and recovery, which delays and undermines a culture of recovery.

Community forensic services

Historically, forensic psychiatry was an almost exclusively institutionally focused subspecialty, originating in prisons and special (high secure) hospitals, later extending to a network of medium secure, and then low secure units. The prevailing model was that patients were detained in hospital until their risk to others, and themselves, was deemed to be sufficiently low for them to be discharged to general psychiatric services in the community. Small numbers of patients discharged from medium and low secure units to the community were kept on as outpatients by their inpatient forensic consultants, but this was the exception rather than the rule; arising often from refusal of general services to accept them.

However, the greater resources given to forensic services from the early 1990s (driven by political and public concern over the risks to the public thought to be posed by mentally disordered patients) allowed for some experimentation in service models, and forensic services began to develop explicit and more substantial community forensic services in many areas; recognising that risk management was potentially much more difficult in the community than in a secure hospital unit.

How are CFTs different from general CMHTs?

In contrast to CMHTs, and even assertive community teams for general psychiatric patients, community forensic teams:
- work assertively with a small caseload[8] of patients;
- expect to treat patients with personality disorder (p.78), comorbid substance misuse, and challenging behaviours (p.108);
- expect treatment to last much longer, and a minority of patients to remain in their care indefinitely, sometimes for regular contact and review of risk and mental state even after all treatment options have been exhausted; and
- expect to deal regularly with other agencies such as probation services (p.584) and the police (p.570), and to take an active role in multiagency public protection arrangements (MAPPA, p.592).

Advantages & disadvantages of community forensic teams

Specialised services allow staff to develop more specialised skills, and confidence in working with high-risk patients and with the criminal justice system. Moreover, having earmarked budgets for such services can permit staff to maintain the small caseloads per staff member necessary for intensive work with certain mentally disordered offenders.

However, a parallel system of services for often-unpopular patients can encourage stigmatisation of those patients, and can lead to pressure for all similar unpopular patients to be referred to, and accepted by that service. As there is no consensus on the entry criteria a mental health patient should meet to enter the care of a forensic mental health team as opposed to a general mental health team, disagreements can be difficult to resolve.

---

8 The Royal College of Psychiatrists and others have recommended a caseload size of ten to twelve patients for assertive outreach and CFT practitioners, as compared with twenty-five to thirty for CMHT practitioners.

Recruitment of staff with skills and enthusiasm in violence risk assessment to specialist services can result in 'de-skilling' of general services. As mental health patients generally only become 'forensic' patients after they have been violent, an ability to assess risk of violence is important for all mental health professionals.

Whether the advantages of CFTs outweigh the disadvantages can depend on the threshold for accepting patents into the community forensic team in a local area, and the degree to which CFTs offers consultation and joint working to other local community teams.

Community forensic service models

- The **integrated model**: staff with special training in forensic psychiatry work within general community mental health teams (CMHTs).
- The **parallel model**: specialist community forensic teams (CFTs) exist separately from CMHTs.
- An **intermediate** between these two models, such as one in which specialist forensic psychiatric staff have their own team base but are managed jointly with CMHT staff.
- The **outreach model**: inpatient staff working at the regional secure unit provide community psychiatric services to their discharged forensic psychiatric patients, maximising continuity of care at the expense of having enough community patients per team to develop into a full CFT.

Many CFTs include elements of both parallel and integrated models, providing case management and treatment for their own forensic community patients as well as consultancy work for general community services, in the form of one-off assessments, advice, and guidance.

Diversion services

Mentally disordered defendants have since time immemorial been excused punishment and/or transferred to hospital in Britain and Ireland, albeit haphazardly: insane (p.620) defendants were sometimes committed to an asylum, sometimes put in the care of their family, and sometimes left to their own devices. After the passing of the Criminal Lunatics Act 1800,[9] defendants found insane were indefinitely committed to Bethlem Royal Hospital and, later, Broadmoor Hospital (p.258).

The diversionary options available to courts (and the police) have grown enormously since then, and now include those listed below, some of which allow legal proceedings to continue.

Pre-court diversion

On arrest, the police may take an apparently mentally disordered person to hospital or another approved place for assessment (see p.494).

At the police station, the police (or designated healthcare professional, p.572) may request a mental health assessment. If admission is then recommended, the custody sergeant[10] may release the person, to be admitted either voluntarily or under section (p.474), in which case there will be no criminal prosecution. Alternatively, they may bail (p.398) them to hospital, whether or not they have also been sectioned, in which case the person may potentially be charged and prosecuted at a later date.

The **prosecutor** (p.566) has discretion to require the police not to charge, or to drop charges already laid, at any pretrial stage, depending on the seriousness of the charge and the public interest (p.347) in prosecution.

Diversion from court

Before or during trial, a court can remand (p.398) a defendant to hospital for assessment (p.498) or treatment (p.500), and may suspend the legal proceedings until the assessment is complete. If the assessed mental disorder renders defendants unfit to plead or stand trial (p.602), they may be admitted to hospital, released, or made the subject of supervision in the community, and prosecution may be discontinued, or suspended until they become fit to plead.

Upon conviction, a court may also remand defendants to hospital for psychiatric assessment and compilation of a presentence report (p.584). It can also sentence (p.500) defendants to detention in hospital instead of punishing them (or in addition to punishing them, in the case of hospital directions and hybrid orders, p.670).

Diversion from prison

If prison staff believe that remand or sentenced prisoners are mentally disordered and require treatment in hospital, they can request transfer to hospital (p.506). Different rules apply depending on whether the transfer is before or after sentence.

---

9 The Act was introduced four days after the trial of James Hadfield, who had attempted to kill George III but was acquitted by reason of insanity. The authorities were worried that he might try again to kill the King and passed the Act to ensure his retrospective detention despite his acquittal.

10 In Ireland, the member of the Garda Síochána in charge of the police station.

Psychiatric liaison & diversion teams

Since 1989, many criminal courts across the UK and RoI have had access to specialist psychiatric teams that can perform brief psychiatric assessments at court, and arrange admission to hospital on behalf of the court, subject to the court's agreement. Some of the courts that do not have a diversion team can 'cross-remand' defendants to another local court that does. In more recent years, such liaison & diversion services have been extended to police custody suites in many areas, where psychiatric staff can conduct initial psychiatric assessments and advise police officers and FMEs (p.572) on diversion.

One Home Office review demonstrated that psychiatric diversion teams can quadruple the rate of detected mental disorder, and reduce the time from arrest to admission by a factor of seven.

There are no generally accepted standards for the composition and functioning of such teams, and they vary from a lone CPN giving oral advice to magistrates, to multidisciplinary teams that can produce instant, authoritative written psychiatric reports and arrange admissions to acute and secure units without delay. Teams with efficient full-time administrators, as well as clinicians with good relationships with local services, have been shown to be far more effective than those without.

Prison psychiatric services

Prisons require psychiatric services because the prevalence of mental illness, personality disorder, substance use, and suicidal or self-harming behaviour are much higher in <u>prison settings</u> (p.578) than in the general population. Prisoners need access to treatment while in prison and may need to be admitted to secure psychiatric services if mentally unwell.

In the UK, the NHS took over responsibility for providing health care in prisons in 2006, aimed at providing services to prisoners that were of an equivalent standard to those in the community. In RoI, healthcare is provided by the Irish Prison Service, which contracts doctors and dentists to provide primary care on a part-time basis; agreements exist for referral to psychiatric services provided by the HSE.

Working in a prison requires good working relationships with prison staff and governors. Prison staff may often take the lead in identifying prisoners who need help. Prisons have a duty of care to prisoners, and there are realistic concerns about how best to prevent deaths in custody.

Reception screening

On arrival into custody new prisoners are usually interviewed by prison staff using a standardised instrument, to identify any obvious mental health needs. The focus is on the risk of suicide and self-harm and reviewing current medication needs.

First night centre and induction wing

The first week in custody is a high-risk period for suicide. The first night centre and induction wing are two initiatives designed to make the experience less stressful. However, they are not provided in all prisons.

Primary care services

The provision of primary care services varies greatly from one institution to the next, with some provided by directly employed prison GPs (often locums), and others by local general practices. Prison psychiatric nurses provide a significant amount of primary care through wing-based triage, clinics, and crisis intervention. Continuity of care between prison and the community is a concern, particularly as many prisoners are not registered with a GP outside prison.

Secondary care services

Not all prisons have a psychiatric inreach team. Most that do not are lower security prisons that in theory only take inmates who have previously been screened in prisons. Mental health inreach teams function as a kind of CMHT for the prison community. They assess prisoners referred by the prison, provide care plans, and allocate CPNs and care co-ordinators, and may also take self-referrals for therapy and support. Some can offer psychological treatment. They play an important role in identifying prisoners who have developed severe mental illness, and arrange their <u>transfer</u> to secure psychiatric services (p.506).

However, prison communities are nothing like general adult community populations. Many prisoners suffer from moderate to severe personality disorder combined with substance misuse problems and the long-term effects of childhood adversity. Inreach teams must be competent at managing people with complex, comorbid conditions: addressing risk to others as well as risk to self. Teams also have a role in supporting prison staff in relation to self-harm and suicide risk management, and in the care of highly disturbed patients in healthcare centres, who may wait a long time for a bed in secure services.

Drug treatment services

Around 75% of prisoners have serious substance misuse problems. Many prisons offer detoxification programmes and then interventions to treat addiction and dependence. These interventions are not based on mental health models of recovery but are peer-led and emphasise motivation. The different models make it difficult for teams to work jointly with the same patients. Clinical drug treatment services are supplemented by nonclinical counselling services, known in prisons in E&W as Counselling, Assessment, Referral, Advice, and Throughcare Services.

Prison inpatient services

Fewer than half of prisons have inpatient psychiatric beds in their health care centres, and these are usually full with prisoners who are either at risk of suicide or are severely mentally ill. The inreach teams provide input into these units.

Nonconsensual treatment in prison

Prison healthcare units are not recognised as treatment settings under mental health law in the UK or RoI, meaning prisoners cannot be treated involuntarily unless they have lost mental capacity (p.532)—or in very limited emergency situations where a common law power (p.542) can be used to treat prisoners in order to prevent significant harm. There are major practical obstacles to using such powers in prisons, which means that, in all but the most severe emergencies, patients refusing treatment remain untreated until transferred to hospital.

Transfer to hospital

For the most seriously ill prisoners, the prison setting is inappropriate, and prisoners are transferred to hospital (p.506) for treatment. In law, any person who could have been admitted compulsorily from the community can be transferred to hospital, but in practice, the threshold is much higher because of limited number of available secure beds.

Relationships between services

Although they are often conceived of as separate services, patients often need to move within forensic services, between forensic and general psychiatric services, or between hospital and prison services, including in the following situations:

• when the risk of harm to others posed by forensic service patients has declined (e.g. through treatment) and they can safely be managed in a lower level of security or an open rehabilitation environment;

• when forensic service patients have been discharged to the community, and there is either no local CFT, p.266), or they have been managed by the CFT for a period of time and their risk of harm to others is now deemed acceptably low;

• when prisoners cared for by a prison inreach team (p.270) are released from prison and require after-care (p.492) in the community;

• when prisoners cared for in a prison healthcare centre (p.271) require transfer to a psychiatric hospital[11];

• when general service patients are convicted of an offence and ordered to a secure hospital by a court, or diverted (p.268) into a secure hospital; or

• when general service patients' behaviour cannot be safely managed on a general psychiatric ward or PICU, and they require care in a secure environment (p.190).

Given the frequency with which patients need to move between services in this way, it is unfortunate that a variety of historical, commissioning, and other factors often combine to produce misunderstanding and discord between forensic and general services, with each raising obstacles to the transfer of the other's patients. It is therefore worth the while of clinicians in all types of service to:

• Make personal contact with clinicians in other services wherever possible, ideally before needing to discuss potentially contentious cases, so as to build trusting relationships.

• Discuss and agree policies and protocols for common scenarios, such as those described above, setting out the mechanisms for assessment, transfer and return of patients, and for joint working where appropriate.

• Discuss disagreements with colleagues and managers at an early stage to ensure that opinions are reasonable and well-grounded, and be ready to consider changing one's opinion if it is unsupported by others.

• Have rapid access to mutually agreeable dispute-resolution mechanisms, such as 'pathways' meetings (at which representatives of various services meet to discuss patient placements and transfers) or binding arbitration procedures.

---

11 Major delays in transfers from prison to hospital used to be commonplace in the UK, and egregious in London. The commissioning of prison healthcare services by the NHS, and improved co-ordination between the MoJ, hospitals, and prisons, have improved transfer processes considerably: the average delay between submitting a valid request for transfer and receiving a warrant authorising it fell from fourteen to three days, until the Covid pandemic. However, occasional long delays still occur, which have led in a few cases to adverse outcomes in prison and subsequent negligence proceedings (p.550) involving the hospital concerned.

Service development

All health and social care services change over time, in response to political priorities (nationally and managerially), the state of the economy,[12] the availability of resources such as suitably trained staff, and the needs of the local population. Successful service developments prioritise quality, safety, and experience of care over a long period (ten years or more); sustain an investment in infrastructure and management processes (despite intervening political and management changes); and embed the systems and processes required in the organisation's culture and way of working. Senior clinicians, especially those with explicit management responsibilities, will periodically be involved in service development.

Needs assessment

Rational planning of future services must include an assessment of the needs of the population (p.276) being served—for example mentally disordered offenders (MDOs) in a specific geographical area.

Person-centred care

Increasingly, healthcare systems try to view the care they provide (and are seeking to develop) from the perspective of the service user, and assess needs holistically as perceived by the person (patient) themselves—which may not be the most convenient form of care for the professionals, or the most financially efficient for the provider organisation. Ideally the needs assessment will be 'co-produced' (i.e. done jointly with patients and carers or their representatives) rather than solely by professionals.

Service evaluation

Assuming that what is planned is not an entirely new service where none currently exists, an important step is to evaluate the existing service, including what works well and how it may be failing. The evaluation should use valid outcome measures (see below) and consider the following:
* inputs such as the service's human and financial resources, its capacity, its structure, its protocols, its information systems, and relevant constraints such as government policy;
* processes such as specific clinical interventions and their frequency and duration, the relationships between clinicians and patients, the movement between service tiers, the service's pathways, waiting lists and bottlenecks, the continuity of care, and efficiency; and
* outcomes, such as reduced reoffending (not a health outcome, but often considered by service commissioners), reduced patient symptoms and distress, and increased social (re)integration.

---

12 This is a perennial concern in the UK and RoI, and leads to repeated changes in service structures, sometimes reversing previous changes (e.g. the current Integrated Care Systems in England greatly undermine the 1990s' Commissioner/Provider split). Although financial pressures pose major problems for health services, debate about more efficient service provision often stimulates innovation (the closure of the asylums and development of community care is a notorious example of both the improvements and harms that can result from such financially-driven innovation).

Outcome measures

For the purposes of service evaluation and development, outcome measures must examine outcomes at the population level, not the level of the individual patient. They should ideally:
- be multidimensional (e.g. combining clinical, social/rehabilitation, humanitarian, and public safety variables);
- examine multiple perspectives (e.g. patient, carer, and society);
- collect data longitudinally (i.e. over time) as well as cross-sectionally;
- be standardised and published, to allow peer review and replication; and
- take costs into account, within a model of cost effectiveness.

Existing outcome measures (used e.g. when <u>evaluating treatment</u>; p.232) rarely live up to these demanding criteria, though certain Patient-Related Experience Measures (PREMs) such as the Individualised Care Scale or FeedbackLive!, and Patient-Related Outcome Measures (PROMs) such as the EQ-5D, attempt to do so to a greater degree than older consensus measures such as the Health of the Nation Outcome Scales (HoNOS).

Population needs assessment

Like those of the individual patient, the needs of the whole population are assessed in order to <u>plan services</u> (p.274). Needs assessment may appear objective, but is heavily value-laden, with different methods offering differing 'perspectives on need'.

Population needs assessment requires:

- Definition of the population, including a threshold of <u>caseness</u> (p.328)—for instance, what is the mental disorder and level of offending behaviour?
- A clear definition of need (e.g. is the need for health or social care, and/ or for reduced offending?)
- Agreement on whose needs are to be responded to, the patient's, society's, or some balance of the two?
- A rigorous, transparent method of measuring prevalence of need.

Methods of population needs assessment

Needs assessment relies upon multiple data sources from different perspectives. These may be summarised as population health needs, normative assessments, and observed outcome.

Population health needs

- Epidemiological surveys
- Sociodemographic indicators (as a proxy for need)
- Community forum/opinion
- Key informants (use of views of stakeholders)
- Rates of people with severe mental illness in prisons (unmet needs)

Normative assessments

- Surveys (either those currently being treated or population surveys)
- International comparisons

Observed outcomes

- Rates under treatment ('met need')
- Negative outcomes
- Hospital key performance indicators (out of area placements, involuntary admissions, discharge to homelessness, and readmission rates)

Cost-benefit analysis calculates the financial cost and monetary value of the benefits of an intervention, then ranks the available interventions by net financial cost. It is frequently criticised for overlooking benefits that cannot be reduced to a monetary value, such as human dignity. **Cost-effective analysis** identifies a given required outcome, without attaching any value to it, and identifies the different costs of alternative ways of achieving that outcome.

Limitations and considerations of needs assessment

- Lack of objectivity—no needs assessment is policy-neutral. Its results are inevitably dependent upon the values underlying the method of assessment and the chosen data sources. Biases due to stigma and cost saving may be subtle (assumption that all community care is better than

hospital care; assumption that all reduced length of stay and absolute liberty is better than restoration of dignity and quality of life).
- Ability to benefit is intimately linked to desired <u>outcomes</u> (p.275); which may be in dispute and difficult to measure.
- Needs assessment amounts to taking a judgment upon available data, or the data selected for use.
- Identified need is arrived at by way of judgment, based upon weighing more than one perspective on a given identified need (each perspective arrived at by its own method).
- If only one method and perspective is utilised, then the need identified will be biased by the method adopted.
- Different social constructions of need are rooted in the philosophical, moral, and temporal contexts within which they sit.

Special forensic issues within needs assessment
- Forensic mental health needs assessment is particularly fraught with definitional and values problems because of services' dual purpose (benefiting both patients and the public).
- The needs of each may often be perceived as in conflict (e.g. the most effective rehabilitation of an offender patient may require granting a <u>leave programme</u> (p.191) which puts the public more at risk than a more cautious leave programme).
- Needs assessment is often pursued in terms of quality-adjusted life years (QALYs). However, forensic mental health needs also involves 'liberty-adjusted life years' (LALYs). <u>Ethical tensions</u> (p.298) may arise in responding to both.
- Identifying alternative responses to need involves comparing service responses, such as comparing treatment within hospital and within the health care services of a prison.

Law can demand an ethical service response in the absence of need. For example, a <u>hybrid order</u> (p.670) served by an offender who has benefited adequately from hospital care cannot be discharged/released because of his underlying prison sentence, forcing the hospital to continue detaining and 'treat' him if his health would suffer from remission to prison.

The ethics of forensic psychiatry

Chapter 9

Ethical decision-making

How to use this part

Clinical ethics is concerned with how we put values into practice in our clinical work. The word *ethical* implies a type of reflective process and discussion. There is rarely a 'right' answer, but there may be more than one justifiable answer.

In this part we explore ethical dilemmas within forensic psychiatry, and ways to address ethical decision-making.

Ethical dilemmas are common in psychiatry because mental disorders can impair autonomy and personhood, because concepts of mental disorder change with time, and because these concepts are used to deprive people of liberty and to enforce involuntary treatment. Psychiatric patients are therefore ethically vulnerable in ways that other patients are not.

Forensic psychiatrists face additional complex ethical dilemmas in clinical and clinico-legal practice for three main reasons:

- They face ethical conflicts at the interface (p.358) with criminal justice and other agencies (p.314), that deal with public risk.
- They often have dual responsibilities, involving a duty of care to a patient and a duty of public protection.
- Giving expert testimony, whether as a professional witness and/or an expert witness (p.652), may challenge their ethical identity as doctor.
- Forensic patients are additionally vulnerable to stigma and to unjust treatment.

Ethics as reflection and dialogue

Ethical dilemmas in medicine usually arise when there is a clash of values between the patient and the doctor or when there is real uncertainty about what a 'good' doctor should do. Ethical decision-making involves both an internal reflective process and external dialogue, about the conflicting values of patients, carers, professionals, and legal processes. Professionals need to develop 'ethical insight'; and an understanding that a good ethical decision is defined essentially by its *process*, rather than necessarily by its outcome.[1]

Raising ethical consciousness

This part is also intended to raise awareness of ethical dilemmas in daily forensic practice. It is a common error for doctors to mistake ethical decisions for clinical ones: that is, to mistake a normative ('should') statement for a positive ('is') statement. A key test question is usually: I **can** do this clinically, but **should** I?

Practice makes better

Good practice of medical ethics requires practice and maintaining awareness of the common ethical dilemmas in forensic psychiatry. This part of the handbook describes some ethical dilemmas in forensic psychiatry and some approaches to ethical reasoning (p.283). It can usefully be read in combination with the worked examples of ethical dilemmas described in the *Oxford*

---

1 There is a direct analogy with clinical negligence law (p.550).

Casebook of Forensic Psychiatry. You might also think of examples from your own practice.

Diligence in ethics

Ethical decision-making involves both a *process* and an *outcome*; both of which may be inherently complex. An 'obvious' answer is likely to have missed out important facts or perspectives. Good-quality ethical decision-making often takes time; anxiety may impel you towards quick, often ethically suspect, solutions. So, if you have an ethical dilemma, take your time, talk to others, gain different perspectives, and make notes of your thinking and discussions, not just the decision arrived at. Put simply, 'show your workings'. Doing so is likely to enhance the quality and clarity of your thinking and, at a later stage (perhaps at an inquiry), demonstrate it to others.

Ethics and data

Good ethical decision-making is dependent upon reliable facts. However, empirical data only help with thinking about the consequences of alternative courses of action; they cannot assist in constructing an ethical analysis of a dilemma.

Ethics and law

Commonly professionals faced with an ethical dilemma ask, 'What does the law say?'. The legal position on any issue may contribute to an ethical reasoning process, and may even offer a legal answer, but this may not be *the most ethically justifiable* answer.

Law and ethics may even be in conflict (as happened to doctors in Nazi Germany, and sometimes to those treating prisoners detained in Abu Ghraib, Guantanamo Bay, and similar facilities) or there may not be any law on the issue available until after the event. In this section we do refer to legal provisions, but mainly in order to view them through an 'ethical prism'.

Approaches to medical ethics

What is medical ethics?

Moral philosophy studies how we decide what is 'good' and 'bad'; medical ethics concerns good and bad medical practice. It involves maximising clinician insight into the ethical implications of alternative decisions and using reflective skills to reach an ethical decision.

Practical medical ethics requires awareness of ethical tensions within a situation, considered within a decision-making process, as well as good reasoning skills, based on established literature and research.

Why do we need medical ethics?

People who are ill or injured are vulnerable, whereas the professionals they seek help from have power and authority because of their specialist knowledge and their social role. With increased power comes increased responsibility, and since the ancient Greek Hippocratic Oath (p.287), doctors have been expected to follow ethical guidance in the exercise of their powers. Sadly, some medical professionals have exploited their power for personal gain, or in pursuit of political agendas; many more can struggle to see that, although something is clinically indicated, it may be unethical.

After the Second World War, the assumption that 'doctor knows best' was increasingly challenged. This followed evidence at the Nuremberg Trials of unethical practice by Nazi doctors, especially in the fields of psychiatry and medical research. It was also challenged by the civil rights movement, which argued that medicine, like the rest of Western society, was a white patriarchy that acted to oppress other groups[2]: which led to demands for autonomy and dignity for all, including patients who had traditionally been treated as unable to make decisions for themselves. A number of seminal legal cases were brought at this time[3] which began to challenge medical authority, arguing that patient rights, choice, and autonomy should be considered alongside medical beneficence.

The development of codes

The Nuremberg Code of Medical Ethics was developed after the Nuremberg Trials, then adopted by the World Medical Association. Most countries have developed their own mandatory professional ethical codes, enforced by their licensing authorities, such as the GMC's Good Medical Practice in the UK.

Codes (p.294) offer general statements which represent particular ethical solutions to types of dilemmas. They are written in very broad terms and do not purport to give unambiguous answers to all potential ethical dilemmas. Codes are not a substitute for ethical reasoning, but offer support to a reasoning process.

---

2 People of colour, women, people with disabilities, nonheterosexuals, trans individuals, and others. Not all doctors necessarily held such views, but they acted within and supported (or did not oppose) the social system they lived and worked within, which suppressed those other groups.

3 For example *Cassidy v Ministry of Health* [1951] 2 K.B. 343; *Roe v Minister of Health* [1954] 2 WLR 915; and *Bolam* (p.748).

Clinical Ethics Committees

Many hospitals in the UK and RoI, including some psychiatric hospitals, have developed Clinical Ethics Committees.[4] They support clinical ethical reasoning by clinicians, but cannot act as substitute decision-makers; also advising services on issues. By contrast, in the USA, some hospitals employ specialist bioethicists to provide solutions to clinical dilemmas.

Research Ethics Committees

Research ethical dilemmas differ from clinical dilemmas because researchers do not generally have therapeutic relationships with research participants. There are complex ethical issues in research involving psychiatric patients, and especially forensic psychiatric patients, because of concerns about patients' freedom to refuse to participate, and the coercive nature of most forensic settings. All such research must be authorised by the relevant licensing body. Research Ethics Committees have a duty to ensure that research is scientifically valid, and protects the welfare of participants, especially those who may be especially vulnerable.

4 There was a burgeoning of clinical ethics committees during, and precipitated by, the Covid-19 pandemic, including many in psychiatric hospitals and services.

Approaches to ethical reasoning

Ethical reasoning is broadly distinguished into those accounts that focus on the likely *consequences* of decisions, and those that focus predominantly on *intentions*. A background assumption to each account is that human societies agree that there are moral rules that should not be broken; and that any challenges to those rules need to be justified in terms of either positive consequences or positive intentions or possibly both.

Utilitarianism

This holds that you should act in ways that maximise the benefit of as many people as possible. Intuitively this is appealing for doctors because it fits with clinical training. However, it carries a risk of assuming that 'the ends justify the means': that you can do something unethical to get a good outcome (e.g. give medication covertly). Utilitarianism also involves assessing the likelihood of different possible outcomes, which is hard to do accurately, and it offers no way of weighing different kinds of benefit. However, it has an important place in medical ethics, especially at the level of community decisions, including reducing risk to the public.

Deontology

This holds that your actions should be based upon intentions that accord with universal principles: famously explicated by Kant, drawing on Judeo-Christian thinking (e.g. the Ten Commandments). It has appeal in medicine insofar as it privileges clinical intention and reason, and provides support for a system of *medical duties*. However, it gives no guidance on what to do when principles or duties conflict.

Kant argued that people were never merely as means to an end. This is important for forensic psychiatry, where practitioners exercise power over patients in the name of public safety, and in research settings where participants may lack capacity to refuse consent.

Liberal individualism

This is a *rights-based* theory, within which respecting others' rights is deemed the proper basis for resolving ethical dilemmas. It appeals to lawyers, as it is rule-based, but it has not been widely applied to medicine. It offers little guidance on what to do when rights conflict nor is it at all clear that a 'right' is meaningful if no other person will respect it.

Communitarianism

This was developed in response to extreme individual rights-based theories. It argues that we are connected to each other through common human values and goals, and that privileging individual rights and choice risks losing sight of the extent to which we are social animals. To some extent, Anglo-Saxon criminal law is communitarian: a crime offends the community as a whole, and the community (not the victim) charges and prosecutes the offender.

Ethic of care

Also known as 'relational ethics', this theory argues that to do the right thing one must understand the network of relationships that affect the patient, including that with the clinician. It has gained wide appeal among nursing staff because it takes account of the feelings of carers, and may have particular relevance for psychotherapists and forensic clinicians who have long-term relationships with patients.

Virtue ethics

This holds that you should develop the character of a good doctor, and pursue the ideal of the virtuous doctor. The assumption is that by trying to be a good doctor, you will think about what a good decision is in the context of your role and identity. This approach places less emphasis on conflicts between consequences and principles, and is particularly appealing in psychiatry, where personal qualities are often crucial to therapeutic success.

The Four Principles

This popular, and dominant account in medical ethics appeals to both *principles* and *consequences*. It states that doctors should pay attention to four principles or duties:

• a duty to respect patient **autonomy**;
• a duty to bring about good consequences—**beneficence**;
• a duty to not cause harm—**nonmaleficence**; and
• a duty to respect **justice**—both to treat people fairly and to engage with the legal system appropriately.

Faced with an ethical dilemma, the doctor considers these duties as a framework for reflecting on the inherent ethical tensions and determining what might be *a* (but not necessarily *the*) right action. Although the four principles are not hierarchically sequenced, there is general acceptance amongst philosophers, and many doctors, that respect for autonomy is most important; although this is effectively challenged within psychiatric practice based upon mental health legislation.[5]

Values-based practice (see p.288) was developed specifically for NHS practice for use in teams where different professionals may 'see' or apply values differently.

Comparing theories

Each theory of ethical decision-making offers a different perspective on, and foundation for, decision-making. Different ethical decisions may be defensible using different models that resolve conflict between duties and outcomes in different ways, and applying different models may give similar or different 'answers'. Together these schools of thought invite decision-makers to be aware of the complexity of ethical decision-making.

---

5 The <u>principles of mental health law</u> (p.466) are emphatically not founded primarily on respect for autonomy.

Values-based practice

Values-based practice (VBP) offers a theoretical skills-based approach to dealing with ethical dilemmas in mental health practice.[6] VBP suggests that such dilemmas arise because different parties (clinicians, patients, and carers) have clashing values perspectives, and these clashes cause anxiety, but are not fully acknowledged or explored. VBP supports resolution of ethical dilemmas using a process of reflection on clashes of values; that includes reflection on law, local policy, and clinical facts. It emphasises resolution of ethical dilemmas by way of a process of reflection on values that are in tension, and not seeking simplistic answers in terms of law, local policy, or clinical facts. All perspectives are important, especially those of the service user.

A values-based approach in practice
- Awareness of the facts and values relevant to the case
- Awareness of the different perspectives of the different players
- Respect for the different values perspectives
- Reflection upon and discussion of these different perspectives
- Resolution by open discussion

VBP in forensic settings
Values conflicts are common in forensic psychiatry because forensic patients may have different values preferences from their treating team, and from society in general. Forensic psychiatrists may have to privilege the value of public safety over their patients' values (e.g. in decisions about leave or discharge), and may have to balance this against the need to make the patient's care their first concern. Team members from different professions bring different values. And when acting as an <u>expert witness</u> (p.652), forensic psychiatrists may indirectly cause the evaluee harm.

VBP may enhance ethical discussions between staff and patients—particularly in relation to risk assessment and management, when anxiety is often high, and can push professionals towards taking decisions quickly and without reflection. VBP can also ensure that the patient's view is not automatically dismissed as unreliable or risky.

> Example: Mr King is detained in a medium secure unit following a violent offence three years ago. He has a diagnosis of schizophrenia and has no current symptoms. He was psychotic at the time of the offence. He has limited insight, and does not accept responsibility for the offence, but has engaged in all treatment. He and his family believe that he should be allowed to live in the community. There is division within the clinical team about this decision because of Mr King's lack of insight and disagreement with the team.

6 It is based upon the work of Professor KWM (Bill) Fulford.

Process in VBP

The discussions in VBP pay attention to different values perspectives. In this example, Mr King values his freedom and may not accept the value of risk reduction in the same way or to the same extent as the professionals, who focus on the value of risk reduction and harm prevention. Professionals who value patient engagement and rapport may advocate for Mr King's view, and Mr King's family may value interpersonal factors that they see as overriding risk. The Ministry of Justice (p.586) may solely value public safety.

Respect and resolution

Respect in VBP means allowing all voices and points of view to be heard, ideally by creating reflective spaces for discussion, where professionals and service users can find common points of reference, as well as clarify areas of difference, especially in relation to risk. Adopting this approach may be particularly helpful for decisions regarding high-risk patients, where anxiety can easily cause conflict between teams.

It is crucial to agree on the available data on which a decision might be based, so that any difference of values applied by different parties is made evident. The alternative of each party selecting facts in support of their value judgment is unhelpful. Within teams, there is often strength in acknowledging uncertainty, and being open about values, particularly when this is done by senior staff, since this is likely to allow less experienced colleagues to do likewise.

Resolution through discussion may lead to a plan of action, but even if not, the reflective process should be recorded, and should include dissenting views. This recording process supports a values-based approach to risk-based decisions which is inclusive and can be scrutinised and reviewed.

Limits of VBP in forensic psychiatry

- Some values may be difficult to respect (e.g. when a patient has values supportive of violence, or hostility to a subgroup of people).
- The values of individuals may be trumped by political, social, or legal values (e.g. anxiety about risk may make senior managers reluctant to support VBP).
- Circumstances of a case may overwhelm attempts at values-based resolution (e.g. the high profile of certain offences may impede balanced consideration).
- In relation to sentencing, expert evidence resulting in a mentally disordered person receiving treatment may be easier to reconcile with values held as a doctor than when it results in indeterminate or extended custodial sentences (p.448).
- In adversarial settings like courts, the sides are likely to pursue values-based narratives which are in conflict, with the court being the arbiter of the outcome.

Ethics and law

The law is a set of rules devised to regulate relationships between individuals, and between individuals and the State, or society as a whole. It evolves over time, including according to circumstance. Although there are some aspects of law that are clear and explicit, often it may be impossible to know exactly <u>what the law is</u> on a given question (p.366). The law may be the codification of a social consensus on an issue, which will commonly express a particular value, or balance between competing values; only rarely, though, does it address questions of value explicitly.

Ethics[7] or morality is also about the relationship between individual parties, and between the individual and the wider social group. However, ethical statements tend to include the words *ought* or *should*. So, for example, under mental health law, it may be legally possible to detain someone, but the ethical question may be Should you?

Ethical questions often involve conflicting moral values (e.g. 'it is good to tell people the truth, but if I tell this patient the truth, he may become angry and violent; so should I tell him the truth?'). The law cannot provide a general answer to this question, although it might set specific rules requiring disclosure or concealment of the truth in specific situations, such as when a patient makes a subject access request under the <u>Data Protection Act</u> (p.736).

Because laws reflect the wishes of society, or at least its rulers, at a given time, it is possible for laws to be ethically incoherent and/or unjust. Consider both the Nazi eugenics laws, and the South African apartheid laws. The Nazi laws allowed doctors to end the lives of those who were disabled, but ignored the basic ethical question of whether one should ever deliberately end the life of another. The apartheid laws, which categorised all subjects as White, Black, Coloured, or Indian, determined where people in the Black (and to a lesser extent, Indian and Coloured) group could live, work, and travel, and even with whom they could interact, and in what circumstances. However, they did not address the fundamental ethical conflict between these policies and the idea of every life having equal value.

Law should follow ethics

It is a good rule that the law should follow ethics, rather than vice versa. Law should have justice as its central value: justice for all, applied fairly and transparently, with equal access. However, if you have an ethical dilemma, while the law may be able to help you with guidance about what acts are *permissible*, it may well not tell you what you should do.

Mental health laws and **mental capacity laws** give powers to certain professionals to detain people for assessment and treatment or to act in their best interests. Because the State should not in general detain individuals who have not broken any law (a tenet of <u>human rights law</u>, p.516),

---

7 The term *ethics* can also mean the philosophical study of morality, and the specific moral codes adopted by a professional group, and the latter is what is usually meant elsewhere in the handbook. However, on this page the reference is to general morality.

there needs to be special powers to detain those who are ill,[8] and/or might benefit from detention for treatment. Mental health legislation empowers professionals to detain: mostly, it does not impose a duty to do so. It cannot answer questions such as How should I balance my patient's personal interests against the public interest in being protected from someone at high risk of violence? For a discussion of this vexed issue, see p.296.

---

8 Not only patients who are mentally disordered: for example, there are powers to detain people with certain <u>infectious diseases</u> for treatment, and to remove <u>persons in need of care and attention</u> (p.542) from their home for treatment.

Chapter 10

Professional duties and personal integrity

Professional guidelines and codes

Professionals' identity or role depends on their specialist knowledge and commitment to that role. Professional identity is achieved by examination of knowledge and competence and reviews of practice. Once accredited, professionals must maintain that identity by:

• continuing professional development of knowledge and skills, and
• adhering to professional standards and guidelines in their practice.

Forensic practitioners will encounter a wide range of types of standards and guidance. These are authoritative statements by the bodies that issue them, covering clinical, legal, professional, or other matters, often with an ethical element.

Legal status

Guidelines, protocols, and codes do not have the force of law, but may be referred to in evidence. They offer courts explicit, albeit contestable, descriptions of relevant standards across a wide range of medical practice, which can be very influential in certain cases (e.g. negligence proceedings, p.550, or inquests, p.560). An unjustified failure to follow them can also result in professional misconduct proceedings (p.552).

Technical protocols versus ethical codes

Protocols give detailed instructions on how to perform a specific clinical procedure. Codes generally provide broad statements of principle about professionals' ethical duties. There may be overlap between them.

Clinical guidelines

In the UK, the National Institute for Health and Clinical Excellence (NICE) regularly publishes treatment guidelines, based on meta-analyses of research; in RoI the Department of Health issues similar guidelines. These help healthcare professionals in their work, but they cannot replace individual professionals' knowledge, skills, and reasoning. Because guidelines rely on aggregate data, they may be of limited use in individual cases, and their recommendations may conflict with the duty to make the care of the specific patient one's first concern (see below).

Where there are published clinical guidelines, it is good practice to consult them, and to record the reasons for any decision not to follow them. Even clinical guidelines are based on ethical theory (e.g. NICE employs cost-benefit analyses based on utilitarianism (p.286) in deciding whether to approve a particular treatment for a particular condition).

Legislative codes of practice

Codes of practice indicate how to apply legislation, most notably mental health law (p.461). These are not ethical codes per se, but may contain matters of ethical substance. The associated law typically requires that the relevant code should be followed unless there is a good reason for not doing so, which should be clearly documented.

Professional codes and managerial policies

Professional ethics must be distinguished from policies and other governance instruments used by employers. Health employers often develop
policies which are explicitly or implicitly ethical in nature (e.g. concerning
participation of employed clinicians in MAPPA, p.592), as may governments that issue directions to those employers. In both cases, there may
be conflict with professional ethical codes, which will be more acute if the
employer would consider disciplinary action (p.557) for contravening the
policy. In general, professionals would be advised to seek advice from a senior colleague, through an employer's governance structure and/or from a
professional association or indemnity organisation, before breaching either
the code or the policy.

Ethical guidelines and codes

Ethical guidelines in medical practice represent codification of professional
consensus. They are informed by the medical ethical literature, as well as by
developments in medical law.

The main sources of ethical guidelines for doctors are the GMC's *Good
Medical Practice* in the UK, and the MC's *Guide to Professional Conduct and
Ethics for Doctors* in RoI. Departures from these guidelines can form the
basis of charges of impaired fitness to practice. The medical defence societies also provide ethical guidance, as well as legal guidance and support.

Codes of ethics in psychiatry

Psychiatry needs a particular frame for ethical decision-making because psychiatric patients are especially vulnerable to abuse, because of the possible
effects of mental disorder on capacity (p.522) and volition (p.24), because
there are historical precedents for misuse of psychiatry (p.520), including
inappropriate treatments and unethical research, and because mental health
law gives unusual power to doctors to enforce treatment.

The World Psychiatric Association, the UK Royal College of Psychiatrists
and the College of Psychiatrists of Ireland each publish their own codes
(p.772) and issue other ethical guidance on specific topics such as commercial interests, expert witness work, and boundary violations.

Codes of ethics in forensic psychiatry

There is no British or Irish code of ethics specifically for forensic psychiat-
rists. In relation to expert testimony, there is some relevant advice in Good
Medical Practice and Good Psychiatric Practice (p.772); also within Royal
College of Psychiatrists, *Responsibilities of Psychiatrists Who Provide Expert
Opinion to Courts and Tribunals*, CR193 (p.774). The American Association of
Psychiatry and Law's ethical guidelines (p.VI, 776) are also useful to consider.

The main ethical duties of an expert witness are not to go beyond one's
competence, always to practise honestly, and not to become aligned with
either side of an adversarial debate. The expert's duty is to assist the court,
and not a particular party or cause, and to guard against bias.

Ethical dilemmas in clinical forensic psychiatry are not well addressed by
current guidelines, particularly in relation to the extent of any duty to protect third parties (p.296) and the harm that may result to the patient, or the
ethical status of forensic psychiatrists who practise only medicolegally and
not clinically.

A duty to prevent violence?

Most psychiatrists accept that they have a duty to treat patients who pose a risk of violence to others in such a way as to minimise that risk. However, there is debate about the extent to which psychiatrists have an ethical or legal duty to go beyond this to protect others from patients' violence.

The argument for a responsibility to prevent violence

Most philosophical accounts of responsibility state that each adult is responsible for their own actions, and no adult is normally responsible for the actions of another. To become the responsibility of another, that person must either:

• be mentally <u>incapable</u> (p.522) of making their own decisions or
• be in the legal custody of the other person.

The latter almost always applies to forensic psychiatric inpatients (the custody being detention under mental health law). Therefore, it is argued, forensic psychiatrists are responsible for their patients' behaviour whilst they either lack capacity or are detained or perhaps even if they are merely subject to legal restrictions in the community.

This appears to have been the UK government's view, in setting up the system of <u>formal inquiries</u> into the actions of services (p.598) whenever a patient commits homicide in E&W. Most forensic psychiatrists can expect to be the subject of such an inquiry in a working lifetime.

The relationship between mental disorder and violence

Where a patient lacks capacity, doctors must act in their <u>best interests</u> (p.334); this could include a duty to prevent them from acting in harmful ways towards others. However, most forensic psychiatric patients do not lack capacity[1] at the time of committing serious violence or homicide (and most violence is committed by people without mental disorder).

It therefore seems unreasonable to hold psychiatrists responsible for the behaviour of their patient when patients are capable or criminally responsible, and where their behaviour was not directly related to mental disorder or to a failure of psychiatric care.

Risk assessment and management

Forensic psychiatrists specifically <u>assess the risk</u> (p.168) of their patients being violent, and construct <u>risk management plans</u> (p.240). It is argued that by doing so they take on additional responsibility for violence if it occurs (certainly, assessing or managing risk inadequately might amount to <u>clinical negligence</u>, p.550).

However, risk assessment is an imprecise process, and cannot <u>predict violence</u> (p.164), partly because violence is a complex behaviour with many determinants, and partly because of the low baseline rate in the population. Only by detaining a very high proportion of forensic patients indefinitely could there be effective prevention of violence in the community by those patients (as opposed to merely reducing the risk of it) using current risk assessment and management techniques. Even if this could be

[1] Or criminal responsibility (that is, they are rarely found not guilty by reason of <u>insanity</u>, p.620)

justified on financial and human rights grounds (p.516), it would not prevent all violence by patients, merely displace some from the community to hospital wards.

A general duty to others

Most philosophical accounts of a 'good life' include duties to others as well as duties to, and responsibility for, oneself. This is often couched as a reciprocal relationship between an individual and society; if we as citizens seek protection and benefit from being a member of group, we have to acknowledge duties to that group. These duties may in some cases be purely moral, with no prospect of legal sanction if they are broken, but they are significant, nonetheless.

What is less clear is how doctors contribute to public health, if 'health' is expanded to include public safety,[2] and patients' liberty may be restricted in that pursuit. One way to look at this has been to argue that where there is no knowledge there is no duty, but as a doctor acquires more knowledge of a dangerous situation, they then have an enhanced duty to do something (although whether this is as a citizen or a professional is debatable).

For example, in relation to child protection and the safeguarding of vulnerable adults (p.590), doctors are expected to participate fully in child protection or safeguarding procedures, even where this may mean breaching the confidentiality of another patient (p.320). The ethical justification is that the duty to a child or vulnerable adult outweighs any duty to a less-vulnerable patient who is more able to protect themselves.

The World Health Organization has argued that violence reduction falls within the work of public health medical practice, and there is some evidence that courts are prepared to examine whether psychiatrists might have duties to third parties who might be harmed by their patients (see p.550). However, there remain debates about the nature of that duty; its scope and how it is to be fulfilled without abandoning the ethical imperative to make the care of the patient your first concern.

Conclusion

Both as citizens and professionals, forensic psychiatrists have duties to do what is reasonable in the circumstances to minimise the risk of their patients doing harm to others. This might include treatments, risk management measures, and sharing information where appropriate (e.g. under the MAPPA, p.592). The scope of these duties is still evolving.

---

2 A lack of public safety can result in injury (damage to health), but to include public safety itself (and therefore crime prevention) as an aspect of public health is excessively to medicalise society.

Competing interests and role conflicts

Competing interests

Competing interests arise in medicine where a clinician is aware of duties, loyalties, or ethical principles that are in conflict one with another. Some arise from conflict between the clinician's different roles. Examples include:

- where one ethical duty conflicts with another in a clinical setting (e.g. where to give adequate pain relief will bring about death, the so-called doctrine of double effect);
- where a clinician has a personal interest in a situation which conflicts with their professional duties, that may reduce their objectivity (e.g. receiving fees from a manufacturer while sitting on a committee that will determine which supplier a hospital buys from);
- where contractual duties conflict with professional ones (e.g. a doctor working for a pharmaceutical company whose executives wish to suppress evidence of harm caused by a new drug);
- where fear of personal consequences affects professional judgment (e.g. reluctance to discharge or grant leave to a patient, for fear of censure if they reoffend, no matter how unlikely that may be); and
- where personal feelings impair professionalism (e.g. jealousy or antagonism affecting neutrality when reviewing a colleague's grant application).

Competing and conflicting interests are inevitable. The key ethical requirement is transparency, and willingness to accept that decisions may be influenced by different sets of values or roles. Conflicts must be declared whenever they arise.

Role conflicts and competing interests in forensic psychiatry

Risk reduction versus rehabilitation

Psychiatrists have to balance duties to the welfare of patients with their duties to public safety, most commonly when considering a patient's needs for leave as part of rehabilitation. The outcome of this balancing process may be biased by the psychiatrists' fear about public scrutiny or disciplinary processes if the patient were to reoffend.

Therapist versus expert for court

It is not uncommon for forensic psychiatrists to be asked to give expert testimony in relation to their own patients. They may be in the best position, in terms of clinical knowledge, to do so, but their therapeutic relationship with the patient may hinder their ability to be objective. Treating psychiatrists are advised not to act as expert witnesses in cases involving their patients, except perhaps in very minor cases.

Professional versus expert witness, versus advocate

When a psychiatrist gives evidence at a mental health tribunal, technically they appear as professional witnesses (p.652) having knowledge of the patient. However, they also provide the tribunal with expert opinion (p.654) about whether the legal criteria for continued detention are fulfilled, including in relation to risk. This situation can be further complicated ethically, in that in some jurisdictions the psychiatrist can cross-examine witnesses and put forward argument on behalf of the hospital, although the hospital's interests may directly oppose those of the patient.

Professional versus contractual duty

Psychiatrists may experience conflict between professional duty and contractual duties to their employer, such as when their employer requires them to participate in multiagency information-sharing regimes such as MAPPA (p.592), but they believe that disclosure of certain information would be an unjustifiable breach of confidentiality (p.320).

Professional versus managerial duty

A specific instance of the conflict above occurs when psychiatrists take on managerial roles within a healthcare organisation, such as clinical director or medical director. Clinicians focus on solving the problems of the individual patient; managers focus on outcomes for a patient group as a whole, and on fair allocation of resources, and have to tolerate numerous problems that cannot yet be solved, political pressures, and the need to prioritise. Managerial priorities, such as financial stability, may conflict with the medical manager's duty to patients (e.g. maintaining patient safety).

Resolution of role conflicts

As with other ethical dilemmas in this part, awareness, articulation, communication, and reflection are crucial steps in a process of managing, if not resolving, role conflicts. Transparency of process is essential so that all views can be heard and considered. The key ethical value here is justice, in terms of fairness of process.

Professional roles and relationships

Professional roles

The scope and nature of the psychiatrist's professional role and duties is set out in:
• general professional <u>ethical standards</u> for doctors[3] (p.295),
• specific professional ethical standards for psychiatrists,[4]
• duties under mental health law, and
• duties agreed in their contract and job plan.

They include a mixture of regulatory expectations, professional expectations, and employment law. All practitioners need to be familiar with the duties, and guidance, from all these sources. The primary professional duties, as set out by the GMC[5] are:
• to make the care of your patient your first concern,
• to provide a good standard of practice and care,
• to take prompt action if patient safety or dignity is compromised,
• to treat patients as individuals and respect their dignity,
• to work in partnership with patients,
• to worth with colleagues in ways that best serve patients' interests,
• to be honest and open, and act with integrity,
• never to discriminate unfairly against patients or colleagues, and
• never to abuse patients' or the public's trust in you or the profession.

Employers cannot require employees to carry out actions that would breach their professional duties if these are clearly and unambiguously relevant to the decision at hand.[6]

Professional roles and relationships in forensic psychiatry

Forensic psychiatrists have the same general professional duties as other doctors and psychiatrists. There are two main contexts in which they may have additional duties:
• in long-stay residential secure care, where much of the care will be delivered by multidisciplinary teams, there is a particular duty to maintain good professional relationships with other clinicians, such as psychotherapists, psychologists and nursing staff; and
• in medicolegal work, care is needed concerning the type of relationship you have with individuals you evaluate for legal proceedings.

Some professionals argue that medicolegal assessments are nontherapeutic processes necessary for the proper administration of justice; others argue

---

3 In the UK, the General Medical Council's *Good Medical Practice* booklets; in RoI, the Medical Council's *Guide to Professional Conduct and Ethics for Doctors*.

4 The Royal College of Psychiatrists' *Good Psychiatric Practice* booklets; the College of Psychiatrists of Ireland's *Professional Ethics for Psychiatrists*.

5 The MC adopts a different formulation: Partnership (trust, patient-centred care, working together, good communication, and advocacy), Practice (caring, confidentiality, patient safety, integrity, self-care, practice management, use of resources, and conflicts of interest), and Performance (competence, reflective practice, acting as role models, and teaching and training).

6 However, the employee cannot simply refuse to comply: they must attempt to clarify or rescind the conflicting instructions from the employer, using its normal governance processes, with support from their professional association if necessary.

that even in <u>nontherapeutic settings</u> (pp.318, 322), doctors are in their professional role, and necessarily utilise therapeutic skills in the assessment.

It is important to be clear with individuals assessed for medicolegal work about the purpose of the assessment, and to whom it will be communicated (see pp.122, 148); this explanation, and the evaluee's consent, should be clearly documented. Because such assessments are often not primarily for the individual's benefit, care should be taken not to confuse clinical and <u>expert witness</u> (p.652) relationships, especially with patients you are also treating (a <u>role conflict</u>, p.298).

Boundary violations

Professional boundaries are determined by the values and behaviours that mark out professional identity, often set out in <u>codes of practice</u> (p.294). Boundary violations occur when professionals cross the boundary between their professional and personal identity; promoting their personal values and feelings, and abandoning their professional stance. They range from the mild and common (e.g. giving a patient a little too much personal information) to the severe and unusual (e.g. borrowing money from or having a sexual relationship with a patient).

By putting their personal interests first, a clinician runs the risk of failing to provide an adequate standard of care and of exploiting the patient's vulnerability, and does harm by bringing the profession into disrepute and breaching public trust in it. Any severe boundary violation therefore usually results in investigation for <u>professional misconduct</u> (p.552) as well as <u>disciplinary proceedings</u> (p.557).

Boundaries in mental health

Mental health professionals are especially vulnerable to professional boundary violations because of the psychologically intimate nature of their work and because the power imbalance is greater than in other areas of medicine (because of the power to detain and treat forcibly).[7] Good mental health work requires personal engagement, so that the boundary between the personal and professional is always under tension. This is especially so in **forensic practice**, where staff may have powerful emotional responses to their patients and their offences, and in **long-stay residential secure care**, where staff and patients spend long periods in each other's company.

To reduce the risk of boundary violations all therapeutic work should be discussed in <u>supervision</u> and <u>reflective practice</u> (p.308).

Nonphysical boundary violations

These most commonly involve the inappropriate disclosure or use of information:

- inappropriate self-disclosure (this rarely results in disciplinary proceedings or other action, but may be the first sign of a loss of professional identity);
- disclosure of <u>confidential information</u> (p.320) without consent or lawful excuse (this can and does result in disciplinary hearings, professional proceedings, or even negligence claims);
- using patient information for personal gain (e.g. undertaking research without consent); and
- having a dual relationship with a patient (e.g. taking tax advice from a patient who is also an accountant).

---

7 Other factors contributing to the power imbalance are that the patient may have to share deeply personal information; the clinician decides what degree of psychological intimacy or physical contact there will be; and the patient may be unaware of what constitutes appropriate professional behaviour in the situation.

Physical boundary violations

The most serious (and commonest) such violations are sexual contacts with patients, which often involve a vulnerable patient unable to protect themselves from a predatory clinician (patients in such relationships may believe they wanted and even that they started the relationship until after it has finished, and they are free to re-evaluate it free of the clinician's influence).[8] They include:

- having a sexual or otherwise improper personal relationship with a patient or former patient and
- inappropriate touching (especially sexual touching) of patients, such as during a physical examination.

Psychiatrists are over-represented amongst doctors who are accused of boundary violations. A 'no-touch' policy is safest in psychiatric settings, with very limited exceptions, such as briefly touching a distressed patient in an appropriate place, such as on the arm or shoulder, to indicate support and concern.

Forensic psychiatrists who evaluate such clinicians for professional proceedings (p.642) should be cautious about bias in favour of doctors, and risk minimisation.

Boundary violations not involving a patient

These are more commonly the subject of disciplinary proceedings (p.557), and may be viewed less seriously, but are nevertheless unacceptable. Examples include:

- theft of the employer's property;
- use of the employer's assets for personal gain without permission (ranging from sending an email relating to a private medicolegal report, to paying for a holiday on a company credit card);
- deliberately giving a false or biased opinion (e.g. giving the opinion desired by those who pay you, as opposed to a genuine opinion);
- allowing your practice to undergo 'baseline drift' over time (through bias in your methods or interpretation of data, your opinions tending to favour a particular side in a case, e.g. prosecution or defence);
- misusing professional knowledge and status for personal gain (e.g. involving oneself in a case without instructions to do so, particularly if this involves something outside one's area of expertise); and
- acting in an unprofessional manner (by e.g. publicly denigrating other clinicians or experts who disagree with your views).

---

8 The predatory nature of the behaviour is rarely perceived by the clinician, who may be under stress or believe themselves 'entitled' to act in this way.

Acknowledging uncertainty

Making good judgments

The ability to make good judgments involves awareness of the nature of the question to be addressed, consideration of the context, and discernment of cognitive and emotional bias; in psychiatry, it requires the application of <u>values-based reflection</u> (p.288) to the available evidence.[9]

The context includes what you do not know, which may include a lot of relevant information (e.g. if <u>consent to assessment</u> (p.148) has been refused by the patient, or an agency has refused to disclose their records)—including information you may not be aware exists. You should consider whether the absence of such information invalidates or limits your conclusions.

Value judgments are applied not only in weighing one outcome against another (e.g. where different courses of action are being compared) but also in determining what level of probability of outcome is acceptable. For example, two clinicians might agree which of two treatment options they value more (for its potential benefit to the patient despite its modest probability of success), but if one clinician is highly risk-averse they may choose the lower-value option, nevertheless.

Despite this, some professionals claim that they always make decisions 'wholly rationally', that is, impartially and dispassionately. However, research evidence on bias contradicts these claims.[10] It is wise to acknowledge that there are always likely to be gaps and errors in our data and reasoning. Acknowledging uncertainty leads to better decision-making.

Uncertainty in clinical forensic psychiatry

Uncertainty in common in forensic psychiatry for several reasons:
- There may be uncertainty in the <u>formulation</u> (p.146) of how the patient's mental disorder affects their risk of harm.
- There is a lack of robust evidence about the efficacy of many treatments in forensic psychiatry, especially in relation to risk reduction.
- Current practice is often based more upon consensus, cultural stereotypes, and tradition than upon an evidence base.
- There is particular uncertainty about the <u>reliability and validity of risk assessment</u> (p.165).

It is ethically crucial to acknowledge these uncertainties and record and reflect on areas of agreement and disagreement. It is also vital to be transparent about the decision that has to be made, the limits of the data available, and the values being applied. Commonly one person or agency may emphasise or ignore particular facts so as to justify their particular position. This is empirically unsound and ethically unjustifiable.

Where there is disagreement, not only the facts but also the values underlying any disagreement must be made apparent. Within teams, acknowledging uncertainty and being open about conflicting values can promote cohesion.

---

9 This topic is explored in detail in Part A of the *Oxford Casebook of Forensic Psychiatry*.

10 A catalogue of the multifarious sources, types and expressions of bias exhibited by doctors and other humans can also be found in Part A of the *Casebook*.

Uncertainty in expert witness practice

In medicolegal practice the <u>adversarial process</u> (p.369) can tend to push experts into expressing greater levels of confidence in their opinion than they might express, for example, in a clinical discussion.

It is therefore important to acknowledge areas of uncertainty, or lack of knowledge, within <u>expert testimony</u> (p.652), and to be honest about the degree of certainty with which a view is held. The <u>duty to the court</u> (p.658) specifically requires that an expert sets out areas of uncertainty in their opinion; and failure to do so risks making the whole of one's testimony appear unreliable.[11]

Failure to acknowledge ignorance or uncertainty can lead to an expert straying outside their areas of competence, with potential for professional <u>fitness to practise proceedings</u> (p.642).

---

11 Research evidence from the USA suggests that juries tend to believe the testimony of experts who express themselves 'about 70% confident' of their opinion over those experts who say that they are 'certain' of their view.

Changing opinions or reports

Proper changes of opinion

In both clinical and medicolegal settings, it is essential to be ready to change your opinion if new relevant information comes to light, or a more appropriate formulation becomes apparent. Good-quality opinions include <u>acknowledgement</u> of uncertainty (p.304) and flexibility of mind. You must therefore always be open to appraising fresh information or evidence, and to acknowledging that there may be a more valid analysis of the available information than the one you have adopted. Doing so is evidence of intellectual integrity and commitment to the goal of objectivity.

Where a previous opinion has been expressed in writing, for example in a report to a court or tribunal, any changes and the reason for them must be obvious to the reader.

When not to change your opinion

In medicolegal practice, lawyers may ask for a <u>change of opinion</u> (p.690) because the report does not support, or undermines, their case. It is clearly wrong to change your opinion in this way, unless new evidence has come to light which does alter your opinion. Your duty is to the court and not to the party that has instructed you.

Removal of information from a report

Alternatively, lawyers may request that you remove certain information from the report (usually the account of your interview with the evaluee or an informant). If the information is wholly irrelevant to your opinion, and to the legal questions to which it is to be applied, then there may be a basis for removal. If the information is legally privileged (e.g. evidence that is inadmissible or past convictions that should not be made known in open court) then it should be removed. However, great caution should be exercised in acceding to the request.[12] If the information is legally inadmissible but clinically relevant then you will be faced with a dilemma, and may have to withdraw from the case.

This holds even if, for example, a report is requested for one legal purpose, and then a request is made for modification for a different purpose (e.g. a report not used at trial but for sentencing). What matters is the use to which it is *now* intended to apply the report, and whether the data are relevant to that new purpose.

When not to give an opinion

Hopefully rarely, instructing solicitors may state that they are seeking an expert opinion that will state or support a particular position, for example after having received an unhelpful report from another expert. You should never take instructions on this basis; to do so would suggest misconduct in expert testimony.

---

12 Indeed, the Court of Appeal has ruled that such behaviour by an expert is usually improper.

Disclosure by the author of a report

Your report technically belongs to those who instruct you, and they may be at liberty not to disclose it. For example, the defence in criminal proceedings and lawyers representing clients at Mental Health Tribunals, but not the prosecution (where the report is automatically disclosed). In family proceedings concerning children, your report belongs to the court, and cannot be shared without its agreement.

Where a report is not used, there is a duty of confidentiality upon the author not to share the contents of the report (including the opinion) with anyone else without the consent of the instructing solicitors. However, disclosure may be both ethical and lawful where it is deemed to be 'in the public interest'; for example in order to reduce a significant risk of serious harm to the public (_W v Egdell_, p.754), or for the administration of justice, such as in relation to proper sentencing of a defendant (_Crozier_, p.752). Such a decision to disclose is complex and may lead to professional scrutiny; you should seek legal advice before disclosure.

Changing your opinion in court

If your opinion changes during court proceedings (e.g. because of new evidence that arises during a trial), you must make this known to those instructing you, and ultimately to the court. On very rare occasions this can occur at such a late stage that it gives rise to legal complications and a professional ethical dilemma.

Supervision, peer review, and reflective practice

All trainees should have access to regular supervision, including concerning report writing and giving evidence (alongside comprehensive training through, for example, psycho-legal workshops[13]). Mentoring is helpful during early senior practice. Any senior clinician should routinely use peer review, including concerning clinico-legal work.

Supervision

The purpose of supervision is to develop knowledge, skills, and professional identity, including by exploring uncertainties, especially about ethical dilemmas. Supervisors should focus on reflection upon clinical and ethical practice. A supervisor will also be a good source of feedback about performance. If the trainee does not feel comfortable with their regular supervisor, it may be sensible to ask for regular supervision elsewhere, or from an additional supervisor.

Supervision is particularly important in psychiatry because psychiatric practice is emotionally demanding. Psychiatrists are over-represented amongst doctors with mental health and substance misuse problems, and as subjects of fitness to practice hearings (p.642). It is therefore very important for all psychiatrists to take their own mind and feelings seriously. Development of the ability to use mentoring and/or a peer group for reflection is a key competence. In training, explicit clinico-legal supervision is necessary (tribunals offer an obviously available focus for both report writing and observed oral evidence).

Peer review and support

Peer review allows for supportive learning and challenge to practice, and may be compulsory towards appraisal and revalidation (p.552). Peer discussion of clinico-legal aspects of work, including both tribunal and court work, is extremely important.

Expert witnesses may receive feedback from instructing lawyers and courts, but this is likely to be biased by case outcome. Peer review of expert witness practice should involve colleagues involved in similar practice. All forensic psychiatrists should ensure that they have access to a forum where their clinico-legal work is reviewed.

Robust peer review can guard against the risk of 'baseline drift' (becoming systematically biased towards the defence, or prosecution), or bias generally. This risk is considerable in forensic psychiatry, with its substantial scope for value judgment, and therefore the intrusion of personal values (p.674) into professional opinions.

13 See *Oxford Casebook of Forensic Psychiatry.*

Reflective practice

This professional group process involves listening and learning from one another, via professionals coming together in a forum where there is no formal agenda, to recall significant events and outcomes in recent practice, to evaluate them critically, and to consider what might be done differently in the future to improve those outcomes.

Reflective practice can encourage teams to share uncertainties as well as different knowledge perspectives. It can be helpful in reducing splitting (p.312) between professional groups, especially in long-stay residential care. It is considered essential for services managing patients with personality disorder (p.78). Within multidisciplinary teams (p.312) reflective practice can be used to pursue values-based practice (p.288) approaches to resolving ethical dilemmas. Research across a range of healthcare settings has demonstrated that a system of reflective practice is very strongly associated with better outcomes for patients.

Chapter 11

Conflicting ethical values

Working in multidisciplinary teams

Professional regulators (p.772) place a duty on professionals to work in teams with other colleagues whenever appropriate. Breakdowns in team functioning can lead to poor communication, which impairs patient care and increases risk. It is therefore essential that all psychiatrists and other professionals understand, and respect, all disciplines which offer care to patients. This is particularly true of forensic psychiatry, where the forensic multidisciplinary team (p.300) is the vehicle for good-quality care, and the repository of both technical and ethical decision-making.

Disputes within teams

It is entirely reasonable that experienced clinicians from different professions will take different views about the management of complex cases, and dissent within a team can be healthy. Often a person who is dissenting holds a perspective or piece of information that needs consideration, however uncomfortable that may be for other team members. All MDT members need to be alert to the potential for blaming a team's difficulties upon one person (scapegoating).

The impact of patients' mental disorder

Working with anyone who is suffering or in pain has a psychological impact on the professional. Where patients have a mental disorder that affects how they relate to others (especially borderline personality disorder (p.84) or narcissistic personality disorder, p.86), their lack of mature skills for managing their emotional distress may result in them unconsciously projecting (p.212) aspects of their distress into certain staff. This can lead to **splitting** within the clinical team, where certain team members, for example, respond to the patients' anger or hatred by wishing to reject them, while others, responding to patients' idealisation of them, wish to go above and beyond to help them.

Maintaining healthy team functioning

It is important that teams have some framework for managing disputes, so as to prevent them from becoming personal and or divisive, and for recognising and managing unhealthy team dynamics, such as splitting. Use of reflective practice (p.308) is beneficial, as is adopting an overall framework of values-based practice (p.288).

Professionals who know the team and its work but who are independent of it, especially those with specific training in understanding organisational dynamics (such as forensic psychotherapists), may be particularly useful facilitators.

Working with other agencies

Agencies commonly encountered

Psychiatry involves working with many different welfare-based professional groups, with differing knowledge bases. These include:
- other branches of medicine,
- <u>social</u> care and chid protection <u>services</u> (p.226),
- housing agencies, and
- charities and other voluntary bodies.

However, forensic psychiatry also deals with justice agencies, whose <u>purposes</u>, <u>values</u>, culture, and methods (p.352) are very different from those of welfare agencies. These include:
- lawyers,
- <u>courts</u> and <u>tribunals</u> (p.372),
- <u>prisons</u> (p.578),
- <u>probation services</u> (p.584),
- <u>police</u> and other criminal investigatory bodies (p.566),
- <u>prosecution</u> agencies (p.566), and
- <u>justice ministries</u> (p.586).

Finally, forensic psychiatrists in the three UK jurisdictions are expected to participate directly in the public management of any risk posed by forensic patients, usually under the auspices of the <u>MAPPA</u> (p.592). This can raise legal and ethical challenges.

What does 'working with' other agencies mean?

Working with an agency usually involves establishing cordial professional relations and channels of communication. Meetings about patients should always identify those present; affirm commitment to duties of confidentiality (which will vary between agencies) and respect for diversity, and set out an agenda. The various professionals may wish to articulate differences of values, conflicts of interest, and limits of what they can say; for example, if a therapist is attending a meeting about a patient, they may state for the record that they will not be able to disclose any material from therapy sessions. Boundary-setting at an early point in a meeting helps other professionals to understand potential conflicts about communication. Minutes of discussions should be kept and checked by all parties before being approved as accurate.

Written reports about the patient's condition, treatment, and prognosis may be requested by any contributing agency. As with any other report, nothing should be committed to paper, or electronically communicated, unless and until the author has established:
- What is the purpose of this report?
- What are the specific questions requested to be addressed?
- Who will see this report and why?
- Can the recipient otherwise guarantee its confidentiality?
- What does the patient think about the request for a report, including does the patient agree to it being written?
- If the patient has refused permission for a report is it possible to justify it without consent?

It is important to remember that just because someone important-sounding asks for a report, or some feedback, does not mean that it has to be given. If in doubt, seek advice.

Disclosure when working with justice agencies

Ethical tension may arise between forensic psychiatrists and justice agencies, particularly in relation to <u>disclosure of confidential information</u> (p.320). Other agencies have different professional agendas and ethical obligations from health agencies, and may insist that psychiatrists help them to deliver them. To maintain boundaries around disclosure, seek the patient's consent wherever possible. Reports written for clinical purposes should not be disclosed to agencies dealing with other purposes without consent; disclosure is often 'justified' on the grounds of time constraints, but it is a breach of governance rules and ethical principles.

Working with other public bodies

Other public bodies

An **agency** provides a service to citizens. In contrast, a **public body** is a publicly funded group established (usually by statute) to contribute to the process of government. Public bodies may be affiliated with a government department but operate with a degree of independence. As other agencies (p.314) that forensic psychiatrists may encounter clinically have been described, this page covers the public bodies they may encounter professionally.

Forensic psychiatrists may be invited to advise or work with:

- NHS/HSE provider bodies, such as Hospitals and Foundation Trusts;
- NHS/HSE commissioning bodies,[1] such as NHS England, Specialist Commissioning Groups, and Health Boards;
- the Law Commission[2];
- the Parole Board;
- healthcare quality regulators[3];
- advisory committees, such as the Sentencing Advisory Panel and Victims' Advisory Panel; and
- professional regulators (p.772).

What does 'working with' public bodies mean?

As with other agencies (p.314), 'working with' usually involves establishing cordial professional relations and channels of communication. Written communication should be kept, and, where discussions are had, notes should be kept and agreed by both parties.

The psychiatrist working with these bodies will usually do so in an advisory or expert capacity, either as an individual or as a representative of their employer or a body such as the Royal College of Psychiatrists. They will usually be invited to provide general information and advice. Where individual clinical material is considered, its use is subject to data protection rules and ethical guidance on confidentiality (p.320).

Research on services may precipitate ethical tension if the results are interpreted differently by the researchers and those who commissioned the research. Researchers may need to gain advice from their professional body in these situations.

Problems relating to commissioning of services

In those countries where there is a split between commissioners and providers of health services (chiefly NI and England), there may be ethical tensions concerning clinical information-sharing, especially where there is

---

1 Scotland and Wales have abolished the commissioner/provider distinction for secondary care, and it has never existed in RoI; in these countries, the same bodies usually both plan and provide care. In England, the development of 'integrated care systems' is blurring the distinction.

2 The Law Commission for E&W, the NI Law Commission, the Scottish Law Commission, and in RoI, the Law Reform Commission.

3 The Care Quality Commission for England, the Healthcare Inspectorate in Wales, the Care Inspectorate in Scotland, the Regulation and Quality Improvement Authority in NI, and the Health Information and Quality Authority in RoI.

'micro-commissioning' of specialist services for named individual patients. Commissioning staff may request detailed information about patients, or seek to approve or not detailed care plans for patients themselves, including adopting their own risk assessments.

Tensions arise because commissioning staff may not have the same clinical or ethical duties to patients as do psychiatrists, and there may be conflict between what is in the patient's interests and what is in the commissioner's interests (e.g. to avoid overspending a budget, or to avoid perceived responsibility for a high-profile offender). Psychiatrists working in commissioning organisations, like those operating as <u>medical managers</u> (p.299), may be particularly affected by such potential conflict.

Faced with potential conflict, or significant concerns about the uses to which a commissioner might put confidential information, it would be wise to seek advice from your defence organisation or professional body, and to present that advice to the commissioner (perhaps via a senior manager within your employer).

Working in nontherapeutic contexts

A nontherapeutic context is one in which there is no individual doctor-patient relationship. This can arise either because the doctor is giving general or aggregate (rather than patient-specific) information, or because they are giving information on a patient to a non-health agency (p.314) or public body (p.316).

Examples

- Giving advice to the Care Quality Commission about services for mentally disordered offenders is working in a *nontherapeutic* context, in that it involves using general professional expertise to assist a public body.
- By contrast, a forensic psychiatrist who discusses a patient's clinical condition with a social worker or housing officer in an effort to find the patient housing is working in a *therapeutic* context, in that the patient's welfare is a key focus of the discussion.
- Giving evidence in relation to diminished responsibility (p.624) during a murder trial involves working *nontherapeutically*, for the purposes of justice (even though the evidence is patient-specific and is partly clinical).
- Even giving evidence to enable court-ordered hospital treatment (p.500) for your patient is *nontherapeutic*, because the purpose of the court is administering justice.
- Particular ethical issues arise in relation to assessment and giving evidence in relation to verdict (p.664) or sentencing (p.670).

Should psychiatrists ever work in nontherapeutic contexts?

Some argue that doctors are always in a therapeutic role because of their training, identity and the skills they apply, and they therefore always owe a duty of care to any individual they assess, whatever the context. If true, psychiatrists could never justify providing courts or tribunals with opinions that might cause harm to an individual (e.g. if the court used their evidence when later finding the defendant 'dangerous', p.672, and imposing an indeterminate sentence, p.448).

If psychiatrists were never to work in nontherapeutic contexts, then public bodies and courts would not be able to benefit from their expertise. Arguably, the professional knowledge that doctors have is acquired for the public good as a whole, and not just for the benefit of individuals. Without good-quality medical opinions, health and welfare provision would be damaged. In relation to the criminal justice process, the lack of such information could itself lead to injustice, which would be harmful to all.

A further argument against working solely within an individual therapeutic model is that psychiatrists often have more than one individual's welfare to consider. For example, a perinatal psychiatrist may decide that the mother's mental disorder may lead her to pose a risk to her baby. The psychiatrist will obviously have to weigh up the risk to the child against the harm of the distress caused by separating mother and child. Under family law principles (p.554), the doctor must put the child's interests above the mother's, even though the baby is not their patient; it is not a situation of competing interests between two of their patients.

Further, some argue that violence reduction is one of the primary tasks of forensic psychiatric practice. If they do not provide risk assessments in nontherapeutic contexts, they will be failing in that task.

Finally, some argue that assisting in public protection by preventing the commission of an offence also prevents patients suffering the harmful consequences of offending. However, this suggestion is not usually applied to people without mental disorder and is therefore arguably discriminatory.

Confidentiality and disclosure

Box 11.1 Ethical bases for sharing information

- Within and between clinical teams providing care, for the purposes of care and audit, providing the patient has not objected ('need to know')
- Where the patient has given informed consent to disclosure
- Where the disclosure will benefit a patient who lacks the capacity to consent to disclosure
- Where the disclosure is required or permitted by law
- Where disclosure is in the public interest, in limited circumstances
- Very occasionally, where disclosure is in a third party's interest

The medical duty of confidentiality is based upon the ethical principle of respect for <u>autonomy</u> (p.331): people should have control over their own personal information.[4] Duties of confidentiality arise because patients need to share information with professionals, for therapeutic purposes, that could make them vulnerable to social shame or criticism.

Disclosure with consent, or within care teams

Informed consent to disclosure is often straightforward to obtain, and this should always be the default requirement for sharing information outside the direct care team. Consent to disclosure within the care teams directly involved can be implied. If a patient with capacity objects to information-sharing the consequences of this (such as not receiving treatment from a team you now cannot refer to) should be explained and a compromise sought; if agreement cannot be reached and disclosure is not legally required or in the public interest, you must respect the patient's wishes. Even when explicit consent is given, the information shared should still be the minimum necessary for the purpose.

Disclosure when the patient lacks capacity

Where the patient lacks capacity and will not regain it soon enough for to make the decision on disclosure, the decision should be based on the patient's best interests[5] (i.e. whether they will benefit overall from disclosure). Patients should be involved in the decision whether to disclose, and their wishes and preferences should be taken into account, along with the views of anyone they ask you to consult or who you know is close to them (or who has a power of attorney or is an appointed deputy or IMCA).

If patients do not agree to disclosure, and cannot be persuaded, you should inform them and any carer before going ahead with disclosure.

---

4 In law, it is based on data protection legislation, and more generally on <u>Article 8 ECHR</u> (p.517). The rules under data protection legislation follow very similar principles to those set out here.

5 In RoI, this remains the explicit guidance from the MC, despite the fact that the concept of 'best interests' is no longer part of Irish law on mental capacity (i.e. the <u>ADMCA</u>, p.534).

Disclosure required or permitted by law

In certain circumstances, there is a legal duty to disclose, such as:

- notification of certain infectious diseases,
- prevention of terrorism or treason,
- investigation of road traffic accidents,
- if ordered by a court (e.g. following a subpoena to give evidence),
- if required or ordered as part of pretrial precognition in Scotland, and
- when required by government agencies, in limited circumstances.

Law in E&W and NI also empowers professionals to disclose information without consent, leaving an element of discretion: only E&W has approved regulations for this purpose, including providing for cancer registries, certain research projects, public health systems, and measures for controlling communicable diseases (including Covid-19).

Disclosure prohibited by law

In the UK, other laws specifically prohibit the sharing of information related to gender recognition and gender history, parentage after sperm donation, and past or current infection with HIV or certain other sexually transmitted diseases. You should seek advice before disclosing such information outside the care team without explicit consent, even if disclosure appears to be legally required.

Disclosure in the public interest

Ethical codes (p.295) allow the patient's interest in confidentiality to be balanced against the harm that would result from nondisclosure. Before relying on the existence of an overriding public interest in disclosure, you should seek consent if possible (unless there is no time, or patients cannot be contacted, or alerting them would defeat the purpose of disclosure, such as preventing serious crime), and you should consider seeking advice before proceeding. You may only share the minimum necessary for the purpose, and should seek confirmation that the person or body to whom you disclose the information will use it properly.

An overriding public interest may exist where there is a significant risk of serious harm to others[6]. This includes:

- abuse of children or vulnerable adults,
- the prevention, detection or prosecution of other serious crime,
- serious communicable diseases,
- unfitness to drive, and
- unfitness to work, if this will place others at risk of serious harm (e.g. air-traffic controllers, surgeons).

Disclosure in the interest of a third party

Patients may request that information is not shared with specific relatives or friends; such requests should be respected unless this could harm that individual. Very occasionally, there may be an ethical duty[7] to consider disclosure to such an individual if they could otherwise suffer serious harm (e.g. from a severe genetic disorder that would therefore go undiagnosed). If you think this might apply, you must seek advice before proceeding.

6 This is also the legal test from W v Egdell (p.754).

7 And, at least in E&W, a legal duty in some cases: ABC v St George's (p.745).

Ethical risk assessment & management

An ethical analysis of risk assessment

Risk assessment is a form of consequential analysis, not a <u>prediction of future events</u> (p.164). It examines the likelihood of scenarios in which harm might occur within a given period. If a patient is assessed as likely to cause serious harm in the near future, this may imply a professional duty to intervene to reduce that risk. Failure to do so may lead to professional criticism, as in the <u>Barrett inquiry</u>[8] (p.780), or even negligence litigation.

Some psychiatrists may wish to try to avoid risk assessment altogether. But risk-taking is unavoidable in psychiatry as in the rest of medicine; choosing to take such risks whilst being wilfully blind to their nature and magnitude is neither ethical nor legally defensible.

However, actions that reduce the likelihood of an offender causing harm may result in conditions that the offender perceives as harmful, such as deprivation or restriction of liberty. The offender may also feel wronged: for example, if uninformed or deceived about the <u>disclosure of confidential information</u> (p.320). Even being known to have been the subject of a forensic risk assessment, whatever the result, can stigmatise patients.

Consent to risk assessment

Doctors may not take actions that could harm a patient without seeking their <u>informed consent</u> (p.332), and can act in the absence of consent only where there is a specific legal power to do so. If a patient has consented in full knowledge of how their interests might be harmed, there is no ethical dilemma in carrying out a risk assessment, and for this reason some advocate seeking explicit <u>consent to risk assessment</u> (p.342). This is, in effect, to treat risk assessment[9] as a technical clinical procedure, akin to an MRI scan, <u>CBT</u> (p.206), or colonoscopy.

Often in forensic psychiatry, either it will be reasonable not to perform the risk assessment if consent is refused, or there will be a legal power that clearly overrides a patient's refusal of consent. However, scenarios such as that presented in Box 11.2 pose serious problems.

In such a case many psychiatrists will proceed with risk assessment on the ground that the benefits to others (e.g. staff and other patients in hospital, or in this case Mr E's children and potentially the children of others) outweigh the possible harm to the patient.

Transparency and joint endeavour

If harm is to be done to the patient (or risked), because the interests of others have been allowed to override the patient's interests, then it is essential that clinicians are honest and open about it, including with the patient.

---

8 The details of this case were more complicated than suggested above: for example, the patient's RMO had believed at the time that he was not at high risk of causing serious harm.

9 *Risk assessment* here refers to a formal process, particularly when carried out by a team using a structured instrument such as the HCR20. If the term is used in the more general sense of 'reaching an opinion on the risk the patient poses', especially a single, personal opinion, then it is not meaningful to seek consent for the forming of that opinion, but consent might be needed before acting on that opinion as part of a risk management plan or disclosing it to others.

Box 11.2 Example: Mr E

Mr E is suspected by the police of a contact child sexual offence, but there is insufficient evidence to prosecute. He is being treated informally for a transient psychotic episode associated with borderline personality disorder. Social services request a formal assessment of his risk of sexual offending in order to decide whether, or under what conditions, he may live with his children. He refuses, fearing loss of contact with his children.

Being open about this process risks damaging the therapeutic relationship in the short-term, but concealing what you are doing risks more serious long-term damage to the relationship, as the patient is likely to discover eventually how they have been deceived.[10] Moreover, building a long-term relationship based upon openness facilitates approaching risk assessment as a joint endeavour with the patient, on the basis of shared decision-making within which different <u>value perspectives</u> (pp.281–291) can be acknowledged and respected, despite being overridden.

Reporting the results of risk assessment

A further ethical dilemma may arise in having to decide whether to disclose a risk assessment to others, including whether to include it in a court report if its conclusions might harm the patient's interest. There may be a specific legal <u>duty to disclose</u> it (p.321). Otherwise, as with the decision to conduct the risk assessment, consent to disclosure should first be sought, and there should only be disclosure after a refusal if that is justified in the <u>public interest</u> (p.321).

Organisational liability and the 'tick-list' mentality

Situations within which a patient's interest in not undergoing risk assessment may be overridden must be considered on a case-by-case basis. It is not acceptable to adopt a blanket policy of risk assessment without consent, particularly if coupled with disclosure, solely in order to discharge or limit the corporate responsibility of the organisation.

---

10 See, for example, <u>RM v St Andrew's</u> (p.766).

Philosophy and ethics of coercion

Mental health legislation in the UK and RoI allows involuntary treatment for mental disorder even where the patient retains the capacity to decide for themselves, and without reference to their <u>best interests</u> (p.334). This remains ethically contentious, given that professionals are usually required to respect patient <u>autonomy</u> (p.331), and coercion may cause harm to <u>treatment acceptance and outcome</u> (p.188).

What is coercion?

Coercion involves putting physical or psychological limits on a person's liberty and freedom to choose. It may be State-sanctioned or institutional; it may involve the use of threats, intimidation, and reward, and may affect a person's agency in terms of exercising choice. Coercion may be <u>objective</u> and/or <u>perceived</u> (p.186) by the patient.

The relationship of coercion to legal compulsion

Involuntary legal status is a poor gauge of perceived coercion: a considerable proportion of detained patients describe feeling *less* coerced than many informal patients. There are doubts about whether it is possible to measure perceived coercion, chiefly because measures cannot assess the influence of social context or interaction. Narrative methods are more likely to provide valid accounts of perceived coercion and may capture contextual and cultural aspects of a patient's story.

The relationship of coercion to agency

Agency is a person's capacity to act: to make choices and then to enact them. Coercion, whether related to legal status or other factors, usually significantly impairs the patient's sense of agency. Just being a psychiatric patient (especially a detained patient or a forensic patient) can inhibit patients' agency, by limiting the choices they believe they are able to make, and the choices other people will respect.

Some argue that a person who is coerced lacks agency completely, whereas other argue that the coercion alters agency by affecting the choices made. For example, offering rewards is seen as less coercive because it is one of many influences on a person's agency; the patient can choose whether to accept the reward. Philosophical consideration of the nature of liberty leads to questions about psychiatric practices, such as making leave or other inducements conditional on compliance with treatment.

There remain debates about whether coercion negates the operation of mental capacity, and conversely, whether incapacity precludes the possibility of coercion.

When is coercion justified?

Justification for coercion depends on a balance between the <u>ethical values</u> (p.286) placed on individual autonomy and on beneficence (to a person) or justice (to others). Most countries have mental health legislation that justifies loss of autonomy in the pursuit of beneficence.

However legally justified, usurping or overriding the will of another is paternalistic, especially when justified on the grounds of beneficence. Coercion into treatment is generally motivated by paternalistic concern for the welfare and safety of the individual, or of others. The harm caused by the loss of individual agency is justified with reference to the potential harm that might occur if the person were not detained; in terms of an overall ethical calculus similar to risk assessment addressing both individual and social risks and benefits. There is a policy assumption that the costs of coercion in terms of deprivation of liberty are outweighed by welfare benefits to patients or society. However, there is less policy attention to proving that coercion actually results in improved mental health outcomes.

Clinical matters raising
ethical issues

Concepts of mental disorder

Forensic psychiatrists use the ICD and DSM, like other psychiatrists. They also work in <u>MDTs</u> (p.312) and with <u>other agencies</u> (p.314), and the latter in particular utilise conflicting <u>constructs</u> (p.354) of mental disorder. They should therefore be very familiar with other concepts of mental disorder in use.

Models used by mental health and social work professionals

The **medical model** of mental disorder assumes that it represents the presence of disease that can be treated by medical interventions (particularly medication) and thereby relieved or even cured. This works tolerably well for mental illnesses such as <u>depression</u> (p.94), but less well for <u>personality disorders</u> (p.78) and developmental disorders such as <u>autism</u> (p.104). The lower the 'fact to values' ratio inherent in a diagnosis, the more room is there for disagreement over whether it is indeed a valid medical diagnosis or whether an individual validly exhibits that diagnosis.[1]

Psychologists and psychiatrists use a variety of **psychological models** of mental disorder (e.g. <u>cognitive-behavioural</u>, p.206; <u>mentalisation-based</u>, p.208; and <u>systemic</u>, p.218), all of which treat individuals as having a greater or lesser degree of a particular trait, dimension, or difficulty. The threshold for 'caseness' is statistical, or arbitrary, and individual <u>formulation</u> (p.146) is essential for understanding *why* a person is now experiencing mental distress.

<u>**Social workers**</u>' (p.226) training focuses on social constructions of distress and dysfunction. Helping patients involves amelioration of an individual's social situation in a holistic way. Social work models do not grant mental disorder any special status relative to other forms of deprivation, and are open to seeing some forms of mental disorder (e.g. <u>ASPD</u>, p.82; or hebephrenic schizophrenia) as purely social constructs, potentially employed so as to disadvantage politically unpopular groups (analogous to the concept of <u>sluggish schizophrenia</u>, p.520, having been misused in the Soviet Union).

Occupational therapists use the **model of human occupation** (p.229) as a basis for recovery. Occupation is seen as essential to a fulfilling life for every person, and occupational therapy emphasises the recovery of personal and social skills (including occupations and activities) that are meaningful and fulfilling to patients.

The **biopsychosocial** model of mind attempts to integrate the strengths of all the above models; it eschews a clear ultimate statement of what mental disorder *is*, in favour of a multifactorial treatment of how it *arises*.

From an ethical perspective, all these models have a clear, unambiguous focus on the welfare of the individual. They explicitly ethically question how justified it is to harm a patient (e.g. through deprivation of liberty) for the benefit of society or individual victims (see p.322).

---

1 See the work of WMK (Bill) Fulford in regard to diagnoses being variously open to values disagreement, as to whether the observed 'difference' inherent in a condition is generally accepted to be 'disadvantageous', and so is 'a disease'.

Legal concepts of mental disorder

In contrast to all mental health professionals, the philosophical starting points for most legal, including criminal justice, professionals are morality (doing what is right) and justice (treating people according to what is fair, due, or owed). Mental disorder is only relevant to justice insofar as it alters what is the right or just response to an offender with such a disorder (e.g. through making available <u>mental condition defences</u>, p.412). This perspective is also respectful of the person with a mental disorder as a citizen, who benefits from a fair justice process.

Justice as fairness is the basis for the State taking action to harm an individual's interest or welfare if they commit an offence. Courts express social condemnation by <u>sentences</u> (p.442) that impose a financial cost or deprivation of liberty. Harm prevention may also be used as a justification for loss of liberty: for example public health laws still allow people who have an infectious disease such as Covid-19 to be quarantined, with loss of liberty, even though they have done no wrong.

Justice processes regulate relations between individuals and society, and by doing so, bind societies together in ways that fosters the dignity and rights of all. Only those professionals who are socially mandated to do so can dispense justice, and it is vital that doctors (especially psychiatrists) do not seek to usurp the role of the courts.

Symptoms, behaviours, and causes

Doctors can mistake behaviours for symptoms, and vice versa.[2] This may be a particular problem when there is a characteristic and close relationship between a behaviour and a disorder—such as between <u>violence</u> (p.44) and <u>ASPD</u> (p.82), or between <u>incompetent stalking</u> (p.52) and <u>intellectual disability</u> (p.110). Conversely, when the underlying disorder is difficult to identify and the behaviour seems intractable, it becomes difficult to see past the behaviour so as to <u>treat the disorder</u> (p.182).

This problem is exacerbated in forensic psychiatry because people are often referred *solely* because of their behaviour: for example, sexually inappropriate behaviour with children, or fire-setting. The referrer wants the behaviour abolished, and will not necessarily easily accept that the psychiatrist can only treat any underlying mental disorder (if there is one[3]), which might or might not affect the behaviour. This problem is particularly acute if the behaviour is not evident during the psychiatric assessment (e.g. during a period of assessment on a medium secure ward) but is expected to recur in the community.

A practical consequence of this is that it is very important to recognise and <u>acknowledge uncertainty</u> (p.304) from the outset, and to be open with referrers and patients about what might, and might not, be achieved by the assessment or treatment that is being offered.

---

2 This problem is not unique to doctors: a social worker, for example, should likewise identify and ameliorate the underlying social deprivation, not the resulting behaviour.

3 In extreme cases, diagnoses may be applied or even defined based upon behaviour alone: for example, a sexually deviant behaviour may be defined as <u>paraphilia</u> (p.102) merely because it conflicts with social values, in the absence of distress or interference with daily life.

Values and diversity in forensic practice

Respect for diversity of values

The rehabilitation and recovery movements of the 1960s and 1990s emphasised respect for the values and views of psychiatric patients, no matter how unwell or disabled they might be. Such approaches are consistent with the ethical principle of respect for <u>autonomy</u> (p.331).

This includes respect for the diversity of experience and identity in human psychological experience. Critics of psychiatric services often argue, with reason, that mental health professionals who have never been mentally ill, or do not otherwise share a patient's experience, cannot fully appreciate their perspective or values. Respect for diversity entails thinking about stereotypes that may be operating in mental health systems, and which may affect professional judgment.

Recognising diversity in psychiatry

Psychiatrists are often asked to comment upon <u>unusual behaviours</u> (p.329). Their assessment of what is unusual may be affected by their own cultural prejudices, or stereotypes of normality, for example:

- age, 'over seventy-five year olds will be too slow to participate in workshops';
- family role, 'normal mothers never hate their children';
- gender identity, 'cis heterosexual men do not dress like that';
- professional role, 'civil servants do not hit their partners';
- ethnicity, 'that black man is psychotic, he must have schizophrenia' (not asking about abnormal mood, or life events; see p.40);
- religious roles, 'Christians do not commit suicide'; 'all devout Muslims reject European value systems';
- educational status, 'she has no qualifications, so she must be stupid'; and
- health status, 'patients will be unable to understand professional views'.

All clinicians must recognise their own prejudices, in order to be able to overcome them in their clinical practice. It is clinically wise, as well as respectful, to treat each patient as an individual, and not make assumptions about their experiences, hopes and aspirations. It is offensive to assume that they will not share ordinary human wants, wishes, and needs because they differ from you in terms of skin colour, sex, or education.

Respect for diversity of values in forensic psychiatry

In forensic psychiatric practice, many service users have antisocial beliefs and attitudes, which conflict with the <u>values</u> of their communities (p.289). They may also not share the values of their treatment team, or the State (e.g. in relation to taking medication that might reduce risk). It can therefore be difficult to respect their personal values.

For many forensic patients, being criminal or antisocial may have been a way to survive trauma and deprivation. Building therapeutic relationships with forensic patients usually requires an empathic understanding of the patient's antisocial stance, and how difficult it feels to give it up.

It is also important to consider the views and values of family members, as they may play a key role in the treatment of the patient. Their value systems may differ from that of the patient.

Autonomy and self-determination

Autonomy means 'self-rule' and entails a sense of 'self' and 'identity'. Autonomy is related to the philosophical concept of agency (p.324). A person's autonomy of action may be impaired (e.g. because they require a wheelchair) but the person may still have autonomy of will and thought.

Most mental disorders impair autonomy, but not all, or at all times, or to the same degree. Loss of identity ('he's not himself') may be the first sign of mental disorder; recovery is often associated with being 'back to their old self'. For many patients, the purpose of psychiatric treatment is to restore autonomy.

Impairment of autonomy is of particular relevance in forensic psychiatry because it can be related to:

• mental disorders that reduce ability to behave pro-socially and in accordance with the law,
• impairment of mental capacity (p.522) affecting legal proceedings, and
• reduction, or lack of criminal responsibility (p.406) for one's actions.

Forensic psychiatric evidence may be called to help the criminal court distinguish a person whose autonomy has been impaired from someone who has chosen to act unlawfully.

The four principles approach (p.287) to medical ethics emphasises respect for patients' autonomy. However, this can be complex in forensic psychiatry because patients' autonomous choices and values sometimes involve exploitation of others or disregard for rules. Respect for one person's autonomy, or freedom of action, must be balanced against respect for that of others (e.g. their potential victims), and considered in the relevant social context. For example, it might be appropriate to restrict a patient's freedom of action in a secure psychiatric unit in a way that would be unacceptable in the community.

Consent to treatment

The ethical requirement of consent is based on the principles of <u>autonomy and self-determination</u> (p.331). The primary focus of consent in mental health is treatment for mental disorder. The <u>law on consent to psychiatric treatment</u> (p.482) and <u>capacity law</u> (p.522) are considered separately.

Patient autonomy

It is an established principle that people with mental capacity can <u>refuse medical treatment</u> (p.336), except where there are specific laws to the contrary. Examples of such laws include compulsory isolation for infectious diseases in the interests of public health, or compulsory treatment for mental disorder in the interests of the health or safety of the patient, or public safety.

Principles of consent

- The individual has the mental capacity to consent or refuse.
- The consent (or refusal) is informed, based upon knowledge of the purpose and nature, risks, and likely benefits of the proposed treatment, and the alternatives to treatment, including no treatment.
- The process of gaining consent involves a dialogue about values that are meaningful to both the patient and the doctor.
- The consent or refusal must be voluntary and uncoerced.

What counts as <u>coercion</u> (p.324) or undue pressure may not be straightforward. In particular, the professionals treating prisoners and detained patients may regard them as having a free choice, but the impact of detention may make that choice feel <u>coerced</u> (p.186) to the person involved.

Process of obtaining consent

The aim is to help the patient understand their role, the options, and all relevant information, and to reach a shared understanding. You must:
- Understand what matters to the patient.
- Explain the diagnosis and prognosis, and any uncertainty about either.
- Explain all options for treatment, including no treatment.
- Explain the likely benefits and chances of success of each option.
- Explain the possible risks and side-effects of each option.
- Explore the value of each option and its possible consequences to patients, based on what is important to them.
- Give patients time to reflect on their decision.
- Point out that consent can be withdrawn at any time.

Methods of giving consent

Express consent involves the patient making an unambiguous consenting statement orally or in writing. In some circumstances the patient and doctor will sign a consent form, but legally the form is merely *evidence* of consent having been given, at a particular time, not the *fact* of consent, and is open to contradiction by other evidence.

Implied consent is deemed to have been given when the patient acts in a manner consistent with having given consent, such as holding out an arm for a blood test; it is only sufficient for minor procedures or procedures with very few risks or side-effects.

Inferred consent refers to the legal notion that consent has been given by an unconscious patient when a treatment is proposed that they are known to approve of, or that 'a reasonable person' would consent to in similar circumstances. This only applies to uncontentious treatments and circumstances, such as changing a patient's bed sheets, except in an emergency. It would be extremely unwise to rely on 'inferred consent' where there is (or could be expected to be) any dispute about the correct course of action. The safest course of action with unconscious or other incapacitated patients is to apply mental capacity law.

Consequences of treating without consent

Unless there is a specific law authorising treatment without consent in the current situation (e.g. a detention under a mental health treatment order), then a doctor who treats a patient without their consent is acting unethically, may be liable in <u>negligence</u> (p.550), and may even have committed a criminal offence such as <u>battery</u> (p.416).

Treatment during incapacity

Incapacity to consent

It is an ethical and legal requirement to obtain <u>valid consent</u> (p.332) be-fore carrying out treatment. However, many mental and physical conditions cause patients to lose their capacity to consent. When treating patients who lack capacity, the following ethical principles must be observed:

- If the patient is expected to regain capacity, and the decision can safely be deferred until then, defer it.
- Arrange circumstances so as to maximise the patient's capacity and ability to participate in the process (e.g. a calm, quiet, warm environment with trusted relatives present).
- Involve the patient in the decision as much as possible.
- Where their wishes and preferences can be ascertained (including based on past statements,[4] evidence from informants, or decisions of <u>deputies</u>, p.534, or those with <u>power of attorney</u>, p.538), respect them.
- Where the law allows you to make a decision on behalf of patients, base it on the patients' **best interests** (i.e. on what appears to be of most value to them).
- Where more than one option would meet these criteria, choose the one which least restricts the patient's rights and future freedoms.

These principles apply whether an incapacitous patient accepts or <u>refuses treatment</u>, but the latter situation presents additional ethical, practical, and emotional difficulties (p.336).

Mental disorder and incapacity

Where a patient lacks capacity because of mental disorder, and does not object to treatment, there will often be power to treat them under both mental health law and mental capacity law. The legal framework whose safeguards are more appropriate to the patient's circumstances should be chosen.

Ethical history

Capacity law's provisions for treating those who lack capacity arose pri-marily from two sorts of poignant human story:

- those with serious (sometimes terminal) illnesses who wanted to ensure they had the treatment they wanted and could refuse what they did not want; and
- those who lacked capacity to consent to or refuse treatment on a long-term basis and needed someone to make treatment decisions for them.

The latter group were sometimes known as 'involuntary informal' pa-tients because they lacked the ability to consent to treatment (which could not, therefore, be described as 'voluntary') but did not need to be detained under mental health law, as they were not refusing treatment.

However, some general mental capacity legislation, particularly in E&W, does not provide legal safeguards for those whose liberty is adversely

---

4 These can be legally binding, including for refusals of psychiatric treatment: see p.536.

affected by their treatment, for instance by being kept indefinitely in nursing homes.[5] The <u>Bournewood case</u> (p.748) provided a high-profile example of the distress (at least to carers and families) that can result, and prompted the development of special safeguards for treatments that involve a <u>deprivation of liberty</u> (p.532).

When patients refuse treatment

Capacity to refuse treatment

Respect for personal autonomy means that patients' decisions about their welfare should be respected. However, doctors may find decisions to refuse treatment difficulty to accept, especially when the result would appear to be life-threatening.

Capacity law (p.522) presumes all people to have capacity, until the contrary has been shown. A person with capacity may legally refuse all treatment[6] no matter the consequences.[7] Making a (medically) unwise decision is not evidence of lack of capacity.

However, treatment refusal, especially if it could lead to death, often triggers a capacity assessment. About half the capacity assessments carried out by liaison psychiatrists are for treatment refusal.

Refusing treatment for physical illness

Most patients who refuse treatment in general hospitals are older men, many of whom have mild cognitive impairments. Only a minority actually lack capacity.

Some of those who do lack capacity may be treated in their best interests under mental capacity law.[8] This can be difficult if the patient is behaviourally disturbed, and can cause distress in family and nursing staff. The psychiatrist can help support both staff and family in these situations. Research suggests that involving family members and friends is often effective, both because they may be able to calm or persuade the patient, and because staff will feel easier about any physical intervention if they have the support of those who know the patient well.

Patients with capacity have the legal right to refuse treatment, and this must be respected, no matter how uncomfortable this may be for staff. It is permissible however to try to find other ways to care for them that they will accept. Many patients refusing treatment change their minds after a psychiatric consultation, whether they retain capacity or not. This suggests that many 'refusals' are really explained by poor communication by medical staff, and by a lack of professional understanding that mild anger and aggression may be signs that the patient is anxious.

Refusing treatment for mental disorder

People with mental illness who are detained may or may not lack capacity to make treatment decisions. Studies of psychiatric patients in the UK have found that between 30% and 60% of inpatients lack capacity. Many of those with capacity are treated under mental health legislation, which allows compulsory treatment of such patients' mental disorder (with variation between jurisdictions: see p.482).

---

6 Although there may be other legal powers to enforce treatment despite their capacitous refusal, particularly under mental health law (p.461), but also public health and welfare laws (p.542).

7 Such as in the English cases known as Miss B and Re C (pp.747, 750).

8 Except in RoI, where staff are bound by patients' known wishes and preferences (see p.536).

Ethical problems

These current legal positions reflect different balances struck between the duty to respect individual <u>autonomy</u> (p.331) *and* the duties to promote the welfare of mentally disordered patients, and to minimise risk of harm to themselves and others.

The ethical dilemma becomes more controversial when considering:

- the long-term compulsory treatment of incapacitous individuals who may be hospitalised for very long periods, sometimes in seclusion (e.g. people with treatment-resistant schizophrenia associated with serious violence) or
- detention for treatment with no proven efficacy, or solely on the grounds of risk reduction (e.g. of patients with severe personality disorders, who retain capacity but pose a high risk of harm to others).

People in the latter group are sometimes <u>transferred to hospital</u> (p.506) shortly before the end of <u>determinate sentences</u> (p.452), meaning they effectively have extended periods of incarceration beyond their prison sentences, for involuntary treatment of doubtful benefit. This issue is a particular problem for high secure services in the UK.

The controversy is still sharper in relation to sex offenders thought to pose a high risk of harm to others through recidivism. In the USA, over forty states have enacted Sexually Violent Predator laws.[9] These allow people convicted of violent <u>sexual offences</u> (p.418) who have a '<u>mental abnormality</u>' (p.354) such as a personality disorder[10] to be detained indefinitely in a secure hospital on the grounds of risk of harm to others.[11] The California SVP programme at Coalinga State Hospital, amongst others, explicitly countenances indefinite detention for the 70%–75% of its inmates who refuse the intensive psychological treatment on offer. Although no equivalent programme currently exists in the UK or RoI, the removal of the exclusion of 'sexual deviance' as a ground for detention under the Mental Health Act in E&W potentially cleared the way for such a programme in the future, despite the lack of evidence that any of the sex offender treatment programmes for offenders are effective.

---

9 Also known by the names of the victims of sexual violence whose high-profile cases led to the passing of the laws, such as Megan's Law and Jessica's Law in California.

10 In California, for instance, the test is a serious mental illness resulting in <u>volitional impairment</u> (p.24), most commonly <u>paedophilia</u> or <u>paraphilia</u> (p.102); there must also be evidence of grooming or otherwise forming a relationship with a potential victim with intent to victimise them.

11 A test that falls well short of that in <u>Article 5 ECHR</u> (p.517), leading the UK to refuse to extradite an alleged child abuser for trial in California, without an undertaking from the US government that he would not be detained after sentence under that law: *Giese (No 1)* [2015] EWHC 2733 (Admin).

What should we treat?

Doctors make diagnoses and treat the pathology that causes symptoms and signs of disorder. Where this is not possible, symptomatic relief, including the relief of distress and pain, is still a reasonable treatment goal (p.182). Psychiatrists are no different from other doctors in this respect.

However, forensic psychiatrists may be explicitly asked to 'treat' the offences their patients commit (i.e. to inhibit or abolish those factors in the patient that increase the risk of offending, particularly violent or sexual offending). Forensic patients detained in secure settings (p.184) are often unable to move on and regain their freedom until their risk to others has reduced, no matter how mentally well they may be.

What is at issue is not whether continued detention in the absence of current symptoms is lawful[12] but whether it is ethically justifiable for doctors to assess and treat for risk (p.322) in the absence of any direct mental health benefit to the patient.

Treating disorders, not behaviours

Arguably, once psychiatrists have improved a patient's mental health, their professional job is over. According to this approach, although managing risk is socially important, it is not a medical matter. However, if the risk of harm is causally related to mental disorder then clearly it is justifiable for psychiatrists to at least contribute to management of risk arising in that way. But it is not the role of forensic psychiatrists to manage the risk of harm arising solely from ordinary criminogenic factors.

The offender/patient confusion

It is easy for a past index offence, and harm done, to loom large in the minds of agencies who have responsibility for public protection like police, government, and MAPPA (p.592) partners. Some mental health staff may also see a patient as a criminal of bad character, who should not be released until after they have been punished (p.354), or pose no risk. Yet using detention in hospital for this purpose is ethically wrong, and a waste of a scarce resource.

Double jeopardy

Offender patients who have complied with treatment and made a good recovery may find themselves facing 'double jeopardy' when they are asked about new and nonpsychiatric motives for offending, which may have a direct effect on decisions about liberty. Forensic psychiatrists should be alert to when the question changes from How ill is he now? to solely How risky is he now? Patients may struggle to show they pose little risk to others, especially if they have been transferred from prison and cannot access prison rehabilitation programmes.

---

12 Though there must be some evidence of benefit in Scotland and RoI (see p.510), and the Wessely review (p.782) has recommended further limits on such detention in E&W.

An ethical position

Even where treatments are aimed at risk reduction, rather than health benefits, treatment must have some connection with mental disorder (as e.g. with psychological treatments for <u>ASPD</u>, p.82) Involuntary treatment can only be ethically justified if there is some prospect of health benefit beyond reduction of the risk of offending.

What counts as treatment?

The problem of deciding <u>what to treat</u> (p.338) is inherently linked with the question, what is treatment? These questions are important in patients with severe <u>personality disorder</u> (p.78) and <u>psychopathy</u> (p.90). Although there are interventions that reduce distress and improve wellbeing, there remain concerns that the patient's condition gives rise to risk of harm to others. Is there any treatment that it may be right to offer?

Forms of treatment

Consider a patient with an amputated limb after a road traffic accident, or a terminal illness such as cancer, where recovery is not an option. They might still be offered the following:

- pharmacological treatments, including antibiotics or chemotherapy;
- surgical treatments, such as resection of a primary tumour, or the fitting of a prosthetic limb;
- psychological treatments;
- habilitation or rehabilitation skills, such as walking with a prosthetic limb;
- personal care, such as assistance to wash or dress;
- social care, such as a residential home, or a 'home help';
- secondary preventive treatments, such as dressing wounds; and
- palliative treatments, such as analgesics.

All these interventions represent treatment, albeit with different aims, and offered by different professionals. Even quarantine for infectious disease is seen as part of treatment[13]; even though it resembles <u>administrative detention</u> (p.467). However, which of the interventions in the list above would it be ethical to administer compulsorily, <u>without consent</u> (p.332), or even in the face of a <u>capacitous</u> <u>refusal of consent</u> (p.336)? And would the answer be different if the primary aim was nontherapeutic, such as public protection? What if the *only* aim was public protection: can detention amount to 'treatment' if there is no discernible benefit to the patient?

The legal definition of treatment

The legal definition of treatment within mental health legislation varies between jurisdictions (see p.482)—but is extremely broad in each, and includes everything in the list above, down to and including social care; moreover, secondary prevention and palliation are accepted as forms of treatment if their intention (not necessarily effect) is to ameliorate or prevent a deterioration in the disorder in question.

However, in E&W the definition is the broadest: 'medical treatment the purpose of which is to alleviate, or prevent a worsening of, the disorder or of one or more of its symptoms or manifestations'. Any treatment under the direction of the responsible clinician counts; it can include treatments aimed at helping the patient cope with, or work around the symptoms of

---

13 Although nonconsensual quarantining cannot legally extend to nonconsensual treatment per se under public health legislation in E&W.

their disorder. In the case of a detained patient with <u>severe borderline PD</u> (p.84), this definition could cover secondary preventive or palliative treatments given in the face of a refusal of consent, such as training in victim empathy, or a mood stabiliser at a low dose.[14]

The intention and likely effect of treatment

Further, in E&W and RoI there does not even have to be any *likelihood* of benefit[15]: merely the *purpose* of alleviating, or preventing a worsening of the disorder, or one or more of its symptoms or manifestations. (The definition in RoI is that treatment includes, but is not limited to, 'the administration of physical, psychological and other remedies … intended for the purposes of ameliorating a mental disorder'.) This presents the psychiatrist with a further ethical challenge: even if there is no evidence base for an intervention, or indeed rationale, with this patient, it can still be given compulsorily— even if it has been tried before and repeatedly failed.[16]

In RoI, patients with personality disorder alone cannot be compulsorily treated at all, which mitigates the effect of the broad definition of treatment somewhat, but in E&W it applies to all patients with mental disorder. The position in Scotland and NI is less clear: the definition of treatment is not based upon intention, but neither is there any requirement to show a likely benefit.

---

14 The former might not alter the patient's personality traits itself, but would hope to prevent or minimise its consequence of victimising others, and the latter would be palliative insofar as it reduced distressing mood swings for the sufferer.

15 In order for a treatment to fall within the definition of 'medical treatment' in the Act. The Upper Tribunal has ruled that a treatment with no realistic prospect of any therapeutic benefit whatsoever would be unlikely to count as 'appropriate treatment' for the purposes of the criteria for detention (*SLL v Priory*, p.768).

16 The Upper Tribunal has refused to adopt any approach that further legally constrains MHTs, indicating that each case is for the MHT to decide on a 'factual' basis.

Consent to risk assessment

Consent to examination, investigation and treatment is essential in all areas of medicine, albeit with exceptions in the absence of capacity, or under the terms of mental health legislation. However, the status of risk assessment as an investigation, or as a prelude to treatment, is uncertain. If there is a therapeutic intention and context, is it part of assessment for treatment, or should it be considered distinct?

The ethics of consent to risk assessment (p.322) therefore relates to:
• situations where there is no right to assess without consent—for instance, when assessing a capacitous defendant prior to sentencing (p.442) in the absence of an order under mental health law;
• clinical situations where risk assessment is for therapeutic purposes with an informal patient, where consent is again required; and
• such clinical situations, but where the patient is subject to mental health or mental capacity law.

The subject of a risk assessment may not understand the potential harm or benefit to them of engaging in the process. This issue is particularly important in forensic psychiatry because of the potential impact of risk assessment upon the individual's liberty. They may not even suspect that assessment which is presented (perhaps intended) as solely for considering treatment in hospital might be used judicially for the purpose of sentencing.

Seeking consent to risk assessment

In seeking consent to risk assessment, the same ethical rules as for consent to treatment (p.332) apply. That is, patients must have capacity to consent; they must be appropriately informed and they must not have been coerced to consent.

A key ethical difficulty for any psychiatrist or psychologist relates to how a risk assessment might in the end be used and therefore what information they should give to the patient. For consent to risk assessment to be valid, the patient must be informed about possible outcomes, including unintended ones (e.g. determining a custodial sentence).

Informed consent to risk assessment

Depending on the circumstances, if consent to risk assessment is sought, some or all of the following information should be given to the patient.
• This process will include an assessment of your risk of harming others.
• It may be helpful for you to avoid further offending.
• It may help healthcare professionals, or other agencies, to support you in managing risks to yourself.
• It may be used by the court to determine your 'dangerousness'.
• It could result in the imposition of a restriction order, or indeterminate or extended sentence, even if that is not the recommendation.

If consent is refused

If the person refuses consent after being informed, but there is a legal power to proceed without consent (and you deem it necessary to proceed), you should explain this. If there is no such legal power, you should explain the likely consequences (e.g. having to write a report that is based solely on available records, and not on an interview) and attempt to persuade persons to change their mind, but if they do not, you must respect their decision.

Consent to risk management

Although consent is not, in so many words, usually sought for risk management, the position is perhaps more straightforward than for risk assessment. Each risk management intervention, such as giving an antipsychotic to reduce command auditory hallucinations to kill, or <u>disclosing information to the police</u> (p.320) about a patient's plans to abuse children, will clearly require either specific consent, or a legal power allowing it to be pursued without consent.

Consent to research and documentaries

Obtaining informed consent is the ethical basis of all research with human subjects, explicitly required by ethical codes (p.285). The NHS Health Research Authority and the Health Products Regulatory Authority in RoI provide guidance on consent from different kinds of participants, including those who may be vulnerable in terms of understanding or exploitation. Applications for research ethical approval must include evidence of how researchers will approach participants, how they will obtain consent, the information they will give participants, and how confidential data will be kept securely.

Participants in research must be free to make their own informed decisions about taking part in research. They must usually have mental capacity (p.522) to give consent. Where potential participants cannot consent, but the research is deemed appropriate and in the interests of the participants by the ethics committee, including being of benefit to similar patients, permission to proceed may be granted, subject to conditions.

Special considerations apply when carrying out research upon detained patients, or prisoners, to ensure that consent is indeed free, and not influenced by any legal coercion or perceived benefit of research participation relating to liberty or special privileges.

Participants should have sufficient knowledge and understanding of what is involved in the research so that they can make informed decisions.

Fully informed consent may not always be possible. However the legal position is that participants must be informed of any significant risks of serious harm that any reasonable person would want to know about, or which the clinician knows or should know this particular person would want to know about.

Research Ethics Committees (RECs) have to balance a range of competing interests, such as the aims of the research, what they consider to be in the best interests of research participants, and the interests of formal and informal gatekeepers, such as bodies funding the research, or employing the researchers.

In practice

- Whenever possible, the investigator should inform all participants of the aims of the research.
- The investigator should inform the participants of all aspects of the research or intervention that might reasonably be expected to influence willingness to participate.
- The investigator should explain all other aspects of the research or intervention about which a reasonable person might wish to know, or they know (or should know) this particular person would want to know.
- Not making full disclosure prior to obtaining informed consent (with ethical approval, because doing so would compromise the study in some way) requires additional safeguards to protect the welfare and dignity of participants.
- Investigators in a position of authority or influence over particular participants (e.g. their students or patients) should not be involved in obtaining consent.

- The payment of participants must not be used to induce them to risk harm beyond that which they would risk without payment in their normal lifestyle.
- In longitudinal research, consent may need to be obtained on more than one occasion.

Consent to research in vulnerable groups

- Children younger than sixteen years old are not automatically assumed to be competent to give consent. However, if a child can be judged to understand what participation in research will involve then parental consent is not necessary. There is a distinction between *consent*, which is a legal term, and infers fully weighing up the decision based upon adequate information, and *assent*, which amounts simply to agreeing to take part. Children need to assent even if parental consent is given.
- In the case of vulnerable incapacitous adults, nobody else can consent on their behalf: they can only participate if the REC has specifically approved the research including willing incapacitous adults, on the grounds of the specific benefit they or others like them might obtain.
- When research is being conducted with detained persons, particular care should be taken over informed consent, paying attention to the special circumstances which may affect the person's ability to give free informed consent.

Consent to taking part in documentaries

There is potential benefit to patients from public engagement concerning forensic psychiatry. When a media team is granted access to a secure setting and its patients they are expected to behave in an ethical manner. The Broadcast Code of the UK media regulator, Ofcom, states that 'vulnerable people' (including those with mental illness) should not be interviewed without the agreement of the person with primary responsibility for their care. Patients should give informed consent for any contributions they make.[17] Forensic psychiatrist may be involved in assessing the capacity of patients to give this content.

---

17 Or others make about them: for example in 2015 journalists and hospital staff were prosecuted in relation to newspaper articles about high-profile patients at Broadmoor Hospital. The journalists were acquitted, as the stories were true and in the public interest, and they had not approached the staff or corrupted them; the hospital staff member was jailed for eight months.

Prosecution of patients

Shift in attitudes

Historically, people with mental disorder were prosecuted just as were other members of society, with the only variation in procedure being that they could be acquitted on the ground of <u>insanity</u> (p.620).

During the nineteenth and twentieth centuries, however, the idea that mentally disordered person should be <u>diverted</u> (p.268) from the criminal justice system into hospital gradually took hold, and by the late-twentieth century it had become commonplace for the police, prosecutors, and courts to **discontinue** proceedings for all but the most serious charges, and to **divert** people they thought to be mentally disordered to hospital for assessment. Police officers and prosecutors became reluctant to charge or prosecute people they thought to be mentally disordered, believing (usually erroneously) that the prosecution would be very unlikely to succeed, because they would be <u>unfit to plead</u> (p.602) or would be unable to stand up to <u>cross-examination</u> (p.714) or would have a mental condition defence or because it was 'pointless' if the person was already under a mental health order.

When is it appropriate to prosecute?

This is governed by the **evidential rule** (does conviction appear more likely than acquittal, based on the evidence) and the **public interest** principle (Box 12.1). There are cases when the decision whether to prosecute[18] appears straightforward: for instance, a floridly psychotic patient arrested for a minor offence (e.g. <u>breach of the peace</u>, p.425) may be diverted and escape prosecution without controversy. Conversely, most professionals would support the prosecution of a patient with antisocial personality disorder alleged to have seriously assaulted or killed someone. In both cases, there should be a focus on ensuring access to treatment. The key question is the balance between the welfare of the patient and society's interest in justice. In less straightforward cases, this involves considering:

The harm to the victim

The seriousness of the offence, and in particular the degree of harm to others that resulted, is important. Victims have a legitimate interest in seeing the person who harmed them tried and, if appropriate, punished: this is one of the key <u>goals of the criminal justice system</u> (p.352).

The nature of the mental disorder

The nature of the patient's mental disorder, and the likelihood that if prosecuted they would be <u>unfit to plead</u> (p.602) or <u>unfit to give evidence</u> (p.606) or would be acquitted because of one of the <u>mental condition defences</u> (p.412) is relevant.[19] Diversion of a patient is more appropriate if any prosecution would be likely to fail on these grounds.

---

18 This section discusses charging & prosecution as if there were a single decision, made by the clinical team. In practice, the clinical team, the victim, the police, and the prosecutor will make a series of decisions: whether to report the alleged offence, whether to arrest the patient, whether to charge them, and whether, finally, to prosecute. The box overleaf summarises the factors weighed up by the Crown Prosecution Service in E&W in making its decision.

19 Police, may request a report, in a short pro-forma style, in which the doctor states whether there is clear evidence at this early stage of unfitness or a relevant incapacity. If the doctor says there is, the police are unlikely to proceed. If there is not, the investigation may proceed, but there will be the opportunity for a formal expert opinion on fitness and mental condition defences at a later stage.

Prosecution as a component of the care plan

Where the risk assessment already indicates a substantial risk of future violence, it may be reasonable to consider supporting prosecution as contributing to objective risk assessment and management. This is most likely to occur with patients with <u>personality disorder</u> (p.78), where it is also important that patients experience consistent consequences of their behaviour.

Box 12.1 Crown Prosecution Service guidelines on the decision to prosecute

Is prosecution required in the public interest?
- How serious is the offence?
- How culpable does the alleged offender appear (based on their involvement, coercion, premeditation, and benefit from the offence)?
- What are the views and circumstances of the victim (e.g. a public servant, or in a relationship of trust/authority with the defendant)?
- What are the alleged offender's circumstances (e.g. age, maturity, mental disorder, and previous convictions)?
- What impact has the offence had on the community?
- Is prosecution proportionate or is an out-of-court disposal (e.g. <u>conditional caution</u>, p.441) more appropriate?

Part IV

Law relevant to psychiatry

The interface between psychiatry and law*

* This part (Chapters 13–16) covers only selected areas within criminal, civil, human rights, mental health, and mental capacity law. For an authoritative treatment of these or other areas of law, you should consult a legal textbook or a professional lawyer.

Objectives of the psychiatric & legal systems

Whether practicing clinical forensic psychiatry or providing psychiatric evidence, it is crucial to appreciate the overall goals of the legal system and how it asks and answers questions in the service of those goals.

The aims of medicine & psychiatry

The primary <u>aim of medical treatment</u> (p.182) is **welfare**: to maximise the quality and duration of patients' lives, individually and at the population level. Psychiatry also aims to reduce patients' risk of harming themselves or others, in the patient's own interests and with their consent wherever possible. However, psychiatrists sometimes override the patient's interests in order to protect others from them.[1]

The aims of the legal systems

There are three interlocking systems, with subtly different aims:
- The legal system, comprising the civil, criminal, and other <u>courts and tribunals</u> (p.372). Its sole aim is the administration of **justice**, by deciding on competing claims by different parties, including the State.
- The criminal justice system (CJS), comprising the criminal courts, the police, prosecution service, probation service, prison service, and government departments overseeing these (e.g. the Ministry of Justice). Its objectives are the prevention, detection, and punishment of crime, and the protection of society as whole.
- The youth justice system is that part of the CJS that deals with children and young people (up to twenty-one years old in some cases). It aims to prevent, detect and punish crime, but in a way that explicitly promotes the welfare and developmental needs of the child or young person.[2]

Psychiatry and law: a two-way relationship

The relationship between the two 'lands' (p.354) of psychiatry and law is bilateral. Psychiatry is *used by law* to assist in answering legal questions, such as when psychiatrists testify as to whether a defendant was capable of forming the requisite <u>intent</u> (p.402) for an offence.

Psychiatry also *uses legal processes* towards therapeutic ends, as when a psychiatrist decides to recommend <u>detention for treatment</u> (p.500) or, as part of their <u>risk management plan</u> (p.238), to recommend a <u>restriction order</u> (p.510) in a <u>report on disposal</u> (p.456). Forensic psychiatrists must be alive to the differences between their own overall objectives and <u>ways of thinking</u> (p.354) about the patient, or litigant, and those of the <u>other agencies</u> (p.314) they deal with as they <u>negotiate the psycho-legal frontier</u> (p.358).

---

1 See the discussion of <u>ethical risk assessment & management</u> on p.322.

2 This aim can be seen clearly in the Scottish <u>Children's Hearings system</u> (p.386), but is less obvious in E&W and RoI, which are more punitive.

Is forensic psychiatry converging on the CJS?

Early in the <u>development of forensic psychiatry</u> (p.14), the discipline approached public protection essentially as an adjunct to, or consequence of, the treatment of patients. Forensic psychiatry operated a 'rescue' system for offenders with mental disorders, who could be diverted from the CJS into mental health care services (in parallel with, or instead of, prosecution).

Increasingly, however, society demands to be kept safe from those it fears, and so expects forensic psychiatrists to minimise the risks posed by mentally disordered offenders, whether or not treatment will benefit the patient. These forces can cause forensic psychiatry to converge on law's public protection function.

Manifestations of convergence

Convergence can be seen in:
- a shift in clinical practice, in the balance between treatment and public protection;
- the widening of definitions within mental health legislation, so as to allow detention of those who may not benefit from treatment[3]; and
- pressure on forensic psychiatrists to give evidence for <u>risk-based sentencing</u> (p.670), particularly in E&W following the <u>Vowles</u> judgment (p.770).[4]

Accepting or resisting convergence

This process has the potential to move forensic psychiatry away from the core objectives and values of medicine. In the UK, forensic psychiatry has experienced a schism in its identity and values. Some have held steadfastly to the 'rescue' approach, resisting involvement wherever there is no treatment benefit to the patient. Others have accepted, even embraced, risk management, on the basis that forensic psychiatrists are best placed in society to assess and manage risk arising from the mentally disordered, and owe a duty to society to assist.

---

3 See p.467. This process has been criticised by the <u>Wessely review</u> (p.782) and by many commentators, and may now be starting to reverse, even in E&W. Notably, however, the recently published government White Paper on reforming the MHA (2021), which responds to Wessely, recommends distinguishing between detention criteria for 'civil' and 'criminal' patients in Part III, so as to continue to emphasise public safety.

4 See also Sentencing Council. Sentencing offenders with mental disorders, developmental disorders, or neurological impairments (Sentencing Council, 2020).

Legal and psychiatric constructs & models

Law and psychiatry as two 'lands'

Law and medicine are like neighbouring countries, each with its own <u>purpose</u> (p.352), processes, discourse, and language, and each with its own regions and districts (within branches of law and specialties of medicine). Communication involves translating the language of one into that of the other; or more properly '<u>mapping</u>' a psychiatric mental state, or <u>formulation</u> (p.146), onto a <u>legal test</u> (p.358), since there almost always is no possible 'translation'; offering many opportunities for confusion and distorted communication.

The problems in the relationship between psychiatry and law differ from those between other medical specialties and law, where the law is interested chiefly in matters of fact (e.g. the nature of an injury and how it could have been inflicted). Psychiatry deals with constructs that appear similar to those of law, such as <u>volition</u> (p.24) in psychiatry and <u>intent</u> (p.402) in law, but which are in fact profoundly different.[5] This can also lead to mutual misunderstanding and, for the psychiatrist, <u>ethical tension</u> (p.298).

Constructs from purposes

The constructs used in a discipline derive from its core purposes. The core purpose of medicine is the amelioration of disease, illness, and suffering, thereby increasing the **welfare** of the individual patient. In contrast, the law pursues **justice**, an abstract concept concerned with what is fair, due, or owed; implicit in which is the idea of balancing the interests (or welfare) of one party against another, or the State.

Compare and contrast, for example, <u>psychosis</u> (p.72) within psychiatry and <u>insanity</u> (p.620) or <u>diminished responsibility</u> (p.624) within law, all of which can involve a loss of reality testing, or of the ability to recognise the true nature of actions, or to control actions. Psychiatry defines psychosis by its symptoms and (sometimes) aetiology, so that it can be reliably identified by different doctors, and classifies it into separate <u>diagnoses</u> (p.144), so as to make a prognosis and facilitate appropriate treatment, not to determine whether the psychotic defendant should be found criminally responsible, or <u>fit to plead</u> (p.602).

To the criminal, law, insanity, and diminished responsibility are artifices constructed to allocate criminal responsibility justly; similarly, law defines fitness to plead in order to determine whether a fair trial is possible. Since the consequence of insanity is to remove responsibility entirely, whereas that of diminished responsibility is merely to reduce it, the law adopts different and mutually inconsistent definitions of the two legal defences.

---

5 For example, one can lack the legal capacity to intend something one has willed (e.g. a psychotic patient deliberately hitting someone they believed to be a devil); whereas one can be deemed to have legally intended something unwilled (e.g. killing people within a house you only wanted to destroy by fire, if their deaths were a 'natural and probable' consequence of the fire).

Disputed models

The picture is complicated further by the fact that psychiatrists and lawyers often disagree about the model their own field should adopt. For example, as to whether the criminal law should be interpreted purely to do what is fair or **just** overall, regardless of the consequences for the individual offender or should focus on what is **proportionate** for that one offender or should include taking account of their **welfare** or should be directed at **deterring** them and others from offending. Hence a homeless teenager convicted of their twentieth minor theft might be <u>sentenced</u> (p.442) to a fine under the proportionality approach, a community order with a residence requirement under the welfare approach, or a short sentence of youth detention under the deterrence approach. Lawyers or judges advocating the welfare approach will be more in favour of <u>diverting</u> (p.268) offenders to hospital than those advocating a pure justice approach.

Lawyers often experience frustration when faced with psychiatric experts with differing diagnostic opinions as to whether a patient suffers from, say, schizophrenia or a transient drug-induced psychosis, conditions which might have different legal consequences. From their perspective, psychiatrists' nuanced disagreements, significant to them in relation to prognosis or treatment, may appear incomprehensible and irrelevant.

Autopoiesis versus reflexivity

Criminal law is highly autopoietic: it employs only its own strictly defined constructs, within a strictly observed discourse, which greatly inhibits adoption of the constructs or methods of other disciplines, and which can seriously distort the meaning of 'alien' constructs given in evidence. It is ultimately preoccupied with ensuring that its procedures (such as the <u>rules of evidence</u>, p.382) are scrupulously fair to defendants and prosecution.

Family law, at the other extreme, is relatively reflexive, being bound by a single and somewhat 'lay' principle, that the welfare of the child is paramount. It can therefore accommodate a wide range of expert evidence and constructs, even at the cost of apparent imprecision and some risk of different courts faced with the similar facts reaching different decisions.

Different uses of information

History versus evidence

Psychiatry and law, because of their different purposes (p.352), regard information in quite different ways:

- To a court, any piece of information is **evidence**, to be admitted or excluded, deemed truthful or false, and given greater or lesser weight, all according to the rules of evidence (p.382). All such evidence contributes to an overall verdict via an *adversarial* process.
- To a psychiatrist, however, the same piece of information forms part of the patient's **history**, to be taken into consideration with much less concern about whether a particular item of information is true (although some assessment of the reliability of the source must still be made). Rather what is addressed, *investigatively*, is the overall pattern (e.g. of symptoms), and whether it is sufficient to make a particular diagnosis (p.144) or formulation (p.146), within which it is to be expected that some symptoms may be absent or even inconsistent with the pattern.[6] This approach implies that consistent information can be mutually reinforcing, in terms of the weight to be attached to each item.

Methods of gathering and selecting information

These also differ between law and psychiatry. Courts will only consider evidence put before them by the parties,[7] and which is deemed admissible (p.382); they will then test each piece of information through cross-examination (p.714). A forensic psychiatrist will actively seek out information from the patient, corroborate or contrast it with that given by the others, and will consider anything available in an investigative fashion.

Implications for forensic psychiatrists

These differences have several consequences for forensic psychiatrists.

- Clinical data within a court report can have legal, as well as medical relevance, including regarding guilt; and its source may be considered legally relevant.
- The sources of all information used by a psychiatrist should be made clear (patient, informant, and records), so that the court can apply its own approach to veracity.
- Some information used by psychiatrists in diagnosis or formulation may be inadmissible in court. This can cause ethical tension for expert witnesses, if their conclusions rely on information they cannot disclose when their conclusions are challenged under cross-examination (so they may need to ask for this to be explained to the judge in chambers). Reports should make clear how conclusions have been derived, with information that may be inadmissible in a separate section of the report that can be withheld if necessary.

---

6 However, if numerous or significant, they challenge the psychiatrist to question whether the perceived pattern (diagnosis, formulation) is correct, or complete.

7 Except in civil law jurisdictions (p.368) where judges and magistrates may actively investigate.

- Information contained within court proceedings, for example witness statements, can be used as data by the forensic psychiatrist (by analogy with informant information in ordinary clinical practice); however, witness evidence may be contradictory, and/or disputed, such that the expert has to make conditional statements ('if the court finds A to be true then the diagnosis of X is reinforced, if B then it is undermined').
- Information received from the CJS should be given great weight if it has been considered and accepted by a court, because it will have been tested against the rules of evidence and been subjected to attempts by one or more parties to disprove it (so convictions should weigh more heavily in a <u>risk assessment</u> (p.163) than allegations, for example).

Negotiating the interface

Forensic psychiatrists work at the frontier between <u>the two 'lands' of medi-cine and law</u> (p.354). Effective, ethical forensic psychiatrists can identify what <u>constructs and models</u> (p.354) arise from each, and keeps strictly to their role. They assist in mapping the language of psychiatry onto the language of law; mapping clinical constructs onto relevant legal definitions. And they must do so in a way that is informed about structure of legal process, and 'how law thinks', including, for example, the 'rules of evidence' even beyond expert evidence, in order to fully and properly tailor their evidence to legal process. That is, they must become a 'frontiersman' (as, from the other side of the border, must become any lawyer who wishes to be an effective advocate in regard to expert psychiatric evidence).

Where is the frontier?

In <u>giving evidence at a tribunal</u> (p.724), or <u>writing court reports</u> (p.677), the frontier is obvious. It is also present in clinical practice, for example when <u>detaining</u> (p.470) or discharging a patient, since the clinical facts must be mapped onto the legal criteria for detention.

Clinico-legal mapping

Dialogue between psychiatrists and lawyers requires each to understand and work with the constructs of the other. In strongly <u>autopoietic</u> (p.355) branches of the law, perfect mapping is impossible: no unidimensional, binary legal construct could adequately capture the subtle variation in the behavioural manifestations of <u>depression</u> (p.94), for example.

Legal definitions vary in their degree of **congruence** with medical constructs (e.g. *insanity*[8] fails to reflect the range of mental state abnormalities potentially relevant to culpability) and **precision**; mapping onto a tight legal definition leaves little room for the exercise of expert discretion, or court interpretation; loose definitions make outcomes less certain. Enacted reform of <u>diminished responsibility</u> (p.624) as recommended by the Law Commission was aimed at enhancing both congruence and precision.

Across regions/districts of both law and psychiatry there are identifiable '**psycho-legal case types**' which 'combine' a given mental state or formulation description with a given legal test, beyond individual case details.

Minimising communication errors

Although a perfect 'translation' is impossible, errors of psycho-legal mapping can be minimised if:

- lawyers ask psychiatrists clear and specific legal questions, especially when giving <u>instructions</u> (p.680);
- psychiatrists understand the precise, potential relevance of the clinical answers they may give to relevant legal questions; and

---

8 In the UK and RoI. The Norwegian Criminal Code, by contrast, defines insanity as identical to the psychiatric construct of psychosis.

- psychiatrists keep to the boundary of their professional expertise and role (and do not attempt, for example, to <u>address the ultimate legal issue</u>, p.664).

Doctors interpreting law

Deciding how the law applies to particular (possibly disputed) facts, and expert opinion, is the core of <u>jurisprudence</u> (p.364); which a court ultimately determines. Yet often clinicians have to operate across the frontier without knowing how the law would view their own interpretation of both the facts and the law.

Hence, <u>mental health law</u> (p.461) allows wide discretion to clinicians in deciding whether or not to use its powers, because of the broad definition of many of its key constructs, such as <u>mental disorder</u> (p.470) or <u>appropriate treatment</u> (p.482). This leaves clinicians free to import their own (mis)understandings of the law, and their own <u>ethical values</u> (p.298), into their clinico-legal decision-making. The psychiatrist therefore holds an ethical duty to promote patients' <u>autonomy</u> (p.331), and to respect their <u>human rights</u> (p.516), in the exercise of their discretion.

Different frontiers for different disciplines

The models adopted by other clinical disciplines may interface differently with the law in a particular context. For example, the categorical psychiatric approach to disorder tends to fit better with binary legal thinking than the dimensional approach of clinical psychology. There may be varying degrees of incongruity, with distinct mapping, between differing mental sciences and law, depending sometimes on the <u>reflexivity</u> (p.355) of the field of law concerned.

Role co-operation not contamination

The proper role of a doctor is to seek to assist justice, not to seek to affect it. However, the inherent bias of psychiatry towards welfare can result in <u>tailoring of opinions</u> (p.674) so as to achieve a result perceived to be in the 'best interests' of the evaluee. This is ethically and legally indefensible— even where the court, usually tribunal, is willing to collude in turning the hearing into 'a glorified case conference'.

Chapter 14

Legal systems

Law in society

Understanding the law in a particular country, as any forensic psychiatrist should, involves recognising Law's place in that country's society. In very early societies, there was no law as such: the only enforceable rules were those that were accepted by consensus in that society (think of taboos, or 'political correctness' in the modern context). Over time, such rules were thought about and seen to have value, and slowly a system developed to consider, enforce, and refine and update them: a system of law.

Law can express orders made by the State or Sovereign, backed by threats of force[1] ; it can express the moral views of the majority, especially a largely homogeneous society[2]; it can be a system of rules that predict whom the State will allow to exercise free choice, and whom it will seek to control or punish. Broadly speaking, earlier societies' laws express orders of the King (sovereign), and modern societies' laws determine whom the State will seek to control or punish (and in what circumstances), in a reliable way that enables citizens to make rational choices.

The rule of law

Everyone in a society governed according to the rule of law (i.e. law ruling over all else) is bound by the law, even those in power and including the Sovereign, if there is one.[3] It acts as a counterweight to the majoritarian tendencies of electoral democracies: the rules of the democracy *authorise* the State to carry out the will of the majority against the will of one or more minorities, but the *legitimacy* of doing so stems from all citizens' acceptance that the process of making the decision was fair and involved everyone on the basis of equal status and equal rights (e.g. an equal right to vote in an election or referendum[4]).

Despite criticism from the socialist and feminist perspectives (that the rule of law ignores inequalities inherent in modern corporate capitalist societies[5]), the rule of law is widely held to be an ideal, with even some societies that do not operate it in practice seeking to claim that they do.

---

1 This was the view of the nineteenth-century <u>positivist</u> (p.662) legal theorist John Austin.

2 This was to some extent the case with English law from the Victorian era until World War 2.

3 Republics vest their sovereignty in the people collectively (e.g. RoI), or a body representing the people collectively (e.g. a Soviet (workers' council) in the pre-USSR Soviet Republics, or the Congress of the United States of America), rather than in an individual person (e.g. the Queen).

4 This was a highly contentious issue in the UK between the 2016 referendum on leaving the European Union and the UK's departure in 2020. To oversimplify somewhat, many 'Leavers' focused on the legitimacy of the majority vote in the referendum, and saw attempts to challenge, delay or frustrate leaving on one or other set of terms as potentially illegitimate; whereas many 'Remainers' focused on the legitimacy of the political system overall, and saw attempts by the majority to force through leaving on one or other set of terms without counterbalancing scrutiny of the terms in Parliament or elsewhere as potentially illegitimate. This led in 2019 to the Supreme Court case <u>*Miller v Prime Minister*</u> (p.VI.2), which settled the constitutional issue in favour of the Remainers' position, and subsequent General Election, which settled the political issue in the Leavers' favour.

5 Such as the unquestioned social privileges of certain groups (e.g. white men, or old Etonians), or being concerned with equality before the law, but not with equality of legal outcome. The feminist position in <u>critical legal studies</u> (p.662) goes further, positing that all law is essentially politics, and the rule of law simply perpetuates the power of the patriarchy and the rich.

Some legal philosophers and commentators argue that the concept of the rule of law is being over-extended in the West, citing two main complaints: that <u>human rights law</u> (p.516) has been inappropriately used to override legitimate democratic decisions[6] ; and that judges have become too ready to interpret law expansively (in effect, to create new law) in an attempt to solve social problems that the legislature and/or executive have failed to address to the court's satisfaction.[7]

The relationship between law and morality

Most citizens, lawyers, and judges believe there to be some kind of relationship between law and <u>morality</u>[8] (see p.662). For example, it has been argued (in increasing order of contentiousness) that:

- The making of laws is influenced by the morality of the group or society from which legislators are drawn.
- The interpretation of laws is influenced by the morality of the group or society from which judges are drawn.
- Laws are legitimate if they meet the moral standard of applying a consistent set of general rules that is intelligible and with which citizens are capable of complying (e.g. because they do not apply retrospectively).
- Law gains authority and legitimacy by being based (or being part of a system based) on generally accepted moral principles—though citizens often obey laws generally perceived to be of questionable morality.[9]
- Laws are only legitimate if they meet 'fundamental' moral standards such as equality before the law (though systems flouting such principles have often flourished for centuries).[10]

And, most contentiously:

- Laws should be retrospectively declared not to have been laws if they failed certain fundamental moral standards, once the political structures that enforced those laws have been overturned.[11]

---

6 For example <u>Hirst</u> (p.757), which forced the UK to grant some prisoners the right to vote, despite this being contrary to the repeatedly-expressed will of Parliament and the electorate at the time.

7 For instance, expansively interpreting the Fourteenth amendment to the US Constitution (which includes a due process clause) as including a right to abortion; or preventing the Attorney General overriding the decision of a senior court despite Parliament expressly giving them the power to do so in cases concerning secrecy of government documents (<u>Evans v AG</u>, p.755).

8 Though they disagree about whether 'morality' means universal principles (e.g. human rights), expressions of society's attitudes and preferences (e.g. on issues of sexuality), or something else.

9 For example paying the community charge or 'poll tax' in E&W in the late 1980s; or complying with racist 'Jim Crow' laws enforcing Segregation in the USA in the late-nineteenth and early twentieth centuries.

10 For instance Islamic Sharia laws setting the evidence of a woman as being worth half that of a man.

11 For example, after 1945, German courts held some areas of pre-1945 (i.e. Nazi) law to be void because of their moral repugnance—as in the postwar 'grudge informer' cases, where people were held criminally responsible for causing the death or imprisonment of others (e.g. unwanted spouses) by accusing them of, for example, criticising Hitler, despite such denunciations being lawful at the time.

Jurisprudence and legal interpretation

Whereas the relationship between law and morality is a question of legal philosophy, how laws should be interpreted and developed by the courts are questions of jurisprudence (which, roughly speaking, means 'the knowledge of law', or 'theory of law'). Sometimes the law very clearly applies to the factual situation (e.g. when a statute, p.732, applies—such as to driving along the motorway at 85 mph, which is clearly in breach of the Road Traffic Act that sets the speed limit at 70 mph); when it does not,[12] jurisprudence guides the court's interpretation of what the law says. See Box 14.1.

> **Box 14.1 Types of disputes between parties**
>
> Disputes between parties can be categorised as:
> - Factual disputes: what is the evidence that A did X to B?
> - Legal disputes: does the law give B a remedy for A doing X to them?
> - Moral disputes: is it just that the law does (or does not) give B such a remedy?

Interpretation of the law

Frequently, a legal case before the courts (or legal advice given before the event) will turn on whether and how one or other law applies in the situation in question. For example, in a judicial review (p.374) of a tribunal's decision to uphold the detention of a patient with autism (p.104) under the Mental Health Act (p.738), the case might turn on whether the Act applied to patients with autism, given that autism and autistic spectrum disorders are not mentioned anywhere within its text.[13]

When judges interpret laws, they adopt one of several approaches:
- The **literal** (or 'black-letter law') approach, usually associated with political conservatives and writers such as Joseph Raz, focuses on the straightforward meaning of the text in question, and minimises the scope for adopting a less obvious meaning in order to reach a 'better' outcome in a situation that the legislators were unlikely to have foreseen.
- The **pragmatic** approach seeks to interpret the law in such a way as to create the most favoured outcome for society. Liberal justices on the US Supreme Court during the 1960s adopted a strongly pragmatic approach that facilitated judicial activism, most notably interpreting the constitution's 'due process' clause to include not only a right to privacy but within that a constitutional right to abortion.

---

12 Such as when there was previously no written statement of the law governing the extent of the prerogative power to suspend Parliament, as in _Miller v Prime Minister_ (p.VI.2).

13 Before the 2007 amendments to the Mental Health Act in E&W, autism was held to be a mental disorder within the meaning of the Act, and could therefore form part of the grounds for detention for assessment (p.474) under section 2, but it was not a mental _illness_ and therefore could not justify detention for treatment (p.478) under section 3 under the rules then in force unless there was also evidence of 'mental retardation' (intellectual disability, p.110). If the _Wessely_ review (p.VI.50) recommendations are implemented, autism will be mentioned explicitly in the MHA in E&W, and powers to detain people with autism will be restricted.

- The **interpretive** approach, most commonly identified with the work of Ronald Dworkin, seeks to interpret the individual law in the given situation in such a way as to give the overall body of law of which it forms a part as much consistency and coherence as possible.

Psychiatrists implicitly adopt aspects of these approaches when interpreting the law for medical purposes, but they also face the additional complications brought by psychiatry's different <u>constructs and models</u> (p.354) and by the need to <u>negotiate the interface with the law</u> (p.358).

Sources of law

What is the law covering this situation?

It can be surprisingly difficult to say. Where a legislature has passed a law that directly relates to the situation in question, and there is no other law to take into account, the answer may be relatively straightforward. Sometimes, however, there will be multiple laws or types of law to take into account. Moreover, some or all of these may require *interpretation* by a judge according to the rules of jurisprudence (p.364) before it is accepted whether and how they apply to a given situation that they do not expressly cover.

Sources of law

The different sources of law or quasi-law, with examples relevant to forensic psychiatry, include:

- National or federal **constitutions** such as the US Constitution: 'super-laws' that overrule all other laws in the country concerned. These tend to cover broad areas of principle rather than narrow situations. For example, the Eighth amendment to the US Constitution bans 'cruel and unusual punishment', and this has been held to prevent the execution of defendants with intellectual disability (p.110).
- **International treaties** such as the European Convention on Human Rights (ECHR),[14] Article 5 of which forced the UK government to allow tribunals to discharge restricted patients (p.510) from hospital.[15]
- Acts of the legislature, otherwise known as **statutes**. Important examples in the UK and Ireland include the MHA, MHCTA, MCANI, and ADMCA (see p.524 onwards). In some countries, especially civil law jurisdictions, statutes are gathered into **codes**, such as the French Code of Commerce law, or the California Code of Civil Procedure. In societies governed by an absolute monarch, proclamations by the King or Emperor with the force of law are also statutes.
- **Common law**, or case law, which is the body of judgments in previous cases by higher courts, both courts applying the **law** and those applying **equity** (originally the Lord Chancellor's power to remedy wrongs ignored by the law). Not all jurisdictions recognise common law (see p.368). In E&W, for example, the common law doctrine of necessity empowered doctors to treat patients who lack capacity (p.522), until the Mental Capacity Act replaced this area of law.
- **Customs** or 'conventions' (in a different sense from international conventions such as the ECHR) can be given the force of law by courts. This is commonest in contract law. For example, if it were customary in a certain area to send a warning letter before taking legal action to recover a debt, and if both parties could be shown to have been aware of and to have accepted that custom when contracting, an action to recover a debt would fail if no warning letter had been sent.

---

14 The convention itself is an international treaty, but many countries have incorporated it into domestic law as a statute. In the UK, this the Human Rights Act 1998. The case that forced the UK to allow tribunals to release restricted patients (*X v United Kingdom*, (1981) 4 EHRR 181) predated the HRA.

15 *X v United Kingdom* (1981) 4 EHRR 181.

- In limited circumstances, the **opinions of academic lawyers**, such as the so-called Institutional Writers of Scotland in the seventeenth century.
- **Guidance** and **codes of practice** can amount to quasi-laws, that is rules whose breach can be taken into account in determining whether a different law has been broken. For instance, breach of important parts of the Mental Health Act Code of Practice in E&W might be held to contribute to a finding of <u>negligence</u> (p.550) by a psychiatrist.

The origins of systems of civil law and common law

Civil law was originally the law (statute law, case law, and customary law) of the *cives*, the citizens of Rome. Roman law was largely forgotten during late antiquity after the fall of the Roman Empire, but it was rediscovered in the twelfth century, and its principles and many of its laws were used to create new legal systems across Europe.

The main exception was England, which by this time had already begun subordinating its patchwork of local customs to a coherent body of national or 'common' law formed by the judgments of the network of royal courts with peripatetic judges established by Henry II in 1166. The influence of re-discovered Roman law was therefore much weaker: Latin terminology and Roman methods of reasoning were imported, but Anglo-Norman procedures and substantive law continued to exist.

The vast majority of legal jurisdictions have developed either from the Roman (civil law) or English (common law) tradition. A few countries' legal systems are founded on religious law (often Islamic Sharia law), but most have since also adopted civil law principles. Lastly, some authors consider 'socialist law' a separate category, distinct from the Western civil law systems they otherwise resemble (most notably because law is subservient to the one-party State, and there is no <u>rule of law</u>, p.362).

Civil law and common law systems

Every jurisdiction's legal system has distinctive features, but most depend on whether it follows civil law or common law principles (Table 14.1). E&W, NI, and RoI are common law jurisdictions; Scotland is a hybrid.[16]

Table 14.1 Features of civil and common law

Feature	Civil Law	Common Law
Codification of laws	Compiled in one 'code'	Many separate laws
Binding nature of judgments (precedent)	Only legislature can make laws (binding decisions)	Higher courts' decisions bind lower courts
Court method	Inquisitorial (judge investigates and decides verdict)	Adversarial (judge is umpire between parties)
Legal reasoning	Deductive (argue from general principles)	Inductive (principles derived from cases)
Standard of proof Criminal trials Civil trials	'personal conviction' 'personal conviction'	Beyond reasonable doubt Balance of probabilities
Rules of evidence	Free evaluation of all evidence, no exclusions	Tightly restricted (e.g. no 'hearsay' in criminal law)
Judicial appointments	Judges form a separate profession with specific training	Judges are selected from experienced lawyers

Codification

Laws in many civil law jurisdictions were rewritten in the nineteenth century to:
- collect them in a single document (or a small number of documents covering different areas of law) rather than a multiplicity of Acts; and
- base them on a coherent set of principles[17] throughout the code, rather than different areas of law being based on different principles.

Precedent

The principle of *stare decisis* ('let the decision stand') found in common law systems means that higher courts' decisions set a precedent: lower courts must reach the same decision in any future such case unless they can **distinguish** it from the precedent (i.e. show that its facts are different in some legally relevant way). Even decisions of lower courts have persuasive authority: courts should only decide differently in subsequent cases if they can explain why. In contrast, courts in civil law jurisdictions are free to use their own interpretation of the legal principles involved.

16 Originally civil law, but many common law features were added after the 1707 union with E&W.
17 This was the goal of many nineteenth-century legislators across the continent, but as codes were updated in the twentieth century to reflect changing social realities, their newer sections tended to embody different principles to the original parts, weakening the overall coherence of the code.

Precedent requires the publication of higher courts' decisions; see Box 14.2.

Box 14.2 Major publications of the decisions of higher courts, and how to cite them

Abbreviation	Law Report Series Name	Jurisdictions
AC	Appeal Cases	UK
AllER	All England Law Reports	E&W
CSIH	Court of Session Inner House	Scotland
ECHR	European Court of Human Rights	UK, RoI
EWCA	England & Wales Court of Appeal	E&W
EWCoP	England & Wales Court of Protection	E&W
EWHC	England & Wales High Court	E&W
FCR/FLR	Family Court Reports/Family Law Reports	E&W
IR	Irish Reports	RoI
JC	Justiciary Cases	Scotland
KB/QB	Kings Bench/Queens Bench (High Court)	E&W
SC	Session Cases	Scotland
SCCR	Scottish Criminal Cases Reports	Scotland
SLT	Scots Law Times	Scotland
UKHL/SC	UK House of Lords/Supreme Court	UK
UKPC	UK Privy Council Judicial Committee	UK
WLR	Weekly Law Reports	UK

Citation: *Complainant v Defendant* [Year] Volume Series Page

e.g. *Gillick v West Norfolk and Wisbech AHA* [1985] 3 AllER 402

Inquisitorial and adversarial methods

Civil law judges are inquisitors: they actively establish facts by questioning witnesses, and in some jurisdictions oversee police investigations. Their high degree of control means that detailed rules for hearings (e.g. <u>rules of evidence</u>, p.382), are not required.

Common law systems are generally adversarial: each party seeks to demonstrate the truth of its own version of events, and interpretation of the law; the judge acts as an impartial umpire, ensuring that each party sticks to the rules and does not gain unfair advantage over the others, including by use of evidence that it would be unfair to admit.

Deductive and inductive reasoning

Civil law systems are characterised by overarching principles, expressed in a <u>constitution</u> (p.366) or in introductory sections of their legal codes. Courts reason by starting with these principles and deducing from them what the outcome should be in the current case.

Conversely, common law courts start with the facts, and make pragmatic decisions by considering relevant precedents from similar cases. Courts rarely state overarching principles explicitly; instead, these are inferred by legal commentators from the verdicts reached.

Courts and tribunals of UK & Ireland

There are three distinct legal systems in the UK, and a separate system in RoI. Their intermixed legal history is in part explained by English rule of Wales from 1283, of Scotland from the 1707 Act of Union,[18] and of Ireland from the 1801 Act of Union until the independence of the southern twenty-six counties in 1922. Wales and England now share a common legal system, and form one jurisdiction; NI is a separate jurisdiction with some independent legal structures, but very heavily influenced by English law; and Scotland has a hybrid legal system, combining earlier Roman and other civil law (p.368) influences with English concepts and structures.

The following is an overview of the types of courts found in almost all jurisdictions; subsequent pages cover each jurisdiction in detail.

Supreme Court

- The highest level of domestic[19] legal court
- The final court of appeal (see below) for all civil and criminal cases—usually only on points of law (as opposed to review of the facts)
- In jurisdictions that permit judicial review (p.374) on the ground of constitutionality, the final arbiter of whether a law is constitutional
- Hearings usually involve five or more judges (so that where there are legitimate differences of view on e.g. questions of interpretation, a majority may prevail)

Appeals Court(s)

- Primarily hear appeals on points of law—that is, claims by a party to a trial that the trial court (see below) mistook, misinterpreted, or misapplied[20] the law
- Review the facts of the case only where the decision of the lower court was unreasonable (p.374) or if there is substantial evidence of a new type which would make the original verdict 'unsafe'; when a retrial by the lower court, or substituted verdict, will be ordered
- Hearings usually consist of three judges

Trial courts

- Also known as *courts of first instance* as they are the first court to hear the substance of the issues in question.
- They are usually divided into courts for **criminal** matters and courts for **civil** matters, with further subdivision of the latter into for example **family**, **administrative**, **general law**, and **equity**[21] courts.

---

18 There is scope for great disagreement over (and this handbook takes no position on) whether Wales, Scotland and NI are still subject to 'English rule', whether the devolution after the 1997 referenda and the 1998 Good Friday Agreement made a material difference; or whether by the twentieth century there was more mutual 'British rule' across all four countries.

19 States may, by ratifying international treaties (p.366), give international courts (e.g. the International Court of Justice in the Hague in relation to, say, disputes over international borders, or the European Court of Human Rights in relation to the ECHR, p.518) and supranational courts (most notably those of the European Union, p.390) supremacy over their domestic courts in relation to issues covered by those treaties.

20 For example, in judicial directions given to the jury.

21 In common law systems, courts of equity (p.366) consider matters that were previously ignored by the law and settled by the Lord Chancellor, most notably issues concerning trusts (not NHS Trusts), where one party holds property on behalf of another and has to use it for their benefit.

- There are often different levels of trial court depending on the seriousness of the matter in question, with the higher-level trial courts sometimes also acting as appeals courts for points of law from the lower-level courts.
- Trial courts rule on the issues before them and make a ruling on guilt and (if guilty) sentence in criminal matters; and on what 'relief' (e.g. damages or an injunction) to grant each of the parties in civil matters.

Tribunals

- Tribunals are similar in function to trial courts for civil matters, but are less formal, act more quickly and at lower cost to the parties.
- Each tribunal (or division of a tribunal) covers a narrow field of law, such as employment law, immigration law, or mental health law.
- They are formed of several members with specialised training and functions (including a legally trained chair), rather than general legal & judicial training.
- For example, Mental Health Tribunals[22] operate to review patients' detention under the MHA and consist of a legal member, a medical member, and a lay member.
- Appeals from tribunals on points of law or by way of <u>judicial review</u> (p.374) go to a senior tribunal in some cases (such as the <u>Upper Tribunal</u> (p.385) in E&W, or to a civil court such as the High Court in others).

---

22 We have used the term *Mental Health Tribunal* (MHT) throughout the handbook (or in the mental health law chapter, simply 'tribunal'). In E&W, tribunals were formerly known as Mental Health Review Tribunals; in Wales they still are, but in England they are now technically the First Tier Tribunal (Mental Health). In Scotland, their formal title is the Mental Health Tribunal for Scotland; in NI, the Mental Health Review Tribunal for Northern Ireland; and in RoI, simply the Mental Health Tribunal.

Judicial review

Judicial review in the UK allows a higher court to cancel the decisions of a body carrying out public functions. In Ireland and other jurisdictions, judicial review is a wider concept, and extends to striking down laws[23] because they conflict with the <u>constitution</u> (p.366).

Judicial review is not an appeal: the 'correctness' of the decision is not examined, merely the procedure by which it was reached; its legality and reasonableness (or, in Ireland, its constitutionality). In this context, a decision is only 'unreasonable' if it is 'so outrageous in its defiance of logic or of accepted moral standards that no sensible person who had applied his mind to the question could have arrived at it'.[24]

The range of public bodies subject to judicial review is very wide, and includes all NHS and HSE organisations (including General Practices) carrying out functions on behalf of the government. For an example see Box 14.3.

Relevance to forensic psychiatry

There may be judicial review in a number of areas in forensic psychiatry:
- decisions made by individual practitioners representing a public body such as an NHS Trust or Health Board (e.g. a decision to refuse <u>leave from hospital</u> ; p.486),
- actions taken by non-NHS bodies that affect patients: for instance, a decision by the Crown Prosecution Service to prosecute (or not to prosecute) a patient, and
- decisions made by Mental Health Tribunals (outside E&W).

England & Wales and Northern Ireland

In E&W and NI, permission for judicial review must first be sought from the Administrative Division of the <u>High Court</u> (p.385). The complaint must be about a public or quasi-public body. Time limits apply to the application. There are three grounds for review:
- Illegality, particularly acting outside the powers granted to the body;
- Unreasonableness; and
- Reaching a decision without following the proper procedure (e.g. a tribunal reaching a decision to discharge before hearing evidence; although, since 2007, the <u>Upper Tribunal</u> (p.385) in E&W has heard appeals on such grounds, removing the possibility of judicial review).

Scotland

The substance of the Scottish law on judicial review is essentially the same as English law, although the procedure is different (e.g. there are no time limits, and applications are heard by the Court of Session rather than a special Administrative Court). Judicial review can apply to any body, public or private, carrying out a public function.

---

23 In the UK, the Human Rights Act 1998 (like the European Convention on Human Rights Act 2003 in RoI) allows higher courts to declare laws incompatible with the ECHR, but the doctrine of Parliamentary supremacy prevents any wider judicial review of the actions of Parliament, and means that incompatible laws remain in effect unless amended by Parliament.

24 These principles are from <u>Wednesbury</u> (p.770), expressed vividly by Lord Diplock.

Republic of Ireland

The High Court and Supreme Court in Ireland can invalidate any legislation that conflicts with the constitution, and can issue injunctions against any public or private body or any individual citizen to prevent them acting unconstitutionally. In addition, some areas of specific concern, such as town planning and immigration, are subject to special statutory judicial review procedures, which can involve consideration of the merits of a decision as well as its legality, constitutionality, and procedural propriety. Applications must be made within six months of the public body's decision.

Remedies after judicial review

Courts exercising powers of judicial review can, if they rule against the decision or action of the body in question:
- quash the decision (in RoI, this includes invalidating legislation);
- order the body (by injunction) to take, or refrain from, certain actions; and
- award damages to anyone who suffered from the original decision or action of the body.

Box 14.3 Judicial Review example

Facts

H was detained at a high secure hospital. There was clear evidence of risk of harm to others and of previous failed discharges. The tribunal discharged him, despite the lack of <u>after-care</u> (p.492) arrangements.

Grounds for review
- The tribunal gave inadequate reasons for its decision (procedural impropriety).
- The tribunal acted unreasonably by discharging the patient in the absence of after-care arrangements, when it could have adjourned to allow time for arrangements to be put in place.

Decision

The Court of Appeal held that the tribunal had decided unreasonably, and that its lack of adequate reasons for its decision was improper, and therefore quashed the decision to discharge H.
R (Ashworth Hospital) v MHRT (see p.746 for full details).

Roles in court

Court personnel have distinctive roles, many of which are established by law and/or long tradition. The following is a summary of those roles, as found in the UK jurisdictions and RoI. Not all personnel will be found in all courts.

Court personnel

- Judge—presides over a court; responsible for ensuring court <u>procedure</u> (p.378) is correctly followed, the law is correctly interpreted and applied, and ultimately that justice is done and seen to be done
- Jury—a body of twelve (fifteen in Scotland) ordinary people (peers of the defendant or litigant) who hear evidence and deliver a verdict, guided by the judge on matters of law
- Court Clerk—responsible for maintaining records, and for giving legal advice to lay magistrates in E&W (who are not legally qualified, unlike District Judges); he or she normally sits at a table in front of the judge/sheriff, facing into the courtroom
- Usher, Court Officer, Macer (Scottish High Court), List Caller—introduces each case by calling parties to the court and telling the court who is representing whom; responsible for ensuring that the comings and goings in the court operate smoothly, and often for arranging the order of cases efficiently, and for maintaining order
- Stenographer—records the proceedings verbatim
- Solicitors—lawyers who deal with most legal matters, but usually only conduct trials (litigate) in lower courts
- Barristers, Counsel,[25] Solicitor advocates (Scotland), Advocates[25] (Scotland)—lawyers who conduct trials in higher courts

The defendant and witnesses are the other parties present in court. The court may also have reporters and the public present as observers.

The judiciary

Heads of judiciary
- Lord Chief Justice—head of the judiciary for E&W
- The Lord President of the Court of Session—head of the judiciary for Scotland
- The Lord Chief Justice of Northern Ireland—head of the judiciary in Northern Ireland
- The Chief Justice of Ireland—head of the judiciary in Ireland

Other judiciary
See Table 14.2.

Tribunal and other roles

- Tribunal Presidents—responsible for the administration of their tribunal
- Tribunal Chairs and Tribunal Judges—appointment based on qualifications for the particular tribunal
- Tribunal Panel members—varies according to the particular tribunal

---

25 Senior barristers and advocates in the UK may be appointed as 'Queen's Counsel' (QC) by letters patent issued by the Queen.

- Notaries Public (Scotland)—solicitors who record certain transactions and sign specific legal documents

Table 14.2 Other judiciary

Court	E&W and NI	Scotland	RoI
Supreme Court	Justices of the Supreme Court	Justices of the Supreme Court	Justices of the Supreme Court
Appeals Court	Lords Justices of Appeal[26]	Lords of Council and Session[27]	Judges of the Court of Criminal Appeal
Senior courts	High Court Judges, Masters, & Registrars	Lords Commissioners of Justiciary	Judges of the High Court
Higher trial courts	Circuit Judges or Recorders[28]	Sheriff Principal Sheriff	Judges of the Circuit Court
Lower trial courts	District Judges or Magistrates[29]	Justice of the Peace	District Judges

Other terms

- The Prosecution—the legal party who presents the case against an individual in a criminal trial, in the name of the Crown in the UK and of the People in RoI
- The Defence—the legal party who represents the defendant
- Claimant[30]/Complainant/Pursuer—the person who initiates a legal action seeking a legal remedy in civil matters
- Defendant/Defender—the person charged with a criminal offence, or the person answering a complaint (in civil courts)

26 These include the Lord Chief Justice, the Master of the Rolls, and from the High Court, the President of the Queen's Bench Division, the President of the Family Division, and the Chancellor (head of the Chancery Division), though not all sit in criminal appeals.

27 Including the Lord President and Lord Justice Clerk. The same people are often both Lords of Council and Session and Lords Commissioners of Justiciary in the High Court.

28 A fully qualified solicitor or barrister sitting as a judge.

29 Magistrates and Justices of the Peace are lay people with basic training (but no legal qualifications) sitting with a legal advisor or clerk.

30 Formerly known as 'plaintiff'.

Court procedures

Court procedures vary depending on the type of court and the jurisdiction. Many aspects will be less relevant to psychiatrists, but it is useful to have some understanding of basic procedures of the <u>criminal justice process</u> as a whole (p.398), those procedures relating directly to <u>expert witnesses</u> (p.652), and a more detailed knowledge of the <u>legal rules</u> (p.654) and <u>codes of practice</u> (p.658) for expert witnesses.

Criminal courts

See also giving evidence in criminal courts (p.718).

- Generally, at the beginning of the case, the charges will be read, and the defendant will be asked to make a plea. If a guilty plea is made the magistrates or judge will hand down a sentence. If a not guilty plea is made, the case will be heard in full.
- The defendant is not obliged to give evidence, however if they do so they will be subject to <u>cross-examination</u> (p.714) by the prosecution.[31]
- Judges in an <u>adversarial system</u> (p.369) like those in the UK and RoI must be impartial and ensure fair play and due process; they decide what <u>evidence</u> (p.382) may be admitted, and other procedural issues.
- In the lower criminal courts (<u>Magistrates' Court</u>, in E&W and NI, p.384; <u>District Court</u>, in Scotland p.386 and RoI p.388), the hearing can take place in a court room, with a gallery for the general public, or in a private room (although people connected to the case such as solicitors and witnesses may be invited to attend). The judge will usually give their verdict immediately at the end of the trial.
- In the higher criminal courts (<u>Crown Court</u> in E&W, p.384; <u>Sheriff Court</u> in Scotland, p.386; <u>County Criminal Court</u> in NI, p.384; and <u>Circuit Court</u> in RoI, p.388), there may also be a gallery for members of the public and the press. The defendant is expected to take a seat on the dock (a raised platform) and to stand when requested. The average trial lasts for a day or so but may extend into weeks and months if the evidence is complex. At the end of the trial the jury will retire to a private room to discuss the case and decide on the verdict. The jury debate is confidential. Once a decision has been made the foreman juror will pass the verdict to the judge before reading it to the court.
- Procedures differ in <u>youth courts</u> (p.384), whether they are wholly separate courts or for example part of a Magistrates' Court. This is also the case when serious youth trials are held in (adult) higher courts. The case is still heard in full but there may be more frequent breaks, and the defendant is given explanations of legal arguments in terms that they can understand. Media coverage and public access is heavily controlled to protect the identity of the defendant.

---

31 If they do not, in the UK the judge may make an **adverse inference direction** entitling the jury to make inferences from the defendant's silence (such as that they wish to avoid incriminating themselves under cross-examination)—unless there is psychiatric evidence that the defendant is <u>unfit to give evidence</u> (p.606) or that their mental disorder makes it 'undesirable' they should give evidence (see *R v Tabbakh* [2009] EWCA where the defendant claimed unsuccessfully that his PTSD inhibited him from controlling his behaviour).

- Following the trial, if defendants are found not guilty (acquitted), they are free to leave the court.[32]
- If defendants are convicted, they will sometimes be sentenced (p.442) immediately; more commonly, the case will be adjourned for pre-sentence reports (p.498) to be compiled, particularly if defendants appear to be mentally disordered.

Civil courts

See also giving evidence in civil courts (p.724).

- The duty of any participant in a civil case is to comply with the Civil Procedure Rules (p.658) in E&W, or equivalents elsewhere.
- In most trials the case is heard by a judge alone; juries are very rare (e.g. in some defamation trials).
- Cases are usually slow to pass through the system (taking months or years), and the vast majority of cases are settled out of court.
- Although the defendant is required to give a statement, this statement is not subject to cross-examination and is not given under oath. However, it is likely to be questioned by the judge.
- In Scotland and NI all witnesses are required to give evidence orally, whether or not they have submitted a report.
- At the end of the trial the Sheriff or judge will usually retire to consider their judgement and will deliver this in writing later.

Tribunals

See also giving evidence to tribunals (p.724).

- Tribunals cover many areas of special jurisdiction including mental health and employment law (p.556).
- Tribunals are usually conducted in private, although the parties may apply for a public hearing (even with Mental Health Tribunals).
- Participants must follow the relevant set of Tribunal Procedure Rules.
- As a witness in a tribunal, you will not be required to take an oath.
- In RoI public inquiries are also often referred to as 'tribunals'.

---

32 Unless, in Scotland, the court makes an order for their urgent detention (p.504) on mental health grounds.

The burden and standards of proof

In any legal proceeding, parties are required to **prove** facts that they wish to rely on. The standard to which they must prove a fact depends on the type of case, and which party is trying to prove it.

The standard of proof in civil courts and tribunals

In all noncriminal court hearings, facts are required to be proved **on the balance of probabilities**,[33] meaning that it is more likely than not to be true, or 'more probable than not'. This is also the standard of proof used in Mental Health Tribunals (p.373), when facts are contested.

This is the case in the UK jurisdictions and RoI, although in civil law (p.368) countries such as France and Germany, the standard of proof in civil matters is the same as in criminal trials, and therefore much higher.

In the USA, the 'balance of probabilities' is usually referred to as the 'preponderance of evidence', but the meaning is the same.

The standard of proof in criminal courts

The general rule in the UK and Ireland is that, in order for the court to convict the defendant, the prosecution must prove that they committed the offence **beyond reasonable doubt**. In cases held before a jury (p.376), the judge should explain that this means that they jury should only return a guilty verdict if they are '**sure**'[34] that the defendant is guilty'.

However, in criminal cases, when the defence is required to prove something—such as the existence of a defence (p.412) to an otherwise criminal act—it usually only has to do so on the balance of probabilities.

Most jurisdictions use the beyond reasonable doubt standard for criminal matters, although it may be phrased differently (e.g. in France as 'a personal conviction' on the part of the judge). However, there are exceptions. For example, in the USA in some circumstances, facts are proven if there is 'clear and convincing evidence', which has been interpreted as just 'substantially more likely than not to be true'.

The standard of 'proof' for prosecution

In making the decision to prosecute, a lower standard of 'proof' is required: the police officer or prosecutor, is not expected to convince themselves that something is the case, merely that it is sufficiently likely to proceed with the investigation, then prosecution.

Some relevant other standards are:
• **Reasonable grounds for suspecting**—the lowest standard, enough to justify a police search of a person or a car for stolen property;
• **Reasonable grounds for believing**—a more demanding standard, enough to justify a police officer entering a private dwelling to look for a specific individual;

---

33 A different phrase may be used: for example, in cases under the Children Act 1989, that the court is "satisfied" of something. This is still taken to mean that it is more likely than not.

34 This means that the word *sure* can have particular weight in evidence: an expert witness (p.652) stating they are not sure about a key point can be enough to result in acquittal.

- **Probable cause**—the US term corresponding to the above, used to justify police searches and arrests (and indictments by grand juries) when there is 'a fair probability' of finding evidence, or of conviction; and
- **Reasonable prospect of conviction**, meaning that conviction is more likely than not—the standard used by prosecution agencies[35] to decide whether to prosecute (see the evidential test, p.346; along with the public interest test, p.347).

The burden of proof

A related issue is which party is required to prove certain matters. In civil matters, whichever party wishes to rely on a fact must prove it. The general rule in criminal cases is that the prosecution must prove all the elements of the offence, otherwise the defendant is acquitted. However, there are exceptions, including the following:

- Where the defendant puts forward certain defences, or partial defence, they must prove the relevant facts (on the balance of probabilities).
- If the defendant claims that they are unfit to plead, p.602, they must prove it (again, on the balance of probabilities).
- In a prosecution for possession of an offensive weapon in a public place, if it has been proved that the defendant was in possession in a public place, they must then prove (on the balance of probabilities) that they had a lawful authorisation or reasonable excuse for this.

There are two different burdens of proof. The first is the **legal burden**, as immediately above: the requirement to prove that something is the case. The other is the **evidential burden**, which means only that a party is required to adduce evidence that something might be the case, which the other party may then have a legal burden to disprove (i.e. effectively the burden shifts). Examples of evidential burdens include:

- The legal justifications (p.410) and the defence of duress (p.634), where the defendant has an evidential burden (e.g. to show that they were threatened), whereupon the prosecution has the legal burden of disproving that (say) the threats were sufficiently serious, or that the defendant had no alternative course of action.
- In a prosecution for handling stolen goods, if it has been proved that the defendant was in possession of stolen goods, they then have the evidential burden of showing that they had a reasonable excuse for doing so; whereupon the prosecution must prove beyond reasonable doubt that their explanation is false.

---

35 In E&W and NI. In RoI, cases where acquittal appears more likely can still be prosecuted if the case is serious enough, provided the chance of conviction is not 'effectively nonexistent'. In Scotland, the test is whether there is sufficient (i.e. corroborated) admissible, reliable, and credible evidence.

Rules of evidence

Rules of evidence govern whether information in a case may be presented, and, when it is presented, in what form. The rules of evidence vary between legal contexts.[36] They are very tightly drawn within the criminal law, less so within the civil courts, and even less so within the family courts. There are subtle variations between jurisdictions, but the concepts are universal.

What is evidence?

Evidence is information that may be presented to a court to prove or rebut a civil or criminal case. The aim of the trial is to test the evidence; a criminal trial will not proceed unless there is a <u>realistic prospect of conviction</u> (p.381). Quasi-judicial bodies such as Mental Health Tribunals do not apply rules of evidence per se.[37] There is therefore greater latitude in what evidence can be presented and when.

Evidence can be:

- Testimony—oral statements;
- Documentary—any paper or electronic records; or
- Real—objects.

Fact, inference, and opinion

There is a distinction drawn between fact and inference derived from fact. Opinion evidence amounts to inference drawn from particular facts. Witnesses who are not expert witnesses may only give evidence of fact, and not inference or opinion. <u>Expert witnesses</u> (p.652) may give evidence of fact, including fact derived through practice of their own professional skills (e.g. a mental state description), and evidence of opinion (e.g. opinion that maps a mental state onto a legal test), drawing inferences from both expertly derived and ordinary facts. Facts may be relevant or collateral, that is, going directly to the legal issue or merely being associated with it.

Relevance and admissibility

Relevant evidence will go some way to showing whether a fact did or did not exist. However, relevant evidence may be inadmissible for example because of perceived unfairness in the way it was collected or presented or because it is more *prejudicial* than *probative*.

In a criminal trial, the jury or magistrates must come to their verdict solely on the facts presented in the case. If they were to use information from outside the trial, it would not be subject to cross-examination.

The law governing what evidence may be excluded makes up much of the law relating to evidence.[38] These rules cover not only what might logically help answer the question but also what it would be fair to include. For example, from the perspective of <u>risk assessment</u> (p.163), a defendant's past

---

36 And even more between jurisdictions: <u>civil law</u> jurisdictions (p.368) have few or no rules on admissibility of evidence, allowing investigative magistrates 'free evaluation' of all the evidence.

37 Tribunals can be criticised as excessively <u>reflexive</u>, (p.355) so lacking in procedural and evidential rules as not adequately to protect patients' rights.

38 This area of law tends to be detailed and prescriptive in E&W and NI, whereas much is left to judges' discretion in Scotland and RoI. See, for example, the admissibility of <u>confessions</u>, p.608.

behaviour might be a strong predictor of having committed the current alleged offence, but it would be unfair to allow a jury to hear such evidence because it might influence their evaluation of the evidence relating to the current alleged offence (similarly, information on past behaviour, including past conviction, is admitted only in very limited circumstances).

Use of evidence

Once evidence is considered admissible, the **weight** attached to it depends on ordinary factors such as:

- support (corroboration) or contradiction by other evidence;
- the status, demeanour, or credibility of the witness; and
- the inherent credibility of the evidence.

Nonexpert witnesses are not permitted to hear the evidence of other witnesses. Expert witnesses are usually encouraged to do so, as the other evidence could affect their expert opinion.

Hearsay

There are rules relating to facts described by a witness arising not directly from their own experience but from what they have heard from others. This kind of evidence is excluded in criminal proceedings unless it is:

- evidence of what a dead, or otherwise unavailable, witness would have said in court;
- a business, professional, or official document providing evidence of what is within the personal knowledge of a potential witness;
- *res gestae*, that is, a statement about a sensation or mental state by someone so emotionally overpowered by an event that the possibility of concoction or distortion can be disregarded;
- information about reputation (e.g. showing the good or bad character of a defendant, in limited circumstances);
- publicly available information; or
- it forms part of the factual basis of an expert witness opinion.

The rationale for this is that the judge or jury cannot properly consider the weight of this evidence if it is not subject to any test of reliability by cross-examination. The strictness of the hearsay rule is much greater within criminal compared to civil proceedings, where hearsay evidence is generally admissible, and where the focus is on the weight of the evidence and not on its admissibility per se.

Voir dire

Prior to a criminal trial commencing there may be an application to **exclude** particular evidence, on the basis that it was unlawfully obtained, or that it would be unfair to include it. Within a *voir dire*[39] the trial judge will hear arguments, sometimes also the evidence itself, as to why the evidence should or should not be admitted.[40] If the evidence is admitted, the same arguments may also be presented during the trial, in terms of whether less than usual weight should to be given to it.

39 Literally, 'let us see what you are going to say [in the trial]'.
40 A common example is in regard to a <u>rebutted confession</u>, (p.V.44) where there is alleged to be evidence of suggestibility and/or compliance.

The court system in England, Wales, & Northern Ireland

The court systems in E&W and NI are separate (apart from the Supreme Court) but almost identical (Figure 14.1).

Supreme Court

- Is the highest appeal court.
- Its role was previously held by (part of) the House of Lords.
- It sits as the Judicial Committee of the Privy Council for appeals from some Commonwealth countries.

Senior courts

- The **Court of Appeal** deals with appeals from other courts or tribunals. The **Civil Division** hears appeals from the High Court and the County Court, as well as some superior tribunals; the **Criminal Division** hears appeals from the Crown Court connected with a trial on indictment. Its decisions are binding on all lower courts.
- The **High Court** comprises the Queen's Bench Division (which includes the Administrative Court, Business & Property Courts, and other specialist courts), the Chancery Division, and the Family Division. The High Court acts as a court of first instance for more serious civil claims; the Queen's Bench also hears appeals from Magistrates' Courts, and the Family Division hears appeals from the Court of Protection (p.535).
- In E&W, the **Family Court** hears almost all cases involving child care and protection, families, and marriage, except for a few specialised cases reserved to the **Family Division of the High Court** (e.g. wardship and child abduction). It is usually co-located with the High Court, county court, or Magistrates' Court.
- The **Crown Court** is a criminal court. It is the only court that has the jurisdiction to try cases on indictment. (i.e. more serious crimes); The **Central Criminal Court**, at the Old Bailey, hears high-profile criminal cases.
- In Northern Ireland, there can be a rehearing of a county court case in the High Court and an appeal from there to the Court of Appeal.

Subordinate courts

- **County courts**: local courts, each one having an area over which certain kinds of civil jurisdiction are exercised, including claims for debt repayment, personal injury, breach of contract, and housing disputes.
- **Magistrates' courts**: These are presided over by a bench of lay magistrates (justices of the peace), or in larger towns in E&W, a legally trained district judge. They hear minor criminal cases.
- In NI, Family Proceedings Court (part of the Magistrates' Court): these hear family law cases including care cases and can make adoption orders.
- **Youth Courts** (part of the Magistrates' Court) deal with almost all criminal cases involving children. The court is served by youth panel magistrates and District Judges. Youth courts are less formal than magistrates' courts, are more open, and engage more with the young person appearing in court and their family. Youth courts are essentially private places, and members of the public are not admitted.

Tribunals

There are statutory tribunals for specialist areas: employment, immigration, social security, pensions, child welfare, and mental health. Appeals are either to appeal tribunals or certain courts, depending on the statute.

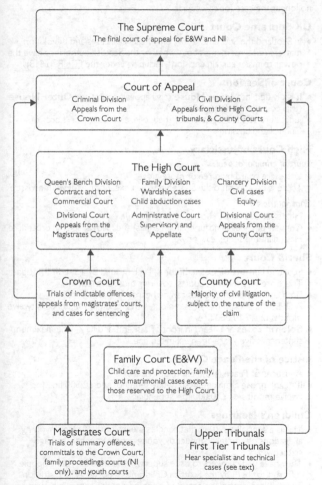

The Supreme Court
The final court of appeal for E&W and NI

Court of Appeal
Criminal Division
Appeals from the Crown Court

Civil Division
Appeals from the High Court, tribunals, & County Courts

The High Court
Queen's Bench Division
Contract and tort
Commercial Court

Divisional Court
Appeals from the Magistrates Courts

Family Division
Wardship cases
Child abduction cases

Administrative Court
Supervisory and Appellate

Chancery Division
Civil cases
Equity

Divisional Court
Appeals from the County Courts

Crown Court
Trials of indictable offences, appeals from magistrates' courts, and cases for sentencing

County Court
Majority of civil litigation, subject to the nature of the claim

Family Court (E&W)
Child care and protection, family, and matrimonial cases except those reserved to the High Court

Magistrates Court
Trials of summary offences, committals to the Crown Court, family proceedings courts (NI only), and youth courts

Upper Tribunals
First Tier Tribunals
Hear specialist and technical cases (see text)

Figure 14.1 The court system in England, Wales, and Northern Ireland

The court system in Scotland

Scotland has a distinct court system, which has <u>developed separately</u> (p.372) from those elsewhere in the UK (Figure 14.2). Notably, criminal courts in Scotland require all evidence to be corroborated by other evidence; this is no longer the case for civil courts.

UK Supreme Court

• In Scotland the Supreme Court only hears civil cases and devolution matters (disagreements about whether the Scottish authorities have the power to make certain decisions, including under the <u>ECHR</u>, p.518).

Court of Session

• It is divided into **Inner House** (civil appeals court) and **Outer House** (trial court for serious civil cases).
• Judges are termed 'Senators of the College of Justice' or 'Lords of Council and Session'.

High Court of Justiciary

Court of criminal appeal
• Cases are heard by three or more judges.
• There is no appeal to the Supreme Court except on a 'devolution issue'.

Criminal trials
• Hears serious cases, such as murder or rape
• Consists of a judge and jury (fifteen adults) and follows 'solemn procedure'
• Has unlimited sentencing powers

Sheriff Court

• Scotland consists of six sheriffdoms, each headed by a Sheriff Principal.
• There are forty Sheriff Courts, covering most districts.
• Both civil and criminal cases can be heard.
• A Sheriff hears summary cases alone—the maximum sentence is twelve months or a £10,000 fine.
• **Solemn cases** are heard in front of a sheriff and jury—the maximum sentence is five years or an unlimited fine.

Justice of the Peace Courts

• A Justices of Peace (JPs) hear minor cases.
• JPs can impose a maximum sixty-day sentence and £2,500 fine (or twelve months or £10,000 for 'stipendiary' JPs).

Children's Hearings

• This is a specialist system that handles the majority of cases involving allegations of criminal conduct by young people younger than age sixteen years.
• They have wide powers to issue supervision orders for young people referred to them by the Scottish Children's Reporter Administration.
• The children's panel is a group of people from the community who are carefully selected and highly trained. The panel members sit on hearings on a rotational basis.
• The Procurator may send serious crimes to the usual criminal courts.

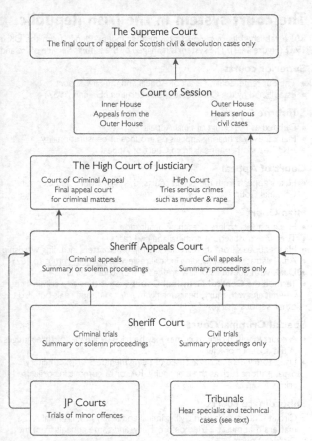

Figure 14.2 The court system in Scotland

The Mental Health Tribunal for Scotland

- This hears applications for, reviews of and appeals against, <u>mental health orders</u> (p.461).
- They also hear excessive security appeals and appeals against the appointment of a named person.
- Any case regarding a restricted patient is chaired by a Sheriff and termed a 'Shrieval Tribunal'.

The court system in the Irish Republic

RoI established its own court system after independence from the UK in 1922 (Figure 14.3). The system is managed by the Courts Service of Ireland.

Superior courts

- The Supreme Court, Court of Appeal and the High Court
- Established by the Constitution (*Bunreacht na hÉireann*, 1937)

Supreme Court

- Defined as the Court of Final Appeal
- Main activity is hearing appeals on grounds of constitutionality
- Also hears other appeals from Court of Appeal

Court of Appeal

- Hears appeals from the circuit courts, the High Court, and Central Criminal Court

High Court

- Has authority to interpret the Constitution
- Tries the most serious criminal and civil cases
- Hears appeals from the Circuit Court in civil matters including wardship
- Administrative law including judicial review and _habeas corpus_ (p.462)
- Deals with questions of law arising from District Courts
- Termed the **Central Criminal Court** when sitting as a criminal court, when it sits with a jury; hears mainly murder and rape trials but also tries other serious charges

Special Criminal Court

- A court in which serious crimes may be tried by a panel of three judges in the absence of a jury
- Used to try defendants accused of being members of paramilitary organisations such as the Continuity IRA, or of committing organised crime

Subordinate courts

- Circuit Court: deals with civil, criminal and family law, criminal matters that must be tried before a jury, and some appeals from the District Courts
- District Courts: deal with criminal matters (predominantly summary matters), lower value civil claims, and many family law matters
- All juvenile cases are referred centrally to the National Juvenile Office, which decides what action should be taken

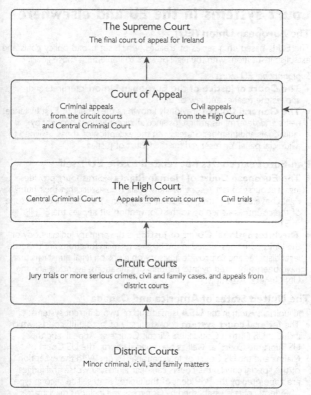

Figure 14.3 The court system in the Republic of Ireland

Court systems in the EU and elsewhere

The European Union (EU)

The EU is based on a series of treaties, which set broad policy goals and establish institutions with the legal powers to implement those goals.

Supranational EU courts
- **The Court of Justice of the European Union** interprets and applies the treaties and law of the EU.
- **The General Court** (previously known as the Court of First Instance) hears and determines at first instance all direct actions brought by individuals and Member States, with the exception of those assigned to a 'judicial panel' or reserved for the Court of Justice.

Pan-European courts not related to the EU itself

- **The European Court of Human Rights** in Strasbourg provides legal recourse of last resort for individuals who assert that their human rights have been violated by a contracting party to the Convention (one of the countries signed up to the Convention). It applies the ECHR (p.518).
- **The International Court of Justice** is the primary judicial body of the United Nations, based in the Hague. Its main functions are to settle legal disputes and to provide advisory opinions on legal questions that have been submitted by international organisations, agencies, and the UN General Assembly.

The United States of America and Canada

The judicial system in the **USA** is made up of two different systems:
- The **federal court system** consists firstly of 'article III' courts, which include: US District Courts, US Circuit Courts of Appeal, and the US Supreme Court, as well as two special courts, the US Court of Claims and the US Court of International Trade. With the exception of the special courts, the courts can hear almost any case and judges are appointed by the President of the United States. The second type of federal court is established by Congress and includes magistrate's courts, bankruptcy courts, the US Court of Military Appeals, the US Tax Court, and the US Court of Veterans' Appeals.
- The **state court system**—no two state court systems are exactly the same. However, most are made up of two sets of trial courts (trial courts of limited jurisdiction and of general jurisdiction), intermediate appellate courts, and the highest state courts. Unlike federal courts, most state judges are not appointed for life but are either elected or appointed for a certain number of years.

The two systems are not completely independent of each other, and they interact, although they are each responsible for hearing certain types of cases. The federal court system deals with issues of law relating to those powers expressly or implicitly granted to it by the US Constitution.

In **Canada**, the court system is a four-level hierarchy from the highest to lowest in terms of legal authority. Each court is bound by the rulings of the courts above them. At the top is the Supreme Court of Canada, then the appellate courts of the provinces and territories, the superior-level courts of the provinces and territories, and finally the provincial and territorial ('inferior') courts. There are also courts at the federal level.

Australia and the Commonwealth

The legal systems in Australia and elsewhere in the Commonwealth is modelled substantially on the systems in E&W, and so are common law jurisdictions. However, many have evolved so they no longer closely resemble the British systems. Australia now has both a state legal system and an overarching federal system with corresponding courts.

Judicial Committee of the Privy Council

Comprising judges of the UK Supreme Court, this court considers appeals for a number of overseas Commonwealth jurisdictions and Crown Dependencies (and very occasionally appeals from ecclesiastical and other courts in the UK). Its particular relevance to forensic psychiatrists is that it often hears final appeals against capital convictions and imposition of the death penalty abroad. The extent of its jurisdiction continues to reduce as former British states establish their own courts of final appeal.

Appeal is to 'Her Majesty in Council' from the following independent nations and other territories:
- The Crown Dependencies of Jersey, Guernsey (which includes Alderney and Sark), and the Isle of Man
- The Commonwealth realms of Antigua & Barbuda, the Bahamas, British Indian Ocean Territory, Grenada, Jamaica, St Christopher and Nevis, St Lucia, St Vincent & the Grenadines, and Tuvalu
- The New Zealand associated states of the Cook Islands and Niue (though not New Zealand itself)
- The British overseas territories of Anguilla, Bermuda, British Antarctic Territory, British Virgin Islands, Cayman Islands, Falkland Islands, Gibraltar, Montserrat, St Helena, Ascension & Tristan da Cunha, Turks & Caicos Islands, and Pitcairn Islands
- The UK Sovereign Base Areas of Akrotiri and Dhekelia in Cyprus

Appeal is directly to the Committee from the following countries:
- The Commonwealth republics of Mauritius, Trinidad & Tobago, and (in limited circumstances) Kiribati

Appeal is to the Head of State (i.e. The Queen) for Brunei in civil cases.

Professional regulatory structures

People working in certain professions in the UK and RoI are subject to a system of obligations and discipline separate from citizens' general obligations under criminal and civil law, and to disciplinary proceedings under employment law. This system of upholding professional <u>standards</u> (p.552) has its own structures that are analogous to courts and prosecutors in the criminal justice system, with appeals to the mainstream legal system. See Figure 14.4.

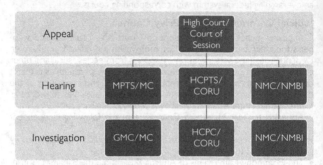

Figure 14.4 Professional regulatory structures in the UK and Ireland
HCPTS/MPTS=Health & Care Professions/Medical Practitioners Tribunal Service; GMC/ HCPC = General Medical/Health & Care Professions Council; NMC=Nursing & Midwifery Council; MC=Medical Council; NMBI=Nursing & Midwifery Board of Ireland. CORU is not an acronym, it comes from the Gaelic for 'fair'.

Broadly speaking, in each country there are three regulators that register healthcare professionals, and investigate complaints against them: one for doctors, one for nurses and midwives, and one for other healthcare professionals (e.g. psychologists, OTs, social workers,[41] art therapists, dietitians, and many others). Whereas in the UK the role of investigating and, if appropriate, prosecuting serious complaints is separated from the role of hearing that complaint and reaching a judgement (to avoid conflicts of interest within the same organisation), in RoI these roles are merged within different parts of the same body. Also, in the UK there is a 'super-regulator', the Professional Standards Authority, which ensures that the individual regulators maintain high standards of performance.[42]

---

41 In England only; social workers in Scotland, Wales, and NI are regulated by the Scottish Social Services Council, Social Care Wales and the Northern Ireland Social Care Council, respectively.

42 Since the case of Dr Bawa Garba, who was convicted of criminal manslaughter in regard to her paediatric care of a child, but was not erased from the Medical Register by the MPTS, against which the GMC unsuccessfully appealed, the government has committed to removing the GMC's right of appeal, in favour of only the PSA having that right (see detailed description of the case in Part C of the *Oxford Casebook of Forensic Psychiatry* addressing different paradigms for critiquing clinical decision making).

Regulatory investigations and hearings

Each regulator operates a process with similar stages:
- Screening of complaints or concerns (e.g. checking whether the subject of the complaint is regulated by the organisation complained to).
- An initial investigation (is there sufficient concern about <u>fitness to practise?</u> p.642)—most complaints stop at this stage.
- An investigation in depth (is there a sufficient case to answer?).
- A solicitor prepares the case for a formal hearing; counsel are instructed.
- The case is heard; determining whether the case is proven.
- The professional is sanctioned.
- There is an appeal to the court.

Available sanctions include a *formal warning*, *giving undertakings*, *having limitations placed on practice*, *temporary suspension* from the register, or *permanent erasure* from the register ('striking off'). Depending on the nature of the allegations there may also be *interim* undertakings or limitations on practice pending the conclusion of the final hearing. Hearings are usually before a panel of three tribunal members, at least one of whom will be from the profession, and one will be independent (a 'lay member').

The <u>standard of proof</u> (p.380) used by the MPTS, NMC, and HCPTS is the balance of probabilities; the <u>burden of proof</u> (p.381) lies with the regulator to demonstrate that the professional fell below the relevant professional standard—the professional does not have to prove anything. However, this does mean a career can be ended despite significant doubt about the truth of the allegations. By contrast, the MC, CORU, and NMBI adopt the criminal standard of proof.

Despite attempts by regulators to minimise the unpleasantness of investigation for practitioners, any complaint that goes beyond initial investigation is usually very stressful, and a hearing usually requires specialist legal skills and expertise. Practitioners are therefore routinely advised to purchase professional indemnity either through a mutual society[43] or insurance contract.

---

43 Such as the Medical Defence Union, Medical Protection Society (both of which cover the UK and RoI) or Medical and Dental Defence Union of Scotland (which covers the UK only).

Inquests and inquiries

Inquests (and Fatal Accident Inquiries in Scotland) are formal factual inquiries into a death that is either violent or unnatural, or which occurred during detention by the State. In E&W eighty-seven Senior Coroners investigate deaths within their jurisdiction; a further three coroners cover NI; in Scotland, the forty Sheriff Courts hold Fatal Accident Inquiries.

Who is involved?

- The coroner, an independent judicial officer who must be a lawyer[44] and has a statutory duty to conduct the investigation and inquest
- A coroner's officer, often a former police officer, who investigates and assists the coroner (in Scotland, staff at the Sheriff's office)
- A jury of between seven and eleven people (except in Scotland)
- Close relatives of the deceased, who are considered 'interested persons' with the right to be notified of the hearing, see relevant documents, and ask questions of witnesses (directly or through a legal representative)
- Any other 'interested person' who (or whose employees) may have caused or contributed to the death
- Witnesses, who submit written statements and may be required to give evidence orally

The jury will make the findings of fact if:
- the deceased died in custody or detention, violently or unnaturally, or from an unknown cause;
- death resulted from an act or omission of a police officer, or a member of a service police force; or
- death was caused by a notifiable accident, poisoning, or disease.

The coroner or jury is responsible for determining who the deceased persons were, when and where they died, and how they came by their death. Neither the coroner nor their jury may make any finding of civil or criminal liability on the part of a named person.

As these are inquisitorial proceedings there are no parties and no pleading or case to answer. All witnesses are selected and first questioned by the coroner.

Psychiatric involvement

Psychiatrists may be involved as witnesses of fact because the deceased was under their care, or as expert witnesses advising the coroner or Sheriff on issues such as the deceased's diagnosis, their intent, or the quality of psychiatric care they received.

Other inquiries

Government ministers and other public bodies may convene a myriad of formal or informal inquiries[45] in a range of circumstances, which occasionally may have relevance for psychiatrists. These include, but are not limited to:

---

44 Or, if appointed before 2013, a doctor.
45 See Part C *Oxford Casebook of Forensic Psychiatry*, comparing and critiquing a variety of legal and nonlegal paradigms for critiquing clinical decisions made.

- statutory public inquiries established under the Inquiries Act 2005 (e.g. into the Grenfell Tower disaster[46]),
- independent government reviews (e.g. the <u>Wessely review</u> into UK mental health law, p.782) not concerned with a particular event,
- <u>homicide</u> <u>inquiries</u> (p.598), and
- independent internal investigations (e.g. a Serious Incident Review or Root Cause Analysis investigation into serious incidents at a hospital).

These inquiries may be chaired by a layperson, a lawyer, another professional, or in more serious cases, a judge. They are usually free to set their own procedure within their terms of reference. They can be held in public or private or have partially public hearings. There is no overarching right of those affected by the events to be a participant or be permitted to question witnesses. Generally the rules of natural justice should be followed, which include a right to know if one is being criticised and be given an opportunity to respond before any adverse findings are made.[47]

---

46 A fire in a tower block in London in 2017, which caused many deaths and raised questions about the practice of 'cladding' older buildings in potentially flammable materials, as well as about the 'stay put' guidance issued by the Fire Service at the time.

47 The right to receive in advance a 'Salmon letter'.

Criminal law

The criminal justice process

Criminal procedure

The main steps in detecting and responding to crime are shown in the flowchart (Figure 15.1). Some details and other possibilities are omitted. For example:

- Suspects do not need to be arrested to be questioned. They may choose to be interviewed voluntarily. Arrests can be authorised by a court warrant; under arrest powers for 'arrestable' offences; for the investigation or prevention of an offence; or for breach of the peace (p.425).
- The decision to charge may be made by the prosecutor, rather than by the police alone. The prosecutor will not proceed unless there is a reasonable prospect of conviction (p.381).
- The first appearance before the lower criminal court[1] ensures there is sufficient evidence to justify a trial, gives the defendant an opportunity to plead guilty, sets the timetable for trial, and considers remand.
- Less serious offences can be tried summarily by the lower criminal court; more serious ones are committed to the higher criminal court,[2] where the trial process is more complex, guilt is usually determined by a jury, and the maximum sentences available are much greater. In a few intermediate cases the defendant may have a choice of court.
- In Scotland, in addition to guilty and not guilty verdicts, there is a 'not proven' verdict that leads to acquittal, but is taken as inferring a strong suspicion that the defendant is guilty.
- Suspects and offenders can be diverted (p.268) into mental health services from the point of arrest to that of sentencing. This might include bail or remand to hospital (p.498). The police, prosecutor or court may then discontinue criminal proceedings, suspend them until the defendant has recovered, or allow them to continue during treatment.

Detention, bail, and remand

During the investigation, police may **detain** the suspect for the times shown in Table 15.1—or give them **police bail**, requiring them to report back and to meet certain conditions (e.g. surrendering their passport, or residing at a specific place)—or simply **release** them **'under investigation'**. After charging, the court can similarly bail the defendant, or **remand** them in custody, usually in a remand prison (p.578) but sometimes in hospital.

---

[1] Magistrates' Court, in E&W and NI, p.384; District Court, in Scotland p.386 and RoI p.388.
[2] Crown Court in E&W and NI, p.384; Sheriff Court in Scotland, p.386; Circuit Court in RoI, p.388.

Table 15.1 Detention times

Detention time limits	E&W	Scotland	NI	RoI[3]
Initial period(s)	24hours	12hours	24hours	6–12 hours
Police can extend to	36hours	24hours	36hours	36hours
Court can extend to	96hours	n/a	96hours	n/a
Terrorist suspects	14days	14days	14days	3–7 days

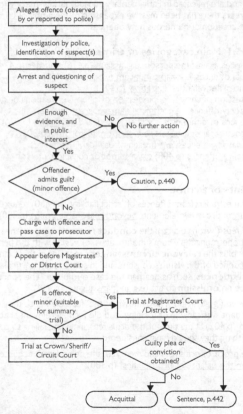

Figure 15.1 Simplified criminal justice process

3 Greater time limits apply in serious cases such as murder and firearms offences.

Elements of a crime

What is a crime?

A crime is any behaviour Parliament[4] or courts have determined should be morally censured and punished. See Box 15.1. By contrast, torts, or 'wrongs', under <u>civil law</u> (p.547) (e.g. libel, product liability, and <u>negligence</u>; p.548) attract less moral disapproval, and the court's action is generally intended to restore the wronged party to their position had there been no tort.

What amounts to criminal behaviour alters over time, as public attitudes change and are reflected in Parliamentary and judicial <u>law-making</u> (p.366). In recent years there has been massive expansion of the ambit of criminal law, with the creation of numerous new offences.

Box 15.1 Main categories of crime

- Offences against the person, e.g. <u>assault</u> (p.416), <u>murder</u> (p.414)
- Sexual offences, e.g. <u>rape</u>, <u>indecent exposure</u> (p.418)
- Public order offences, e.g. <u>affray</u> (p.424)
- Possession offences, e.g. possession of offensive weapons or drugs
- Property offences, e.g. <u>criminal damage</u>, <u>arson</u> (p.422)
- Offences of dishonesty, e.g. <u>theft</u>, <u>fraud</u>, and <u>deception</u> (p.426)
- Offences against the state, e.g. <u>treason</u>, <u>terrorism</u> (p.430)
- Regulatory offences, e.g. breach of bail, driving offences
- <u>Inchoate offences</u> (p.408) e.g. attempt or conspiracy to rob

---

Elements of a crime

Most crimes (apart from offences of 'strict liability', p.IV.50) require that the prosecution prove two elements <u>beyond reasonable doubt</u> (p.380):

- *Actus reus* ('wrongful act'): the **conduct** relevant to the offence (e.g. penetrating the victim's mouth, anus, or vagina with the penis in rape); plus the **relevant circumstances**,[5] meaning in this example the absence of the victim's consent, and in some cases, particular **consequences**, such as death in the case of murder. The conduct can also be an **omission** to act (e.g. in <u>manslaughter</u>, p.414).

- *Mens rea* ('guilty mind'), also known as the 'fault element': the defendant was capable of forming, and did form, a relevant **state of mind** (p.402) at the time of the *actus reus*, including failing to consider something they should have considered.

Despite proof of *actus reus* and *mens rea*, the defendant is acquitted if they prove <u>on the balance of probabilities</u>[6] (p.380):

---

4 Dáil in RoI.

5 These include the status of the defendant: for example, children under the <u>age of criminal responsibility</u> (p.406) cannot be prosecuted for conduct that would otherwise be wrongful.

6 Or, in some cases, if they raise evidence of the defence and the prosecution fails to disprove it beyond reasonable doubt, as with duress.

- An excuse or **justification** for their conduct (e.g. self-defence, prevention of crime; see p.410) or
- A **defence** to the prosecution for their conduct (e.g. duress; necessity, p.634; insanity, p.620; or automatism,[7] p.612).

---

7 In can be argued that the 'defence' of automatism actually reflects incapacity to form the necessary state mens rea 402.

The mental element of crime

The mental or 'fault' element of a crime, its *mens rea* ('guilty mind'), is the state of mind necessary for wrongful conduct to amount to the particular criminal offence. Fault is not required for some crimes of strict liability (see below).

Some crimes are graded as being of greater or lesser severity depending on the fault element. For instance, arson with *intent* to endanger life is more serious (with a greater maximum <u>sentence</u>, p.442) than arson being *reckless* as to whether life is endangered, which is more serious than *simple arson*.

There may be more than one fault element, relating to different aspects of the offence: for example <u>fraud</u> (p.427) requires, amongst other things, *knowledge* that a statement made is false, plus an *intention* to gain personally from making the false statement.

Intention

To a philosopher, *intention* refers to what persons wish to bring about (i.e. the purpose of their actions). However, law refers to this concept as **motive**.[8] For most offences motive is irrelevant, except as potentially probative of intent or as a <u>mitigating</u> or <u>aggravating factor</u> in sentencing (p.638).

Generally, someone is said to intend something they decide to do,[9] whatever their reason. Imagine A wishes to save B from choking, and slaps his back; whereas C wishes to hurt D, and similarly slaps him. Despite different motives, the law views both A and C as having intended to slap.

Intent is central to the <u>inchoate offences</u> (p.408) such as attempt, conspiracy, and aiding and abetting, in which defendants do not themselves cause the harm (the offence is incomplete or 'inchoate'). The essence of their crime is their intent to bring that harm about through a failed attempt (e.g. attempted murder) or persuading another to act (e.g. counselling to cause an explosion).

Oblique intent

Often no direct evidence shows that a defendant intended a particular harm. Deciding whether they had intent may involve inference from other evidence (e.g. witnesses' descriptions of their behaviour). Oblique intent applies where the harm is a virtually certain (or 'natural and probable') consequence of an action (e.g. B would be virtually certain to die if A set fire to her house with her inside). In these circumstances, courts[10] may infer that the defendant intended the harm.

---

8 The legal use of the word *intention* defies robust definition. Courts use the word slightly differently from one offence to another, reflecting policy considerations about who should be held liable to conviction for that offence.

9 As courts cannot know exactly what someone decided (not having direct access to their mind), judges infer that someone intended something when they 'acted so as to bring it about'.

10 A common law rule, amended by s8 Criminal Justice Act 1967 to require evidence from which to infer. The rule does not apply in Scotland, NI, or RoI, where *intention* is less strictly defined and can include or exclude oblique intent as necessary.

Basic and specific intent

Some crimes require that one intends not only one's actions (**basic intent**), but also certain consequences. For example, <u>GBH with intent</u> (p.416) requires a **specific intent** to cause serious injury. Imagine A and B deliberately push C, fracturing C's pelvis. If A intended serious injury but B was only play-fighting, A and B might both be convicted of GBH, but only A can be convicted of GBH with intent.

Crimes of specific intent include possession of a drug with intent to supply, <u>arson with intent to endanger life</u> (p.422), and <u>indecent exposure</u> (p.419, which requires intent to be seen). Whether an offence is deemed to require specific or basic intent is not based upon coherent criteria.

Psychiatric evidence supporting <u>incapacity to form intent</u> (p.610) may serve to negate specific intent, but can very rarely support negation of basic intent, at least in E&W.[11] The issue arises most commonly in regard to self-induced intoxication, but the bar is set extremely high (<u>DPP v Majewski</u>, p.761),

Recklessness

Recklessness refers to the defendant's subjective awareness of a genuine risk of harm, even though no harm is intended. However, if the defendant does not foresee the harm at all, there is no offence, even if the risk should have been obvious. For example, in <u>R v Stephenson</u> (p.768), a defendant with schizophrenia slept in a haystack and made a small fire to keep warm, setting the haystack on fire. Medical evidence suggested that, because of his disorder, he could not have foreseen the risk of fire. He was therefore acquitted.

Negligence

Negligence is analogous to *recklessness* in that it refers to situations in which the harm is foreseeable. However, whereas recklessness is subjective,[12] requiring the defendant to have foreseen the harm, negligence is objective, requiring only that a reasonable person would have foreseen it. There are degrees of negligence: <u>manslaughter</u> (p.414) requires gross negligence; dangerous driving a standard 'far below' that of a competent and careful driver; and careless driving just ordinary negligence.

Knowledge and belief

Some offences require the prosecution to prove that the defendant knew of circumstances relevant to the *actus reus*. For example, the offence of <u>fraud</u> (p.427) committed by making a false statement requires that the defendant knew that the statement was (or might be) false. For other offences, such

---

11 Consider a person with dementia who leaves a bookshop with a book he forgot to pay for, and then accidentally drops it in a puddle, ruining it. Psychiatric evidence that he did not have the capacity to form intent would, if accepted, prevent conviction for theft (an offence requiring specific intent to deprive the owner of the item permanently), but would not prevent conviction for simple criminal damage to the book (an offence of basic intent).

12 In relation to who needs to be aware of the risk. There are other, objective, elements, as with any offence.

as handling stolen goods, the defendant need only **believe** the goods to be stolen, meaning that they can be convicted of attempted handling even if by chance the goods are legally in their possession.

Mistaken belief

Some offences allow a mistaken belief to negate an element of the offence, such as criminal damage, where a defendant's mistaken belief that the damaged property was their own will prevent conviction. In other cases, an objective standard is applied, and only *reasonable* knowledge or belief suffices. For instance, nonconsensual penetrative sex is not *rape* (p.418) if the defendant believed the victim consented, provided that belief was reasonable in the circumstances.[13] See also mistake (p.412).

Lesser degrees of knowledge

In wilful blindness, also called 'connivance', the defendant realises that the relevant circumstances might exist, and deliberately avoids finding out (i.e. the defendant is reckless as to whether they exist). This has been held to be sufficient for conviction of offences such as driving an uninsured or dangerously loaded vehicle. *Constructive knowledge*, on the other hand, refers to a situation where the defendant did not contemplate the existence of the circumstances, but had reasonable cause to believe they might exist (i.e. the defendant was negligent), such as in an unauthorised, albeit unintended, disclosure of information protected by the Official Secrets Act.

Subjective and objective approaches

A conviction may hinge on whether the law applies a subjective test (e.g. recklessness,[14] mistaken belief) or an objective test (e.g. negligence, constructive knowledge). However, there is no coherent general principle determining when one or the other applies. A further complication is variation between jurisdictions: the most notable being that, in Scotland, defendants are sometimes held to an objective standard for offences of recklessness, making them effectively indistinguishable from offences of negligence.[15]

Objective tests favour victims and public welfare at the expense of individual autonomy (p.331), and they disadvantage mentally disordered defendants in particular. Some argue that the 'reasonable person' in objective tests should be a reasonable person with the same mental capabilities as the defendant, but others argue that this would introduce a slippery slope allowing, for instance, criminals of low IQ to escape conviction.

---

13 In E&W, an earlier case (*DPP v Morgan*, p.753) had held that the mistaken belief that the victim had consented prevented conviction for rape. The requirement for belief in consent to be reasonable was introduced by the Sexual Offences Act 2003.

14 Some argue that recklessness is a hybrid concept because there must objectively be a genuine risk that it is unreasonable to take, in order for there to be something for the defendant to be subjectively aware of.

15 This was also the case in E&W from 1982, after *Caldwell* (p.750), until 2004, when that authority was overturned by the House of Lords in *R v G* (p.756).

Strict liability

Many 'regulatory' offences, and a small number of others, have no mental element, and are known collectively as offences of strict liability. Examples include unlawful parking, fishing (or watching TV) without a licence, and <u>outraging public decency</u> (p.420). For defendants to be convicted, they need only to be shown to have done the acts or omissions concerned.

Capacity and criminal responsibility

Incapacity due to youth

Children under the **age of criminal responsibility** are deemed to lack the capacity to commit crime, as they may be insufficiently capable of moral reasoning (though they will often still be held responsible, and punished, by their parents, teachers, and others). From a purely utilitarian perspective, an age of criminal responsibility of up to twelve years accords with evidence (p.36) that children do not commit behaviours amounting to criminal offences against society[16] in significant numbers until age elven to twelve. However, a general age of criminal responsibility ignores the fact that children develop at different rates, and that some under the age will be capable of being held criminally responsible, whereas some over the age will not (and some aspects of brain maturation relevant to moral reasoning continue into adulthood; see p.36).

In E&W and NI, the age of criminal responsibility is ten years; in RoI it is twelve (but with the possibility of trying ten and eleven year olds for serious offences including murder and rape), and in Scotland twelve[17] (although younger children can still be dealt with through the Children's Hearings system, p.386). In other countries it ranges from seven to ten in the USA, to eighteen in Belgium and Argentina.

The European Commissioner on Human Rights has recommended that the UK adopt an age of criminal responsibility in line with the European norm, on the grounds that children younger than twelve years old cannot have sufficient consciousness of the nature and consequences of their actions to be held criminally responsible as their cognitive abilities and capacity for self-control may not be sufficiently developed[18]; and they may be particularly susceptible to peer pressure.

Protections for child defendants

Each jurisdiction has its own youth justice systems (see pp.384–389), which attempts to balance the youth and inexperience of the defendant against the interests of their victims and of society. These systems tend to be more informal and less frightening in style, to allow relatives and friends to support the young defendant, to make less use of remand procedures (p.398), to detain young offenders in smaller institutions such as secure children's homes (p.580) with access to schooling, and to employ less-punitive sentences (p.442), with a stronger emphasis on promoting healthy, pro-social development.

There used to be an additional rule, called *doli incapax*, that children younger than fourteen could not be convicted of a crime unless the

---

16 As opposed to hitting (assaulting) each other and taking toys and other items (stealing), which is rife amongst toddlers in particular.

17 In addition, children younger than sixteen years old can only be prosecuted in Scotland (as opposed to being dealt with under the Children's Hearing system) with the consent of the Lord Advocate.

18 However, the British government does not accept this, as evidenced by its refusal to follow the Law Commission recommendation for E&W of including 'developmental immaturity' as a ground, for example, for diminished responsibility (p.624).

prosecution had shown that they knew that what they were doing was wrong. This rule was abolished in E&W and NI in 1998, and in RoI in 2006; it has never applied in Scotland.

Incapacity due to mental disorder

As with other forms of <u>mental capacity</u> (p.522), adults and children over the age of criminal responsibility are presumed capable of committing crime; that is, capable of forming the relevant *mens rea*. However, some will in fact be incapable in some way, because of mental disorder, and this is recognised by the law in different, albeit limited, ways.

- Mental disorder **at the time of legal proceedings** may render a defendant <u>unfit to plead</u> and stand trial (p.602). For example, a person with severe Alzheimer's dementia might be unable to concentrate on or comprehend the proceedings.
- Mental disorder **at the time of the alleged offence** may:
  - prevent the defendant forming the necessary *mens rea* (p.402) for the offence, particularly <u>intent</u> (p.610) or
  - less definitively, give rise to a <u>defence</u> (p.412), such as <u>insanity</u> (p.620), <u>automatism</u> (p.612), or the partial defence of <u>diminished responsibility</u> (p.624).

Incapacity due to intoxication

Intoxication with alcohol or drugs can alter one's criminal responsibility for one's acts and omissions. However, the law on whether and how intoxication affects liability in a given case is highly complex. A broad principle is that unintended intoxication (e.g. your drink being spiked) is a defence, whereas voluntary intoxication is not. (See detail on pp.614–617.)

Who is a party to the offence?

If A hits B, A can be charged with assault; if A dishonestly takes B's money, A can be charged with theft. However, what if C is involved, but without hitting B or taking B's money?

In criminal law A is the **principal**; C may be an **accessory** (secondary party).

Inchoate offences

These offences are 'incomplete' in one of the following ways:

- **attempting** to commit the offence (e.g. attempted robbery: threatening the victim with a weapon but not obtaining anything);
- **aiding and abetting** (e.g. providing A with a weapon, knowing they will murder B with it);
- **inciting**, counselling, and procuring (e.g. inciting terrorism: training A as a terrorist); and
- **conspiring** (e.g. to defraud: planning with A to defraud B, even if B is not eventually defrauded).

The <u>mental element</u> (p.402) of an inchoate offence is often different from that for the main offence. For instance, an intent merely to cause grievous bodily harm suffices for murder, but only intent to kill suffices for attempted murder. Defences such as <u>duress</u> (p.634) apply in the usual way (e.g. if a violent husband coerces his wife into assisting in the offence, she may have a defence).

Encouraging or assisting, and joint enterprise

Before 2013 in the UK

The common law principle of joint enterprise[19] generally meant that if C and A carried out a crime together, they would both be responsible for each other's actions during the joint criminal enterprise: not only agreed actions, but also actions that C foresaw A might take.

For example, A and C jointly commit burglary, intending no-one to be hurt. During the offence A kills B. If C foresaw the killing (i.e. knew A had a knife, or believed A had a gun when A had a knife), C could be convicted of murder with A.[20] Only if A's killing was 'fundamentally different' from anything foreseen by C, would C be acquitted of murder.

Since 2013 and in RoI

The Supreme Court reviewed the case law in <u>R v Jogee</u> (p.758) and concluded that a legal misunderstanding meant that 'foreseeability' was being treated as equivalent to intent. It held that the prosecution still had to demonstrate that C intended to assist or encourage A, not only in the original plan but also in A's further crime. Under this rule, C from the example above would only be found guilty of burglary.

---

19 Set out in the leading case <u>R v Chan Wing-Siu</u> (p.751). Although old law, it remains relevant for appeals against convictions before 2013.

20 As controversially occurred in <u>R v Bentley</u> (p.747).

In practice, foreseeability remains relevant, as evidence from which intent may be inferred. Psychiatric evidence may be relevant, to determine for example whether C was capable of foreseeing what A went on to do.

However, controversially, convictions under the law prior to 2013 will rarely be overturned by the Court of Appeal: those convicted would first need to demonstrate 'substantial injustice'.

In RoI, the law never took the 'wrong turn' of joint enterprise and has followed principles almost identical to *Jogee* throughout.[21]

Entitlement to control

The common law has sometimes held C liable for A's actions, in the absence of an inchoate offence or assisting & encouraging, where C was 'entitled to control the actions' of A and failed to do so. Examples include:

- a passenger held liable for the driver's dangerous driving because he could have stopped the driver;
- a publican held liable for customers' illegal drinking outside licensed hours as he could have prevented them; and
- a haulage company found liable for failing to stop its drivers falsifying their tachograph records.

The rule on 'entitlement to control' represents a breach of the general principle that people are not responsible for what they do not do. Its extent is unclear. It could in principle be applied to a party host who walks in on a guest raping another and does nothing. Or, applying it more widely, to a homeowner who looks out on their garden and sees one stranger assaulting another but does not intervene. These possibilities have not yet been tested in the courts.

---

21 From the earlier (pre-*Chan*) English case *R v Anderson; R v Morris* [1966] 2 QB 110, where the test, rather than foreseeability, was whether A had 'departed completely from the concerted action of the common design'.

Self-defence and other justifications

Legal justifications apply to all offences and excuse conduct that would otherwise be unlawful—in contrast to <u>defences</u> (p.412), which allow the defendant to escape conviction (or receive a lesser conviction, in the case of partial defences). Five justifications are recognised[22] :

- defending oneself against attack (self-defence),
- defending another person against attack (public defence),
- preventing an offence,
- apprehending an offender, and
- preventing serious damage to property.

Necessity

The conduct must have been necessary[23]: that is, the aim of defending oneself or apprehending an offender for example could not reasonably have been achieved another way (e.g. by running away in the case of self-defence).

Reasonable force and proportionality

The degree of force used must have been reasonable in the circumstances,[24] and proportionate to the harm that could otherwise have occurred. For instance, considerable force, possibly resulting in the death of the attacker, may be justified in defending oneself or one's children against a potentially fatal attack, but little or no force be justified in preventing someone damaging property by daubing graffiti on a wall.

Objective and subjective tests

The test of 'reasonableness' is objective: would a reasonable person have used that type and degree of force in those circumstances, bearing in mind the difficulty of making such a judgment in the heat of the moment?

The circumstances are addressed subjectively, as the defendant believed them (reasonably or otherwise) to be.[25] For example, whether the defendant was committing an offence (e.g. burglary) or whether he initially provoked his attacker or struck the first blow or sought revenge, any of which will make it more difficult to claim justification. The location of the attack is also relevant: it is easier to claim self-defence, for example, if one is attacked in one's own home.

---

22 There are different mixtures of common law and statute in each jurisdiction; the rules are similar, but there are minor differences (e.g. that in RoI, public defence applies only to family members in certain cases, and that the common law duty to retreat or escape if possible before using force in self-defence still applies in RoI and Scotland but has been abolished in E&W and NI). RoI enacted legislation in 2011 which specifically covers justifiable use of force against a trespasser reasonably believed to be intending to commit a criminal act.

23 The necessity and proportionality requirements are particularly important in homicide cases, where they balance the victim's <u>right to life</u> (p.516) against that of the self-defending attacker.

24 s3(1) Criminal Law Act 1967 for E&W, s3(1) Criminal Law (NI) Act 1967, and common law for Scotland and RoI. In E&W, s76 Criminal Justice & Immigration Act 2008 defines 'reasonable force', and states that in the case of a householder, only 'grossly disproportionate' force is unreasonable.

25 Unless that belief resulted solely from voluntarily induced <u>intoxication</u> (p.616). At least in E&W, a genuinely held mistaken belief is sufficient for self-defence, whether or not it is 'reasonable': s76 Criminal Justice and Immigration Act 2008.

Burden of proof

Once the defendant has put forward sufficient evidence to raise the justification, the <u>burden of proof</u> (p.381) is on the prosecution to prove beyond
reasonable doubt that the justification does not apply.

Relevance of mental disorder

The role of psychiatric or psychological evidence is limited to how mental
disorder might have affected the defendant's perception of the circumstances, and is not permitted in relation to the objective test of whether
force was reasonable in those circumstances.[26]

In _R v Martin (Anthony)_ (p.762), the defendant's misperception of risk due
to his <u>paranoid personality disorder</u> (p.88) and depression has been held irrelevant to the objective test; even florid psychosis has been held irrelevant
(_R v Jason Cann_, _R v Oye_, pp.758, 764).

---

26 In contrast to the partial defences of <u>provocation</u> and <u>loss of control</u> (p.630) and <u>diminished
responsibility</u> (p.624), which allow mental disorder to be considered to a limited extent. The difference is because successfully pleading a justification results in acquittal, and if mental disorder
were allowed within the objective test, that would prevent the State protecting the public from
people who had seriously harmed others.

Defences and partial defences

The term *defence* is often used to refer to anything that defendants may argue to rebut a charge or to show that their actions were justified (p.410). However, strictly speaking a defence relates only to matters that, if proven, reduce or negate the defendant's criminal liability. Full defences result in acquittal; partial defences result in a lesser conviction. Psychiatric evidence is frequently relevant.

The defences on this page are counted as 'special defences' in Scottish law, meaning that in solemn cases (p.386), the defendant must give notice at least ten days before trial that the defence will be pleaded.

Full defences

The **insanity** defence allows that the defendant's mental disorder prevented them bearing criminal responsibility for their actions, because they did not understand the true nature of what they were doing. See p.620.

Automatism is a state in which the defendant acts without exercising conscious control, often because of a psychiatric or medical condition. See p.612.

Duress (also known as **coercion** or necessity in Scotland) occurs when a defendant commits a crime only because another person threatens to harm them or someone else if they do not (duress by threats), or because of their situation (duress of circumstances). See p.634.

Partial defences

Each of the following applies only to murder (p.414), and if successfully pleaded, reduces the offence to manslaughter or culpable homicide (p.414).[27]

Diminished responsibility (p.624) partially excuses responsibility by way of mental disorder (of a lesser degree than required for insanity)

The essence of **loss of control** (in E&W and NI) or **provocation** (in Scotland and RoI) is that the defendant was provoked into killing by something that another person did or said. See p.630.

Deliberately killing a person who wishes to die is murder, but if there is a **suicide pact** (where the defendant had intended to kill themselves afterwards), this reduces the conviction to manslaughter in E&W and NI.[28] Unlike other partial defences, the defendant bears the full burden of proof (p.381) of demonstrating the existence of the pact.

Mistake

A mistake by a defendant does not, of itself, give rise to a defence. However, it may have a similar effect if it negates an element of the offence (e.g. where a defendant mistakenly believes the victim to have consented

---

27 The partial defences are anomalous, in that they exist only because of the strict definition of murder and because of the desire to avoid passing the mandatory life sentence (p.448) on more 'deserving' defendants. Infanticide (p.414) is also a partial defence as well as an alternative offence in E&W, NI, and RoI.

28 In RoI & Scotland, the defendant can in theory be convicted of murder but is more likely to be charged with manslaughter (culpable homicide in Scotland) or assisting suicide.

to assault or indecent exposure[29]) or if it amounts to a belief in facts which, if true, would give rise to a defence or justification (p.410), such as where a defendant assaults someone, mistakenly believing that they are defending themselves.[30] This is particularly relevant to psychiatrists where the mistaken belief arises from mental disorder.

Potential defences

Killing persons in order to end their pain and suffering is not a defence in any UK jurisdiction or RoI, despite proposals that it should be. However, mentally disordered people who have perpetrated an apparent **mercy killing** have been found guilty of manslaughter, or culpable homicide, by reason of diminished responsibility.

There have been proposals in E&W and RoI for a partial defence to murder of **excessive force in self-defence** (i.e. where the defendant believed they were using reasonable force, but objectively it was unreasonable, so the claim of self-defence (p.410) therefore fails). Where the result is merely injury, a lesser sentence can be given, but if death results the current outcome is a mandatory life sentence.

---

29 For instance *Kimber* (p.759). The same principle was applied to rape in *DPP v Morgan* (p.753); in E&W the Sexual Offences Act 2003 introduced the requirement that the mistaken belief be reasonable.

30 This is arguably the same point as that about negating the offence, as persons who believe they are acting in self-defence do not intend to commit assault (i.e. to hit someone unlawfully).

Homicide offences

Homicide is the killing of another person. It is not necessarily an offence.

In most jurisdictions, there are at least two homicide offences: one indicating intentional, culpable killing (murder), and another indicating less intentional or culpable killing (manslaughter). Manslaughter may be voluntary (as a result of successfully pleading a partial defence to murder) or involuntary (resulting from recklessness or criminal negligence).

Definitions

Murder—In E&W, NI, and RoI, to kill a person unlawfully with the intention (p.402) of killing them or doing them serious harm; in Scotland, to kill a person unlawfully with 'wicked recklessness (p.403) or intent'. 'Unlawfully' in this context refers to the absence of a justification (p.410) such as self-defence, or being an active soldier in a legally declared war.

Manslaughter—In E&W, NI, and RoI, to kill a person recklessly or grossly negligently (p.403) or through an otherwise unlawful and dangerous act. In Scotland, the equivalent offence of culpable homicide is to kill a person with intent only to assault them nonfatally, or through a grossly negligent act.[31] Grossly negligent medical care resulting in the death of a patient has resulted in doctors being convicted of manslaughter.

Infanticide—Many cultures treat the intentional killing by the mother of a child aged up to twelve months (i.e. infanticide, p.46), differently from other homicide offences. In E&W, NI, and RoI, infanticide is both a specific offence and a partial defence to a murder charge; the same penalties are available as for manslaughter. The court must be satisfied that 'the balance of the mother's mind was disturbed by the childbirth or lactation'. In Scotland, the same mother would be convicted of culpable homicide by reason of diminished responsibility, with the same effect.

There are a number of other specific homicide offences in some of the jurisdictions, including causing death by dangerous driving, child destruction (to which being a registered medical practitioner performing an authorised abortion is a defence), and assisting suicide.

Defences specific to murder

Most of the partial defences (p.412) are only available on a charge of murder. If a partial defence to murder is accepted by the prosecution or court, the defendant will be convicted instead of voluntary manslaughter or culpable homicide. The current partial defences are:
- diminished responsibility (p.624),
- loss of control (p.630) or provocation (p.630),
- infanticide, and
- killing in pursuance of a suicide pact (p.412).

---

31 A Culpable Homicide Bill is under consideration by the Scottish Parliament at the time of writing, to change the law so that persons in large organisations do not escape prosecution for deaths caused recklessly or by gross negligence. This is part of a larger Scottish parliamentary project that aims to put common law principles into explicit statutory terms for 'fair labelling' of offences.

HOMICIDE OFFENCES 415

Sentencing guidelines for murder

As murder carries a mandatory <u>life sentence</u> (p.448) in all four jurisdictions, <u>sentencing guidelines</u> (p.442) have been developed to take into account the seriousness of the killing. A minimum term or <u>tariff</u> (p.448) is set by the trial judge (from twelve years for a child defendant with no aggravating factors, to a whole life tariff in extreme cases); it is open to appeal. A <u>hospital disposal</u> (p.500) is not a sentencing option, but it is possible for prisoners to be <u>transferred to hospital</u> (p.506) after sentencing.

Attempted murder

In E&W, NI, and RoI, this consists of an act which is more than merely preparatory to an unlawful killing, with intent to kill. In Scottish common law, attempted murder differs from murder only in that death did not result.

The partial defences do not apply to attempted murder, creating the anomalous situation where a defendant may be in a more advantageous position, in terms of pleading a partial defence, if the victim dies. The maximum penalty is a life sentence.

Assault and other violent offences

Assault is a nonfatal violent crime committed against another person. Other violent crimes include homicide offences (p.414), robbery (p.426), and sexual offences (p.418). In E&W and NI there are many separate offences, classified by method, severity of injury, and intention; in Scotland, there is only really one offence, that of assault, with an extraordinarily wide range of sentences.

Assault offences in E&W and NI

In order of diminishing severity, the main offences[32] are:

- **Wounding with intent to cause GBH** (grievous or 'really serious', bodily harm), and **causing GBH with intent**; sometimes referred to as 'section 18 GBH'. Defined as intentionally or recklessly wounding (causing an injury that breaks the skin) or causing GBH, with specific intent (p.402) to cause someone (not necessarily the victim) GBH, or to resist or prevent arrest or detention.[33] Maximum life imprisonment.
- **Unlawful wounding** and **inflicting GBH**. Sometimes referred to as 'section 20 GBH' or just 'GBH'. Intentionally or recklessly (p.403) wounding or inflicting GBH. Maximum seven years' imprisonment (five in E&W).
- Assault causing **actual bodily harm** (ABH). Any hurt or injury calculated to interfere with the health or comfort of the victim, which is not transient or trifling. Maximum five years' imprisonment.
- **Battery**. Charged as 'assault by beating'. Intentionally or recklessly touching or applying unlawful force (e.g. pushing) to another person. Maximum six months' imprisonment.
- **Common assault**. Causing a person to fear an immediate touching or application of unlawful force, or actually doing so. Maximum six months' imprisonment (two years in NI).

Aggravated assaults.

A group of specific offences wherein an aggravating factor (p.638) is present, and the maximum sentence is therefore greater. They include assault with intent to rob, racially aggravated assault, and religiously aggravated assault.

Assault offences in RoI[34]

- **Causing serious harm**. Intentionally or recklessly causing another person, not necessarily by assaulting them, a substantial risk of death, serious disfigurement, or substantial loss or impairment of mobility or function. Maximum life imprisonment.

---

32 Mostly offences under the Offences Against the Person Act 1861. There are also a number of rarely used specific offences such as poisoning or causing bodily injury by gunpowder. More commonly used are a series of specific offences of assaulting police and prison officers or emergency workers.

33 The commonest relevance of mental disorder to a charge of section 18 GBH is where it is pleaded as evidence that the defendant was not capable of forming the specific intent (p.610).

34 Under the Non-Fatal Offences Against the Person Act 1997. There are also, as in E&W and NI, a number of more specific offences (see previous footnote).

- **Assault causing harm**. Intentionally or recklessly assaulting another person, causing harm to body or mind (including pain and unconsciousness). Maximum five years' imprisonment.
- **Assault**. Intentionally or recklessly directly or indirectly applying force or impact to another person, or causing them reasonably to fear immediate force or impact. Maximum six months' imprisonment.

The offence of assault in Scotland

Scotland has one general offence of **assault** under common law, although charges often use additional words to indicate the nature or severity of the assault, such as *serious assault, assault to injury, or assault to the danger of life*. It has been defined as intentionally or recklessly directing an attack to take effect physically on the person of another, whether or not actual injury is inflicted. It includes threats of attack. Assaulting a police officer is a separate offence[35]; and domestic abuse is the subject of specific legislation,[36] which augments the general offence of assault.

Assault is usually charged as 'serious assault' if the victim's injuries require inpatient treatment in hospital, or involve fractures, internal injuries, severe concussion, loss of consciousness, or lacerations requiring sutures which may lead to impairment or disfigurement.

The maximum penalty for assault in Scotland is life imprisonment.

---

35 Police and Fire Reform (Scotland) Act 2012.
36 Domestic Abuse (Scotland) Act 2018.

Sexual offences

Different jurisdictions define and classify sexual offences differently, based partly on social attitudes towards <u>sexual behaviour</u> (p.54). Sexual offences are often separated into 'contact' and 'noncontact' offences; some apparently nonsexual offences may have a sexual motive or component. Table 15.2 summarises the definitions, mostly statutory, of the more common sexual offences in the UK and RoI.

Other offences

Other sexual offences, often with definitions that differ in detail between jurisdictions, include **incest** and related offences, abuse of trust offences against children or vulnerable adults, offences related to prostitution and trafficking, and offences related to the production and possession of pornographic images, especially of children.

Historic offences

Sexual offences, particularly against children, are often prosecuted many years after they allegedly occurred. Offences committed before new Acts came into effect are tried under the law in effect at the time. Allegations based on '<u>recovered memory</u>' (p.V.102) are profoundly problematic.

Table 15.2 Summary of definitions of the more common sexual offences in the UK and RoI

	E&W and NI	Scotland	RoI
Primary legislation	Sexual Offences Act 2003; Sexual Offences (NI) Order 2008	Sexual Offences (Scotland) Act 2009	Criminal Law (Rape) Act 1981; Criminal Law (Rape) (Amendment) Act 1990; Criminal Law (Sexual Offences) Act 2017
Rape	A penetrates B's vagina, anus, or mouth with his penis; B does not consent; A does not reasonably believe that B consents (Note that B can be male or female in UK jurisdictions)	Without B consenting; Without reasonable belief that B consents; A penetrates B to any extent, either intending to do so or reckless as to whether there is penetration by his penis	A has unlawful sexual intercourse (penile penetration of mouth or anus, or penetration of vagina by penis or any object) with B who does not consent, knowing that B does not consent, or being reckless as to whether B consents

Table 15.2 (Contd.)

Sexual assault (Indecent assault)	*Assault by penetration* A intentionally penetrates the vagina or anus of B with part of their body or anything else; the penetration is sexual; B does not consent; A does not reasonably believe that B consents *Sexual assault* A intentionally touches B; the touching is sexual; B does not consent to the touching; A does not reasonably believe that B consents	Without B consenting Without reasonable belief that B consents: *Sexual assault by penetration* … A penetrates B to any extent, either intending to do so or reckless as to whether there is penetration with body or anything else *Sexual assault* … A intentionally or recklessly: sexually penetrates B; or touches B sexually; or has any other form of sexual activity; or ejaculates semen, or sexually emits urine or saliva, onto B	*Sexual assault* Any indecent assault (defined by courts as 'conduct that right-thinking people would consider an affront to the sexual modesty of a woman') *Aggravated sexual assault* A sexual assault that involves serious violence or the threat of serious violence or is such as to cause injury, humiliation, or degradation of a grave nature to the person assaulted
	E&W and NI	**Scotland**	**RoI**
Indecent exposure	A intentionally exposes his genitals, and intends that someone will see them and be caused alarm or distress	A exposes his genitals in a sexual manner to B with the intention that B will see them; obtaining sexual gratification thereby; and humiliating, distressing or alarming B	A exposes his genitals with intention to cause fear, distress, or alarm

(Continued)

Table 15.2 (Contd.)

Sexual offences against society	*Outraging public decency*	*Public (shameless) indecency*	*Offensive conduct of sexual nature*
	A public act of such a lewd, obscene, or disgusting nature as to amount to an outrage to public decency, whether or not it tends to deprave and corrupt those who see it	A lewd act in public that offends a witness to it *Lewd, indecent, or libidinous practices* As for shameless indecency, but without the requirement of a witness being offended	Sexual intercourse, buggery, or masturbation in a public place Offensive conduct of a sexual nature in a public place: likely to cause fear, distress, or alarm
Child offences	Unlawful sexual intercourse and other offences against a child younger than thirteen years old (most serious) Similar offences against a child older than thirteen Offences of inciting or arranging sexual activity involving children	Unlawful sexual intercourse and other offences against a 'young' child Similar offences against an 'older' child Intercourse of person in a position of trust with a child younger than sixteen years old	Sexual act with child younger than fifteen years old Sexual act with child younger than seventeen Child trafficking & sexual exploitation

Arson and criminal damage

Arson and criminal damage

These offences relate to destroying or damaging property, wilfully or recklessly. Arson or fire-raising involves causing damage by setting fires (setting a fire that causes no damage might not be an offence, but might still be a behaviour of clinical interest, p.50). The act is further classified as to whether there was an intention to endanger life, or recklessness concerning life.

Many judges routinely request an expert psychiatric report in cases of arson because of the perceived association with mental disorder.

Typology of arson and criminal damage

Both arson and non-fire-related criminal damage have been classified into four broad categories:
- youth disorder—young children (accidental), vandalism;
- malicious—using fire as a weapon, malicious damage;
- psychological—communication of frustration, pain, or hostility; and
- criminal—covering up evidence of other crime, fire for financial gain.

The offences

In E&W, NI, and RoI, the relevant statutes[37] are broadly similar (Box 15.2).

> ### Box 15.2 Criminal damage and arson
> - **Criminal damage**: a person who without lawful excuse destroys or damages any property belonging to another intending to destroy or damage any such property shall be guilty of an offence
> - **Arson**: destroying or damaging property by fire is charged as arson
>
> *The mental element*
> - **Intending** to destroy or damage any property **or being reckless** as to whether any property would be destroyed or damaged
> - Aggravating factors (p.638): intending by the destruction or damage to **endanger the life of another** or being reckless as to whether the life of another would be thereby endangered

The effect of the aggravating factors is to create three arson offences: arson with intent (to endanger life), reckless arson; and simple arson. The specific intent (p.402) can be difficult to prove, so that defendants charged with arson with intent are often convicted of reckless arson.

In Scotland, vandalism is defined by statute (Box 15.3), but it excludes fire-raising, which remains a common law offence.

---

37 The Criminal Damage Act 1971, Criminal Damage (Northern Ireland) Order 1977, and Criminal Damage Act 1991 respectively.

Box 15.3 Scottish offences

- **Vandalism**: without reasonable excuse, wilfully or recklessly destroying or damaging any property belonging to another
- **Wilful fire-raising:** the raising of fire, without any lawful object ...

The mental element:

- Wilful fire-raising requires the **deliberate intention** of destroying certain premises or things
- Wicked, culpable, and reckless fire-raising requires only **recklessness** as to the risk of destruction

Public order offences

Public order offences are intended to penalise the use of intimidation or violence by groups or individuals, particularly if it could pose a threat to the State, and can generally be committed in private as well as public places. They can be controversial because of the scope for misuse in order to suppress legitimate political protest. For common examples, see Table 15.3.

Table 15.3 Common public order offences

	E&W	NI	RoI
Primary legislation	Public Order Act 1986; Common law	Public Order (NI) Order 1987; Common law	Criminal Justice (Public Order) Act 1994
Riot	Using unlawful violence as part of a group of twelve or more, using or threatening unlawful violence for a common purpose, where the group's conduct would cause a person of reasonable firmness present[38] to fear for their personal safety	Where three or more persons assist each other in carrying out acts of violence, which alarms or terrifies at least one person	Using unlawful violence as part of a group of twelve or more, using or threatening unlawful violence for a common purpose, where the group's conduct would cause a person of reasonable firmness present to fear for their or another's safety
Violent disorder (Riotous & disorderly behaviour in NI)	Where three or more people together use or threaten unlawful violence and their conduct would cause a person of reasonable firmness present to fear for their personal safety	Where a person in any public place uses disorderly behaviour or behaviour whereby a breach of the peace is likely to be occasioned	Where three or more people together use or threaten unlawful violence and their conduct would cause a person of reasonable firmness present to fear for their or another's safety
Affray	Where a person uses or threatens unlawful violence towards another, and their individual conduct would cause a person of reasonable firmness present to fear for their personal safety	Affray involves the fighting of two or more persons, which alarms or terrifies at least one person	Using or threatening unlawful violence to another person (who uses or threatens violence) where the joint conduct would cause a person of reasonable firmness present to fear for their or another's safety

38 In all the E&W and RoI offences, no person of reasonable firmness need actually be present.

Table 15.3 (Contd.)

	E&W	NI	RoI
Threatening, abusive, or insulting[39] words or behaviour, or displaying signs	Using or threatening such words, signs, or behaviour: (1) with intent to cause fear of immediate violence or (2) with intent to cause (or (3), unintentionally causing) harassment, alarm, or distress	Using such words, signs, or behaviour in a public place or at a public meeting, or procession, with intent to cause a breach of the peace, or by which a breach of the peace is likely	Using or engaging in any such words, signs, or behaviour in a public place with intent to provoke a breach of the peace, or being reckless as to breaching the peace
Disorderly conduct or intoxication in a public place	Behaving in a disorderly fashion while drunk in a highway or other public place	Where a person in any public place uses disorderly behaviour, or behaviour whereby a breach of the peace is likely to be occasioned	Engaging in any unreasonable behaviour in public at night likely to cause serious offence or annoyance, or being intoxicated in public to such an extent as would give rise to a reasonable fear endangering oneself or others nearby

Breach of the peace

This common law concept applies across the UK and in RoI. A person may be arrested or removed to prevent a <u>breach of the peace</u> (p.543) (i.e. to prevent the violence or disorder). It is not an offence as such, but those arrested may be 'bound over' for a period, meaning that they must pay the court money that they lose if they later offend.

Scotland

There are only three public order offences in Scotland:

Mobbing and rioting, where a group convenes for an illegal purpose, or to carry out a legal purpose by illegal means (e.g. violence or intimidation);

Threatening or abusive behaviour[40] likely to cause a reasonable person to cause fear or alarm, intending or being reckless as to causing fear or alarm; and

Breach of the peace, which is also an ordinary offence in Scotland covering conduct that is 'genuinely alarming and disturbing' to any reasonable person.

Additional public order matters

- All jurisdictions have laws relating to public processions and meetings. These are particularly clearly defined in NI legislation. Most relate to the risk of stirring up hatred or arousing fear.
- Wilful obstruction of people or vehicles, especially those of emergency services, can be a public order offence.

39 In E&W S57 Crime and Courts Act 2013 removed the word *insulting* from the definition, in response to campaigns citing freedom of speech.
40 Contrary to s38 Criminal Justice and Licensing (Scotland) Act 2010.

Acquisitive offences

Acquisitive offences occur where offenders derive material gain from the crime, by obtaining something that is of direct benefit to them, or that can be used to obtain what they want (such as drugs).

In E&W, NI, and RoI these offences are almost entirely defined in statute, with the wording shown or summarised in Table 15.4. In Scotland, most offences exist only in common law (p.368) and do not have precise wording. The focus of psychiatric evidence is often the mental element (p.402) of the offence.

Table 15.4 Acquisitive offences

	E&W and NI	Scotland	RoI
Primary legislation	Theft Act 1968; Theft Act (NI) 1969 Fraud Act 2006	Common law; Civic Government (Scotland) Act 1982	Criminal Justice (Theft and Fraud Offences) Act 2001; Criminal Justice (Public Order) Act 1994
Theft	Dishonestly appropriating property belonging to another with the intention of permanently depriving the other of it	The taking and appropriating of property without the consent of its rightful owner or other lawful authority	Dishonestly appropriating property without the consent of its owner and with the intention of depriving the owner of it
Burglary (Theft by house breaking in Scotland)	Entering a building as a trespasser with intent to steal, or by stealing after entering a building as a trespasser No distinction in definition between burglary of dwellings or other premises but distinction in sentencing Other forms of burglary exist, e.g. with intent to commit criminal damage or GBH	Theft by housebreaking occurs whenever the security of a 'house' is overcome, and an article is abstracted or removed for the purpose of being carried off Housebreaking with Intent to Steal— person breaks into 'house' with the intention of stealing property	Entering a building or part of a building as a trespasser and with intent to commit an arrestable offence Or Having entered a building or part of a building as a trespasser, commits or attempts to commit any such offence therein
Robbery	When stealing, and immediately before or at the time of doing so, and in order to do so, using force on any person or putting or seeking to put any person in fear of being then and there subjected to force	The felonious appropriation of property by means of violence or threats of violence	When stealing, and immediately before or at the time of doing so, and in order to do so, using force on any person or putting or seeking to put any person in fear of being then and there subjected to force

Table 15.4 (Contd.)

	E&W and NI	Scotland	RoI
Blackmail/ Extortion	Blackmail—the making of an unwarranted demand, reinforced by menaces, with a view to making gain or inflicting loss	Extortion—obtaining money or any other advantage by threat	Blackmail—the making of an unwarranted demand, reinforced by menaces, with a view to making gain or inflicting loss
Handling stolen goods (including those obtained by fraud etc.)	Dishonestly receiving or arranging to receive stolen property, or undertaking, or assisting, or arranging to retain, remove, dispose of, or realise it, knowing or believing it to be stolen	With intent to deprive the owner, to receive and keep property knowing that it has been appropriated by theft, robbery, embezzlement, or fraud (known as 'reset' in Scottish law)	Dishonestly receiving or arranging to receive stolen property, or undertaking, assisting, or arranging to retain, remove, dispose of, or realise it, knowing or believing it to be stolen
Other related offences	Fraud by false representation; Fraud by failing to disclose information; Fraud by abuse of position; Obtaining services dishonestly; Making off without payment	Falsehood—false representations by words, writing or conduct; Fraud—intention to deceive or defraud; Wilful imposition—the cheat designed has been successful to extent of gaining benefit or advantage or of prejudicing or tending to prejudice the interests of another	Making gain or causing loss by deception; Obtaining services by deception; Making off without payment; Unlawful use of a computer; False accounting

Juvenile offences

Recorded rates of cautions or sentences for people aged ten to seventeen years have decreased by 83% in the last ten years in E&W (although sentences are longer). The common assertion that rates of offending are high amongst adolescents is complex. Ten years ago, this may have been backed by data, but now perpetrators of violence are most likely to be twenty-five to thirty-nine. Of first-time entrants to the youth justice system, 80% are male.

The proportion of Black children being cautioned or sentenced has increased over the last ten years. People from mixed ethnic backgrounds are also over-represented on a purely statistical proportionate basis of the population ignoring complex socioeconomic factors.

There are some differences in data reported from Scotland with estimates suggesting a higher proportion of crime committed by children than in E&W. This may be due to differences in data collection or how lower severity antisocial behaviour is handled. The variation in the <u>age of criminal responsibility</u> (p.406) also complicates comparisons in juvenile offending rates.

Type of offences

A distinction can be made between status offences and index (or notifiable) offences.

- **Status offences** refer to acts that would not usually be illegal if committed by an adult. They are relatively trivial (e.g. truancy, drinking alcohol, and driving a motor vehicle under legal age), and rarely result in conviction.
- **Index offences** refer to all other offences (e.g. murder, rape and sexual assault, burglary, arson, and robbery) where the age of the offender is irrelevant to determining the crime.

The number of status offences committed each year by juveniles greatly exceeds the number of index offences committed. In both cases, most offences are minor enough to be tried summarily (p.398). Possession of weapons is the only offence category clearly increasing in children.

Police decision-making in relation to young offenders is discretionary, and structured by the cautionary guidelines and local arrangements for dealing with young defendants. Decisions to charge must include detailed inquiry into the accused's circumstances, and there are crimes for which a person younger than eighteen years old would not be prosecuted whereas a person older than eighteen would be. For example, an adult may be charged with ABH following an assault on a peer whereas a ten year old would not.

Juvenile offences are usually managed in the <u>youth justice system</u> (p.352) and youth courts, except in very serious offences which may be tried in adult courts with modifications.

Terrorism and treason

Both are crimes with a political aim, using means that harm others. **Terrorism** is defined in the UK and RoI as[41] committing or threatening a seriously violent, dangerous, or disruptive act with the intention of influencing, destabilising, or destroying a government organisation, or intimidating the public, to advance a political, religious, racial, or ideological cause. Treason is more specific (see Box 15.4). It can be an offence to fail to give information to the police about acts of terrorism or treason.[42]

Because many terrorist acts are international, but States where they are committed may refuse or be unable to prosecute, the UK and RoI adopt extra-territorial jurisdiction, meaning their nationals can be convicted of terrorist offences committed entirely abroad, unlike other offences.

Governments often limit, suspend, or even break <u>human rights laws</u> (p.516) when combating terrorism and treason; the resulting measures such as indefinite detention without trial[43] can cause mental disorder.

Box 15.4 Treason in RoI and the UK

In RoI, under the Treason Act 1939 and article 39 of the Constitution:
- Levying war against the State, or conspiring, assisting, or inciting it
- Conspiring, inciting, or attempting to overthrow the government

In the UK, under the Treason Act 1351:
- Conspiring, inciting, or attempting[44] to kill the King, Queen, or heir
- Violating (sexually assaulting or raping) the Queen, the King's unmarried daughters, or the wife of the heir to the throne
- Levying war against the King, or adhering to, aiding, or comforting the King's enemies
- Killing the Lord Chancellor, Treasurer, or royally appointed judges

---

Categories of terrorist offences

The criminal law on terrorism has undergone a major shift since the 1980s, moving from broad but often temporary 'catch-all' offences focused on membership or support for certain terrorist organisations,[45] to large

---

41 Under the Terrorism Act 2000 and Criminal Justice (Terrorist Offences) Act 2005, respectively (see p.740). The RoI definition does not include the requirement for the advancement of a cause.

42 See p.400. Failing to report information on possible treason is known as 'misprision of treason'.

43 In the UK, for example, the Anti-Terrorism, Crime & Security Act 2001 allowed effective detention ('house arrest') without trial of suspected terrorists on the order of a government minister, until it was ruled <u>incompatible</u> (p.516) by the House of Lords in 2004, and earlier laws allowed detention without trial ('**internment**') of suspected IRA terrorists in NI during the 1970s.

44 The actual language of the Act is 'compassing or imagining'.

45 For example, the Prevention of Terrorism (Temporary Provisions) Acts 1974-89 criminalised belonging to proscribed organisations such as the Irish Republican Army and the Irish National Liberation Army, or financing or demonstrating in support of them, and created 'exclusion orders' prohibiting people entering Great Britain from Ireland (RoI or NI). The law gave the government discretion to decide what should be proscribed, with no appeal against exclusion orders (only judicial review of grounds for thinking the order 'expedient' and 'appropriate').

numbers of specific offences designed in response to shifting behaviour by terrorist groups, intended to bring this area of law into compliance with human rights law. This process is further advanced in the UK than in RoI.

The main categories of terrorist offences are as follows (those not in bold do not apply in RoI):

- '**Convention offences**'[46] including offences of using or attempting, inciting or conspiring to use explosives, biological weapons, chemical weapons or nuclear materials, or to take hostages or hijack aircraft or ships, or otherwise kill people, for terrorist purposes.
- Intentionally using, possessing, providing, receiving, or inviting the provision of 'terrorist property' (money or items likely to be used for terrorism, or the proceeds of terrorist acts), or in RoI, **financing terrorism**.
- Failing to disclose information to the police about terrorist property.
- **Possessing an article or information**, or collecting or accessing information, for a terrorist purpose.
- **Making, possessing, or using radioactive devices or materials** for terrorist purposes or making related threats.
- **Providing**, receiving, or inviting the receipt of **training** in the use of weapons, explosives, or radioactive material for a terrorist purpose.
- Providing or receiving training for terrorism more generally, or doing acts preparatory to terrorism.
- Entering or remaining in an area overseas designated as representing a risk of terrorism, unless for journalism or humanitarian or similar work.
- Inciting terrorism overseas or encouraging or inducing terrorism more generally or disseminating terrorist publications.
- **Directing** the activities of **a terrorist organisation**.
- **Belonging to a proscribed terrorist organisation** (with a right of appeal against proscription).
- **Inviting financial or other support** for a proscribed organisation.
- **Demonstrating** (e.g. by wearing uniform) for a proscribed organisation.
- Breaching an order restricting the freedom of a terrorist suspect.[47]

Relevance to forensic psychiatry

Forensic psychiatrists may become involved in assessing and treating alleged or convicted terrorists. They have also in the past been involved, along with psychologists, in cases claiming that indefinite detention, detention without trial, or repeated retrials (all of which have occurred in terrorist cases in the UK) are disproportionate under human rights law (p.516) in part because of their effect on the alleged terrorists' mental health. Lastly, forensic psychiatrists and psychologists may be asked to give expert opinion on whether the extreme beliefs (see p.42) of an alleged terrorist were related to mental disorder, or whether a particular individual was vulnerable to radicalisation (p.42) because of mental disorder or traits such as suggestibility or compliance (p.160).

46 Offences listed in the UN International Convention for the Suppression of the Financing of Terrorism 1999 and its annexes (related conventions on non-financial international offences).

47 A Terrorism Prevention and Investigation Measure (TPIM), an order for up to two to three years restricting where a suspect can reside or travel, what they can do or own or pay for, and whom they can contact; or a Temporary Exclusion Order, prohibiting a suspect from entering the UK.

Stalking and harassment

The essence of this group of offences is deliberately acting in a way that causes significant fear, alarm, or distress—for example through threats, abuse, multiple unwanted communications, or intrusive approaches (Table 15.5). Psychiatric evidence of psychological harm to the victim may be relevant.

Table 15.5 Stalking and harassment

	E&W and NI	Scotland	RoI
Primary legislation	Protection from Harassment Act/Order (NI) 1997; Serious Crime Act 2015; Criminal Justice and Courts Act 2015.	Protection from Harassment Act 1997; Domestic Abuse (Scotland) Act 2018; Abusive Behaviour and Sexual Harm Act 2016.	Non-Fatal Offences Against the Person Act 1997 S10; Domestic Violence Act 2018.
Harassment: offence	Pursuing a course of conduct which amounts to harassment of another, and which one knows or ought to know amounts to harassment of the other. Up to six months' imprisonment.	No specific offence, but civil court may grant damages for harm (including anxiety) experienced as a result of the harassment.	Harassing another by persistently watching, following, pestering, besetting, or communicating with the person without lawful authority or reasonable excuse. Up to seven years' imprisonment.
Harassment: civil[48] or criminal injunction	To prevent repeated or anticipated harassment. Both civil and criminal available. Criminal court may issue injunction even if it has *acquitted* the defendant. Up to five years' imprisonment for breach.	To prevent anticipated harassment. Civil available, plus criminal on conviction of an offence causing alarm or distress, (e.g. assault, threats, and abuse). Up to five years' imprisonment for breach.	Not to communicate or approach the person or their place of residence or employment. Criminal only, on conviction *or acquittal*. Up to seven years' imprisonment for breach.

48 Civil injunctions against harassment, and those issued on acquittal, raise the same issues of civil liberty as do ASBOs (p.458) and other noncriminal injunctions regulating behaviour that can result in imprisonment on the basis of an order made on the lower civil standard of proof.

Table 15.5 (Contd.)

	E&W and NI	Scotland	RoI
Stalking[49]	The harassment involves following, contacting, monitoring, loitering for, watching or spying on a person, or publishing material about (or appearing to be by) them, or interfering with their property. (E&W only) Up to ten years' imprisonment if put in fear of violence or caused serious alarm or distress.	The harassment involves following, contacting, monitoring, loitering for, watching or spying on a person, or publishing material about (or appearing to be by) them, or interfering with their property. Up to five years' imprisonment.	No separate offence, but harassment offence provides penalties of equivalent severity.
Putting in fear of violence	The harassment causes the victim to fear, at least twice, that violence will be used on them. Up to ten years' imprisonment (seven years in NI).	No equivalent offence.	No equivalent offence.
Domestic abuse (coercive control)	Repeatedly or continuously engaging in behaviour to a someone personally connected (in an intimate relationship, family, or living together) that causes serious alarm or distress or fear of violence (E&W only).	A course of behaviour which is abusive[50] of a partner or ex-partner, intended to cause (or reckless as to causing) physical or psychological harm.	Knowingly and persistently engaging in behaviour that is controlling or coercive and causes serious alarm or distress or fear of violence.

(Continued)

---

49 In addition, in E&W reasonable grounds for believing stalking is taking place allows courts to grant police additional powers to enter and search the alleged stalker's property.

50 Violent, threatening, or intimidating; or intended or likely to cause dependence, isolation, control, monitoring, regulation, loss of freedom, fear, humiliation or degradation, or punishment.

Table 15.5 (Contd.)

	E&W and NI	Scotland	RoI
Malicious communications	Sending a letter, electronic communication or anything else conveying a threat, false information, or grossly indecent or offensive message, to cause distress or anxiety.	No equivalent offence, though such conduct, if repeated, could be covered by the stalking offence above.	No equivalent offence.[51]
Revenge porn	Disclosing a private sexual photograph or film without consent, to cause distress.	Disclosing an intimate photograph or film without consent, to cause distress.	No equivalent offence.
Upskirting	Photographing beneath the clothing without consent, with the intention of observing underwear, genitals, or buttocks for sexual gratification, alarm, humiliation, or distress.	Observing, recording, or photographing a private act for sexual gratification, alarm, humiliation, or distress.	No equivalent offence.

In general, these offences do not require the defendant to recognise the likely impact on the victim: the fault or <u>mental element</u> (p.402) is simply negligence (i.e. that the defendant ought to have known the likely impact).

Mental disorder is common in people charged with these offences (see p.62); they should routinely be considered for psychiatric assessment.

51 The RoI government introduced the Harmful and Malicious Communications Bill in 2015 that would have introduced such an offence, but it was not passed by the Dáil.

Other offences relevant to psychiatry

Offences involving the care of children

Where there are concerns about the care of children, the social services authority will bring care proceedings against a parent or carer, and the police will bring criminal charges (e.g. neglect or cruelty to a child, or child sexual exploitation). Psychiatrists who are asked to give expert opinion need to be clear about what proceedings they are being asked to provide testimony for, and aware that a report in one context may be used in the another.[52] Ordinary <u>psychiatric defences</u> (p.412) may be raised to criminal charges of violence against a child.

Offences involving the care of psychiatric patients

It is an offence for care staff to assault, or to have sexual contact with, a detained patient. Conviction can result in imprisonment, as well as professional sanctions such as being struck off the professional register.

Slavery

Historically, slavery—being able to acquire other persons as property—and forced labour were overt and in many jurisdictions lawful; after being internationally banned,[53] they have continued as secretive practices, albeit on a smaller scale. Many people are trafficked from poor countries to work in rich ones, some forced to work indefinitely (e.g. in prostitution) for the benefit of their masters in conditions that amount to slavery, others in lawful employment but forced to pay back a very large debt to the criminals who trafficked them before they earn their freedom. It is an offence to enslave, traffic, or exploit another person. People with mental disorders are often particularly vulnerable to being trafficked and enslaved. The Modern Slavery Act has been used to prosecute adults in the exploitation of children by 'county lines' drug supply gangs.

False imprisonment

This is the restraint of a person in a bounded area without justification or consent. A person convicted criminally of false imprisonment can be punished by probation, heavy fines, or imprisonment. Civilly, they can be liable for punitive damages related to pain and suffering.

Making threats to kill

Making a threat to kill is an offence, if the defendant intends the victim to fear that it will be carried out. It does not matter whether it is premeditated or said in anger. Although the normal maximum sentence is ten years in E&W and NI, offenders thought to present a 'significant risk' of 'serious harm' to the public can receive a <u>life sentence</u> (p.448). The offence in RoI includes threats to cause serious harm. Making threats to kill is notoriously

---

52 For example a diagnosis of personality disorder made in a psychiatric report for criminal sentencing purposes might be used by a social services authority in family proceedings as evidence that parent poses a continuing risk of harm to the child.

53 The first comprehensive ban was the 1926 International Convention to Suppress the Slave Trade and Slavery, but large-scale overt slavery had been greatly diminished by bans in the British Empire and elsewhere during the nineteenth century.

difficult to prove, as there is rarely clear evidence that the defendant intended the victim to believe the threat would be carried out.

Poisoning

Criminal poisoning occurs when an individual or group deliberately attempts to harm someone using a toxin. Historically, poisoning cases have proved difficult to assess, investigate, and prosecute, even if death results (in which case the more common charge is murder). The methods of delivery may be highly sophisticated and subtle. Poisoners are often hard to detect.[54]

Cybercrime

This term refers to a group of offences of 'hacking' (gaining unauthorised access to) computer systems, or using computer systems to commit other crimes, such as fraud, deception, or harassment ('cyber bullying'). People with autistic spectrum disorders, particularly Asperger syndrome (p.104), are over-represented amongst such hackers, and victims of cyber bullying are more vulnerable to anxiety and depression.[55]

Contempt of court

This occurs when an individual disobeys a court order or is disrespectful of the court's authority, such as by showing disrespect for the judge, by disrupting the proceedings through poor behaviour, or by publication of material deemed likely to jeopardise a fair trial. This may result in a fine or imprisonment. Mental disorder is a possible cause of such behaviour.

54 An example of a high-profile case is that of the serial killer Dr Harold Shipman, a GP in Hyde near Manchester, who killed over 200 of his patients in the 1980s and 1990s through poisoning them with overdoses of morphine and other drugs before he was caught.

55 Extradition requests (p.559) for cybercrime offences, for example, hacking, are not uncommon, and may involve psychiatric assessment in regard to whether the defendant is fit for extradition (p.648).

Crimes under international law

Criminal law is country-specific, albeit with much similarity between countries with similar cultures. Since the beginning of the 20th century a body of international jurisprudence has arisen[56] which criminalises certain very serious behaviours.

Prosecutions under international law are rare. However, psychiatrists may be called upon to examine defendants and give evidence in such cases, which may be brought at the International Criminal Court in the Hague, specifically convened tribunals or in national courts of countries such as the UK that recognise 'universal jurisdiction' for such crimes.

Genocide

Defined by a series of acts which violate the right to life or physical or mental safety of a group 'with intent to destroy, in whole or in part, a national, ethical, racial or religious group'. Conspiracy, incitement, complicity, and attempted genocide are all crimes.

Crimes against humanity

These crimes are committed when an individual, as part of a 'widespread or systematic attack directed against any civilian population, with knowledge of the attack', commits any of the following, amongst others:

- murder,
- extermination (mass killing, directly or through, say, starvation),
- enslavement,
- deportation, or forcible transfer of population,
- illegal imprisonment or 'disappearance' (secret abduction),
- torture, and
- rape, sexual slavery, enforced prostitution, and related offences.

War crimes

War crimes are crimes committed by agents of an aggressor state against individuals, including that state's own citizens, and include using unlawful weapons, such as poison gas; mistreating civilians, the sick and wounded, and prisoners of war; and causing destruction not warranted by military or civilian necessity.

Crimes of aggression

Crimes of aggression, the most recently enacted crimes in international law, have been ratified by the fewest states; they allow the prosecution of leaders responsible for waging illegal wars.

---

56 The Hague Conventions of 1899 and 1907 (after the Boer War) and the Geneva Conventions (which were revised and expanded after the First and then the Second World War), all setting out war crimes, and the Charters setting up the Nuremburg Tribunal 1945; tribunals in Tokyo 1945, Yugoslavia 1993, and Rwanda 1994; and that of the International Criminal Court 2002 (The Rome Statute), which developed international human rights law.

Cautions and warnings

For minor offences where there is evidence of guilt and the offender admits it, a senior police officer and/or the prosecutor may give a **caution** (or 'recorded police warning'[57] in Scotland), instead of charging them. In RoI the adult caution scheme is only available for certain specified minor offences.[58] This speeds the administration of justice, can reduce a backlog of trials, and avoids the expense and distress of a trial when the likely sentence would be minor (e.g. a conditional discharge, p.456).

Requirements for a caution or warning

- The offender is aged older than eighteen years (older than sixteen in Scotland)
- Sufficient evidence of guilt, such as a reasonable suspicion of guilt, coupled with reasonable grounds to believe that further investigation will reveal enough evidence for a reasonable prospect of conviction
- An offence and consequences that are sufficiently minor[59]
- A clear and reliable admission of guilt by the suspect
- No overriding public interest in prosecution
- Belief that the caution will be effective: for example, it will usually be inappropriate to issue repeat cautions
- The offender's consent to the caution (which may include signing a formal admission and record of the caution and any conditions)

Effects of a caution

Cautions are not convictions, and therefore appear separately (or not at all) on criminal records. However, the admission of guilt may be taken into account in sentencing for any future offences, as evidence of 'bad character', and some jobs involving work with vulnerable individuals may require applicants' cautions to be disclosed. A caution accepted by a doctor, for example, must be reported by them to the General Medical Council and could lay the foundation for a finding of professional misconduct.

Cautions are recorded as a successful detection of an offence for the purposes of police statistics, giving police and prosecutors an incentive to use cautions where possible.

Youth cautions

In E&W, Scotland, and RoI, young offenders are eligible for youth cautions instead of ordinary cautions or police warnings; in NI, the equivalent is an 'informed police warning' (or in more serious cases a 'restorative caution', which involves meeting victims with their parents to apologise). In RoI a caution can only be administered to a young person at the discretion

---

57 *Caution* in Scotland refers to a financial bond that insures an incapable adult's estate against mismanagement by a guardian.

58 For example, being drunk and disorderly, theft of less than €1,000, minor assault, or minor criminal damage.

59 For example, in E&W a caution is not permitted for indictable-only offences (p.398); in Scotland a recorded police warning cannot be given to someone on a compulsory supervision order (p.454), meaning that they are in the care of the local authority.

of the National Juvenile Office. The requirements are the same as for a caution, except that an appropriate adult or other suitable person must be present—and in the UK, controversially, that young offenders or their parent/guardian do not need to consent to the youth caution or informed warning.[60] See Table 15.6 for approximate frequencies.

Unlike a caution, a youth caution or informed warning usually involves referral to the Youth Offending Team (YOT, p.585) or in RoI, Juvenile Diversion Programme. If young offenders fail to co-operate with the YOT/JDP there are no immediate consequences, but their noncooperation may be taken into account in any subsequent prosecution.

Table 15.6 Approximate frequencies of cautions and youth cautions, E&W 2018[61]

Age group, years	
Children 10–17	32%
Young adults 18–20	13%
Adults older than 21	5%

Fixed penalties and other direct measures

For certain specific offences, police officers and others such as traffic wardens in E&W and the Procurator Fiscal in Scotland have discretion to give a fixed penalty notice to an offender as an alternative to prosecution. Relevant offences vary from one jurisdiction to another, but include road traffic and cycling offences, public disorder, theft, antisocial behaviour, and minor environmental offences such as littering. In Scotland the Procurator Fiscal's discretion to use such 'direct measures' applies to a much wider range of offences, and includes power to agree compensation offers, 'fiscal' unpaid work offers, warnings similar to police recorded warnings, and counselling or psychiatric treatment.

Conditional cautions

In E&W and Scotland (and possibly in the future in NI[62]), the prosecutor has discretion to give adult and child offenders a caution or youth caution with conditions that, if breached, result in the original prosecution resuming. The conditions may include paying a financial penalty, attending particular places, or conditions aimed at rehabilitation or reparation. The offender (including young offenders) must consent to the conditional caution or youth conditional caution.

---

60 This appears to be a breach of the ECHR (p.518), and might be ruled incompatible (p.516) by the Supreme Court (p.384) in future.

61 These rates and the averages presented in the table on p.446 are not comparable because the latter includes within 'cautions etc.' other out-of-court disposals such as fixed penalty notices, and because they break down age groups differently.

62 Conditional cautions were legislated for by the NI Assembly in the Justice Act (Northern Ireland) 2011, but the relevant sections of the Act have never been brought into effect.

Principles of sentencing

Sentences are passed by courts after conviction—that is, after the individual's criminal responsibility has been established.

Purposes of sentencing

Sentences may attempt to serve a number of incompatible purposes[63]:

- punishing them (giving them their 'just deserts', p.355);
- deterring them and others from future offending;
- reforming them (e.g. through changing their attitudes and moral views);
- rehabilitating them (e.g. by teaching new skills);
- incapacitating the offender (protecting the public from them);
- making reparation to the victim and/or society (e.g. through compensation or community service: the 'restorative justice' approach);
- treating them (e.g. for drug misuse) to improve their welfare (p.355); and
- obtaining retribution on behalf of the victim and/or society at large.

Sentences in the UK and RoI focus on different purposes depending on the legislature's view of the nature of the offence. For example, sentences of imprisonment (p.448) focus on incapacitation, retribution, punishment, and deterrence[64]; fines (p.456) focus on retribution and reparation; community orders with a drug testing requirement (p.454) focus on reform; and hospital orders (p.500) focus on treatment.

Process of sentencing

In deciding the appropriate sentence, judges take the following steps[65]:

- applying statutory mandatory or automatic[66] sentences (e.g. the mandatory life sentence (p.448) for murder) if they apply; and otherwise—
- determining the seriousness of the offence (the harm caused, and the offender's degree of responsibility for that harm);
- considering aggravating factors (p.638) such as committing the offence whilst on bail, being motivated by racial or religious hatred or hatred of a sexual orientation or disability, or certain past convictions;
- considering mitigating factors (p.638) such as having been provoked, offending because of a genuine misunderstanding, having mental disorder, showing remorse after committing the offence, admitting the offence to police, or making an early guilty plea (p.398);

---

63 In E&W, courts are required to have regard to the first six purposes in the list, except when considering a psychiatric disposal or mandatory or automatic sentence.

64 Many prisons (e.g. 'training' prisons in the UK) also have facilities that attempt to rehabilitate and reform the offender.

65 These steps are taken from the Sentencing Council guidelines in E&W, and draft guidance from the Scottish Sentencing Council. There are no equivalents (other than certain decisions of higher courts) for NI or RoI, but judges may informally follow a similar process.

66 The distinction is that there are no exceptions to mandatory sentences, but automatic sentences (e.g. imprisonment for a third domestic burglary) can be overridden in exceptional circumstances.

- if relevant to the sentence, considering whether it should be extended because of the <u>dangerousness</u> (p.672) of the offender, or reduced because of time already spent in custody <u>on remand</u> (p.398);
- considering orders <u>ancillary</u> to the sentence (p.457), such as a compensation order or binding over to keep the peace; and
- reviewing the 'totality' of the sentence that results from this process to ensure it is just and proportionate.

Pre-sentence reports

Judges frequently request reports from probation officers before making a decision on sentence and may[67] also request them from others including psychiatrists, psychologists, schools, and social work departments where relevant. Psychiatric <u>reports on disposal</u> (p.456) usually address whether a mental health disposal is recommended (e.g. admission to hospital, or compulsory outpatient treatment), but may also be used in <u>mitigation</u> (p.638); a psychiatric <u>risk assessment</u> (p.163) may also be taken by a court as evidence of <u>dangerousness</u> (p.672) giving grounds for an increased or <u>indeterminate</u> (p.448) sentence, which can pose <u>ethical problems</u> (p.318) for the assessing psychiatrist.

Sentencing guidelines

In **E&W**, criminal courts are required to consider prescriptive guidelines issued by the Sentencing Council,[68] as well as directions issued by the <u>Court of Appeal</u> (p.384) and the <u>Lord Chief Justice</u> (p.376). Offences are mostly defined by statute, with maximum sentences and some rules on the purposes of sentencing.

The same general process is followed when sentencing mentally disordered offenders as others, although the fact of the mental disorder may make treatment the primary purpose of the sentence p.670. Recent guidance requires the judge to 'state clearly their assessment of whether the offender's culpability was reduced (by impairment or disorder) and, if it was, the reasons for, and extent of, that reduction'. This runs the risk of experts being asked to address culpability directly; rather than restricting their evidence to the causal contribution of their disorder to commission of the offence.

---

67 In some cases, the law requires them to do so (e.g. in E&W, after conviction for <u>arson</u>, p.422).
68 Such as on corporate manslaughter, sexual offences, and health & safety offences.

In **RoI** and **NI**, the superior courts have produced a substantial body of case law that establishes general principles of sentencing, the most notable in RoI being that the sentence must be proportionate to the gravity of the offence and the circumstances of the offender. Offences are mostly defined by statute, with maximum sentences, and in NI, some rules on the purposes of sentencing. Guidelines issued by the E&W Sentencing Council are sometimes of persuasive authority in the NI courts.

In **Scotland** the judge's sentencing discretion is almost entirely unfettered. Offences are mostly defined only in case law, with few or no maximum sentences. The High Court has made only a few decisions on sentencing principles, and there are very few statutory sentences except for a mandatory life sentence for murder. A Scottish Sentencing Council was established in 2010 but has been very slow to create sentencing guidelines, with no case-specific guidelines yet having moved beyond the draft stage.

Sentencing children and young people

The sentences applicable to convicted children, and in some cases also young adults (aged eighteen to twenty-one), differ from those for adults (Table 15.7). For example, they cannot be sentenced to <u>life imprisonment</u> (p.448), but receive an alternative form of indeterminate sentence; instead of imprisonment, they are subject to <u>detention</u> (p.449) with a substantial educational or training element, usually in a special institution[69] instead of a prison; and their <u>community sentences</u> (p.454) are usually more focused on rehabilitation than on other <u>aims of sentencing</u> (p.442), such as punishment.

Principles of sentencing young people

Whereas society is usually content to see adults as capable of choosing whether to offend, it regards children as less able to do so. The first purpose of sentencing children is, in general, not to punish but to prevent offending; in E&W, this 'principal aim' is enshrined in law,[70] and the Youth Justice Board operates the principle 'child first, offender second'.

In E&W, NI, and RoI, if it appears to the court that a first- or second-time young person charged with a minor offence can be better dealt with informally rather than by sentencing them, it may offer them a <u>referral order</u> (E&W) or <u>diversionary youth conference</u> (p.458). The law in E&W[71] requires judges in the Youth Court to give all children there for the first time a referral order if they plead guilty (the only exception is if the charge is very serious, and the Youth Court commits the defendant for trial in the Crown Court as an adult).

The system in Scotland goes considerably further, and its de facto principal aim is to rehabilitate and reform children in the interests of their welfare. This is done most notably by diverting the vast majority of children out of the criminal justice system and into the <u>Children's Hearings</u> system (p.386), but even within the Scottish youth justice system the culture opposes punitive sentences for children.

Table 15.7 Differences in sentencing between all ages and children and young people

Sentence type	All ages, 2019		Children & YP, 2018	
Total	1,406,827	100%	39,215	100%
Cautions etc.	215,045	15%	11,282	29%
First-tier sentences*	983,167	70%	19,134	49%
Community sentences	91,948	7%	6,794	17%
Custodial sentences	116,667	8%	2,005	5%

* Conditional and absolute discharges, fines, bind-overs and other orders (including mental health disposals), plus for children, referral orders.

69 Such as a secure children's home, secure training centre, or <u>Young Offender Institution</u> (p.580).

70 In s37 of the Crime and Disorder Act 1998; s142A of the Criminal Justice Act 2003 adds that the second consideration is children's welfare, followed by punishment, reform & rehabilitation, protecting the public, and making reparations.

71 LASPO 2012 (p.737), which also increased the use of precourt options like cautions.

The use of custody

There is a presumption against the custody for children, on remand or conviction, and detention is used less frequently than for adults. The table above shows this for E&W, where custody for children has been declining steadily.

Life and indeterminate sentences

Sentences of imprisonment can be <u>determinate</u> sentences (p.452), of a fixed maximum length; or indeterminate sentences such as 'life' sentences, which end only after the offender has served a defined 'tariff' and can show they are fit for safe release. Indeterminate sentences form a small proportion of prison sentences (Table 15.8).

Table 15.8 Numbers of people sentenced to immediate custody* in E&W in 2018/19

Total prison sentences	76,776	100%
Determinate sentences	76,331	98.60%
Life sentence	445	0.40%

* i.e. excluding suspended sentences of imprisonment

Life sentences

In the UK and RoI, there are three types of life sentence for adults:
- The **mandatory** life sentence applies only to <u>murder</u> (p.414), and in RoI, to treason; the judge has no discretion to pass any alternative sentence.
- **Automatic** life sentences in E&W apply to adults' convictions for a second specified serious or violent offence unless the judge decides there are particular circumstances that would make this unjust.
- **Discretionary** life sentences are available for serious offences ranging from <u>manslaughter</u> (p.414) to aggravated <u>burglary</u>. (p.IV.72)

Minimum terms (tariffs)

Before being considered for release, life sentence prisoners must serve a minimum term, known as a 'tariff' in NI, and as the 'punishment part' of the sentence in Scotland. The minimum term is set by the trial judge[72] but can be increased or reduced on appeal. In the most serious cases, the minimum term can be the whole of the offender's life. In RoI, the Parole Act sets a default minimum term of twelve years.

Release on licence

After serving the minimum term, offenders can apply to the <u>Parole Board</u> (p.582) to be released from prison. If their application is granted,[73] they remain liable to recall to prison to serve the rest of their sentence, if they breach the conditions of their licence or reoffend. Like other offenders on licence, they must report regularly to their <u>probation officer</u> (p.584).

---

72 The Home Secretary (in RoI, Minister for Justice) used to set the tariff, often based on political considerations in high-profile cases, until in 2002 this was held to breach the <u>ECHR</u> (p.518).

73 In RoI, a decision of the Parole Board to release a prisoner must be approved by the relevant Minister.

Indeterminate sentences

Whereas offenders sentenced to life remain in prison or on licence until their death, other indeterminate sentences can in principle end. Indeterminate Custodial Sentences (ICS) in NI,[74] and Orders for Lifelong Restriction (OLR) in Scotland apply to convictions for serious sexual and violent offences where the maximum sentence is over ten years, and the court deems the offender <u>dangerous</u> (p.672), in Scotland under a <u>risk assessment order</u> (p.504).

ICSs and OLRs comprise a minimum term of imprisonment and a period of licence (of at least ten years for ICSs; lifelong for OLRs). Offenders under ICSs can apply to the Parole Board for their licence to be revoked once per year after the first ten years.

Corresponding sentences for children and young adults

The life and indeterminate sentences described above cannot be imposed on children (and, in some cases, young adults). Instead, there are a variety of specific alternatives, as shown in Table 15.9. Only small numbers of children receive such sentences, even in E&W: fewer than twenty-five people younger than twenty-one years old each year are detained at Her Majesty's Pleasure or sentenced to custody for life.

Table 15.9 Indeterminate sentences for under twenty-one year olds

Age (years) & sentence	E&W	Scotland	NI	RoI
Under 18 Life	Detention during Her Majesty's Pleasure	Detention without limit of time	Detention during the Secretary of State's pleasure	None unless tried as adult[75]
18–20 Life	Custody for life[76]	Detention for life	Life imprisonment as for adults over 21	Life imprisonment as for adults over 21
Under 18 OLR	N/A	Order for Lifelong Restriction	N/A	N/A
18–20 ICS/OLR	N/A	Order for Lifelong Restriction	ICSs as for adults over 21	N/A

74 ICSs (known there as IPPs) were also available in E&W between 2003 and 2013, when they were replaced with automatic life sentences (which had been abolished when IPPs were introduced).

75 In RoI, children as young as ten (i.e. below the usual age of criminal responsibility) can be tried in adult court for very serious offences such as murder and rape, and receive adult sentences.

76 Custody for life was abolished and replaced with life imprisonment as for adults by the Criminal Justice and Court Services Act 2000, but this provision has never been brought into effect.

Death

Although abolished in the UK and RoI, the death penalty is available in several Commonwealth and related jurisdictions that use the Judicial Committee of the Privy Council (p.391) as their court of final appeal; determining that not only forensic psychiatrists from those jurisdictions but also UK forensic psychiatrists can be involved in giving expert evidence within appeals.

Within countries that use the Privy Council, the established sentencing criteria for imposition of the death penalty (where it is discretionary rather than mandatory) are that it should be applied only to cases that are 'the rarest of the rare'/'worst of the worst', and then only if the defendant is deemed to be 'beyond reformation' *Trimmingham v The State* (St Vincent & The Grenadines) [2009] UKPC 25. The defendant must also not suffer from mental retardation or not have the mental capacity to understand the punishment given. All of these tests are clearly susceptible to expert psychiatric or psychological evidence, including about the treatability of any condition, and whether any mental disorder may have influenced the severity of the offence, making it 'the worst of the worst' when otherwise it might not have been.

Fitness for execution

Once an offender has been sentenced to death, the sentence can only be carried out if they are 'fit' for execution. The test of fitness for execution in common law jurisdictions relies upon the USA case of *Ford v. Wainwright* 477 U.S. 399 (1986).

The test is based upon the notion that execution should only be applied to individuals who are aware of the nature of the punishment and why they have been sentenced to it, including having moral comprehension of 'culpability' and 'retribution'. And if, for example, the perpetrator is not able to make a moral connection between the crime and the punishment, then such punishment is considered necessarily to fail in its retributive function.

A mental health expert may be asked to comment upon a person's capacity to comprehend the nature of the death penalty and why it has been imposed upon them as well as upon the significance of any mental disorder for such ability.

The American Bar Association test might assist in understanding the possible purpose, and focus, of mental health evidence: A convict is incompetent to be executed if, as a result of mental illness or mental retardation, the convict cannot understand the nature of the pending proceedings, what he or she was tried for, the reasons for the punishment or the nature of the punishment. A convict is also incompetent if, as a result of mental illness or mental retardation, the convict lacks sufficient capacity to recognise or understand any fact which might exist which would make the punishment unjust or unlawful, or lacks the ability to convey such information to the court.

The clinical interview should consider, therefore, all these different facets in relation to any diagnosed medical or psychiatric condition, and specifically the convict's:

- understanding of the reasons for punishment;
- understanding of the nature of the punishment itself, including its finality;
- ability to reason and weigh up matters relevant to their current legal situation; and
- ability to provide instructions to legal representatives.

Determinate prison sentences

'Determinate' prison sentences run for a fixed maximum period, unlike <u>life sentences</u> (p.448). Numbers and proportions are shown in Table 15.10.

Table 15.10 Numbers of people sentenced to immediate custody in E&W in 2018-19

Total prison sentences	76,776	100%
Up to 3 months	27,645	36%
3 months to 1 year	20,690	27%
1 to 5 years	23,462	31%
Over 5 years	4,534	6%
Life sentences	445	0.40%

Ordinary determinate sentences

The length of an ordinary determinate sentence is intended to be proportionate to the seriousness of the offence, and to reflect the culpability of the offender in terms of the current offence and any past offending.

Short sentences, particularly those of three months or less, provide little or no opportunity for training, rehabilitation or reform, whilst still interfering with offenders' employment and family responsibilities, and are discouraged by law in Scotland and in sentencing guidelines in E&W.

Parole and release on licence

Prisoners can often apply for release before the end of their sentence or may be released automatically. The rules vary between jurisdictions, and the details have changed repeatedly over time. In general, those in E&W and NI, and those in RoI on sentences of up to eight years, are released automatically on licence at the PED, whereas those on longer sentences in RoI may apply to the <u>Parole Board</u> (p.582) for release from their PED, and if unsuccessful are released automatically on their NPD. See Table 15.11.

In Scotland, the trial judge sets a 'custody part' of half to three-quarters of the sentence, after which the prisoner is automatically released.

Table 15.11 Acronyms related to parole

PED	Parole Eligibility Date (halfway through sentence*)
EDR	Expected Date of Release (varies depending on parole decisions)
NPD	Non-Parole release Date (two-thirds point; automatic release**)
SED	Sentence Expiry Date (latest point of release from prison)
LED	Licence Expiry Date (same as SED except for extended sentences)

* Or after seven years in RoI if the sentence exceeds fourteen years. In E&W, the Minister can release well-behaved prisoners sentenced to four years or less on curfew up to 135 days before the PED.

** Automatic release is subject to good behaviour in prison. The NPD is at the three-quarter point in RoI, though prisoners may apply to the Minister for discretionary nonparole release ('enhanced remission') from the two-thirds point.

Extended sentences

In E&W, Scotland, and NI, those convicted of serious sexual, terrorist, or violent offences who are regarded as <u>dangerous</u> (p.672) by the court may receive an extended licence period of up to five years (eight for serious sexual or terrorist offences; ten years in both cases in Scotland), provided this does not exceed the maximum sentence for the offence.

In Scotland, ministers can prevent prisoners' release after the custody part of their sentence, if they deem them likely to cause serious harm to the public; unless they appeal successfully to the Parole Board, they will not be released until their SED.

Determinate sentences for children and young adults

The corresponding sentences shown in Table 15.12.

Table 15.12 Determinate sentences for under twenty-one year olds

Age (years) & sentence	E&W	Scotland	NI	RoI
Under 21 Ordinary	Detention and training order (DTO)[77]	Detention in YOI	Juvenile Justice Centre Order	Children detention order[78]
Under 21 Extended	Extended DTO[79]	Extended detention in YOI	N/A	N/A

Other forms of imprisonment

Several variations are found in some or all of the jurisdictions:
- Ordinary determinate sentences (e.g. sentences of twelve months or less in E&W) can be **suspended**, meaning that the offender does not have to serve the sentence unless they reoffend within a specified period or breach any conditions of the suspension.
- In **intermittent custody**, previously piloted in E&W but not continued, the offender spends for example the weekend in prison but can continue their employment on licence during the week.
- **Custody plus** combines prison and a <u>community sentence</u> (p.454); it was part of the law in E&W in 2003–2012 but never brought into effect.
- Eligible prisoners may be released up to 135 days early on **home detention curfew** in E&W and NI, during which period they are tagged and monitored by the probation service.

---

77 DTOs last up to two years; however, children convicted of certain very serious offences with maximum adult sentences of fourteen years or more may be sentenced to detention up to the adult maximum. These are known as 'section 91 PCCSA' sentences.

78 Children Detention Orders last for up to three years; however, children convicted of very serious offences may be sentenced as adults.

79 The extension periods are the same as for adults: up to five years, or eight for serious sexual or terrorist offences.

Community sentences

Community sentences impose a variety of requirements on offenders rather than, like imprisonment, depriving them of their liberty.

The details of community sentences vary between jurisdictions, and between the adult and youth justice systems, and some orders and requirements are available in some jurisdictions but not in others.

- In **E&W**, there is a single order for adults, the Community Order, and one for children and young people, the Youth Rehabilitation Order.[80] Unless the relevant law specifically provides for an adult Community Order, one can only be made if the offence carries a potential sentence of imprisonment. At least one requirement must be for the purpose of punishment. See Box 15.5 for examples.
- **Scotland** has individual probation, community service, community reparation, and restriction of liberty orders applicable to both adults and children that together allow for most of the requirements in the box. In addition, children dealt with through the Children's Hearing system rather than prosecuted in adult courts can also be made subject to more welfare-focused orders such as the compulsory supervision order.
- In **NI**, there is a similar range of orders covering similar requirements (reparation, community responsibility, community service, probation, drug treatment and testing, combination, youth conference, attendance centre, and juvenile justice orders).
- There is more reliance on short custodial sentences in **RoI**, and fewer community sentences. Probation and community service orders are available for adults (the latter for those older than sixteen years who would otherwise have received a prison sentence of a year or less), and in addition for children there are youth conferences, mentoring, day centre, and restriction orders. There are also restriction on movement orders that are similar to curfew and exclusion requirements in E&W and NI.

---

80 The Criminal Justice and Immigration Act 2008 also introduced the 'Youth Default Order', allowing for unpaid work, attendance centre, or curfew requirements instead of detention or other penalties for young people who default on fines, but it has never been brought into effect.

Box 15.5 Examples of Community Order requirements
- unpaid work
- activity (e.g. helping at an old persons' home)
- programme (e.g. probation-run offending behaviour group)
- prohibited activity (e.g. not carrying an otherwise legal firearm, or not associating with a particular person)
- curfew
- exclusion (e.g. not to enter certain streets or areas)
- fine
- residence
- mental health treatment
- drug rehabilitation (including drug testing)
- alcohol treatment
- supervision (e.g. attending appointments with probation officer)
- attendance centre (e.g. attending the centre during football matches)
- reparation (e.g. having to meet, talk to and apologise to the victim)
- education
- electronic monitoring (e.g. with a 'tag')
- intensive supervision and surveillance (ISSP)
- fostering

Fines and other sentences

See Table 15.13.

Fines

A fine is a payment to the court intended as punishment. Failure to pay can result in bailiffs seizing the offender's property, or imprisonment for <u>contempt of court</u> (p.437). Parents are responsible to pay fines if their children do not.

Conditional discharge and binding over

A **conditional discharge** imposes no immediate punishment, but if the person reoffends during the specified period, they will be sentenced for the original offence as well as the new one. Conditional discharges can last from six months to three years.

Binding over is available where the court believes offenders may be violent in future.[81] It requires them to refrain from acts specified in the order (e.g. visiting the home of their victim) for a certain period, and to make a recognisance (i.e. pay a sum of money) which they lose if they breach the order. The parents or guardians of child offenders may also be bound over.

Absolute discharge and admonition

An order for **absolute discharge** means that the offender receives no punishment, although the conviction will remain on their criminal record.

In Scotland, the offender may also be dismissed with an **admonition**, a reprimand from the judge.

Mental health disposals

Convicted offenders suffering from a mental disorder may be:
- sent to hospital (e.g. for treatment under a <u>hospital order</u>, p.500);
- required to accept outpatient treatment (e.g. under a <u>compulsion order</u>, p.500, or a <u>Community Order with a mental health treatment requirement</u>, p.454); or
- given an order combining hospital treatment and possible imprisonment (e.g. a <u>hybrid order</u>, p.504).

Table 15.13 Offenders sentenced in 2018-19 in E&W

Total	1,406,827	100%
Fines	914,113	65%
Conditional or absolute discharge	43,870	3%
Mental health & other	16,404	1%
Cautions etc.	215,045	15%
Community sentences	91,948	7%
Suspended sentence	39,890	3%
Imprisonment	76,776	5%

81 That is, they may 'breach the [Queen's] Peace', in the original <u>common law</u> (p.368) terminology.

Ancillary orders

On passing sentence, courts may make additional orders, often intended to fulfil different sentencing purposes (p.442). These ancillary orders are listed below; some are unavailable in some jurisdictions.
- **Compensation order**—this requires the offender to pay the victim to make up for the loss the offender has caused (e.g. to pay for the replacement of damaged property).
- **Drinking banning orders** and **football banning orders** prevent relevant offenders visiting specified premises where alcohol is served, or attending specified football matches. In the case of overseas football matches, offenders may have to surrender their passports. More general banning requirements may be imposed under the broader **Criminal Behaviour Order**. Breach of the order may result in a fine (p.456), or in the case of football banning orders, a short sentence of imprisonment (p.452).
- An order for **confiscation**, **deprivation**, or **forfeiture** allows the state to remove the means and proceeds of crime, by seizing specific assets (forfeiture,[82] particularly of weapons or drugs), by depriving the offender of specific items (e.g. a car) used in the offence, or by seizing property of a certain value (confiscation). In E&W and NI in 2018-19 £217m was seized.
- Offenders convicted of driving offences can be **disqualified from driving** for a period (or have 'points' added to their licence, which cumulatively lead to disqualification). Likewise, company directors can be disqualified from future directorships if they commit fraud (p.427) or related offences.
- **Parenting orders** require the parents or carers of a young offender to undergo counselling, guidance, or a parenting course for up to three months, and may impose conditions for up to a year (e.g. attending school meetings, or ensuring their child is at home at certain times or is not in certain places unsupervised.) Failure to comply is an offence.
- Orders for **restitution** require an offender convicted of theft (p.426) or related offences to return specified property, or assets of equivalent value, to the person it belongs to.
- **Restraining orders**, and in the UK Sexual Harm Prevention Orders, Serious Crime Prevention Orders and Violent Offender Orders are civil injunctions (p.458) which courts can impose, usually[83] after conviction for serious violent or sexual offences. The injunction typically bars offenders entering certain places at specified times, or from contact with certain people, especially former victims.
- Terrorist and sex offenders can be placed on a **register** that requires them to inform police of their address at all times, and to be monitored by police under the MAPPA (p.592). Registration can be for a fixed period, or for life, and failure to comply with monitoring requirements is an offence.
- Lastly, all courts can make **costs orders** requiring one party to pay some or all of the other party or parties' costs, as well as their own.

---

82 *Forfeiture* originally meant the automatic loss of property in cases of treason or murder, particularly rules preventing killers inheriting their victim's property. Weaker forfeiture rules still exist in the UK and RoI, distinct from forfeiture orders.

83 Controversially, it is possible to receive such a criminally-enforced civil order without being convicted. The House of Lords ruled in *McCann* (p.VI.3) that such orders, despite their potential impact on liberty, are not criminal proceedings and not covered by the presumption of innocence in article 6(2) of the ECHR (p.518). See also ASBOs (p.458).

Civil orders and quasi-punishments

Referral orders and diversionary youth conferences

In E&W, referral orders, and in NI & RoI, diversionary youth conferences,[84] allow the court or prosecutor to refer children to community panels instead of trying them. The victim is often invited, as well as the child and their parents. If the panel and child agree an alternative to prosecution that is acceptable to the court, the case can be suspended. If the child breaks the agreement, the prosecution can resume.

Civil measures for antisocial behaviour

An **Acceptable Behaviour Contract** in the UK or **Good Behaviour Contract** in RoI is an agreement between a young person, their parents, the police, and (in the UK) a Youth Offending Team (p.585). It involves a signed promise by the young person not to engage in certain antisocial behaviour. It is not a sentence, and breaking the contract does not directly give rise to criminal penalties, but the breach can later be used in evidence.

Anti-Social Behaviour Orders (ASBOs) are civil orders obtained by local authorities in the UK or RoI against young people or adults because of their past antisocial behaviour, if it caused or was likely to cause harassment, alarm, or distress. The order requires the person to do or not do certain things, such as not to enter a certain area. As a civil order, the antisocial behaviour need only be proved on the balance of probabilities (p.380), but breaching the order can result in imprisonment. ASBOs are therefore, in effect, suspended criminal punishments imposed without the safeguards of a criminal trial (e.g. excluding hearsay evidence, p.383, or requiring proof beyond reasonable doubt, p.380), which has caused much controversy.[85]

Domestic Violence Protection Orders in the UK and **Safety Orders** in RoI are civil injunctions obtained by the police to protect victims of domestic violence while evidence is gathered to charge the alleged perpetrators or while the victim moves home or seeks a longer-term injunction.[86] They last for fourteen to twenty-eight days and can prohibit alleged abusers from being in contact with victims, or force them to leave a shared home.

Other civil measures

In E&W, **Local Child Curfews** allow children younger than sixteen to be banned from entering public places during prescribed hours unless they are with a responsible adult. As a civil order, it includes children younger than ten.

A **Child Safety Order** applies to children younger than ten in E&W who have acted in a way that could have resulted in conviction had they been over the age of criminal responsibility (p.406). It allows the child to

---

84 The Children's Hearings (p.386) system in Scotland allows for similar outcomes.

85 They have been found lawful in the UK nevertheless (see e.g. *McCann*, p.VI.3). This is the same position as with SHPOs, SCPOs, and VOOs on p.457, but whereas those are usually issued as orders ancillary to a sentence following criminal conviction, ASBOs are often stand-alone orders (albeit for people who tend to have multiple prior convictions for minor offences).

86 Such as a restraining order in the UK, or a more specific protection order or barring order in RoI.

be supervised for a set period by a social worker or an officer of the Youth Offending Team. In Scotland, <u>Children's Hearings</u> (p.386) can make similar orders, such as Compulsory Supervision Orders, to protect children.

Lastly, most courts have a general <u>equitable</u> (p.366) power to issue orders, known in most cases as **injunctions**, to individuals and organisations. Some injunctions are now regulated by statute (e.g. the <u>SHPO</u> and <u>Violent Offender Order</u>, p.457). Injunctions requiring a party to do a specific thing may be referred to as 'mandamus', and those requiring a party to refrain from doing a specific thing as 'certiorari'.

Chapter 16

Mental health and mental capacity law*

---

* The intention of this chapter is not a comprehensive and definitive rehearsal of all mental health law across the UK and RoI, but to show in broad terms how the law operates, and its relationships with other branches of law that affect those with mental disorder. It assumes that all law enacted at the time of writing will be brought into effect (most notably the MCANI).

Historical development

For a considerable period after the recognition of mental disorder as an entity in its own right, there was no specific mental health law: mentally disordered people were treated informally, with or without their consent[1] (especially if they were rich enough to have a <u>personal physician</u>, p.12), or were dealt with under general laws for the poor and destitute.

In the UK & Ireland, this amounted to the Poor Laws and the <u>Vagrancy Acts</u> (p.740), under which mentally disordered people unable to support themselves would be placed in an almshouse; those able to work would do so in a workhouse; and those deemed idle would be confined in a House of Correction or prison. From the seventeenth century, they could also be confined in the new private 'madhouses'. If detained unwillingly (on the order of a magistrate or relative, or under a medical certificate), inmates could only force their release under the law of *habeas corpus*,[2] if their detention was illegal (e.g. because the madhouse was not registered).

Lunacy Acts

The first specific mental health law[3] in the UK was the <u>Criminal Lunatics Act 1800</u> (p.268). This diverted mentally disordered offenders into lunatic asylums, but did not affect the vast majority of mentally disordered patients. They had to wait for the Lunacy Act 1845 and associated legislation, which established a network of county asylums across E&W (and later Scotland and Ireland) and instituted a system of inspection of institutions by Commissioners who could order minimum standards of treatment and the release of patients. The right of appeal to the courts was removed, however. The Act was the product of the therapeutic optimism of the period, the belief that patients could recover if given 'asylum' from harsh social conditions, and the advent of the railways, which made a national supervisory regime possible. At the same time, public fear of 'dangerous lunatics' such as Daniel McNaughten (p.620) made it politically possible to pay for a new generation of asylums.

There was eventually an outcry against the abuses that arose because any person purporting to be a doctor could commit someone to an asylum or madhouse, and because there was no legal mechanism for challenging the truth of statements made in the doctor's certificate. A series of amendments culminating in the Lunacy Acts 1890 & 1891 required specialist magistrates to authorise all admissions, allowed leave, permitted 'boarding out' with friends and relatives, and restricted admission to patients with serious mental disorder.

---

1 Informal treatment without consent usually meant being forced into treatment by your family.

2 *Habeas corpus* is a writ requiring any person detaining any other (e.g. in prison) to bring the detainee before the courts and to show that they had the legal power to detain them. In practice, it was only available to the wealthy who could afford solicitors.

3 Discounting feudal laws that gave the King custody of the land and property of lunatics and idiots, and eighteenth-century Acts regulating private madhouses.

Mental Deficiency and Mental Treatment Acts

Until the twentieth century, so-called idiots and mental defectives (broadly speaking, people with <u>intellectual disability</u>, p.110) were cared for by relatives, or were placed in workhouses or lunatic asylums. However, at the turn of the century there was public fear of being 'overrun' by people with intellectual disability, who were perceived to have many children. The Mental Deficiency Act 1913[4] set up specific institutions for their care and control, with a Board of Control to inspect them, modelled on the Lunacy Commission. The system then expanded to take in the many victims of the encephalitis lethargica epidemic of 1919–1930.[5] At first, it was seen as progressive despite its origins, but concern grew in the 1940s at prevalent abuses, including using patients as cheap labour.

The Mental Treatment Act 1930[6] began a gradual process of liberalisation and deinstitutionalisation. Patients could be admitted and treated voluntarily (i.e. without compulsory powers); all institutions were renamed Mental Hospitals; and outpatient and <u>after-care</u> (p.492) services were developed. At the same time, the first genuinely effective (though still poor, and overused) treatments for mental disorder, including <u>ECT</u> and <u>psychosurgery</u> (p.198), allowed many more patients to be discharged.

Mental Health Acts

The first Mental Health Acts[7] marked a decisive break with the legalism of the Lunacy Acts, continuing the processes of liberalisation and medicalisation. Doctors were given the leading role in making decisions on compulsory, as well as voluntary, treatment, and courts were replaced by less formal <u>tribunals</u> (p.512). However, such trust was placed in this benignly paternal system that the Lunacy Commission and other independent inspectorates were abolished; a fresh round of public scandals led to their re-creation under new names in the 1960s.

Divergence in mental health law

Mental health law in the UK and RoI remains true to many of the principles of the first Mental Health Acts, particularly medical dominance within the legal process. However, the details have diverged in the four jurisdictions, and the current laws reflect each nation's different emphasis on individual freedom, paternalism, legalism, and public protection: see p.466.

---

4 The Mental Deficiency and Lunacy (Scotland) Act 1913 brought in similar provisions for Scotland, but there was no special system for people with intellectual disability in Ireland, partly because the debate over its autonomy ('Home Rule') overshadowed any other legislative developments.

5 Widely thought to be a postviral syndrome related to the 1919 influenza pandemic. Many fear that a similar postviral 'long Covid' syndrome has begun to spread at the time of writing, in the wake of the SARS-Cov-2 pandemic.

6 In NI, The Mental Treatment Act (NI) 1932; there was no corresponding Act in Scotland. By this time RoI was an independent country, and later passed the Mental Treatment Act 1945, which went much further and abolished the need for judicial orders for any patients.

7 The Mental Health Act 1959 for E&W, the Mental Health (Scotland) Act 1960, the Mental Health (NI) Act 1961, and the Mental Treatment Act 1961 in RoI.

Relationship with other areas of law

Mental health law should not be viewed in isolation from the values and principles (p.466) of the society it serves, or from other law with which it coexists. In these different areas of law, mental disorder is constructed in a variety of different ways, because of the different social aims or goals (p.352) of each area of law, and therefore the effect of a given type of mental disorder on the outcome of a case will vary considerably depending on the field of law concerned.

Informal treatment under mental health law

The pages that follow describe the compulsory powers[8] available under mental health law in each jurisdiction. The same law also governs 'informal' or voluntary treatment. In E&W, s131 MHA (like article 127 MHNIO) states that mentally disordered patients may be admitted to hospital without any compulsory legal processes[9]; s244 and s291 of the MHCTA imply the same for Scotland.[10] In RoI, S2 MHA limits informal admissions to capacitously consenting patients.

Mental capacity law

Whereas mental health law governs the compulsory treatment of people with mental disorder for that disorder, mental capacity law (p.522) provides rules for determining who lacks capacity (because of mental disorder, or other causes such as brain injury) to make decisions regarding a variety of acts, including those with legal consequences such as buying and willing property, marrying, voting, and accepting or refusing medical treatment (where mental health law does not apply).

   Medical treatment in the absence of consent can be lawfully authorised under both laws, but (except in NI) on very different grounds, reflecting profoundly different ethical principles. Some authors have argued for unification of the two areas of law within in a single mental capacity law applicable to treatment for both mental and physical disorder, as is now the case in NI, and as was considered in the Wessely report (p. 782) for E&W.

Family and social care law

Both mental health law and mental capacity law are specific examples of a broader field of public law that aims to protect the rights and interests of potentially vulnerable members of society. This includes laws on child protection and safeguarding of vulnerable adults (p.574), laws prohibiting discrimination on the grounds of disability and other characteristics, health and safety law, social security laws (the successors to the Poor Laws, p.462), and social welfare law (p.542).

---

8 Strictly speaking, in NI, the protections from liability for acting under the MCANI.

9 Adults, plus sixteen and seventeen year olds who capacitously consent (parental consent alone is insufficient). The section implicitly allows informal treatment of adults lacking capacity. The Wessely report (p.782) recommended requiring admissions of incapacitous patients to be under DoLS/LPS if they do not object, or MHA compulsory powers if they do.

10 For example by providing for rules to be made to require authorisation for certain informal patients, such as children.

Criminal law

Criminal law (p.397) is concerned with regulating behaviour through punishing and/or reforming individuals who behave in socially unacceptable ways. Unlike mental health law, which is paternalist in approach, criminal law assumes that individuals are able to make rational choices about their behaviour, and that they are therefore responsible for those choices. However, it overlaps with mental health law to the extent that it recognises several exceptions to the rule of personal responsibility based upon mental disorder (e.g. insanity, p.620), and it allows for mentally disordered offenders to receive psychiatric treatment, either in conjunction with or instead of, a penal sentence (p.442). It also takes mental disorder into account as a factor indicating risk of harm to others that may justify some form of indeterminate sentence (p.448) for public protection, and as a factor relevant to mitigation (p.638).

Which branch of law should do what?

The relationship of the purposes of mental health law to the purposes of other fields of law raises the following questions, amongst others:

- Should there be similar principles, or separate law dealing with treatment for mental and physical disorders?
- What rights to treatment, if any, should be granted specifically within mental health legislation, by comparison with other law?
- Should mental health law allow preventive detention directed towards public protection, as an alternative, or in addition to, use of the criminal law?
- How should the boundary between criminal and mental health law be drawn?

Should we have mental *health* legislation, directed solely at individual mental health and welfare, or mental *disorder* legislation, directed effectively also at the control of mentally disordered individuals for the public good? One answer is provided by the new 'fusion' legislation for NI in the MCANI, which provides a largely unified framework for treatment for mental and physical disorder, with a focus on individual health and welfare. It remains to be seen how this will work in practice when brought into effect.

Principles of mental health laws

Ethical principles underlying law

The law regulates relationships between individuals and the State (public law), and between individuals or groups in different types of relationship (private law). Laws embody society's views on questions such as:

- What should society do about a 'dangerous' individual?
- Should we help a citizen who doesn't want to be helped in that way?
- When should we allow one group of citizens to use force against another, and in what circumstances?
- When is it right to detain or treat someone against their will, if ever?

Mental health laws provide specific answers to these questions in relation to mentally disordered individuals, and set out who has the power to detain or force treatment on them, and in what circumstances.

Intention, capacity and paternalism

Criminal law (p.397) and much of the civil law (p.547) assume that, generally, individuals have the 'capacity' to make rational, voluntary decisions about their actions, and their consequences; hence, the primary basis of criminal liability is an individual's intention (p.402) to commit crime. However, mental health laws recognise that mental disorder may impair the capacity to avoid crime or to seek treatment. From this perspective, mental health laws are based on one of two principles[11]:

- protection of those who lack the capacity to desist from crime or seek treatment (mental health law as an extension of capacity law, p.522) and
- protection of others from those deemed 'objectively' to need treatment, and/or to pose an unacceptable risk of harm (p.163) to themselves or others.

In E&W, the MHA, as emphasised by its 1995 and 2007 amendments, ignores capacity in determining whether a person can be detained (although capacity is relevant to treatment, p.482), and focuses heavily on **protection of the public** and of the individual. In Scotland, and even more in NI,[12] by contrast, mental health law requires evidence of impaired capacity before allowing civil detention, even in emergencies (p.476).

The law in RoI falls between these two extremes. Since the MHA in RoI allows detention without reference to capacity, but in more restrictive circumstances than in E&W: for example, detention cannot be for treatment of personality disorder alone[13]; the risk of harm to the patient or others must be serious and imminent; and there must be evidence that the proposed treatment is likely to materially benefit the patient's condition.

---

11 There is also a third principle, ignored in this debate, of mental health law assisting those who are capable of seeking treatment, but are actively unwilling to do so (against their own best interests).

12 This is the eventual position in NI, though at the time of writing the law is in transition between the old MHNIO (based very closely on the E&W MHA), and the new MCANI. Even after the MCANI is fully in effect the old rules will apply to those younger than eighteen.

13 Reflecting the very different diagnostic status of the condition.

Dichotomising physical and mental health

Except in NI, there is a legal distinction drawn between nonconsensual treatment for physical and mental disorder. The former can occur only where the patient **lacks capacity**, and treatment is in their **best interests**; or (in very limited circumstances) where there is a risk to public health (p.542). Even the Scottish capacity-based mental health law is distinct to some degree from general capacity law, with a less stringent test of incapacity ('significant impairment' of capacity) in the MHCTA than in the AWIA. Dichotomising physical and mental health is not only open to ethical challenge; it also can create practical difficulties or anomalies where the patient has a condition that is both physical and mental in its nature or manifestations ('which bit of the patient am I treating under which law?').

Rights of the individual

Both under the Lunacy Acts (p.462) and the midtwentieth-century Mental Treatment Acts, there were very few protections for patients against abuse (p.520) by those detaining and treating them. Public scandals arose frequently. Modern mental health laws have been repeatedly amended, partly in response to human rights law (p.516). They include:

* legal definitions (p.470) of key concepts, limiting discretion;
* procedures (p.470) requiring two or more professionals from different disciplines to agree on the need for compulsory treatment;
* built-in reviews of detention and treatment;
* rights of appeal (p.512) to independent tribunals or courts; and
* restrictions on long-term or irreversible treatments (p.482).

As much ethics as law

Mental health law represents a significant intrusion by the State into an individual citizen's private life. It allows for people to lose their liberty and have their movements controlled without having been convicted of a crime—known as **administrative** (i.e. noncriminal) **detention**. It allows people to be forced to do things, and have things done to them, against their will. It places great power in the hands of those approved by the State to utilise these laws. These intrusions are ethically justified by the future benefits that people are expected to perceive when restored to health; the benefits to society of caring for the vulnerable; and public protection.

However, the wide discretion allowed to clinicians under such loosely drawn laws creates the possibility for abuse (p.520), and requires enormously careful ethical decision-making (p.281). Many patients may be legally 'detainable'; but the ethical question will be 'should I recommend detention?' For those who use these laws, it is important to ask oneself, 'If I, or someone I love, became mentally unwell, would I be comfortable with the use of these laws on me or them?'[14]

---

14 This principle is now the basis of the 'Friends and Family Test' used by all mental health services in England to assess service quality.

Roles of professionals and relatives

A variety of individuals have legally defined roles under mental health law. The following is a glossary of roles across the UK and RoI.

Medical or clinical roles

Appointed Doctor/Approved Medical Practitioner (NI): a doctor appointed by the Secretary of State under the MHNIO or MCANI respectively to issue recommendations for admission, or to give second opinions on treatment.

Approved Clinician (AC, E&W): a mental health professional approved by the Secretary of State to exercise powers under the MHA associated with being in overall charge of a patient's care.

Approved Medical Practitioner (AMP, Scotland): a doctor with appropriate training and experience approved by a Health Board under s22 of the MHCTA.

Clinical Director (CD, RoI): a doctor in charge of an Approved Centre.

Designated Medical Practitioner (DMP, Scotland): a doctor appointed by the Mental Welfare Commission (MWC) to give second opinions under the treatment (p.482) provisions of the MHA, who is independent of the hospital concerned.

Responsible Clinician (RC, E&W): the AC with overall responsibility for the patient's case.

Responsible Medical Officer/Practitioner (RMO, Scotland; RMP, NI): the doctor with overall responsibility for the patient's care.

Section 12 approved doctor (s12 doctor, E&W): a doctor, usually a GP or a psychiatrist, approved by the Secretary of State as having special expertise in the assessment or treatment of mental disorder.

Second Opinion Appointed Doctor (SOAD E&W): a doctor appointed by the Secretary of State to give second opinions on treatment under the MHA, who is independent of the hospital concerned.

Social work and related roles

Approved Mental Health Professional (AMHP, E&W): a mental health practitioner (other than a psychiatrist; usually a social worker) who has undergone special training in working with mentally disordered patients and their relatives.

Approved Social Worker (ASW, NI) or **Mental Health Officer** (MHO, Scotland): a social worker with appropriate training and experience who has been approved under s32 MHCTA or under the MHNIO/MCANI.

Relatives' and others' roles

Independent Mental Health/Capacity Advocate (IMHA/IMCA, E&W, and NI): a person trained in advocacy appointed to support and advise people detained under mental health and/or mental capacity law.

Named/nominated person (Scotland & NI): a person nominated by patients (subject to their consent) under MHCTA/MCANI to protect their interests, and in certain circumstances to receive information and make decisions on their behalf.

Nearest relative/default nominated person (E&W, Scotland, & NI): the relative deemed to be closest or most significant to the patient, and able in limited circumstances to apply for their detention or discharge (Box 16.1).

Box 16.1 Nearest relative (default nominated person), in order of priority

The nearest relative is usually the first of those in this list who is adult, alive, and resident in the UK. Where two or more people are of equal priority, the nearest relative is usually the oldest of them. Preference is given to those who live with or care for the patient.

- carer (NI only)
- spouse or civil partner, or person lived with as a spouse for at least six months
- son or daughter (biological children before step-children)
- father or mother
- brother or sister (full siblings before half- or step-siblings)
- grandparent
- grandchild
- uncle or aunt
- nephew or niece
- cohabitee (NI only)

Organisational roles

Approved Centre (RoI): a mental hospital approved and registered with the Mental Health Commission (MHC) for the detention and treatment of patients under the MHA.

Care Quality Commission (England), **Healthcare Inspectorate Wales**, and **Regulation & Quality Improvement Authority** (RQIA, NI): three healthcare inspectorates, whose duties include the inspection of mental health facilities to ensure that they and their staff comply with their duties under mental health & mental capacity law.

First-Tier Tribunal (Mental Health) (FTTMH, E&W): a special Tribunal (p.372) to which patients (and in some instances their nearest relatives) can appeal or be referred (p.512) for release from hospital detention.

Mental Health (Review) Tribunal (MHT/MHRT, NI,& RoI): an appeals tribunal analogous to the FTTMH in E&W.

Mental Health Tribunal (MHT, Scotland): a tribunal like the FTTMH in E&W, but with broader powers to make and renew Compulsory Treatment Orders in the first instance, as well as to hear appeals.

Mental Health Commission (MHC, RoI) and **Mental Welfare Commission**, (MWC, Scotland): bodies with wide-ranging powers to ensure compliance with mental health law and supervise its operation.

Procedures for using civil powers

UK and RoI procedures for using civil powers to detain and treat patients all have the same main elements: an application,[15] supported by one or more medical recommendations, which meet a definition of mental disorder. There may also be urgency or necessity criteria, capacity tests, risk criteria, and treatability or proportionality tests.[16]

The application

The process of compulsory detention begins with a person who knows the patient, or a suitable professional, recognising that they appear to be mentally unwell and in need of treatment that they are thought likely to refuse. In E&W and RoI certain relatives can apply (and in NI in certain circumstances), but in Scotland only doctors can do so, although they need the consent of a specially-trained social worker.

The recommendations

Except in <u>emergencies</u> (p.476), the application must come with a recommendation from one or more doctors (often specially approved), certifying that the requirements below are met.

Definition of mental disorder

The law defines *mental disorder* so as to limit discretion and reduce the scope for <u>abuse</u> (p.520). However, the definitions are broad and reflect social views on the circumstances when forced treatment is appropriate: for example, none allows detention for alcohol or drug dependence alone[17]; in RoI personality disorder alone is insufficient, as is sexual deviation[18] in RoI and Scotland.

In E&W, the broad definition of mental disorder ('any disorder or disability of the mind') is qualified by the requirement that, in the case of intellectual disability, there must be 'abnormally aggressive or seriously irresponsible conduct' in order for treatment to continue after an initial assessment period. A requirement for such conduct is also incorporated in the definition of 'significant intellectual disability' in RoI.

The mental disorder must also cross a qualifying threshold in E&W: it must be of a nature (its type and past history) and/or of a degree (its current severity) sufficient to warrant the use of the particular compulsory power in question. The NI threshold is that the disorder must make the person incapable of deciding on treatment.

---

15 In the case of patients before the criminal courts, the 'application' is in fact a court order.

16 These terms are not generally used in the legislation, but are adopted here to enable analysis and comparison of the rules in the different jurisdictions. The term 'treatability test' appeared in the E&W MHA until 2007, but had a more limited meaning than used here.

17 However, the MCANI would allow this if the person lacked capacity and safeguards were met.

18 In E&W and NI, the exclusion for sexual deviancy was removed in 2007 and 2016, respectively: if it amounts to a diagnosable mental disorder, it can justify detention and treatment.

Risk criteria

Suffering from mental disorder is not enough to justify compulsory detention and/or treatment; there must also be grounds for believing that, without treatment, harm would result. This usually means harm to the patient's health, welfare, or personal safety, or harm to other people.

In Scotland and RoI, where there is no threshold for mental disorder, there is instead a threshold for the risk criterion such as that the harm to the patient's health or safety must be 'significant'.

Urgency and necessity criteria

In order to use the simplified procedures available in emergency situations or with <u>patients already in hospital</u> (p.476), there must be some reason why the situation is urgent and the normal, longer procedure cannot be employed. Similarly, for treatment beyond an initial assessment period to be authorised, there must be some reason why compulsory powers are necessary: for example because the patient continues to refuse treatment in E&W, or because treatment is in the patient's best interests in NI.

Capacity tests

There is no requirement in E&W of any loss of capacity. The <u>basis of mental health law</u> (p.466) in NI is now that the patient lacks capacity. In RoI 'impaired judgment' is a basis for detention as an alternative to risk of harm; in Scotland 'significantly impaired ability' is a general criterion for the use of compulsory powers; and in all jurisdictions capacity after admission is relevant to justifying <u>certain treatments</u> (p.482).

Whether the capacity tests in RoI and Scotland rule out compulsory admission of all patients with capacity, or whether some patients who met the test for capacity under <u>mental capacity law</u> (p.522) could nevertheless be deemed to have 'impaired judgment' or 'significantly impaired decision-making ability', has not been legally tested.

Treatability and proportionality tests

Concerns about the risk of <u>administrative detention</u> (p.467) of people who have committed no crime but are deemed to pose a high risk of harming others, yet for whom there might be no effective treatment, have led to use of various forms of 'treatability' test before compulsory treatment beyond an initial assessment period can be authorised. These range from a requirement that treatment is 'likely to benefit or alleviate the condition' in Scotland and RoI, to a vaguer requirement that 'appropriate treatment is available ... the *purpose* of which' is amelioration of prevention of deterioration in E&W. There is no treatability test in the MHNIO; the

MCANI introduces instead the test that the treatment (or other measures) must be a 'proportionate response' to the likelihood and severity of harm to the patient or others.

Tables 16.1–16.21 set out the details of the main powers in each jurisdiction. The NI columns refer to the MCANI; as the MHNIO still applies there for children but is almost identical to the E&W MHA, it is referred to in the E&W columns.

Civil admission for assessment

Relevant legislation

- E&W: MHA s2 (article 4 MHNIO) admission for assessment
- Scotland: MHCTA part 6 s44 short-term detention order
- NI: MCANI schedule 2 short-term detention for examination
- RoI: MHA ss9–14 application for involuntary admission (only allows for assessment, not for subsequent treatment like the longer UK orders)

Table 16.1 Grounds for admission for assessment

	E&W (and MHNIO)	Scotland	NI (MCANI)	RoI
Mental disorder definition (physical or mental in NI)	Any disorder or disability of the mind, of sufficient nature or degree	Any mental illness, personality disorder, or intellectual disability, however caused or manifested	Any illness or suspected illness (including any injury, disorder, or disability requiring treatment or nursing)	Mental illness, severe dementia, or significant intellectual impairment (i.e. **not** personality disorder alone)
Risk criterion	In the interest of patient's own health or safety or for the protection of others (substantial likelihood of serious physical harm to patient or others in NI)	Significant risk to the patient's health, safety, or welfare, or to the safety of others	Serious harm to patient or serious physical harm to others	Serious likelihood of the patient causing immediate and serious harm to themselves or others (*alternative* to capacity test)
Proportionality test	None	None	Detention is a proportionate response to likelihood and seriousness of harm	None
Capacity test	None	Significantly impaired ability to make decisions about medical treatment	Patient lacks capacity in relation to whether they should be detained (and treated)	Judgment so impaired that without compulsory treatment a serious deterioration would be likely
Necessity test	None	None	In patient's best interests to be detained	None

Table 16.2 Process of admission for assessment

	E&W (and MHNIO)	Scotland	NI (MCANI)	RoI
Recommendation(s)	One recommendation from s12/appointed doctor plus a second (knows patient or s12 in E&W; given on admission in NI)	Approved medical practitioner	One report by doctor who has consulted NP/ IMCA if practicable; second report by RMP or specified doctor on admission	Doctor not working at the approved centre where the patient is to be admitted
Applicant	Nearest relative or AMHP/ASW (who in NI must consult nearest relative if practicable, plus another ASW if NR objects)	No application as such, but the doctor must obtain the consent of a MHO to the order, who must interview the patient if practicable	Appropriate healthcare professional, either an ASW or a designee of hospital managing authority	Spouse or relative, an authorised officer (of the Health Board), a Gard (police officer) or any other adult with no conflict of interest
Maximum duration	28 days, or 7 days in NI (48 hours if the second doctor was not the RMO or an approved doctor)	28 days	14 days (2 days if the second doctor was not the RMP or prescribed type of doctor, unless such a doctor makes a report within those 2 days)	The recommendation lasts for 7 days, but detention is authorised for only 24 hours to allow assessment for an admission order
Renewal	Cannot be renewed in E&W; in NI, one further occasion of 7 days, on the order of the RMO	Cannot be renewed; can be extended for 3 days to allow an application for a compulsory treatment order to be made, plus a further 5 days once the application has been made	One further period of 14 days following a report by the RMP or another prescribed doctor	Cannot be renewed

Emergency civil procedures

These comprise simpler, more rapid emergency assessment procedures (not required in NI and RoI, where the main procedure is itself simple and quick), and procedures for patients already in hospital voluntarily.

Table 16.3 Grounds for emergency admission for assessment

	E&W (and MHNIO)	Scotland	NI (MCANI)	RoI
Mental disorder definition	Any disorder or disability of the mind, of sufficient nature or degree	Any mental illness, personality disorder, or intellectual disability, however caused or manifested	N/A— must use short-term detention for examination (see p.474)	Mental illness, severe dementia, or significant intellectual impairment (i.e. **not** personality disorder alone)
Risk criterion	In the interest of patient's health or safety or for protection of others (substantial likelihood of serious physical harm to patient or others in NI)	Significant risk to patient's health, safety, or welfare, or to the safety of others	N/A	(*alternative* to capacity test) Serious likelihood of patient causing immediate and serious harm to themselves or others
Urgency criterion	s4, urgent necessity to avoid undesirable delay; s5, immediately necessary to stop patient leaving (in NI, immediate attendance of a doctor not practicable)	Urgent necessity, and s44 would involve undesirable delay; for s299, immediately necessary to stop patient leaving hospital	N/A	None—merely that the patient indicates they wish to leave
Capacity test	None	For s36 only, significantly impaired ability to make decisions about medical treatment;	N/A	Judgment so impaired that without compulsory treatment, serious deterioration likely

Relevant legislation

- E&W: MHA s4 emergency admission, s5 (art.7 MHNIO) holding power
- Scotland: MHCTA s36 emergency detention, s299 nurse holding power
- NI: MCANI schedule 2 (see p.474) must be used
- RoI: MHA s23: power to prevent patient leaving approved centre

Table 16.4 Process of emergency admission for assessment

	E&W (and MHNIO)	Scotland	NI (MCANI)	RoI
Recommendations	For s4, one medical recommendation, by a doctor who knows the patient or by a s12-approved doctor None for s5/art7	For s36, one medical practitioner	N/A	None
Applicant	For s4, an approved Mental Health Professional or nearest relative; for s5(2), the doctors or AC in charge of treatment or their nominee; for art7(2) a doctor on the hospital staff; for s5(4)/art7(3) a mental health nurse	For s36, no application as such, but the doctor should if practicable obtain the consent of a MHO to the order; for s299, a mental health nurse	N/A	Consultant psychiatrist, doctor or registered nurse on the staff of the hospital
Maximum duration	72 hours for s4, s5(2) 48 hours for art7(2) 6 hours for s5(4)/art7(3)	72 hours, or 3 hours in the case of s299	N/A	24 hours
Renewal or extension	s4 cannot be renewed, but when converted to s2 will then last for a total of 28 days if a second doctor completes a recommendation s5/art7 cannot be renewed/extended	Cannot be renewed or extended	N/A	Cannot be renewed or extended, but can be converted into an admission order (p.478) if a second consultant psychiatrist makes a recommendation

Civil admission for treatment

Relevant legislation

- E&W: MHA s3 (article 12 MHNIO) detention for treatment
- Scotland: MHCTA part 7, s57 compulsory treatment order
- NI: MCANI schedule 1 authorisation for detention & treatment
- RoI: MHA s15 admission order

Table 16.5 Grounds for admission for treatment

	E&W (and MHNIO)	Scotland	NI (MCANI)	RoI
Mental disorder definition (physical or mental in NI)	Any disorder or disability of mind (in NI, mental illness or severe mental handicap only), of sufficient nature or degree	Any mental illness, personality disorder, or intellectual disability, however caused or manifested	None (treatment can be for any condition)	Mental illness, severe dementia, or significant intellectual impairment (i.e. **not** personality disorder alone)
Risk criterion	In the interest of patient's health or safety or for protection of others (in NI, substantial likelihood of serious physical harm to patient/others)	Significant risk to patient's health, safety, or welfare, or to safety of others	Serious harm to patient or serious physical harm to others	Serious likelihood of patient causing immediate and serious harm to themselves or others (*alternative* to capacity test)
Treatability or propor tionality test	Appropriate medical treatment is available (none in NI)	Available treatment likely to prevent disorder worsening or alleviate its symptoms or effects	Detention & treatment is a proportionate response to likelihood and seriousness of harm, appropriate treatment is available	Likely to benefit or alleviate the condition of that person to a material extent

Table 16.5 (Contd.)

	E&W (and MHNIO)	Scotland	NI (MCANI)	RoI
Capacity test	None	Significantly impaired ability to make decisions about medical treatment	Patient lacks capacity in relation to whether they should be detained and treated	Judgment so impaired that serious deterioration likely without compulsory treatment
Necessity test	Cannot otherwise be treated (in NI, other methods inappropriate)	Making of CTO is necessary	In patient's best interests to be detained and treated	None

Table 16.6 Process of admission for treatment

	E&W (and MHNIO)	Scotland	NI (MCANI)	RoI
Recommendations[19]	One recommendation from s12-appointed doctor, plus another in E&W	Two medical recommendations (one must be approved under s22)	One report by doctor who has consulted NP/IMCA if practicable	Consultant psychiatrist
Applicant	Approved Mental Health Professional or nearest relative (N/A in NI)	MHO, who has a **duty** to apply	Appropriate healthcare professional, either an ASW or a designee of hospital	N/A (see p.474 for details of the initial application and recommendation process)
Maximum duration	6 months	6 months, or 28 days for interim CTOs	6 months	21 days
Renewal	6 months then annually	6 months then annually (or for one further period of 28 days for interim CTOs)	6 months then annually, with agreement of ASW or designee of hospital	6 months, then annually

(Continued)

19 In E&W and Scotland, the second recommendation must be either from a registered medical practitioner who knows the patient (e.g. their GP) or from a second approved doctor.

Table 16.6 (Contd.)

	E&W (and MHNIO)	Scotland	NI (MCANI)	RoI
Additional Info	art12 MHNIO only applies if first detained under art4 (p.474) / art7 (p.476)	Authorisation granted by tribunal. CTOs can authorise <u>community treatment</u> (p.488) and inpatient treatment	Authorisation granted by three-member panel, and can include <u>attendance</u> and <u>residence requirements</u> (p.488); treatment without detention can be enforced without authorisation unless it would/might have serious consequences	Only applies if first detained under ss9–14 (p.474), s12 (p.494), or s23 (p.476)

Consent to treatment

The patient's consent (p.332) is required for all medical treatment except where it is given under a specific legal power to treat without consent. Powers to detain patients[20] for treatment generally include power to give certain treatment, subject to the safeguards below. There are very different rules for treatment without consent under mental capacity law (p.522).

The detained patient

Although mental health law addresses the patient's mental capacity to make treatment decisions, in E&W and Scotland it ultimately allows the overriding of a patient's refusal even when they retain mental capacity. There are safeguards for the use of compulsory treatment, such as independent second opinions, but it still raises important philosophical (p.324) and ethical (pp.288, 351–359) issues.

What counts as treatment?

Except in NI, the proposed treatment must be for mental disorder, or its symptoms or consequences (e.g. refeeding is accepted as a treatment for severe anorexia[21]). In NI the treatment can be for any condition.

In E&W, the definition of treatment shown in the table is arguably broad enough to encompass some forms of administrative detention (p.467) despite the ethical objections. The ethics of these various definitions are discussed on p.340.

Mental health laws and consent to treatment

Table 16.7 shows the legal position in each jurisdiction. Accompanying codes of practice provide guidance on consent. In all cases, consent can only be a valid basis for treatment if the patient has capacity to consent.

---

20 Unlike in prison, where consent for treatment is always required (*Freeman*, p.756).

21 Because psychological treatment alone is ineffective, partly due to depressive cognitions and rigidity of thought caused by starvation.

Table 16.7 Legal position by jurisdiction for consent to treatment:

	E&W (and MHNIO)	Scotland	NI (MCANI)	RoI
Relevant law	Part IV (ss56–64K, arts62–69)	MHCTA part 16 (ss233–249)	MCANI part 2 (ss16–23)	MHA part 4 (ss56–61)
Treatment definition	Medical treatment including nursing care, psychological intervention, and specialist mental health habilitation, rehabilitation, and care	Medical treatment including nursing care, psychological intervention, habilitation (including education & training), and rehabilitation	Treatment including any examination, procedure (diagnostic or otherwise), and any therapy	Treatment including administration of physical, psychological, and other remedies for care & rehabilitation of a patient under medical supervision
Purpose	To alleviate, or prevent a worsening of, the disorder or its symptoms or manifestations	Likely to prevent disorder worsening or to alleviate its symptoms or effects	Which is appropriate in that person's case	Ameliorating a mental disorder
Default position	Inpatient treatment may be authorised by AC/RMO without consent. Under CTO, need capacity and consent; if lacks capacity, need authorisation under MCA or passive assent	Treatment may be authorised by RMC without consent	Treatment only with consent, unless patient lacks capacity and treatment does not have serious consequences, patient does not resist and is not subject to any other order, or treatment is authorised under sch1 (p.478) or sch2 (p.474)	Treatment only with consent unless patient lacks capacity and treatment necessary to save life, restore health, alleviate condition or relieve suffering

(Continued)

Table 16.7 (Contd.)

	E&W (and MHNIO)	Scotland	NI (MCANI)	RoI
Restricted treatments	Psychosurgery (need consent and a second opinion) ECT, or medication after three months (need consent or a second opinion, or both for a child)	Psychosurgery (need three second opinions and either consent or a court order) ECT or medication after two months (need consent or best interests)	Psychosurgery (need consent) Treatment with serious consequences (e.g. serious side-effects) including medication after three months (need consent or second opinion)	Psychosurgery (need consent and tribunal authorisation) ECT, or medication after three months (need consent or if lacks capacity, a second opinion)
Overridden by	For ECT, any valid applicable advance decision (p.536) or decision of a donee (p.538), or deputy (p.534)	None	Any effective advance decision (p.536) or decision of a donee (p.538) or deputy (p.534)	None
Exceptions	Treatment immediately necessary to save life, or nonirreversible, nonhazardous treatment immediately necessary to prevent serious deterioration, serious suffering, or violence	Urgent treatment to save life, or nonirreversible, nonhazardous urgent treatment to prevent serious deterioration, serious suffering, or violence	To delay until the safeguard is met would create an unacceptable risk of harm to the patient	None

Leave from hospital

For the vast majority of patients in <u>secure care</u> (p.258), periods of <u>therapeutic leave</u> (p.191) outside the secure environment are a cornerstone of <u>rehabilitation</u> (p.264). However, for patients detained under mental health law,[22] and particularly for patients subject to <u>special restrictions</u> (p.510), there are legal procedures that must be complied with before such leave may be taken.[23] See Table 16.8.

Leave versus suspension

Whereas the laws in E&W and RoI use the concept of leave from hospital (and in NI the related concept of permitted absence), Scottish law employs an alternative concept, that of the temporary suspension of measures. The latter is considerably more flexible, as it not only allows the leave of absence from a place of detention subject to certain conditions, but also allows for other aspects of an order—such as requirements to accept a particular treatment, or reside in a certain place—to be lifted temporarily. In NI, similar flexibility comes from rules allowing the RMP to vary <u>attendance requirements</u> and <u>community residence requirements</u> (p.488).

Leave for restricted patients

Leave outside the hospital or unit to which a patient is admitted or transferred from court or prison can only be granted to patients subject to <u>restriction orders</u> or <u>restriction directions</u> (p.510) with the consent of the relevant government department (e.g. the Ministry of Justice in E&W). In such situations, it is important to consider what the court or department has defined as the 'hospital' or 'unit' in the order or warrant authorising the patient's admission. For example, if the order specifies a single ward, then the patient cannot go outside the ward without a leave application being approved. Conversely, if the order specifies an entire hospital, then the patient may be permitted into the grounds of that hospital at the discretion of the treating team. However, if the grounds of the hospital are not within a secure perimeter, and the patient would be in prison if not in hospital, it may be unwise for the treating team to authorise this, particularly if the patient is unescorted.

Revocation of leave and recall to hospital

Once leave or permission has been granted, or suspension has been authorised, it can be revoked at any time by the RC, RMO, RMP, or consultant psychiatrist who granted it, provided the necessity criterion has been met; this automatically recalls the patient to hospital.

---

22 The arrangements for leave under other laws, notably <u>mental capacity law</u> (p.522) are very much simpler.

23 If they are not complied with, the leave is legally <u>unauthorised</u> (p.179).

Table 16.8 Leave by jurisdiction

	E&W (and MHNIO)	Scotland	NI (MCANI)	RoI
Relevant law	MHA s17/ MHNIO art15	MHCTA ss41, 53, 127, 179, 221, and 224	MCANI ss25, 27, 187, 195, and 202	MHA s26
Leave authorised by	RC/ Responsible Medical Officer	Responsible Medical Officer	Responsible Medical Practitioner or (under ss25–27) any designee of the hospital or care home management	Consultant psychiatrist responsible for patient's care
Nature of leave	Indefinite (E&W only) or on specified occasions or for any specified period (may be extended)	A period (not exceeding 200 days): the duration of an event or series of events, plus associated travel	A specified occasion or a specified period (may be extended)	For any period less than the unexpired period of the admission order
Criteria	Leave for more than 7 days can only be authorised if a CTO (p.488) is considered first. In NI, RQIA must be informed of leave over 28 days	Leave for more than 28 days must be notified to the Mental health officer, GP, and others first, and to the MWC within 14 days	RQIA must be informed of leave over 28 days	None
Custody during leave	May be kept in custody of authorised person if necessary for patient's health/ safety or to protect others	Patient may be kept in the charge of any authorised person	May remain in custody of authorised person if necessary for patient's health/ safety or to protect others	No specific provision Could be made a condition
Leave conditions	Any necessary in the patient's interests or to protect others	Any necessary in the interests of the patient or to protect others	Any necessary for patient's health or safety or to protect others	Any the consultant psychiatrist considers appropriate
Recall: necessity criterion	For patient's health/safety or to protect others	For patient's health or safety or to protect others	For patient's health/safety, to protect others or if not receiving proper care	In the patient's interests

Civil community treatment

Relevant legislation

- E&W: MHA s17A Community Treatment Order, s7 (art18 MHNIO) guardianship
- Scotland: MHCTA part 7, s57: compulsory treatment order
- NI: MCANI schedule 1 authorisation for attendance requirement or community residence requirement (with treatment measure)
- RoI: No powers to enforce community treatment

Table 16.9 Grounds for compulsory community treatment

	CTO E&W	Guardianship E&W MHNIO	Scotland	NI (MCANI)
Mental disorder definition (physical or mental in NI)	Any disorder or disability of the mind, of sufficient nature or degree	Any disorder or disability of mind (in NI, mental illness, or severe mental handicap only), of sufficient nature or degree	Any mental illness, personality disorder, or intellectual disability, however caused or manifested	None (treatment can be for any condition)
Risk criterion	In the interest of the patient's health/safety or for to protect others	In the interests of the patient's welfare or (in E&W) to protect others	Significant risk to the patient's health, safety or welfare, or to the safety of others	Serious harm to patient or serious physical harm to others (or for attendance, if patient would probably not otherwise be treated)
Treatability or proportionality test	Appropriate treatment can be provided without continuing detention in hospital	None	Available treatment likely to prevent disorder worsening or to alleviate its symptoms or effects	Requirement is a proportionate response to likelihood and seriousness of harm; appropriate care available

Table 16.9 (Contd.)

	CTO E&W	Guardianship E&W MHNIO	Scotland	NI (MCANI)
Capacity test	None	None	Significantly impaired ability to make treatment decisions	Patient lacks capacity in relation to imposing the requirement
Necessity test	Power of recall is necessary (considering risk of relapse)	Guardianship is necessary	CTO is necessary	Requirement in patient's best interests

Table 16.10 Process of enforcing community treatment

	CTO E&W	Guardianship E&W MHNIO	Scotland	NI (MCANI)
Recommendations	Supporting statement from AMHP	Two medical (one must be s12/ appointed), plus in NI one from ASW	Two medical recommendations (one must be approved under s22)	One report by doctor who has consulted NP/ IMCA if practicable
Applicant	Responsible Clinician	Nearest relative or AMHP/ASW	MHO, who applies with a care plan to the Tribunal	Appropriate healthcare professional, either ASW or designee of hospital
Maximum duration	6 months	6 months	6 months, or 28 days in the case of interim CTO	6 months

(Continued)

Table 16.10 (Contd.)

	CTO E&W	Guardianship E&W MHNIO	Scotland	NI (MCANI)
Powers available	Attendance for examination, and any condition necessary or appropriate for ensuring treatment, for health/ safety or for protection of others	Residence; attendance at appointments for medical treatment, education, occupation or training; access for visits	Giving treatment; attendance to receive treatment or community care services; residence; and access for visits	Residence; attendance at appointments for treatment, education, occupation or training; access for visits
Enforcement provision	Recall to hospital for 72 hours if treatment required and risk criterion applies, then revocation (meaning detention under s3 or s37) if s3 criteria met	Reasonable force can be used to ensure compliance	Reasonable force to ensure compliance and/ or 72 hours' detention in hospital in the event of noncompliance	Any act to secure compliance that is in patient's best interests, including use of reasonable force, if patient at risk of harm and act is proportionate
Renewal	6 months then annually	6 months then annually	6 months then annually	6 months then annually
Additional Info	Patient must be under s3 (p.478) or s37 (p.500) for CTO to be available. Conditions must not amount to a deprivation of liberty	The guardian may be the local social services authority, or its nominee Conditions must not amount to a deprivation of liberty	CTOs can authorise inpatient treatment (p.478) as well as community treatment Conditions must not amount to a deprivation of liberty (p.532)	Authorisation granted by three-member panel Renewal requires agreement of ASW or designee of hospital

After-care

Historically, mental health care was provided solely in institutions such as the asylum (p.462) and the madhouse; when inmates left such institutions, they were expected to be ready to cope with the outside world. However, from the late-nineteenth century it became clear that many people released from mental institutions needed support to adjust to life in the community. In the UK charities such as the Mental After-Care Association were formed to provide it. Eventually the UK government recognised a duty to ensure that patients who needed it received after-care.[24]

Table 16.11 summarises the after-care provisions across the different jurisdictions.

Accepting a duty to provide after-care can represent a significant financial burden. There has been much argument and litigation in England in particular about exactly which health or social services authority is responsible for certain patients.[25]

After-care should not be confused with the Care Programme Approach (CPA) in the UK. All patients detained for treatment in E&W are entitled to after-care,[26] but only those with greater needs are treated under the CPA.

The Republic of Ireland

Chiefly because of its separate historical development, the mental health system in RoI has never had a duty to provide after-care. Many public and private hospitals provide community and after-care services on a discretionary basis. There is debate about whether there should be a duty to provide after-care to children leaving State care services at the age of eighteen years, including mental health after-care, but there are no proposals for a general duty to provide mental health after-care.

---

24 There is no clear conceptual distinction between 'after care' provided on discharge from hospital, and treatment provided in the community without any hospital admission, but the concept of after-care persists because of the specific legal duties to provide it.

25 Following _Sunderland v South Tyneside_ (p.768) and other cases, the rule in England is that the responsible local social services authority (LSSA) is determined by the patient's 'ordinary residence' (in essence, where they see themselves as living), and services should be provided by the NHS Trusts and LSSA that cover that area. The costs of providing the NHS-funded components of those after-care services should be charged to the CCG responsible for the GP with whom the patient is registered (or the CCG covering the area in which they are ordinarily resident if they are not registered with a GP).

26 Even those that do not fall within s117 (e.g. because they were only detained for assessment under s2) still have a right for assessment of their needs under other legislation such as s9 of the Care Act 2014, but they do not have the automatic right to free provision of services to meet those needs that they would have under s117.

Table 16.11 After-care provisions across the different jurisdictions.

	E&W	Scotland	NI
Relevant law	MHA s117	MHCTA ss25–27	MHNIO arts112–113 MCANI s281
Application	Patients detained under s3 (admission for treatment, p.478), ss37, 37/41, 45A (court-ordered admission for treatment, p.500) or ss47, 48 (transfer from prison, p.506)	All persons not in hospital who have or have had a mental disorder	Patients in general (there is no specific duty to provide specific services to individual patients)
Responsible bodies	Clinical Care Groups (England)/ Local Health Boards (Wales), and local social services authorities, based on the patient's ordinary residence	Local Authorities, in co-operation with health bodies and voluntary organisations	Health and Social Services Boards, and Health and Social Care Trusts
Nature of the duty	Provide, with voluntary organisations, after-care services	Provide care and support services: services to promote well-being, social development, and associated travel assistance	Make arrangements to promote mental health, prevent mental disorder, and promote treatment, welfare, and care of people with mental disorder
Specific powers (not associated with a duty)	N/A	Provide residential accommodation; social, cultural, recreational activities; training; employment support; to provide similar services to inpatients	Pay inpatients personal expenses; financial assistance to those on leave (p.486) if needed for treatment/ resettlement; contribute to maintenance of those with residence requirements (p.488); provide education, training, and occupation
Extent of the duty	Until satisfied the person is no longer in need (or under CTO p.488)	Indefinite; to minimise the effect of mental disorder and promote normal life	Indefinite
Notes	Charges may not be made (in contrast to identical services provided otherwise than under s117)	Charges possible for some services	All subject to the approval of the NI Department of Health

Police powers under mental health law

Frequently, the first professionals to have contact with mentally disordered people are the police. A person may be known to be suffering from a mental disorder and need immediate assistance, but be on private property where staff do not have permission to enter.

Table 16.12 Powers available in public places under mental health law

	E&W (and MHNIO)	Scotland	NI (MCANI)	RoI
Relevant law	MHA s136 MHNIO art130	MHCTA s297	MCANI s139	MHA s12
Power held by	Police constable	Police constable	Police constable	Gard (police officer)
Criteria for removal	Appears to be suffering from mental disorder and be in immediate need of care or control	Reasonable suspicion of mental disorder and are in immediate need of care or treatment	Unable because of impairment/ disturbance of mental functioning to decide, in immediate need of care or control, removal in best interests	Reasonable grounds for believing they suffer from mental disorder
Risk and pro portionality criteria	In the interests of that person or for the protection of others	In the interests of that person or for the protection of others	Serious physical or psychological harm to person, or serious physical harm to others, removal is proportionate	Serious likelihood of the patient causing immediate and serious harm to themselves or others
Removal to	Place of safety (can include some private premises except in NI, and for adults, a police station)	Place of safety (can only include police station if nowhere else available)	Place of safety (hospital or police station)	Into custody

Table 16.12 (Contd.)

	E&W (and MHNIO)	Scotland	NI (MCANI)	RoI
Detention period	24 hours, or 36 if extended by a doctor due to patient's condition (48 in NI)	24 hours	24 hours	No maximum
Purpose of detention	Assessment by AMHP/ASW and doctor, making arrangements for treatment/care	Assessment by doctor, making arrangements for treatment or care	Assessment by ASW and doctor	Assessment by doctor for an admission order (p.478)

Table 16.13 Powers available in private places under mental health law

	E&W (and MHNIO)	Scotland	NI (MCANI)	RoI
Relevant law	MHA ss135(1)[27] MHNIO art129	MHCTA s293	MCANI s292	MHA s12
Power held by	Justice of the Peace (magistrate)	Sheriff or (if urgent) a Justice of the Peace	Magistrate	Gard (police officer)
Applicant	AMHP (in NI, constable or health staff)	Mental Health Officer	Constable or health staff	N/A

(Continued)

---

27 s135(2) in E&W, s292 in Scotland, and art129(2) MHNIO also provide a power like that of s292 MCANI, when a constable or other person authorised to take a patient to hospital etc. applies to a magistrate stating that they believe the patient to be on certain private premises and that permission to enter has been or would be refused. No AMHP or doctor is involved in this case.

Table 16.13 (Contd.)

	E&W (and MHNIO)	Scotland	NI (MCANI)	RoI
Criteria for forcible entry and removal	Reasonable cause to suspect that a person believed to be suffering from mental disorder is ill-treated, neglected, or not kept under proper control, or lives alone and is unable to care for themselves	Over 16-year old has mental disorder, is at risk of neglect, ill-treatment, property damage, or lives alone and is unable to care for themselves; serious harm likely if not removed	Reasonable cause to believe that a person who could be detained under the Act is on premises and access would be refused, and warrant is reasonable	Reasonable grounds for believing they suffer from mental disorder, are in premises, and serious likelihood of causing immediate and serious harm to themselves or others
Conditions on forcible entry and removal	Constable must have warrant & be accompanied by doctor (and AMHP in E&W)	Constable must have warrant & be accompanied by MHO and doctor	Constable must have warrant & be accompanied by doctor	None
Removal to	Place of safety (can include some private premises except in NI, and for adults, a police station)	Place of safety (can**not** include police station)	Any place named in warrant	Into custody
Detention period	24 hours, or 36 if extended by a doctor due to patient's condition (48 in NI)	Up to 7 days	N/A (detention authorised by existing or new measure, e.g. under sch.2)	No maximum

Court-ordered pre-sentence assessment

Relevant legislation

- E&W: MHA ss35,36 (arts42–43 MHNIO) remand to hospital
- Scotland: CPSA ss52A–52U assessment and treatment orders, s200 pre-sentence report
- NI: MCANI s162 remand to hospital
- RoI: CLIA ss4(6), 5(3): committal for examination. (Note dramatically narrower legal grounds compared to the UK.)

Table 16.14 Grounds for pre-sentence admission

	E&W (and MHNIO)	Scotland	NI (MCANI)	RoI
Mental disorder definition (physical or mental in NI)	For s35, reason to suspect mental disorder (art42, mental illness or severe mental impairment); for s36/art42, any such disorder of sufficient nature or degree	Any mental illness, PD or LD, however caused or manifested; for assessment order and s200, reasonable grounds for believing such disorder is present	Reason to suspect any disorder	No specific requirement, but presumably the court must suspect that a doctor might diagnose mental disorder
Risk criterion	None	Significant risk to patient's health, safety or welfare, or others' safety (not s200)	None	None
Necessity test	Impractical to obtain medical report on bail	Detention necessary for assessment; or for treatment order, that available treatment is likely to prevent deterioration or alleviate symptoms	Proper assessment impracticable if remanded in custody but practicable in hospital	None
Purpose	For s35/art42, a report on mental condition; for s36/art43, treatment	Assessment and treatment; for s200, inquiry into mental condition required to decide sentence	Report ought to be made on person's mental or physical condition	For examination by an approved medical officer, for the court to decide whether to make order for treatment (p.500)

Table 16.15 Process of pre-sentence admission

	E&W (and MHNIO)	Scotland	NI (MCANI)	RoI
Stage of legal proceedings required for order to be considered	Charged with offence punishable with imprisonment; and for s36/art43, be in Crown Court[28]	In Sheriff Court charged with imprisonable offence (including if committed by District Court under s52A)	Offence punishable with imprisonment, either in Crown Court or convicted (or found to have done the acts) by magistrates	For s4(6), meets criteria for <u>unfitness to plead</u> (p.602); for s5(3), meets criteria for <u>insanity</u> (p.620)
Evidence (medical recommendation)	Written or oral evidence of a s12-appointed doctor (and a second doctor for s36/art43, plus evidence from hospital representative that a bed will be available within 7 days	For assessment order and s200, written or oral evidence of a doctor; for a treatment order, one approved and one other doctor; in all cases, evidence that a bed will be available within 7 days	Oral evidence of a doctor with special expertise in diagnosing or treating disorder (an approved doctor if mental disorder), plus written or oral evidence of a second doctor; evidence of arrangements made for detention	None
Applicant	N/A	Prosecutor or Scottish Ministers (not s200)	N/A	N/A
Maximum duration	Up to 28 days	Assessment order, 28 days; s200, 3 weeks; treatment order until disposal	Up to 28 days	Up to 14 days
Renewal	Can be renewed by request of the AC/RC/RMO up to 12 weeks	Cannot be renewed. Assessment order can be extended once for 14 days, s200 once for 3 weeks	Can be renewed at RMP's request up to 12 weeks	S4(6) (unfitness to be tried) cannot be renewed; s5(3) (insanity) can be renewed up to 6 months

28 For the magistrates' court in E&W or NI to remand a person under s35/art42, it must have convicted them, or have satisfied itself that they did the act or omission charged (i.e. the *actus reus*, p.402) or they must consent to the remand.

Court-ordered sentence of treatment

Relevant legislation

- E&W: MHA ss37–38 (interim) hospital order (arts44–45 MHNIO)
- Scotland: CPSA s53 and s57A: (interim) compulsion order
- NI: MCANI s167 public protection order
- RoI: CLIA s4(3)–(5) and s5(2): committal for treatment. (Note dramatically narrower legal grounds compared to the UK.)

Table 16.16 Grounds for court-ordered sentence of treatment

	E&W (and MHNIO)	Scotland	NI (MCANI)	RoI
Mental disorder definition	Any disorder or disability of mind (in NI, mental illness, or severe mental handicap only), of sufficient nature or degree	Any mental illness, personality disorder, or intellectual disability, however caused or manifested	Impairment or disturbance in functioning of mind or brain	Mental illness, severe dementia, or significant intellectual impairment, or for outpatient treatment if unfit to plead, any disease of the mind
Risk criterion	None (but for ID in E&W, need abnormally aggressive or seriously irresponsible conduct)	Significant risk to patient's health, safety, or welfare, or to safety of others	Serious physical or psychological harm to others (linked to mental disorder)	For inpatient treatment, serious likelihood of patient causing immediate and serious harm
Treatability or proportionality test	For hospital order, appropriate treatment available (E&W only)	Available treatment likely to prevent disorder worsening or to alleviate its symptoms or effects; for interim order, reasonable grounds for believing this	Detention is a proportionate response to likelihood and seriousness of harm, appropriate care or treatment for patient is available	For inpatient treatment, likely to benefit or alleviate the condition of that person to a material extent

Table 16.16 (Contd.)

Necessity test (capacity test in the case of RoI)	For interim order, a hospital order might be appropriate/warranted	Medical treatment can only be given if detained in hospital (unless compulsion order is only for community treatment)	Public protection order is most suitable way of dealing with the case	For inpatient treatment (as *alternative* to the risk criterion) Judgment so impaired that without treatment serious deterioration likely

Table 16.17 Process of court-ordered sentence of treatment

	E&W (and MHNIO)	Scotland	NI (MCANI)	RoI
Stage of legal proceedings required for order to be considered	Convicted (or, in magistrates' court, found to have done the act/omission) of imprisonable offence	Convicted of imprisonable offence	Convicted of imprisonable offence	For s4, meets <u>unfitness to plead</u> (p.602) criteria; for s5, meets <u>insanity</u> criteria (p.620)
Evidence (medical recommendation)	Oral evidence (or written in E&W) of S12/appointed doctor, a second doctor, plus evidence that a bed will be available within 28 days	Written or oral evidence of one approved doctor and a second doctor, plus evidence that a bed will be available within 7 days, plus report from a mental health officer	Oral evidence of approved doctor, plus written or oral evidence of a second doctor; evidence that arrangements have been made for detention	None
Maximum duration	6 months (12 weeks for interim order)	6 months (12 weeks for interim order)	6 months	Indefinite

(Continued)

Table 16.17 (Contd.)

	E&W (and MHNIO)	Scotland	NI (MCANI)	RoI
Renewal	For 6 months and then yearly; for interim order 28 days at a time up to a year	For 6 months and then yearly; for interim order, up to 12 weeks at a time, up to a year	For 6 months and then yearly	No necessity for renewal, but the order must be reviewed by Review Board at least every 6 months
Additional information	S37 and art44 authorise guardianship. Need an ASW in NI to authorise guardianship	Compulsion order, like compulsory treatment order (p.478), can compel community treatment. An order for lifelong restriction (p.449) is automatically available as an alternative sentence	Does not authorise treatment—can only treat with consent or by using civil powers under part 2 MCANI simultaneously (e.g. sch1 authorisation, p.478)	Review Board can terminate order, or restart legal proceedings

Other court orders

Urgent detention of acquitted persons

Generally, if a court acquits a person it has no further power to deal with them. In Scotland, however, if the court has written or oral evidence from two doctors that the defendant is suffering from a mental disorder of a type required for a <u>compulsion order</u> (p.500), and the risk criterion and treatability test for that order are met, and it is not immediately practicable for a doctor to examine the person to consider making a <u>short-term detention order</u> (p.474) or <u>emergency detention order</u> (p.476), it can order that the person be taken to a place of safety and detained there for up to six hours to enable such an examination to take place.

Risk assessment order

All three UK jurisdictions have a system for <u>extended</u> (p.453) or <u>indefinite detention</u> (p.449) of people convicted of serious violent or sexual offences who are thought by the court to be <u>dangerous</u> (p.672). Whereas in E&W and NI the court may make its assessment of dangerousness based on whatever conviction and other information is before it, in Scotland the court must usually make a risk assessment order, requiring the <u>Risk Management Authority</u> (p.594) to compile a risk assessment report.[29]

Hybrid order and hospital direction

The UK government has been concerned about offenders, especially those with personality disorder, receiving hospital orders but proving untreatable and having to be released, possibly many years earlier than they would have been released from prison. The **hospital and limitation direction** in E&W (known as 'the hybrid order'), and the hospital direction in Scotland and NI, were created in response, as well as in order to include an element of punishment. The order allows anyone tried in a criminal court in NI, in the Crown Court in E&W, or Sheriff Court or High Court in Scotland eligible for a <u>public protection order</u>, <u>hospital order</u>, or <u>compulsion order with restrictions</u> (p.510) to be given a prison sentence but initially directed to hospital. Should treatment prove unsuccessful, they can be remitted to prison to serve the remainder of their prison sentence. Case law in E&W requires judges to consider a hybrid order first, whenever a hospital order is possible,[30] and restricts the use of interim hospital orders in these circumstances (see also <u>sentencing</u> (p.442).

Supervision and treatment order

This order is available throughout the UK (known as a supervision order in E&W and a supervision & assessment order in NI), and applies only to those found <u>not guilty by reason of insanity</u> (p.620) or <u>unfit to plead</u> (p.602), where neither admission to hospital nor an absolute discharge (nor, in Scotland, guardianship) would be appropriate. It makes the

---

29 Twenty-one such orders were made in 2019-20.

30 *Vowles* and *Edwards* (pp.754, 770); the latter includes detailed guidelines. Five or fewer hybrid orders a year were made in E&W before 2010 (compared with around 300 restricted hospital orders); following *Vowles*, this quintupled, to twenty-eight in 2016 and twenty-five in 2017.

defendant subject to the supervision of a social worker or (in E&W and NI) probation officer[31] for up to three years (two years in E&W), during which time they must take any prescribed medical treatment for mental disorder, under medical supervision. There is no appeal to a tribunal (p.512) against this order; appeals must be made to the relevant court.

Guardianship orders and intervention orders

Guardianship is available in E&W and under the MHNIO as an order for mentally disordered persons, both as civil guardianship (p.488), and as a variant on a hospital order (p.500). However, in Scotland, court-ordered guardianship (p.534) and the associated intervention order (p.534) are available only for defendants who lack capacity (p.522). A similar result can be obtained under the MCANI if the court makes a supervision & assessment order with a residence requirement.

Detention in excessive security

The MHCTA in Scotland allows patients to appeal to the court on the ground that they are being detained in conditions of excessive security. If the court agrees, the Health Board has a limited period to transfer the patient to a lower security unit.

Courts-martial

Military courts trying members of armed forces have limited powers to order treatment for mental disorder.

In the UK, defendants who have been found unfit to plead (p.602) or not guilty by reason of insanity (p.620) can be given an **admission order** authorising detention and treatment in hospital, a **supervision and treatment order** equivalent to the order described above, or a **guardianship** order. In each case, the defendant is then treated as if a criminal court had made the order.

In RoI, if a court-martial finds a member of the defence forces unfit to plead or insane at the time of the offence, the defendant is transferred to a designated centre for treatment as if they had been committed for treatment (p.500) under the CLIA.

---

31 Home Office guidance states that it should be an approved social worker (i.e. an AMHP in E&W). Strictly speaking, the NI order only requires submission to treatment if that is separately authorised under schedule 1 of the MCANI (pp.478, 488).

Transfer from prison for treatment

These are not court orders, but directions issued by the government department that runs the <u>prison service</u> (p.578).

Relevant legislation

- E&W: MHA s47–48 (urgent) transfer of prisoner (arts53–54 MHNIO)
- Scotland: MHCTA s136: transfer for treatment direction
- NI: MCANI ss211–224 hospital transfer directions
- RoI: CLIA s15: transfer of prisoner

Table 16.18 Grounds for transfer from prison

	E&W (and MHNIO)	Scotland	NI (MCANI)	RoI
Mental disorder definition (physical or mental in NI)	Any disorder or disability of mind (in NI, mental illness or severe mental handicap only), of sufficient nature or degree	Any mental illness, personality disorder, or intellectual disability, however caused or manifested	Any disorder requiring treatment	Mental illness, mental disability, dementia, or any disease of the mind
Risk criterion	None	Significant risk to patient's health, safety or welfare, or to the safety of others	Serious physical or psychological harm to the offender or serious physical harm to others	None
Treatability test	Appropriate treatment is available (E&W only)	Available treatment likely to prevent disorder worsening or alleviate its symptoms or effects	Appropriate care or treatment is available in hospital	None
Necessity test	In the public interest, and expedient in all the circumstances; and for s48/art54, in urgent need of treatment	Transfer for treatment direction is necessary	Hospital transfer direction is appropriate, considering alternatives	Cannot be afforded appropriate care or treatment in the prison where they are detained

Table 16.19 Process of transfer from prison

	E&W (and MHNIO)	Scotland	NI (MCANI)	RoI
Stage of legal proceedings required for order to be considered	Convicted, sentenced to imprisonment (or for s48/ art54, detained for civil or criminal trial or deportation)	Convicted, serving sentence of imprisonment, or detention under immigration law	Convicted, serving custodial sentence; or if urgent treatment required, any other detainee	At any stage
Evidence (medical recommendation)	Reports by a s12-appointed doctor, and by a second doctor	Reports by approved doctor and a second doctor, plus evidence that a bed will be available within 7 days; consultation with MHO if practicable	Reports by a doctor with special expertise in disorder (an approved doctor if mental disorder), and a second doctor; evidence of arrangements for detention	Report by two doctors, or one doctor with patient consent
Maximum duration	Until <u>EDR</u> (p.452), after which detention continues under 'notional' <u>hospital order</u> (p.500)	Until <u>custody part</u> (p.453) of sentence ends	Until <u>EDR</u> (p.452)	Until no longer a prisoner
Return to prison	At any time, if RC/RMO or Tribunal states that treatment no longer needed or no further effective treatment available	At any time (or at annual reviews), if RC and MHO, Scottish Ministers or Tribunal no longer think conditions met	At any time, if doctor or tribunal states that treatment no longer needed or no further effective treatment available, or harm would no longer result if remitted	If prisoner refuses treatment (unless two doctors certify they should stay in hospital); or if CD or Review Board concludes conditions not met

(Continued)

Table 15.19 (Contd.)

	E&W (and MHNIO)	Scotland	NI (MCANI)	RoI
Additional information	In practice, s49/art55 restrictions (p.510) are always applied for s47/art53; they are mandatory for s48/art54	Prisoners on remand can only be treated under an assessment or treatment order (p.498)	Can only treat with consent or using civil powers under part 2 MCANI simultaneously (e.g. sch1 authorisation, p.478)	Detention reviewed by Review Board at least every six months

Restriction orders and directions

In the UK, the philosophy underlying court orders and transfer directions is that where offenders or potential offenders are assessed as suffering from treatable mental disorder, they should be <u>diverted</u> (p.268) to hospital (or occasionally to the community) for treatment. Where the offence is relatively minor and/or the offender's <u>risk assessment</u> (p.163) suggests they are not a <u>danger to society</u> (p.672), that is usually the end of the matter. However, if they are charged with or convicted of a serious sexual or violent offence, or deemed 'dangerous' for another reason, they will usually be treated in <u>secure services</u> (p.258), and will be subject to restrictions that limit the treating clinicians' powers.

In RoI, there is no general power to sentence offenders to treatment, and no order under which offenders can be treated in an unrestricted fashion. All court treatment orders and transfers from prison are automatically subject to what in the UK would be regarded as restrictions.

Orders and directions to which restrictions can be applied

Orders marked with an asterisk* below either require that restrictions be applied automatically, or imply restrictions by having no mechanism for the RC/RMO/CD to discharge, transfer or grant leave to the patient.

Sentences of treatment
- Hospital order (E&W, MHA s37–41; NI, MHNIO art44–47)
- Compulsion order (Scotland, CPSA ss57A–59)
- Public Protection order (NI, MCANI s167)
- Committal for treatment (RoI, CLIA ss4–5)*

Other court orders
- Hybrid order (E&W, MHA s45A)*
- Hospital direction (Scotland, CPSA s59A; NI, MCANI s197)*

Transfer directions
- Transfer of prisoner (E&W, MHA s47; NI, MHNIO art53/ MCANI s211)
- Urgent transfer (E&W, MHA s48; NI MHNIO art54/MCANI s214-220)*
- Transfer for treatment (Scotland, MHCTA s136)*
- Transfer of prisoner (RoI, CLIA s15)*

Criterion for making a restriction order

Where the court or relevant Minister[32] has discretion over whether or not to apply restrictions, it may do so if the restrictions are **necessary for the protection of the public from serious harm**,[33] having regard to the offence they have been convicted of, their past criminal record, and any available risk assessment.

Where a court considers making a restriction order, it must hear oral evidence from at least one of the doctors recommending admission.

32 The government minister or department responsible for running the prison service: the Ministry of Justice in E&W, the Scottish Ministers, or the Secretary of State in NI. See p.586.
33 'The public' includes a known individual.

Restrictions when in hospital

During the period that the restrictions apply, the RC/RMO/CD cannot:
- Grant leave (p.486) from hospital (or suspend detention in Scotland).
- Transfer the patient to another hospital or unit outside the boundaries of the hospital or unit named in the order.
- Discharge the patient from hospital.

Instead, the CD, RC, or RMO must apply to the relevant Minister, who will decide whether or not to transfer the patient, or grant leave, or in the case of sentences of treatment, discharge the patient; in other cases, discharge is not usually possible, but the Minister may decide to return the patient to prison.

The order cannot expire and therefore does not need renewal; it lasts until restrictions are lifted by the relevant Minister or a tribunal or (in the case of transfer directions, hybrid orders, and hospital directions) until the patient would have been released from prison had they not been transferred, after which it may end completely or continue as an unrestricted form of the order (see pp.498–508 for details).

Restrictions after discharge from hospital

Patients treated under a restricted hospital or compulsion order (or committed for treatment in RoI) can be **conditionally discharged** by a tribunal (UK) or Review Board (RoI); or in E&W and NI, by the relevant Minister. After a conditional discharge, if they relapse or breach conditions (with evidence suggesting risk of relapse), the Minister can recall (p.589) them to hospital to continue treatment under the original order; the patient must be told why.

Common conditions include residing in a mental health hostel, accepting treatment, accepting drug testing, and attending appointments with the RC/RMO, social supervisor (p.589), or others. The conditions may be varied at any time by the relevant Minister. They cannot amount to a deprivation of liberty (p.532; see *MM and PJ*, p.762) unless a power to impose a DoL is granted for example under the High Court's inherent jurisdiction (for a capacitous, consenting patient, see *AB*, p.745) or under MCANI or by the Court of Protection (for an incapacitous patient).

Where a tribunal in E&W, Scotland, or NI grants a conditional discharge, it may **defer** it taking effect until whatever arrangements it thinks necessary (such as obtaining funding for a placement) have been made.

Reporting requirements

When restrictions apply to patients, the law requires the RMO/RC to keep the relevant Minister informed of developments in their care and treatment. This includes an update on their condition whenever the RMO/RC/RMP applies for leave, transfer, or discharge, and:
- Annual review for patients in Scotland.
- Annual Statutory Report on inpatients in E&W and NI.
- Quarterly reports on conditionally discharged patients in E&W and NI.

Appeal against detention & treatment

The cornerstone of the protection of patients' rights under mental health law is the role of the tribunal[34] (p.469), which independently reviews the use of detention and compulsory treatment. See Table 16.20.

Civil detention and treatment

A tribunal can review detention and treatment automatically, before the relevant order comes into effect; if the patient appeals against the order; and if the order is referred to it by hospital managers, the MHC/MWC, or the relevant Minister (p.586). There is no appeal against or review of emergency civil detention (p.476) because the detention is so brief.

Table 16.20 Appeal against detention & treatment in civil detention

	E&W (and MHNIO)	Scotland	NI (MCANI)	RoI
Review prior to order	None	CTO only made or varied if tribunal approves	None (but authorisations require panel approval, p.482)	None
Appeal against assessment	Within first 14 days of s2 order only (6 months in NI)	Any time under short-term detention certificate	Within 28 days of admission	None
Appeal against treatment or guardianship	Within 6 months of s3, guardianship or CTO starting, plus once in every renewal period	If RMO extends unvaried CTO (which does not need tribunal review); or three months after making, varying or extending order	Within 6 months of sch.1 authorisation being given (28 days if interim authorisation), plus once in every renewal period	Once in each renewal period (but not in the first 3 months of the first renewal)
Referral to Tribunal	At discretion of Minister; and by hospital managers at 6 months then every 3 years (2 in NI), if no appeals	MWC can also revoke short-term detention, interim CTO or CTO, as well as to refer CTO to Tribunal	At discretion of Minister; and by hospital managers every 2 years if no appeals	By MHC on making or renewal of admission order

---

34 The First-Tier Tribunal (Mental Health) in E&W, the Mental Health Tribunal in Scotland and NI, and the Mental Health Review Tribunal in RoI. This is in addition to associate hospital managers' reviews of applications and renewals in E&W, which can include a hearing and lead to discharge.

Court-ordered treatment and transfer from prison

See table 16.21 on the next page. There is no appeal against or review of a court order for <u>pre-sentence assessment</u> (p.498).

The review process

Review by a tribunal (or the Review Board for offenders in RoI) involves the following stages:

- examination of the patient by the RMO/RC and a care co-ordinator, social worker, or social supervisor, and, if requested by patients or their solicitor, an independent psychiatrist or other appropriate professional, each of whom must submit a <u>report</u> (p.692);
- in E&W, examination of the patient by the medical member of the tribunal, if the patient desires it[35];
- representation of the patient by a publicly funded solicitor;
- an oral hearing, usually in private, before the tribunal panel[36];
- <u>giving of evidence</u> (p.720) and cross-examination of each party;
- the tribunal giving written reasons for its decision; and
- the opportunity for patients to appeal against the decision,[37] but in the UK only by <u>judicial review</u> (p.374) or on equivalent grounds.

Powers of tribunals

Tribunals must immediately discharge all patients absolutely from detention and treatment if the criteria for the order under which they are detained and/or treated are no longer met, and have an additional discretionary power to discharge any unrestricted patient. In the case of certain restricted patients,[38] the effect of the tribunal finding that they should be absolutely discharged is that they will return to prison. There is no power for tribunals to discharge *unrestricted* patients subject to conditions. Tribunals in the UK can take further actions as follows.

Unrestricted patients[39]

- Order a **delayed discharge** in E&W or under the MHNIO, that is, a discharge that is to take effect on a specified future date.
- In E&W or NI, make a **recommendation** to the RC/RMO/RMP that the patient for example be granted leave, be transferred to another hospital, or be subject to a different order, and reconvene if it is not followed.
- In Scotland and NI, uphold the CTO, unrestricted compulsion order or schedule 1 authorisation but **vary measures** authorised by it.

---

35 Or the tribunal directs it, or it is an appeal against s2, and the patient does not object.

36 Comprising an independent consultant psychiatrist, a lay member (often a retired ASW or AMHP in E&W and NI), and a legally qualified president (a high court judge or equivalent in RoI and for restricted patients in E&W); the hearing may be held online.

37 In E&W, to the <u>Upper Tribunal</u> (p.385); in Scotland, to the <u>Sheriff Principal</u> or <u>Court of Session</u> (p.386); in NI, the <u>Court of Appeal</u> (p.384); and in RoI, to the <u>Circuit Court</u> (p.388).

38 That is, prison transfers; hybrid orders, in E&W; or hospital directions in Scotland and NI.

39 Except patients subject to <u>short-term detention certificates</u> in Scotland (see p.474).

Table 16.21 Appeal against detention & treatment in court-ordered treatment

	E&W (and MHNIO)	Scotland	NI (MCANI)	RoI
Appeal against treatment, PPO or guardianship	After 6 months of unrestricted hospital order (or within 6 months for guardianship) then once in every renewal period	If unrestricted compulsion order, tribunal must approve extension or variation; appeal 3 months after making, varying, or extending order	Within 6 months, then once in every renewal period	None, except to appeal court against the finding of unfitness to plead or insanity
Appeal against transfer from prison	If unrestricted s47/art53, within 6 months plus once in every renewal period; otherwise, as for restriction order	During first 12 weeks, then after 6 months, then yearly	Within 6 months, then in next 6 months, then yearly	None
Restriction orders (including hospital directions)	After 6 months, and then yearly (plus within first 6 months in NI)	After 6 months, and then yearly; plus within 28 days of recall	Within 6 months, then in next 6 months, then yearly	None
Appeal against conditional discharge	After 12 months, and then 2 yearly (1 in NI)	Yearly, plus within 28 days of variation of conditions	Yearly	None
Referral to Tribunal	At discretion of relevant Minister; and by the Minister every 3 years (2 in NI) if no appeals, plus within a month of recall	At discretion of relevant Minister, and by the Minister every 2 years if no appeals	At discretion of Minister; and by hospital managers every 2 years if no appeals, plus within a month of recall	Automatic review by Review Board at least every 6 months, plus at discretion of relevant Minister or Board

Patients sentenced to treatment with restrictions
- Discharge the patient **conditionally**[40] (including in RoI; see p.511).
- Direct that the patient be conditionally discharged, but **defer** this taking effect until necessary arrangements have been made (or in NI delay it until a future date), and reconvene if they are not made.
- Uphold the restriction order in Scotland, while **varying** the measures authorised by the associated compulsion order.
- In Scotland, **revoke** the restriction order, but uphold the (now unrestricted) compulsion order.
- For conditionally discharged patients, uphold the restriction order but **vary** conditions of discharge, or discharge them **absolutely**.

Prison transfers, hybrid orders, and hospital directions
- **Direct** the relevant Minister in Scotland or NI to revoke the hospital direction or transfer direction, in which case the patient will be returned to prison[41]; or
- Make a **recommendation** in E&W to the <u>relevant Minister</u> (p.586) that the patient be conditionally or absolutely discharged; the relevant Minister may then authorise conditional or absolute discharge within ninety days, after which the patient is otherwise remitted to prison unless the tribunal has recommended they remain in hospital.

Relationship with Parole Boards

A small number of patients detained in hospital in the UK under hybrid orders or hospital directions or after transfer from prison will have received <u>life sentences</u> or other <u>indeterminate sentences</u> (p.448). They cannot be released into the community unless authorised by the <u>Parole Board</u> (p.582).

In Scotland and NI, if the tribunal directs that the hospital direction or transfer direction should be revoked for a patient who has received such a sentence, they return to prison, and the normal procedure for consideration of their release by the Parole Board will apply.[42]

In E&W, if the tribunal recommends conditional or absolute discharge, and states that the patient should remain in hospital in the meantime, and if the patient is eligible for parole (because they have passed their <u>tariff</u>, p.448), the Parole Board may then meet at the hospital and allow the patient to be discharged directly into the community.

---

40 Absolute discharge of a patient sentenced to treatment with restrictions without an initial period of conditional discharge is also possible in the UK, but only if the tribunal is satisfied that liability to recall is inappropriate.

41 In NI it is also possible for the Minister to order, in effect, that they be released directly from hospital.

42 As above, release directly from hospital is also possible in NI.

Human rights law

In the UK and RoI, the <u>European Convention on Human Rights</u> (ECHR, p.518)[43] has been incorporated into domestic law. This means that courts must take the Convention (and judgments of the European Court of Human Rights) into account in reaching verdicts; that public bodies must exercise their powers in ways that conform with the Convention; and that courts undertaking <u>judicial review</u> (p.374) can declare acts of public bodies, and domestic laws themselves, incompatible with the ECHR.

Rights under the ECHR can be *absolute* (e.g. the prohibition of inhuman and degrading treatment under article 3) or *qualified*, meaning they can be interfered with to uphold the rights of another person (e.g. where one's article 10 right to freedom of speech conflicts with another's article 8 right to a private life). Other rights can be limited in certain circumstances (e.g. the article 5 right to liberty can be removed provided that a lawful procedure has been followed). Articles are written in extremely broad terms; individual countries are allowed a 'margin of appreciation': a degree of flexibility in the interpretation of an article to fit their domestic law.

Incorporation has had a significant impact on the detention and compulsory treatment of patients under mental health law. The articles of the Convention and associated case law with the most significant impact on practice are outlined below.

Article 2—right to life

The death of a person in the State's custody, such as someone detained under mental health law, may contravene article 2. The courts have held that the State has a positive duty to safeguard the lives of prisoners (*Edwards v UK*, p.754) and others in its custody, not merely not to kill them. Moreover, if aware of a real and immediate risk to life, State agents have a specific 'operational duty' to take reasonable steps to safeguard that life, through police protection (*Osman v UK*, p.764) and, in hospital, from suicide (*Savage, Rabone*, pp.765, 767).

The State's positive duty is not absolute: for example if a hospital or prison takes all *reasonable* and *proportionate* steps within its powers to guard against a patient's suicide (e.g. with systems of <u>observations</u>, p.190), the patient's suicide despite these steps will not be a breach of article 2 (*Powell v UK*, p.765). Conversely, if reasonable and proportionate steps are not taken, the State may be liable even if death does not result, but there was a 'material risk' of death.

The courts have also held that article 2 gives rise to a 'procedural duty' of the State to proactively investigate deaths of people in its custody (or for whose safety it is responsible, such as in a high-speed police chase), and to conduct independent investigations promptly, impartially with public accountability and sufficient involvement of the next of kin.

---

43 To be distinguished from the United Nations Convention on the Rights of Persons with Disabilities (CRPD), article 12 of which is highly relevant to capacity law (see p.522), and from conventions associated with the European Union (meaning that the UK's departure from the EU has not affected its membership of the ECHR).

Article 3—prohibition of torture and degrading treatment

Whether a certain treatment is 'inhuman' or 'degrading' depends on the circumstances of the case, the treatment's duration, its purpose, and its cumulative effect on the patient. Holding a person with schizophrenia in overcrowded conditions without daylight or adequate lighting or ventilation, alongside people with infectious disease and with parasitic insects, was held to breach article 3, as was force-feeding a patient when the alternative of parenteral nutrition was available.

The courts have held that the feelings of inferiority and powerlessness often associated with mental disorder create a need for vigilance to ensure article 3 is complied with.

Article 5—right to liberty and security

This right is limited, and does not prohibit detention of 'persons of un-sound mind'. Many cases have concerned the scope of this right: what amounts to detention and when detention is authorised, for how long, and in what circumstances. Rulings include that in a tribunal (p.373) the burden of proof (p.380) is on the hospital to show that detention continues to be justified, not on the patient to show it is not; that tribunals, not Ministers, must be free to discharge restricted patients (p.510) absolutely; and that undue delays in implementing detention powers or holding tribunals are un-acceptable. Compliance with article 5 was also the reason for creating the Deprivation of Liberty Safeguards (DoLS, p.532) in E&W, after *Bournewood* (p.748).

A possible future target for litigation under article 5 is the inability to ap-peal against specific conditions of a Community Treatment Order (p.488) in E&W (as opposed to appealing against the entire order).

Article 8—right to private and family life

This has been interpreted very widely by the court, and imposes positive obligations on States to uphold the rights, not merely negative obligations not to interfere with them. An excessive delay in providing necessary med-ical treatment was held to be a breach, as were unnecessarily disclosing a person's HIV status during court proceedings, and disclosing a private psychiatric report to a GP without consent. The E&W MHA had to be amended when it was found to be in breach by restricting too greatly who could act as a patient's nearest relative (p.469).

Other decisions have held that the following are all lawful under the Convention:

• compulsory antipsychotic treatment causing unpleasant side-effects,
• limited disclosure of HIV status to protect prison staff,
• closing a residential home or day centre on financial grounds,
• restricting day care services to local residents, and
• health authorities' decisions on which treatments to fund.

And, in high-security hospitals (p.258):
• randomly monitoring 10% of telephone calls,
• refusing to supply condoms,
• refusing to allow a patient to cross-dress, and
• imposing a smoking ban.

European Convention on Human Rights

The main text of the key articles of the Convention for the Protection of Human Rights and Fundamental Freedoms is in the box below, along with the articles from the first and thirteenth protocols that apply in the UK and RoI, and the articles of the fourth protocol that apply in RoI. The relevance of certain articles to forensic psychiatry is discussed on p.516 p.IV.144.

> **Article 1** The High Contracting Parties shall secure to everyone within their jurisdiction the rights and freedoms [below].
>
> **Article 2** Everyone's right to life shall be protected by law. No one shall be deprived of his life intentionally … [except] when it results from the use of force which is no more than absolutely necessary in defence of any person from unlawful violence; in order to effect a lawful arrest or to prevent escape of a person lawfully detained; or in action lawfully taken for the purpose of quelling a riot or insurrection.
>
> **Article 3** No one shall be subjected to torture or to inhuman or degrading treatment or punishment.
>
> **Article 4** No one shall be held in slavery or servitude. No one shall be required to perform forced or compulsory labour.
>
> **Article 5** Everyone has the right to liberty and security of person. No one shall be deprived of his liberty save in the following cases and in accordance with a procedure prescribed by law:
> - lawful detention after conviction by a competent court [or for contempt of court];
> - lawful arrest or [remanding in custody before trial]; …
> - lawful detention for the prevention of the spreading of infectious diseases, [or] of persons of unsound mind, alcoholics or drug addicts, or vagrants;
> - lawful arrest or detention to prevent unauthorised entry into the country or with a view to deportation or extradition.
>
> Everyone who is arrested shall be informed promptly, in a language which he understands, of the reasons for his arrest and the charge against him.
>
> Everyone who is deprived of his liberty by arrest or detention shall be entitled to take proceedings by which the lawfulness of his detention shall be decided speedily by a court and his release ordered if the detention is not lawful.
>
> Everyone who has been the victim of arrest or detention in contravention of the provisions of this article shall have an enforceable right to compensation.
>
> **Article 6** Everyone is entitled to a fair and public hearing within a reasonable time by an independent and impartial tribunal.
>
> **Article 7** No one shall be held guilty of any criminal offence on account of any act or omission which did not constitute a criminal offence under national or international law at the time when it was committed.
>
> **Article 8** Everyone has the right to respect for his private and family life, his home, and his correspondence.

Article 9 Everyone has the right to freedom of thought, conscience, and religion.

Article 10 Everyone has the right to freedom of expression.

Article 11 Everyone has the right to freedom of peaceful assembly and to freedom of association with others.

Article 12 Men and women of marriageable age have the right to marry and to found a family.

Article 13 Everyone whose rights and freedoms as set forth in this Convention are violated shall have an effective remedy before a national authority. [Directly applicable in RoI, but not in UK.]

Article 14 The enjoyment of the rights and freedoms set forth in this Convention shall be secured without discrimination on any ground such as sex, race, colour, language, religion, political or other opinion, national or social origin, association with a national minority, property, birth, or other status.

Article 15 In time of war or other public emergency threatening the life of the nation any High Contracting Party may take measures derogating from its obligations under this Convention.

1st Protocol Article 1 Every natural or legal person is entitled to the peaceful enjoyment of his possessions. No one shall be deprived of his possessions except in the public interest and subject to the conditions provided by law.

1st Protocol Article 2 No person shall be denied the right to education... [which should be] in conformity with their own religious and philosophical convictions.

1st Protocol Article 3 The High Contracting Parties undertake to hold free elections at reasonable intervals by secret ballot, under conditions which will ensure the free expression of the opinion of the people in the choice of the legislature.

4th Protocol Article 1 No one shall be deprived of his liberty merely on the ground of inability to fulfil a contractual obligation [RoI only].

4th Protocol Articles 2, 3, and 4 guarantee freedom of movement and prohibit the expulsion of national citizens or the collective expulsion of foreigners [RoI only].

13th Protocol Article 1 The death penalty shall be abolished. No one shall be condemned to such penalty or executed.

Misuse of mental health law

Mental health law allows the State to detain people without having to prove that they have committed an offence, and without the need for a trial. Across the UK and RoI, tens of thousands of orders for compulsory detention and treatment are made yearly, as shown in Table 16.22. The detainee may appeal to a tribunal (p.512), but this is not available under some orders, and it may be weeks or even months before the hearing occurs. The potential for abuse (p.462) is obvious, and mental health laws in all jurisdictions have gradually evolved to include progressively greater safeguards (p.467) to protect patients' interests. Nevertheless, there continue to be occasional claims that mental health law is used improperly. The potential for misuse is greater where the law is vague or broadly drawn.

Table 16.22 Frequency of detention under mental health law, 2018

Order Type	E&W[44]	Scotland	NI	RoI
Civil assessment	34,202	2,859	No data	N/A[45]
Civil treatment	9,589	1,421	No data	1,825
Civil emergency	5,489	3,867	No data	610
Court-ordered	213	24	No data	0[46]
Total orders	49,551	8,171	1,010	2,435
Orders per 100,000 people	84	151	54	50

Misuse for political purposes

The most egregious and well-known examples of using mental health law to detain political prisoners occurred in the former Soviet Union from the 1940s to the 1970s, ultimately in organised fashion, with the creation of a network of psychiatric prisons under the control of the secret police. The Serbsky Institute in Moscow defined a form of schizophrenia unrecognised

---

44 The UK Statistics Authority stated that these figures are underestimates, because not all providers yet supply reliable MHMDS data. This particularly applies to court orders. The estimated total from a different reporting process in 2016 was 63,622, including 1,696 court orders.

45 There are no separate data for civil assessment orders (p.474) for RoI because the same order, the admission order, serves both assessment and treatment functions.

46 In RoI, there is no general power for courts to make hospital disposals: only transfers from prison (p.506) and hospital treatment for insanity (p.620), diminished responsibility (p.624), and unfitness to plead (p.602) are available. Figures for the numbers of these are not published.

in the West, **sluggish schizophrenia**, in which the only symptoms were changes in social behaviour, most notably 'ideas about a struggle for truth and justice ... formed by personalities with a paranoid structure'. Many hundreds of dissidents were incarcerated by psychiatrists on the grounds that they suffered from sluggish schizophrenia, in some cases with psychiatrists consciously acting on behalf of the State (a grave breach of their professional ethics, p.295); other psychiatrists naively believed they were correctly diagnosing genuine mental illness. Once detained, dissidents were given antipsychotic medication and other unnecessary treatments or medical procedures, and sometimes subjected to torture masquerading as treatment, including electric shocks, radiation exposure, and beatings.

Similar political abuse occurred on a lesser scale in East European countries under Communist rule during the same period, and some authors claim that it continues today in Russia and China. Although such gross abuse is not believed to occur in the UK or RoI, some provisions of mental health law imply a recognition of the possibility (e.g. by requiring special procedures before Members of Parliament can be detained).

The focus on dangerousness

As discussed elsewhere (e.g. pp.293–347), there is a continual tension within forensic psychiatry between the duty to act in the patient's best interests and the need to protect the public. Some authors regard it as an outright misuse of mental health law to use it with any purpose other than the patient's best interests, and argue against ethical risk assessment and management (p.322) being a legitimate possibility. Others accept 'double effect': that detention for public protection is justifiable, but only if there is some benefit to the patient (other than merely the avoidance of future offending and incarceration).

The antipsychiatry position

Since the 1960s the antipsychiatry movement has argued that psychiatry, far from being a legitimate medical specialty, is nothing more than a form of social control. Szasz cited previous mainstream psychiatric views, later discredited because social views had changed (such as regarding masturbation, homosexuality, or transsexuality as signs of mental disorder) as proof that psychiatry is not objective science but merely reflects the views of powerful social groups. From this position[47] any use of mental health law to detain or treat a person involuntarily is by definition a misuse of State power.

---

47 A development of this position is Fulford's concept of the 'fact-to-value' ratio of medical diagnoses. Some such as Alzheimer's disease, have a clear factual biological basis; others, such as personality disorder, are much less clearly biologically defined, and more subject to the incorporation of value judgments that can lead to abuse.

Principles of mental capacity law

The legal term *capacity*[48] refers to the mental ability to make a decision for oneself in relation to a legal matter, such as making a will, marrying, selling property, and consenting to treatment (p.482).

Historical development: the basis for incapacity

Capacity law developed from property law, determining when individuals could decide how they managed and disposed of their property. Initially, certain groups such as children, women (in some circumstances), 'lunatics' (people with mental illness), and 'idiots' (people with intellectual disability) were deemed incapable for all decisions (a **status** approach).

As recognition spread after the Enlightenment that mental disorders could change, status approaches declined, except for childhood. Instead, often those with mental disorder who made foolish or incomprehensible decisions were thought incapable: that is, it was the **outcome** of their decision-making process that indicated their incapacity.

Modern mental capacity law, however, takes a **functional** approach: what matters is not the wisdom of the decision, but the process by which it was reached. Only if a person lacks the functional ability to make a decision (e.g. by being unable to understand relevant information) are they incapable of making such a decision.

General principles of capacity law

- Capacity relates to a specific decision at a specific time: a person may lack capacity for one decision on one day (e.g. selling their home), but have it for another decision (e.g. making a small gift), or have it on another day (e.g. after recovery from illness).
- Every adult is presumed to have capacity unless shown to lack it.
- Courts determine mental capacity on the balance of probabilities.[49]
- Nobody lacks capacity merely because they make an unwise decision.
- Nobody can be determined to lack capacity unless reasonable efforts have been made to facilitate their decision-making (e.g. calming anxiety, presenting information simply).
- Decisions must be made jointly with people who lack capacity, or according to their wishes and preferences (RoI) or in their best interests (E&W, NI) or be 'reasonable in the circumstances' (Scotland).
- Decisions must be those that least restrict the person's future freedom.
- Decisions must take into account advance statements (binding or not) and the views of carers, relatives, nominees, donees, and deputies.

These principles are explicitly stated in the MCA, MCANI, and ADMCA; the latter four are explicitly stated in the AWIA. The purpose of these laws is to provide a legal framework for acting with, for or (in the UK) on behalf of, people lacking capacity.

---

48 The term *competence* is sometimes used in medical and philosophical literature to refer to the same mental ability in a more general sense (i.e. without reference to any specific legal rules).

49 Except in criminal proceedings involving the capacity of the alleged victim to consent (e.g. sexual offences), where the prosecution must prove incapacity beyond reasonable doubt (see _R v A_, p.745).

Definition of mental capacity

The legal definitions of mental capacity (or incapacity) are shown in the table on the following page. They comprise the following elements:

A cause of incapacity

Except in RoI, there must be an identifiable reason for the alleged mental incapacity; under the AWIA this must be mental disorder or (in inability to communicate) physical disorder, whereas the MCA and MCANI allow any impairment or disturbance of mental functioning.[50]

Comprehension and appreciation

The person must be able to understand relevant information: not every detail, but the essence of it. In some definitions,[51] this goes beyond an intellectual understanding to include being able to see its relevance to themselves and their situation (to 'appreciate' it). For example, a young person or someone with intellectual disability might understand the notion of death but be unable to appreciate that their own death could result.

Using information

They must be able to make use of the information in coming to a decision. This includes

- retaining the information in memory for long enough to make the decision (this might be a short time for, say, a decision on what meal to order, but a much longer time for a complex financial transaction);
- believing it as appropriate (e.g. accepting that one has a heart condition requiring treatment, rather than having grandiose delusions that one is invulnerable); and
- weighing up different pieces of information 'in the balance' (i.e. within a reasoning process[52]) so as to arrive at a decision.

Communication

If a person is unable to communicate their decision to others (explicitly, by speaking, writing, or signing or implicitly, by acting in a particular way) or to act for themselves they are in effect incapable.

---

50 The boundaries of 'mental functioning' are uncertain. A mentally healthy young adult might be so emotionally overwhelmed by a life-or-death decision that they cannot comprehend, appreciate, or use the information. They would have capacity under AWIA but perhaps not the other Acts.

51 The MCANI explicitly includes 'appreciation', whereas the MCA in E&W does not. The Supreme Court in Victoria, Australia ruled in 2018 that the Victorian statute, which used an identical definition to that in E&W, did not permit a tribunal to rule that two patients lacked capacity to consent to ECT solely because they did not agree with their diagnoses and therefore could not apply the information to their own circumstances (*PBU v Tribunal*, p.764).

52 Reasoning distorted by mental disorder can result in incapacity. For example, a depressed person's hopelessness may lead them to undervalue continued life. More controversially, a patient with severe PD who over-valued the pleasure of manipulating of others as a factor in decision-making was found potentially incapable because of 'distorted' reasoning (*R v Brady*, p.749).

Differences in mental capacity law

Table 16.23 Differences in mental capacity law between jurisdictions

	E&W	Scotland	NI	RoI
Relevant law	Mental Capacity Act 2005 (MCA)	Adults with Incapacity (Scotland) Act 2000 (AWIA)	Mental Capacity (Northern Ireland) Act 2016 (MCANI)	Assisted Decision-Making (Capacity) Act 2015 (ADMCA)
Permitted causes of incapacity	Impairment of, or disturbance in the functioning of, the mind or brain	Mental disorder or physical disability	Impairment of, or disturbance in the functioning of, the mind or brain	Any
Definition of incapacity	Unable to understand relevant information; retain that information long enough to make a decision; use or weigh that information as part of the decision-making process; communicate the decision	'Incapable' means incapable of acting; making decisions; communicating decisions; understanding decisions; or retaining the memory of decisions	Unable to understand relevant information; retain that information for the time required; appreciate the relevance of and use and weigh that information; communicate the decision	Unable to understand relevant information; retain information long enough to make voluntary choice; use or weigh that information as part of the decision-making process; communicate the decision
Age limit, years	Over 16	Adult (over 16)	Over 16	None (over 18 for advance healthcare decisions)
Result of finding of incapacity	Decisions taken by others in person's best interests	Decisions taken by others in person's best interests	Decisions taken by others in person's best interests	Decisions assisted, co-decided or made by representative
Safe guards	Involvement Consultation Overriding Restraint/DoL	Consultation Overriding Certification Force/DoL	Involvement Consultation Overriding Certification Second opinion Restraint/DoL Authorisation	Involvement Consultation Overriding Restraint/DoL Agency principle

Table 16.23 (Contd.)

	E&W	Scotland	NI	RoI
Appeal against finding of incapacity	To Court of Protection or by judicial review (p.374) of assessor's decision	To Court of Session, by the person or anyone with interest in their property	To the Tribunal against authorisations; otherwise to the High Court	To the Circuit Court (High Court in limited circumstances)

Fluctuating capacity

A person may have capacity for one decision, but not another (e.g. which requires more complex information to be understood for longer). Even in relation to the same decision, a person may have capacity one day and not another, because of confusion, pain, anxiety, drugs, or alcohol, or the variable symptoms of mental disorders such as Alzheimer's disease.

If a person with fluctuating capacity loses capacity temporarily, those acting for them may rely on consent given when they had capacity, or if practicable delay the decision.

Emergency situations

It is a common misconception that special rules apply in emergencies. This is not the case. The only difference is that there may not be time to assess a person's capacity, give relevant information, or comply with the full range of safeguards (p.528). In this situation, urgent treatment necessary to save life or prevent major deterioration can be given.

Advocates

In addition to friends and relatives, people who lack capacity often benefit from the advice and support of a trained advocate who understands the issues involved. In Scotland and RoI such advocates are available informally; in E&W and NI, there is a statutory system of IMCAs, whom doctors are required to consult for major treatment and welfare decisions (in E&W, if no appropriate relative or friend is available, in NI if the patient has not declined an IMCA).

International perspective

The principles of UK capacity laws represent uneasy compromises between two principles:

- decision support (promoting the ability of the person to exercise their legal capacity) and
- decision substitution (allowing someone else to make decisions on behalf of the mentally incapacitated person, neither appointed by the person nor bound by their will and preferences).

By contrast, the legislation in RoI does not allow decision substitution.

The **UN Convention on the Rights of Persons with Disabilities** promotes decision support without (quite) outlawing substituted decision-making. Article 12 states that all persons with disabilities have the right to recognition everywhere as a person before the law, and enjoy legal capacity on an equal basis with others in all aspects of life, and that States must support people with disabilities to exercise their legal capacity and must provide appropriate safeguards (respecting the rights, will, and preferences of the person, free from conflict of interest and undue influence, proportionate and tailored to the person's circumstances and the effect on the person's rights and interests, for the shortest time possible, and subject to regular competent, independent, and impartial review).

Safeguards within mental capacity law

Each legal regime provides safeguards against abuse when people lack the capacity to act for themselves. Safeguards in the MCA and AWIA are substantially weaker than in more recent Irish and Northern Irish legislation. The Scottish government is consulting on reform of the AWIA at the time of writing, and a similar process is likely in E&W as part of the forthcoming UN review of compliance with the CRPD.

Involvement

The most direct safeguard is to require that patients participate in the decision-making to the greatest extent the possible. E&W and NI require this before a decision is made on behalf of the person; RoI requires all decisions to involve participation of the incapacitated person (with, in extreme cases, a decision-making representative acting for them, bound by their previously expressed wishes and preferences).

Consultation

All jurisdictions require some consultation with others who might know what that person would want—for example carers, nominees, and advocates. Under the MCANI and ADMCA, every decision has to involve appropriate consultation (except in emergencies where there is no time). The MCA requires consultation if 'appropriate'. The AWIA only requires consultation with guardians, attorneys, or other formal court appointees.

Overriding

All jurisdictions allow a decision made by the person when they had capacity, or by someone they chose to decide for them, to override a potential decision by someone else (e.g. a healthcare professional—but not a court). For example, a doctor cannot make a decision for a patient that conflicts with a valid, applicable advance decision (p.536), or with a decision by the donee of an applicable power of attorney (p.538).

Certification

To treat persons without capacity under the AWIA in Scotland, doctors must complete a form certifying that they lack capacity in relation to the treatment decision. The MCANI requires certification of a formal capacity assessment for any treatment or intervention with serious consequences (e.g. serious side-effects). Under the MCA in E&W, no special forms are required; it is advisable, however, to document any capacity assessment and actions taken in the patient's medical notes. The ADMCA requires certification of decision-support arrangements rather than individual supported decisions.

Second opinion

Because the MCANI covers treatment decisions that in the other jurisdictions are made under mental health law, it provides for second opinions to be given by independent professionals for the same kinds of treatment as require second opinions under mental health law, most notably psychosurgery, ECT, and longer term medication with serious side-effects.

Limits on force, restraint, or deprivation of liberty

Where an act for persons who lack capacity involves restraint or force, detaining them or otherwise depriving them of liberty, all UK jurisdictions require an additional test, balancing the act against the risk of harm without it. The test in RoI is more stringent. See p.532 for details.

Authorisation

This safeguard requires more intrusive acts, or those with more serious potential consequences, to be authorised in advance by a special panel,[53] given that they can be done to the person without their involvement and against their will (which would be impossible in RoI under the ADMCA, though it would be possible for acts governed by the MHA). Equivalent interventions can only be done under mental health or other noncapacity-based legal frameworks in the other jurisdictions, which incorporate safeguards similar to authorisation.

Agency principle

The most radical innovation in the ADMCA, and the reason it alone amongst the jurisdictions is fully compliant[54] with the UN CRPD (p.525), is that even when persons cannot participate at all (e.g. when in a coma), their decision-making representative is their legal agent and is bound by the person's known or likely will or preferences, rather than being free (as in the UK) to make a decision that seems to them to be in the person's 'objective' best interests.

---

53 Or the Court of Protection in E&W (outside the MCA framework, under its inherent jurisdiction).

54 This is a disputed point—many in the UK argue that the substituted decision-making regimes in the MCANI (and perhaps even the MCA in E&W) provide safeguards that sufficiently respect the rights, will, and preferences of the incapacitated person, to count as complying with the CRPD.

Capacity in children and adolescents

The same general <u>principles of capacity law</u> (p.522) apply to children as to adults, but with two significant variations:

• Children younger than sixteen are presumed to *lack* capacity in the UK.
• In some cases, children under this age can be shown to have capacity (referred to in this context as *competence*) if certain criteria are met.

Table 16.24 shows how these variations apply in each jurisdiction.

Table 16.24 Capacity in children and adolescents by jurisdiction

	E&W	Scotland	NI	RoI
Relevant law	MCA; Family Law Reform Act 1969; *Gillick* (p.756)	Age of Legal Capacity (Scotland) Act 1991	Age of Majority (NI) Act 1969; *Gillick* (p.756)	Advance Decision-Making (Capacity) Act 2015
Under 16s presumption	Lack capacity	Lack capacity	Lack capacity	**Have** capacity
Definition of capacity	If they have sufficient understanding and intelligence to understand fully what is proposed	If they are capable of understanding the nature and possible consequences of the treatment	If they have sufficient understanding and intelligence to understand fully what is proposed	Same as adults—able to understand and retain relevant information; use or weigh it to make decision; communicate decision
16-17 year olds	Have capacity for all purposes	Have capacity for all purposes	Have capacity for medical treatment	Have capacity for all purposes except advance directives
If parents and child disagree	A competent child can give consent even if parents refuse it, but parents can also give consent if child refuses it	Parents cannot override consent or refusal by a competent child	A competent child can give consent even if parents refuse it, but parents can also give consent if child refuses it	A child with capacity can give consent even if parents refuse it, but parents can also give consent if child under 16 refuses it
Additional information	MCA applies to 16 and 17 year olds High Court can overrule both competent child's and parents' refusal of consent	All under 16 year olds have legal capacity to make 'reasonable' transactions 'of a kind commonly entered into' by children	MCANI explicitly excludes children A further review of this area of law will occur after its implementation	s23 Non-Fatal Offences Against the Person Act 1997 governs treatment of 16 and 17 year olds

Despite the legal presumption in the UK that children younger than sixteen years old lack mental capacity until they are shown to have it, in practice many CAMHS services assume that twelve-to-sixteen-year-old children have capacity, unless there is a reason to doubt it, or it needs to be confirmed for legal purposes.

The ability of parents in E&W and NI to overrule a competent child's refusal of consent (even for sixteen and seventeen year olds) may contravene human rights law (p.516). This has not yet been legally tested.

The Scope of Parental Responsibility (SPR)

This concept, also known as the 'zone of parental control', was developed by the European Court of Human Rights (p.390). It is helpful for considering whether it is appropriate to assist parents or others with parental responsibility (e.g. a local authority in the case of a child in care) in overriding the decision of a competent child. A decision within the SPR is one which:
• the parents appear able to make in the child's best interests, and
• other parents would normally make for a child of that age.

The E&W MHA Code of Practice suggests that doctors should only rely on parental consent in the absence of the child or young person's consent for the treatment of mental disorder if the decision is within the SPR, and the young person lacks capacity. Otherwise, consider using mental health law (p.461) if it applies, or applying to the Court of Protection.

Advance statements, powers of attorney, and court powers

These options for managing the affairs and personal welfare of adults who lack capacity are generally not available for children younger than sixteen (eighteen in RoI). Instead, those with parental responsibility can decide for them, or others can be appointed to manage their affairs or welfare under child protection legislation.[55]

Criminal prosecution

The mental capacity law described here does not apply, by and large, to criminal proceedings. Instead, there is a separate age of criminal responsibility (p.406) and related rules of the youth justice system (p.352).

---

55 Principally the Children Act 1989, Social Work (Scotland) Act 1968, Children (NI) Order 1995, and Child Care Act 1991 in RoI. For a discussion of the complex field of Child Welfare and Child Protection Law, readers are advised to consult a textbook of child psychiatry or child & family social work.

Powers in mental incapacity

Mental capacity law means that acts on behalf of people who lack capacity do not amount to torts or crimes such as battery, conversion, or false imprisonment, as they would if done without consent. This protection is not absolute: applicable safeguards (p.528) must be complied with, and there are limits on the use of force and detention.

Restraint and the use of force

In order to restrain or otherwise use or threaten force to compel a person to comply with the act done on their behalf, this must be justified: as immediately necessary and for the minimum time (Scotland); necessary to prevent harm to the person (E&W, NI) or in exceptional emergency circumstances, necessary to prevent an imminent risk of serious harm to the person or others (RoI); except in Scotland, the act must also be a proportionate response to the likelihood and seriousness of harm.

Detention

The European Court of Human Rights has ruled that any detention or other 'deprivation of liberty' amounts to a breach of article 5 of the Convention (p.517) unless it follows a legal procedure, and the patient has access to a court or tribunal to challenge it.

What amounts to a deprivation of liberty?

There is no simple rule for determining whether measures amount to a deprivation of liberty. The ECtHR and the Supreme Court have ruled[56]:

- the distinction between a (lawful) **restriction** of liberty and a potentially unlawful **deprivation** of liberty is 'merely one of degree or intensity, not one of nature or substance';
- factors suggesting deprivation include restraint and control of social contacts, residence or movement for a significant time—the 'acid test' is being under complete supervision and control, not free to leave; and
- factors such as compliance or not objecting, the normality of the setting, and benevolence of purpose are irrelevant.

Authorising a deprivation of liberty

Beginning in 2008,[57] all four jurisdictions have developed legal regimes that can be used to authorise a deprivation of liberty in a way that complies with article 5. They all follow the principles in Box 16.2.

In Scotland, the relevant orders are an intervention order or guardianship order (p.534); in NI, the authorisation procedure described on pp.478, 488 is used, and in RoI an assisted decision-making or co-decision agreement or representative decision-making order can be used (p.534).

---

56 These tests come from _HL v UK_ (p.758) and _Cheshire West_ (p.751).

57 The first were the DoLS in E&W, described above. These followed the House of Lords' ruling in Bournewood (p.748) that up to 11,000 'involuntary informal' patients in care homes and elsewhere were unlawfully deprived of their liberty.

Box 16.2 Principles guiding authorisation of a deprivation of liberty

Measures amounting to a deprivation of liberty are only permissible if:
- they are <u>ordered by a court</u> as part of a decision on behalf of the person lacking capacity or a minor (p.534) *or*
- they apply to someone resident in a hospital or care home and special authorisation has been obtained (see below) *or*
- they are necessary to give treatment to sustain life or prevent a major deterioration, while a declaration is sought from the court.

In E&W a separate procedure exists under the DoLS/LPS[58] for a responsible body[59] to authorise a deprivation of liberty[60] if an independent assessor/AMCP certifies that it is for care or treatment, and the person:
- is over eighteen (over sixteen when LPS in effect) and has mental disorder;
- lacks capacity for the decision to accept care or treatment;
- under LPS, has been consulted (and their carers if appropriate), or under DoLS, does not refuse the care or treatment (including by <u>advance decision</u>, p.536, an <u>attorney</u>, p.538, or <u>deputy</u>, p.534);
- is not covered by other safeguards such as under the MHA; and
- the deprivation is necessary to prevent harm and a proportionate response to the likelihood and severity of harm (and under DoLS, in the person's best interests).

A right of appeal exists to the Court of Protection.

Research

Research on subjects who lack capacity, who cannot <u>consent</u> (p.482) to the risks involved, requires special permission from a research ethics committee, and is only appropriate if it could not be carried out on subjects with capacity. There must be a chance of the research benefiting the subject, and the costs of participating (e.g. the time taken and the risk of discomfort or pain) must be reasonable when balanced against the possibility of benefit. Alternatively, if there is no personal benefit, unintrusive research carrying a negligible risk of harm can go ahead if it is likely to increase knowledge about the subject's condition or a related condition.

---

58 Deprivation of Liberty Safeguards (DoLS) have been criticised as unwieldy, bureaucratic, expensive, and underutilised. The Mental Capacity (Amendment) Act 2019, when it comes into force in 2023, will replace them with less complex Liberty Protection Safeguards (LPS).

59 A CCG/LHB or Local Authority, or (under LPS) an NHS hospital's management. Under DoLS, the treatment must be in a hospital or care home.

60 There is no power under DoLS/LPS to authorise the most extreme forms of treatment against the patient's will. An order from the Court of Protection is required: <u>NHS v FG</u> (p.756).

Court powers in mental incapacity

Intervention orders

In Scotland, anyone with an interest in the personal welfare or property of persons without capacity (or those person themselves) can apply to the Sheriff Court for an intervention order. This can authorise anything that persons would have been able to do themselves if they had capacity. It can include appointing someone to perform specific acts or make specific decisions on their behalf.[61]

A criminal court can also make an intervention order as an alternative to another <u>sentence</u> (p.456) if the defendant lacks capacity and it believes this to be the most appropriate disposal.

Decisions, deputies, and representatives

In E&W, NI, and RoI, the Court of Protection, High Court or Circuit Court (but not criminal courts) can make decisions on behalf of persons lacking capacity, or appoint a deputy ('representative' in RoI) to make a specific health, welfare, or financial decision or class of decisions for them. This is analogous in E&W and NI to the Scottish intervention order. In RoI the representative is bound by the known wishes and preferences of the persons and cannot make their own 'objective' decision for them.

Assisted decision-making and co-decision-making

In addition to reforming powers for courts to make decisions for people lacking capacity, and to appoint decision-making representatives, the ADMCA in RoI also introduced assisted decision-making agreements and co-decision-making agreements. These agreements, which do not need the involvement of a court if other formalities are complied with, provide legal recognition of the role of a trusted friend or advisor who obtains and explains information, facilitates the persons making a decision, and relays their decision to others, or who makes decisions jointly with them.

Guardianship orders in Scotland

In E&W and NI, <u>civil guardianship</u> (p.488) is a form of community treatment for mental disorder under mental health law, and does not require evidence of incapacity. By contrast, in Scotland a guardianship order[62] can only be applied to a person who lacks capacity, although that incapacity need not be due to mental disorder. As with intervention orders, a guardianship order can be made by a criminal or civil court. They are oft-used; in 2018, 13,501 orders were in force.

Anyone with an interest in the personal welfare or property of someone without capacity (or, as with an intervention order, that person themselves) can apply to the Sheriff Court for a guardianship order, on the grounds that the person's long-term incapacity means they cannot

---

61 The court can require appointees to pay a deposit, (to 'find caution'), which they forfeit if they act improperly or cause loss to the person. It may also require a guardian to do this.

62 Before the AWIA, there was a similar form of guardianship for those under eighteen and (loosely) those who lacked capacity, known as curatorship; the guardian was known as the 'curator bonis'.

safeguard their own interests adequately. Additionally, the local authority is under a duty to apply for one if it thinks these conditions are met.

A guardianship order can last for any period, the default being three years, and can be renewed by the court. The guardian can be any appropriate relative or friend, or a social worker in the case of a guardianship order on the grounds of personal welfare alone. The guardian is required to visit the patients regularly, investigate their affairs, and report to the Public Guardian and/or the local authority on their actions every month.

As with a <u>welfare power of attorney</u> (p.538), a guardian appointed on the grounds of personal welfare may (if the guardianship order permits it) consent to medical treatment, but cannot consent to treatment for mental disorder against the person's will.

The Court of Protection

In E&W, the Court of Protection was for centuries responsible for managing property and financial affairs of those lacking capacity, exercising the king's so-called *parens patriae* ('father to the country') jurisdiction on his behalf. The Court was revised and reconstituted by the MCA, and now deals with financial and personal welfare matters in respect of those who lack capacity (e.g. decisions about residence and care, writing a statutory will, or the appointment of deputies). Only specially designated judges may sit.

Advance statements

Anyone can make a statement in advance about what they would like or not like to happen in a given situation in the future. Such advance statements can be relevant to deciding how to treat persons who have subsequently lost capacity to decide for themselves.

Binding advance decisions

In E&W, advance decisions by adults to *refuse* treatment are binding on doctors (and the courts) in specific circumstances. To be binding, an advance decision must be **valid** and **applicable** (Box 16.3).

Box 16.3 Criteria for validity and applicability of advance decisions in E&W

An advance decision is valid if, at the time of the proposed treatment:
• It has not been withdrawn while the patient still had capacity.
• It has not been superseded by a relevant <u>lasting power of attorney</u> (p.538).
• The patient has not done 'anything else clearly inconsistent' with it remaining a 'fixed decision' (e.g. requesting a blood transfusion after making an advanced decision to refuse all life-preserving treatment).

An advance decision applies if, at the time of the proposed treatment:
• The patient lacks capacity.
• The proposed treatment is specified.
• The current situation is envisaged.
• There are no 'reasonable grounds for believing' that the patient would not have made the advance decision if they were in the situation that has now arisen.

Advance decisions can only allow a refusal of life-sustaining treatment if they contain an explicit written, signed, witnessed statement that they apply to such treatments.

A valid, applicable advance decision to refuse treatment overrules a decision made by the donee of a <u>lasting power of attorney</u> (p.538).

Generally, valid and applicable advance statements are overridden by the MHA—the major exception is <u>ECT</u> (p.198), which can be refused in advance (see p.484).

The ADMCA in RoI likewise makes advance decisions to refuse treatment that meet its criteria legally binding. The criteria are those in the box above, except that the decision must have been made voluntarily and must be in writing. There are additional rules for situations such as pregnancy, and the law requires advance directives requesting (rather than refusing) certain treatments to be considered. Written reasons must be given by the doctor if they are not followed.

In NI, common law requires doctors to accept 'effective' advance decisions refusing treatment. What counts as 'effective' in the relevant common law[63] is unclear, but includes that the person making the decision must have been over eighteen and have had capacity at the time, and to be clear and specific in what it covers. The MCANI requires the government in NI to review the common law on advance decisions within three years, with a view to enacting a statutory rule like that in E&W.

Nonbinding advance statements

A variety of provisions of mental capacity and mental health laws require doctors and others to consider previously expressed wishes of patients, before they make a decision in the patient's best interests—this obviously includes any advance statements.

The MHCTA in Scotland requires psychiatrists to consider any written, signed, and witnessed advance statement when they make decisions on treatment for mental disorder under the Act. Likewise, the AWIA states that 'account must be taken' of wishes expressed in such statements, including in relation to life-sustaining treatment.

Answers to the questions below may help in deciding whether a nonbinding advance statement[64] should be taken into account in a given situation.

- Does the statement clearly envisage the current situation? For example, a statement refusing resuscitation in the context of terminal cancer would not apply for resuscitation after a myocardial infarction.
- Is the course of action in the statement both legal and clinically justifiable? For example, an advance statement, no matter how specific and clearly drafted, cannot justify a decision to give a drug to cause death,[65] or to give amphetamines for bipolar disorder.
- Has the patient since done anything to withdraw the statement, or that is inconsistent with it, or suggests they have forgotten it or consider it to have been withdrawn?
- Is the statement consistent with what relatives and friends say the patient would have wanted? (If it differs, that does not necessarily invalidate it, but it may reduce the weight given to it.)

---

63 For example _F v West Berkshire_ (p.755).

64 Some authors believe that article 8 (p.517) of the European Convention on Human Rights (p.518) makes at least some advance statements of the kinds listed in this section directly binding, despite not being made so by capacity law. This has not been tested in court.

65 At the time of writing, euthanasia is illegal throughout the UK and RoI, although there have been debates in E&W in particular about not prosecuting those who assist in euthanasia for terminally ill relatives.

Powers of attorney

What is an attorney?

An attorney is someone appointed to take decisions on behalf of someone else. Originally, in an age before the rapid communication made possible by the telephone and the internet, people travelling abroad for several weeks or more might appoint a trusted attorney to take decisions on business or financial matters that could not wait until their return.

The basic form of the power of attorney can be revoked by the donor (the person who appointed the attorney[66]) at any time. The power can only apply to decisions involving financial matters or other property—not to health or personal welfare decisions. As the attorney can only make decisions or exercise power that the donors could themselves have exercised, if the donors lose capacity (and therefore cannot make such decisions themselves), the attorney's power also ceases.

A power of attorney puts the donee in the position of making decisions as if made by the donor. There are no rules relating to what decisions should specifically be made.

Enduring, continuing, and lasting powers of attorney

Recognising the limitations of the original power of attorney in common law, governments have legislated to create the Enduring (or Continuing) Power of Attorney (EPA/CPA), and the more extensive Welfare Power of Attorney (WPA) and Lasting Power of Attorney (LPA). Table 16.25 shows which forms apply in each jurisdiction. In E&W and NI, EPAs made under older laws remain valid, but the table only lists the newer and more extensive LPAs.

Like simple powers of attorney, the donor must be over eighteen (or over sixteen in Scotland) and have capacity when granting the power. The donor can grant a general power, or one limited to specific decisions or types of decisions. It would almost always be inappropriate for a treating psychiatrist or other similar professional to be the donee of an LPA or WPA covering health, welfare, or personal care decisions.

---

66 Therefore, the attorney is sometimes known as the *donee*: that is, the person who has been given the power. In Scotland, the donor may be called the *granter*, and the donee the *grantee*.

Table 16.25 Forms that affect powers of attorney in different jurisdictions

	E&W	Scotland	NI	RoI
Name of the power	Lasting Power of Attorney	Continuing or WPA	Lasting Power of Attorney	Enduring Power of Attorney
Relevant law	Mental Capacity Act 2005	Adults with Incapacity (Scotland) Act 2000	Mental Capacity Act (Northern Ireland) 2016	Assisted Decision-Making (Capacity) Act 2015
Decisions covered	Personal welfare, property and affairs	Property and financial affairs (CPA); personal welfare (WPA)	Care, treatment, personal welfare, property, and affairs	Personal welfare, property, and affairs
Conditions on making welfare decisions	Donee must reasonably believe donor now lacks capacity	Donee must reasonably believe donor now lacks capacity	Donee must reasonably believe donor now lacks capacity; no conflicting effective advance decision	Donee must consult family and act in accordance with what donor was likely to do
General restrictions on donee	Must act in best interests of donor	Must be satisfied act will benefit donor, and is least restrictive option	Must act as common law fiduciary (in donor's interests & for their sole benefit)	Must act in best interests of donor
Restrictions on welfare power	Cannot restrain[67] donor unless restraint is necessary, and proportionate to the harm prevented	Cannot authorise treatment for mental disorder against the will of the donor	Cannot authorise deprivation of liberty and can only restrain donor if necessary and proportionate to likely harm	Cannot restrain donor unless an emergency, and necessary and proportionate to imminent risk of serious harm
Other information	LPA must be registered with the Public Guardian before it has effect	CPA or WPA must be registered with the Public Guardian before they have effect	LPA must be registered with the Public Guardian before it has effect	EPA must be registered with the Directorate when donor loses capacity

67 In this context, *restraint* refers to using force or the threat of force, or restricting the donor's liberty or movement.

Mental capacity and other social roles

Marriage

A person must have mental capacity in order to marry. A decision to marry[68] cannot be taken on their behalf by anyone who would be able to take other decisions on their behalf, such as an <u>attorney</u> (p.538) or a <u>deputy</u> (p.534).

However, the test of capacity has a low threshold that in E&W requires only a 'rudimentary' understanding of the marriage contract, including that there may be financial consequences, plus capacity to decide to engage in sexual relations.

Conducting legal proceedings

A complainant or defendant in civil law proceedings must have adequate mental capacity to conduct proceedings, even with professional legal representation. The general test of capacity (e.g. under the <u>MCA</u> in E&W, p.522) applies. If they lack capacity, despite adjustments to the process to assist them, their interests will be represented instead by an Official Solicitor from the Office of the Public Guardian.

In criminal law, defendants currently face a quite different test of ability, known in E&W as the *Pritchard* criteria: see p.602.

Entering into contracts

People with mental disorder can make valid contracts. However, if a contractor lacks mental capacity at the time, then under common law the contract is invalid if the other party knew at the time that the person lacked capacity.[69] In addition, a contract may be set aside by a court if they consider it sufficiently 'unconscionable' or 'improvident', which might be the case if it appeared to exploit the vulnerability of a person without capacity.

Wills and testamentary capacity

Disputes may arise over the making of a will. A psychiatrist may be requested to provide an opinion on whether the testator possessed testamentary capacity, defined as follows:

- **E&W** and **NI**—ability to understand the nature of the act and its effects, to understand the extent of the property being disposed, and to appreciate the claims of others to which one ought to give effect; not being inhibited in any one by mental illness.[70]
- **Scotland**—the person must comprehend what a will is and what would be the consequences of making one.
- **RoI**—The person must have 'understanding and reason' and not suffer from mental conditions such as 'delusion, insane suspicion, or aversion'.

---

68 The same applies to decisions on other family matters such as divorce and adoption, and to a decision to consent to sexual acts.

69 The MCA in E&W and the MCANI require that even in this situation a person lacking capacity must pay 'a reasonable price' for the supply of any 'necessary' goods or services.

70 See *Banks v Goodfellow* (1869-70) LR 5 QB 549; *Key v Key* [2010] EWHC 408 (Ch); *Walker v Badmin* [2015] WTLR 493.

Voting

The law is unclear on whether electors must pass a test of mental capacity to be allowed to vote, especially in E&W. Old common law rules disenfranchising prisoners and people with mental disorders have been abolished; in RoI, all prisoners may vote, and in the UK people on remand (p.398) or detained under civil mental health law (p.478) may vote, if necessary using the hospital or prison as their address.[71] Electoral Commission guidance is that people who lack capacity probably cannot be stopped from voting, but that they do need capacity if they wish to appoint a proxy to vote on their behalf.

Jury service

Considerable restrictions on jury service affect those with mental disorder.[72] In RoI, anyone who suffers from mental disorder and is still receiving treatment cannot be a juror. In NI, anyone with a diagnosis of mental disorder is automatically excluded. In E&W only psychiatric inpatients, those subject to guardianship or a CTO, and people lacking mental capacity are disqualified; in Scotland, only *detained* inpatients and those subject to guardianship are excluded.

Driving

Complex rules govern fitness to drive in the presence of various mental (and physical) disorders. In the UK, the Driver and Vehicle Licensing Agency (DVLA), and in RoI the Road Safety Authority (RSA), must be informed of any medical condition that might affect fitness to drive. This means a doctor may be required to breach confidentiality (p.320) and inform the DVLA or RSA if the patient refuses to do so. The DVLA's rules relating to mental disorder currently forbid the following from driving, amongst others:
- a person who is currently psychotic,
- a person with bipolar disorder who has had more than three episodes in the last year, unless that person has been well for six months,
- a person with epilepsy who had daytime seizures in the last ten years,
- a person with severe intellectual disability, and
- a person with dementia who has poor short-term memory, disorientation, and lack of insight and judgment.

---

71 The ECtHR ruled in *Hirst* (p.757) that all prisoners should be allowed to vote. The UK refused for twelve years to implement this ruling, but in 2017 agreed to re-enfranchise prisoners on temporary release and home detention curfew, in addition to remand prisoners. This was accepted as within the margin of appreciation (p.516) of article 3 of the first protocol to the ECHR.

72 In addition, persons who have been convicted of a serious offence usually cannot serve on a jury until five to ten years after their sentence ends (or at all, if they receive a life, indefinite, or extended sentence in the UK).

Other powers to detain or treat

Powers to access or remove persons in need of care

In Scotland,[73] local authorities may remove <u>vulnerable adults</u> (p.574) from their home for their health or safety or that of others.[74] A psychiatric assessment may be requested. Certain people who have intimidated, exploited, or endangered them may be denied contact. This is a more extensive, enforceable system than is available under the statutory <u>safeguarding of vulnerable adults</u> (p.590) guidance in E&W. No equivalent exists in NI or RoI.

Police powers

Police have powers to protect vulnerable people, including those with mental disorder. In E&W and NI, these include powers to enter and search premises to arrest someone for provoking violence, retake someone liable to be detained in prison (even if transferred to hospital), or save life and limb or prevent serious damage to property.[75] In Scotland and RoI, police have a common law power to enter property if they detect a 'disturbance' or hear cries for help or of distress.

Infectious diseases

All jurisdictions provide[76] for a magistrate to order persons with a serious infectious disease to be detained in hospital if they refuse treatment or otherwise act in a way that makes the spread of the infection likely. This might be relevant to patients with mental disorder who also have conditions such as Covid-19 or tuberculosis, who cannot be treated for it under <u>mental health law</u> (p.461).

Common law emergency powers: the doctrine of necessity

In the UK there is a general common law power to 'take such steps as are reasonably necessary and proportionate to protect others from the immediate risk of significant harm', a power that 'applies whether or not the patient lacks capacity to make decisions for himself' (_Munjaz_, p.763). Another case (_Black v Forsey_, p.748) added that all private individuals have a legal power to restrain or detain 'in a situation of necessity, a person of unsound mind who is a danger to himself or others'. The power was held in _Munjaz_ to permit seclusion of informal patients, and could be considered by extension to include a power to give treatment in prison or other settings outside hospital, if that is 'reasonably necessary and proportionate' to the 'immediate risk of significant harm'.

However, the UK Supreme Court subsequently ruled (_Sessay_, p.767) that the common law doctrine of necessity does not apply where mental

---

73 This power was abolished in E&W by the Care Act 2014 (see p.734), though there and in NI it is possible (though expensive and unwieldy) to apply to the High Court for a similar order, or an order allowing social workers or others to gain access to someone at risk.

74 Under s14 of the Adult Support and Protection (Scotland) Act 2007. A court order is required before the person may be removed from their home.

75 PACE S17(1) (c)(iii), (cb), and (e), respectively; PACE art 19(1)(c), (ca), and (e) in NI.

76 Under s37 of the Public Health (Control of Disease) Act 1984 in E&W, s39 of the Public Health etc (Scotland) Act 2008, s3B of the Public Health (Northern Ireland) Act 1967, and s38 of the Health Act 1947 in RoI.

health or capacity law are available. Hospital staff cannot detain or treat a patient in hospital under common law, even in an emergency, except as an interim measure while MHA or MCA processes are followed, and providing that there is no 'undue delay'.

It is likely that courts in RoI would recognise similar common law emergency powers, but this too has not been tested in court.

Making an arrest and preventing crime

In addition to the general common law emergency power above, criminal law[77] provides a power to members of the public to 'use such force as is reasonable in the circumstances in the prevention of crime, or in effecting or assisting in the lawful arrest (p.571) of offenders or suspected offenders or of persons unlawfully at large'. This enables restraining and secluding an inpatient, whether informal or detained, if necessary to prevent them committing an offence (e.g. assaulting another patient or member of staff) or restraining someone in the community who has absconded from detention in hospital.[78]

Preventing a breach of the peace

The common law provides every citizen, not just police officers, with a power to use reasonable force to prevent a breach of the peace (p.425), meaning the use or threat of violence or disorder. In the leading case (*Laporte*, p.760), the House of Lords ruled that 'every citizen enjoys the power and is subject to a duty to seek to prevent, by arrest or other action short of arrest, any breach of the peace occurring in his presence, or any breach of the peace which (having occurred) is likely to be renewed, or any breach of the peace which is about to occur'. This enables a nurse or doctor in a hospital or a CPN or social worker in the community to restrain a person or patient whose abusive or threatening behaviour is likely to provoke imminent violence.

---

77 Specifically, s3(1) of the Criminal Law Act 1967 for E&W, and s3(1) of the Criminal Law (NI) Act 1967, which are identically worded. S4(1) of the Criminal Law Act 1997 in RoI, which allows for citizen's arrests (p.571), implies a similar power to use reasonable force. In Scotland, a similar rule applies under common law.

78 This is in addition to statutory powers under mental health law to retake such patients. Technically, the power to use reasonable force in these circumstances does not apply to people meeting the legal test for insanity (p.620), at least in E&W; the power in *Black v Forsey* above could apply in such cases.

The rights of victims of patients

Victims' rights in general

The <u>prosecution service</u> (p.566) is meant to promote the interests of victims as well as the Crown (or the People in RoI). However, there have been calls for increased recognition of victims' experience. In practice, crime victims can expect assistance:

- at the time of any criminal trial where they are witnesses and
- at the time of any offender's discharge where they may be affected.

Standards of support for victims

Victims Charters are in place in E&W, NI, and RoI that indicate standards of service provision that victims of crime can expect to receive from the CJS. These services are not founded on a legal right of the victim (beyond the legal rights to information and to make representations referred to below); the charters take a 'needs-based' approach to victim services and distinguish between those victims who are eligible for special service provision and those who are not.

The Code of Practice for Victims of Crime 2015 sets out requirements for various agencies within the CJS; these include the <u>police</u> (p.570), <u>Probation Service</u> (p.584), <u>Prison Service</u> (p.578), Witness Care Units, HM <u>Court Service</u> (p.372), and <u>Youth Offending Teams</u> (YOTs, p.585). It represents a minimum standard of service and aims to ensure that victims are provided timely, accurate information about their case at all stages of the criminal justice process. The victims may choose not to receive services, or request modification of the services they receive.

In Scotland, the Executive has produced National Standards for Victims of Crime, including the rights to information, support, and participation. The Victim Notification Scheme provides the victim with information about offenders sentenced to custodial sentences of more than eighteen months.

Victim support services

Victims of crime in E&W and NI may also be supported by Victim Support, independent charities which offer free assistance, including advice and help for psychological and emotional needs, as well as practical help. Other charitable victim groups include Support After Murder and Manslaughter. Similar organisations exist in Scotland and RoI. These charitable organisations have turned their attention towards a 'rights-based' approach to victim's needs. The USA has used this latter approach for some time and has introduced the Victim's Rights Act across different states as statutory legal requirements affording rights to a range of victims.

Victims' rights under mental health law

In the UK and RoI, victims of crime by a mentally disordered offender who has committed a serious sexual or violent offence (or in RoI, any offence resulting in <u>committal for treatment</u>, p.500) have the right to information about the offender's detention in (or transfer to) and release from hospital, and (in the UK) to make representations about those issues, whether or not the patient is subject to a <u>restriction order</u> (p.510).[79] In Scotland, the law applies to offenders sentenced to imprisonment, or compulsion orders with restrictions, or transfer directions. These are shown in Box 16.4.

The law in E&W and NI places a number of statutory duties on the Probation Service (and their Victim Liaison Officers) and on hospital staff, tribunals, and other bodies, all of whom have a duty to consider victims' views. In inpatient facilities, the MDT <u>social worker</u> (p.226) will often take on the statutory role of liaising with past or potential victims in order to assess their needs and rights.

Mental Health Tribunals have addressed cases on whether to admit victims' testimony into evidence, and to what extent information from MHTs may be shared with victims.

Box 16.4 Rights of victims of mentally disordered offenders in the UK and RoI

To make representations (in the UK) about:
- whether any discharge or release should be subject to conditions or supervision requirements if applicable (e.g. under a restriction order or a licence) and
- if so, what those conditions should be.

To be informed about:
- when the patient is to be discharged or released from hospital,
- what conditions or supervision requirements (if any) they will be subject to after discharge or release, and
- in RoI, about the escape or death of the patient or their recall to hospital.

In Scotland & NI, the law also allows victims to make representation and to receive information about leave from hospital and its conditions.

---

79 Relevant laws are the Domestic Violence, Crime and Victims Act 2004 (DVCVA) for E&W and NI, the Criminal Justice (Scotland) Act 2003 and Mental Health Scotland Act 2015, and the Criminal Justice (Victims of Crime) Act 2017 in RoI.

Chapter 17

Civil law

Tort law and negligence

Tort law deals with breaches of general duties to others, as opposed to breaches of duties to society (crimes, p.400), or of a duty arising from an agreement with a specific individual (breach of contract).

Tort law aims to restore victims (claimants or pursuers) to the position they would have been in had the tort not occurred, through monetary compensation ('damages') by the defendant. In a few cases, equitable remedies (p.366) such as 'specific performance' may be applied.[1]

Major categories of tort are shown in Box 17.1.

> ### Box 17.1 Major categories of tort
> - Negligence
> - Nuisance (e.g. noise or pollution)
> - Libel (written) and slander (spoken)
> - Intentional torts[2] (e.g. battery, false imprisonment, trespass, and conversion)
> - Economic torts (misrepresentation, restraint of trade)
> - Statutory torts (competition law, product liability etc.)

Only negligence is of relevance to psychiatrists, apart from occasional evidence on mental state and capacity in intentional tort cases.

Negligence

The law of civil negligence is built upon the principle of **neighbourship**: that we each have a legal duty to consider the welfare of those 'near' us. Where you fail to act as a good neighbour, and that failure causes harm, the law requires you to pay damages equivalent to the harm. Key questions are:

- Who is my neighbour? (To whom do I owe a **duty of care**?)
- What is the standard of being a good neighbour in this case? (What amounts to **breach** of that duty?)
- What harm (**damage**) did my neighbour suffer?
- Did my being a bad neighbour **cause** the harm to my neighbour?
- How will the amount (**quantum**) of damages be calculated?

Duty of care: who is my neighbour?

In simple terms your neighbour is anyone you ought to have in mind when you do something. Examples include:

- individuals who occupy adjacent property—neighbours in a literal sense;
- the user of a product or service;[3] and
- the client of someone claiming to have special expertise or knowledge, for example the patient of a doctor (see clinical negligence, p.550).

---

1 For example in the tort of conversion, where the defendant (the 'tortfeasor') has used the claimant's property as their own, and the property is of great sentimental value to the claimant but little monetary value, requiring the tortfeasor to return the property instead of paying damages.

2 Many intentional torts are similar to crimes. In tort, however, the claimant sues for compensation for the harm suffered, whereas the State prosecutes crimes and inflicts punishment.

3 Not merely the purchaser who is owed a duty in contract law: _Donoghue v Stevenson_ (p.753).

For a person to owe a duty to another, they must be 'so closely and directly affected' by the person's acts that it is reasonable to expect the person to take them into account (i.e. there must be **proximity**); harm must have been **reasonably foreseeable**; and it must be **fair, just, and reasonable** for a duty to exist.[4]

What amounts to breach of duty?

- Someone who knowingly exposes their neighbour to a substantial risk of harm is in breach of their duty to the neighbour (this is analogous to recklessness in the criminal law, p.403).
- Someone who fails to realise that they are exposing their neighbour to a substantial risk of harm is still in breach of duty if a **reasonable person** would have foreseen the potential harm.[5]

Causation: did my actions cause the harm?

This underlying principle is simple: would the harm have resulted if the defendant had not acted as they did? This 'but for' test can be complex and often rests on expert evidence (including psychiatric evidence where the harm is psychological):

- If a **new event intervened** before the harm occurred, and was not reasonably foreseeable, the defendant did not legally cause the harm.
- If the harm was **too remote** from the defendant's actions, they have not legally caused it (this is similar to saying the harm must be reasonably foreseeable). For example, depression caused to bystanders who witness an accident is too remote.
- If it is impossible to establish the cause (e.g. because medical science cannot separate possible causes in a complex clinical negligence case), then a different standard of material contribution (p.551) may be used.

Quantum: how much must I pay in damages?

The aim is to restore the claimant to the position they would have been in had the breach not occurred, so far is practicable. It can be difficult and arbitrary to assign monetary values to harms such as pain, the loss of a limb, or psychological trauma; though loss of employment arising from them may be easier to calculate. Courts use schedules of standard values for harms such as amputation, blindness, or paralysis.

If there are several defendants—all of whom owed a duty, breached that duty, and caused the harm—the quantum will be shared between them. If the claimant is deemed to have **contributed** to the harm by their own negligence, the quantum will be reduced.

Expert evidence on prognosis, treatment, or support needs may be relevant to quantum.

4 This is the 'threefold test' laid down by the House of Lords in *Caparo v Dickman* (p.751).

5 If defendants hold themselves out as having special knowledge or experience, the test involves being a 'reasonable' member of that profession: for example the *Bolam* test (p.748) for doctors.

Clinical negligence law

Claims can arise from any aspect of a clinician's professional interaction with a patient: not merely technical procedures (e.g. <u>ECT</u>, p.198) but also for example not giving all relevant information in seeking consent, or unreasonably failing to recommend <u>detention for treatment</u> (p.478).

The usual elements of a claim for <u>negligence</u> (p.548) apply: the doctor must owe the claimant a **duty of care**; they must have **breached** that duty; and that breach must have **caused the harm** the claimant suffered, in order for a **quantum** of damages to apply.

Gross clinical negligence can occasionally result in criminal charge of <u>gross negligence manslaughter</u> (p.414).

When clinicians owe a duty of care

Medical and other practitioners owe duties of care to:
- a patient they have treated personally,
- a potential patient to whom they have offered their services,
- a patient reasonably referred to them who they failed to assess or treat,
- a patient treated by someone for whom they are responsible (e.g. a trainee supervised by them),
- a relative of a patient who might be harmed by nondisclosure of information about the patient, in the exceptional circumstance that the relative has a relationship of 'close proximity' with the clinician.[6]

What amounts to a breach of duty

The courts have adopted a 'peer review' approach to clinical negligence: would the allegedly negligent practice be accepted as proper by a responsible body of clinicians from the same profession (the *Bolam* principle, p.748)?

However, the following caveats apply:
- The opinion of the responsible body of clinicians must have a logical basis (*Bolitho*, p.748).
- When disclosing information prior to seeking consent to treatment, all 'material' risks[7] must be disclosed, not merely those that a responsible body of clinicians would disclose.
- Where there is no relevant body of clinicians, the standard is that of an averagely competent and well-informed person performing the relevant function in that setting (e.g. a receptionist in A&E: *Darnley*, p.752).

Breaches by trainees

The law holds all professionals, including trainees, to the same standard of care. However, those who are not experts in a particular field (because they are in training, or they normally practice in another field) are expected to know their limitations and to seek advice when needed. A supervisor can be liable for the negligence of a trainee, if consulted by the trainee.

---

6 For example where the relative has often taken part in discussions with the clinician and patient, or has been a participant in family therapy with them: *ABC v St George's* (p.745).

7 Risks that, in the circumstances, a reasonable person in the patient's position would think significant, or that the doctor knew (or should reasonably have known) that particular patient would think significant: *Montgomery v Lanarkshire* (p.762).

Causation in clinical negligence

Establishing the 'chain of <u>causation</u>' (p.549) in clinical negligence cases is often more complex than in other cases, because:

- There may be multiple negligence claims, one relating to the genesis of the medical condition (e.g. a workplace or road traffic accident, or an industrial disease), and another relating to allegedly negligent treatment.
- It may be unclear what harm would have resulted from the underlying medical condition with non-negligent treatment.
- There may have been many different practitioners from multiple professions involved in the care provided, and it may not be possible to disentangle the effects of breaches of duty by one or more of them.

In cases where (perhaps because of the second and third points above) it cannot be established whether it was more likely than not that the harm would have occurred 'but for' the breach of duty, the court may apply an alternative test of whether the breach 'materially contributed' to the harm (<u>Bailey v MoD</u>, p.747).

Clinicians as employees and as private practitioners

Clinicians who practice privately are wholly liable for any negligence claims. However, those who are employees will share liability for negligence with their employer, who is **vicariously liable** for the employees' actions.

In the NHS, this brings the clinician both advantages and disadvantages:

- Cases will often be managed, and damages will usually be paid, by NHS Resolution[8] under NHS indemnity.
- NHS indemnity may even cover self-employed clinicians (e.g. locum GPs) if their status is deemed 'akin to employment' by the court.[9]
- The interests of the employer may be different from those of the clinician (e.g. the NHS might want to settle a claim out of court, whereas a doctor might want to defend it, to preserve their reputation).
- If the claim relates to any work the clinician does outside their contract of employment, it will not be covered by NHS indemnity: the clinician will be personally liable for the proceedings and any damages.

For these reasons clinicians, especially doctors, are strongly advised to maintain personal medical defence cover, even if they undertake no private practice, so that they can be independently legally represented if necessary, and can continue proceedings in their own name if the NHS wishes to settle its part of the claim. Cover is also necessary for situations where the employer takes action against the doctor, for example under employment law, in relation to <u>inquests</u> (p.560), or in <u>professional conduct</u> proceedings (p.552).

---

8 This runs the NHS Clinical Negligence Scheme, which helps NHS employers learn from past negligence cases and avoid acting (or having employees who act) in ways that may be negligent. For example, it produces advice on safe record-keeping and good communication, failures in which are two of the most common reasons for being unable to defend a negligence claim successfully.

9 <u>Whetstone v MPS</u> (p.770).

Professional regulatory law

Complaints to professional regulators can run in parallel with civil and criminal actions. For example, a professional who drinks heavily at work and is later apprehended driving home may be subject to:
- an action in civil negligence (p.550) by any patient harmed by professional decisions they took whilst intoxicated,
- a criminal charge of driving whilst intoxicated,
- disciplinary action (p.557) by their employer, and
- fitness to practise proceedings (p.642) by the regulator (p.294).

Professional standards

In general, professional regulators uphold the following standards:
- Standards of conduct and performance (e.g. being honest; not having sex with your patient).
- Standards of competence or proficiency (e.g. undergoing regular appraisal and revalidation,[10] keeping accurate, contemporaneous records).
- Standards of continuing professional development (e.g. keeping your knowledge up to date, developing your skills).

Common scenarios

Psychiatric practice circumstances that most often result in a finding of **unfitness to practise**, according to medical defence organisations, include:
- poor-quality clinical care, for example prescribing and failing to change an antipsychotic (p.200) that then produces severe tardive dyskinesia;
- missing a diagnosis, particularly organic conditions (p.116) with psychiatric presentations, and coincidental comorbid conditions;
- breaches of confidence (e.g. through inappropriate disclosure, p.320, at a MAPPA meeting, p.592);
- sexual boundary violations (p.302); and
- inadequate risk assessment (p.163) or management (p.237), leading to suicide, escape, or harm to others.

Professional liability for the actions of patients

Persons under your control—The UK courts have held that there is a duty of care towards those who might reasonably foreseeably be harmed by the actions of those under your control, if you fail to exercise proper control (_Home Office v Dorset Yacht Co_, p.758). Whilst this could not be applied to patients treated in the community (since the patient is not 'under your control'), it is possible that a court could hold a doctor or hospital liable for harm caused by detained inpatients over whom it negligently failed to exercise proper control. This might even extend to a duty to prevent them acting violently (p.296).

---

10 Revalidation is a periodic (usually five-year) process of the regulator ensuring the practitioner has undergone sufficiently rigorous appraisal, including (where appropriate) reviewing mortality and other data. It was introduced in the UK in response to the Shipman inquiry (p.782), and is now operated by the GMC, NMC, and HCPC, but with requirements varying depending on the degree of risk posed by the profession concerned. There is no equivalent system in RoI.

Duty to warn or to protect others—In the USA, courts have ruled that psychiatrists and therapists have a legal duty to protect identifiable third parties who are at risk from patients under their care, by warning them, notifying the police, or taking other reasonable protective steps (*Tarasoff*, p.769). For many years, courts in the UK avoided laying down such a duty in cases where they might have decided otherwise,[11] but the High Court has recently ruled that there may be a duty to disclose such information to a relative with whom the doctor has a relationship of 'close proximity'.[12]

Duty to the patient—Doctors and hospitals owe a duty of care to their patients to diagnose and treat them adequately, and in certain cases will be liable for consequent harm if they fail to do so (e.g. for the pain and suffering caused by a missed diagnosis). However, they are not liable to their patient for failing to prevent them offending: a patient cannot base a claim for negligence upon their own offending behaviour (*Clunis*, p.751).

---

11 See for example *Palmer v Tees*; *Surrey v McManus*; and *K v Home Office*, pp.764, 769, 759.

12 *ABC v St George's* (p.745): this concerned the nondisclosure of genetic information, but contained *obiter dicta* that a risk of violence to that relative would also be covered.

Family law

Family law deals with conflicts and disputes that arise in the context of close and enduring relationships. It is more <u>reflexive</u> (p.355) and less adversarial in process than criminal law and other areas of civil law.

Matters which come before family courts typically involve the break-up of personal relationships and the care and protection of children. Examples include contested divorces, adoption, child abduction, wardship (where the court supervises a child's care), child protection, parental responsibility, and children's residence and contact with parents.

Who are the parties?

There are usually at least three parties in child welfare proceedings, and often more. They may include:
• the mother;
• the father;
• the children, represented by (for example) a Guardian ad Litem;
• other relatives who seek to be involved in the children's care; and
• the State, most often the local council responsible for child protection.

Principles

Where children are involved, the court is bound by the <u>family legal principle</u> (p.355) that the welfare of the child is paramount; the role of the family court is to determine what is in the 'best interests' of children. Other potential aims, such as doing justice to the parents and other parties, are subservient.

Private and public law proceedings

Legal disputes concerning children may be matters of private law (concerning disputes between individuals), and/or of public law (where the State intervenes to protect children). The differences and interactions between the two can be complex, and have a significant impact on those involved. For example, a local authority can usually only remove children from their mother's care under public law if there is evidence of significant harm arising from that care; whereas if the grandmother with whom the mother and children live applies for a special guardianship order,[13] which is a private law matter, the mother could lose the care of her children if the court considers the grandmother a more suitable guardian—a much lower threshold than 'substantial harm'.

Family courts

Family courts may seek expert evidence on a range of matters, including psychiatric evidence addressing the mental health of children and young people, and evidence concerning the impact of any parental mental disorder on their provision of care, and any risk to children. Psychiatrists who work in CAMHS, perinatal services, and forensic services are more likely to have the kind of expertise that is helpful to the family court.

---

13 Or its equivalents in Scotland, NI, or RoI.

E&W has a specialist <u>family court</u> (p.384); in NI, hearings may take place in County Courts, Family Proceedings Courts, or the High Court. In Scotland, the majority of hearings take place in the Sheriff Courts. In RoI, hearings take place in the District or Circuit Court.

Legislation

There are a number of relevant statutes: the following is a nonexhaustive list.
- Family Law Act 1996, Children Acts 1989 & 2004 in E&W
- Family Law (Scotland) Act 2006, Children (Scotland) Act 1995
- Children (Northern Ireland) Order 1995
- Family Law Act 1995, Children Acts 1997 & 2001 in RoI

Employment and equality law

Employment law deals with complaints by employees of being unfairly or wrongly dealt with by employers, including wrongful dismissal (p.646), and maltreatment during employment (causing, for instance, psychological harm). This is relevant to forensic psychiatrists instructed to prepare reports in relation to the effects of adverse treatment or work conditions, including disciplinary proceedings and dismissal.

Equality law is concerned with eliminating unlawful discrimination. It places responsibilities on employers and others[14] to prevent or avoid discrimination. Most employees with mental disorder are eligible for the protection offered by the legislation described below; psychiatrists may be involved in demonstrating how the disorder places the claimant in a protected group, or how alleged discrimination might have affected them.

Specific legislation

Equality Act 2010 (UK), 2004 (RoI)
These almost identical acts implement EU law (p.390). The UK Act replaced the Disability Discrimination Acts, and consolidated others such as the Race Relations Act and Sex Discrimination Act.

In broad terms the relevance to people with mental disorder is that the Act protects anyone who has, or has had, a disability (along with seven other 'protected characteristics': age, gender reassignment, marriage or civil partnership, race, religion or belief, sex, and sexual orientation). Disability includes people who have **any substantial mental impairment** if it has a substantial and long-term adverse effect upon their ability to perform normal day-to-day activities. The prohibited forms of discrimination and examples are shown in Box 17.2.

Box 17.2 Prohibited forms of discrimination

Direct discrimination
Refusing to serve a person in a shop because they are Black.

Indirect discrimination
Requiring all prospective employees to be at least a certain height, as this will prevent many more women obtaining a job than men.

Discrimination arising from disability[15]
Evicting a tenant with schizophrenia who has sublet their property in breach of the tenancy agreement, if the symptoms of schizophrenia made it harder for them to control his behaviour and adhere to the rule prohibiting subletting.

---

14 Such as those running businesses or providing services to the public.

15 This disability-specific third form was added in order to reverse the decision of the House of Lords in *Lewisham v Malcolm* (p.760), which was thought wrongly unfavourable to disabled persons.

Health & Safety Acts

These Acts[16] place duties upon employers to their employees, including people with mental disorder, to ensure a safe workplace and safe working practices. There is also a duty to protect the mental health of employees.

Tort law

Separately, the common law provides remedies for damage to mental health caused by employers' negligence (p.548):

- If psychiatric harm has occurred when such harm to the individual concerned was reasonably foreseeable (p.549). Foreseeing harm relates to both the nature of the job and any known individual vulnerabilities.
- Employers must take reasonable preventive action if harm is foreseeable.

Employment tribunals

These independent judicial bodies determine disputes between employers and employees. They consist of three members, including a legally-qualified chair. The Employment Appeals Tribunal is the higher tribunal. In RoI, an employee can present a complaint to the Rights Commissioner Service, with referral on to the Employment Appeals Tribunal. Complaints under equality legislation are heard by an Equality Tribunal.

Disciplinary proceedings

These are conducted by the employer and relate solely to the doctor's contract of employment; although they may run in parallel with professional regulatory (p.552) or negligence proceedings (p.548).

The grounds for dismissal in the NHS Consultants Contract are shown in Box 17.3; those in trainee doctors' contracts are very similar. Terms in non-NHS contracts may differ significantly.

> **Box 17.3 Grounds for termination of employment in the NHS consultants' contract**
>
> - Conduct
> - Capability
> - Redundancy
> - Failure to maintain registration with the GMC etc.
> - Failure to comply with a relevant statute
> - Any other 'substantial reason in a particular case'

16 Health & Safety at Work Act 1974 in the UK; Health & Welfare at Work Act 2005 in RoI.

Immigration and extradition law

Immigration law deals with the rights of noncitizens to enter and stay in the UK and RoI. Relevant to psychiatric practice are:

- Asylum seekers—who have lodged an application for asylum.
- Refugees—who have had their asylum claim accepted.
- Mentally disordered offenders with no right to remain in the country.
- Defendants facing trial in foreign courts and subject to extradition requests.

People may have no right to remain because of illegal entry, overstaying, or breaching conditions (e.g. engaging in paid employment without permission). Unless the matter is dealt with as a criminal offence, the usual outcome of breaches of immigration law is removal[17] to the country of origin. Direct appeals to **immigration appeal tribunals**, and further appeals to courts under human rights law (p.516), are available but may take months or years to complete. Psychiatric evidence may be relevant to fitness for deportation or extradition (p.648).

Law relating to deportation

In the UK, anyone who receives a prison sentence of a year or more is automatically deported unless an exception applies, or it would breach their human rights. In RoI, there are far fewer deportations, and deportation is not automatically considered following conviction.

Appeals against deportation on human rights grounds usually relate to article 2 or 3 rights (alleging that the person would be killed or subject to torture or inhuman or degrading treatment or punishment in the country concerned) or article 8 rights (alleging that deportation would breach their right to a family life, by separating them from parents, children, or other relatives). In the UK, statute law[18] sets a high threshold for article 8 claims for serious 'foreign criminals': courts can only allow a claim if:

- they have been resident for most of their life, are socially and culturally integrated, and face obstacles to integration in the new country;
- they have a partner who is British or has indefinite leave to remain, or a child who is British or has lived in the UK for seven years, and the impact of their deportation on the partner or child would be 'unduly harsh'; or
- there are other 'very compelling' circumstances.

Access to mental healthcare

Those who are not citizens of the UK or RoI are, in general, not entitled to the benefits of citizenship,[19] such as free healthcare from the NHS or HSE, or social care from local authorities, or benefit payments. A major exception is compulsory treatment provided under mental health law (p.461),

---

17 Removal is termed 'administrative removal' when the right to remain has expired, and 'deportation' when it follows criminal conviction (or a decision of the Minister).

18 s117A-D Nationality, Immigration and Asylum Act 2002 (inserted by the Immigration Act 2014).

19 Those with certain immigration statuses such as 'indefinite leave to remain' are entitled to healthcare and other benefits of citizenship. Citizenship of certain other countries, especially former countries of the British Empire, may confer some benefits of UK citizenship when that person is in the UK. Others have the right only to urgent treatment which stabilises their condition.

for which no person can be charged. In E&W and Scotland this also means that noncitizens can be provided with free NHS <u>after-care</u> (p.492), although this does not extend to social care or housing (i.e. accommodation that does not count as 'continuing healthcare').

Removal of mentally disordered people

The deportation or removal of mentally disordered people is permitted under human rights law, subject to the following:
- Convicted offenders who receive mental health disposals (including <u>hybrid orders</u> (p.504)) are exempt from automatic deportation in the UK, but may still be deported if the Secretary of State deems this 'conducive to the public good'.
- However, convicted foreign offenders who receive mental health disposals count as 'foreign criminals' for the purposes of the restrictions on article 8 claims described above.
- If a person has no, or only minor, criminal convictions, or was found unfit to plead (or is in RoI rather than the UK), then the restrictions on article 8 claims do not apply. However, a **proportionality assessment** will still be carried out and the effect of removal on their health will be weighed against the 'public interest' in removal, including any criminal or immigration history.
- The relevant minister may lawfully order a restricted patient be discharged from hospital in order to facilitate deportation.[20]
- Detained patients can also be repatriated under mental health law by being transferred as an inpatient to another country which has undertaken to continue their treatment.

Extradition

Extradition law allows a foreign country to request the surrender of an individual to face trial. The rules vary depending on the extradition treaties individual countries have signed with each other. Neither the UK nor RoI extradite those suspected of political offences or where the country requesting extradition applies the death penalty to the alleged offence (unless a commitment not to apply the death penalty is made).

Inquest law

Most deaths do not require any legal inquiry by a coroner or (in Scotland) Procurator Fiscal: the cause of death will be clear, uncontested, natural, and involve no suspicious circumstances, and so a doctor may issue a death certificate. However, a death must be reported[21] if any of the following apply:

- The cause of death or identity of the deceased is unknown.
- The deceased died in custody or State detention.
- The doctor suspects the death was due to:
  - poisoning or exposure to a toxic substance;
  - the use of a medicine or psychoactive substance;
  - violence, trauma or injury, or self-harm;
  - neglect including self-neglect;
  - treatment or a procedure of a medical or similar nature; or
  - an injury or disease attributable to employment.
- The death was otherwise unnatural.
- There is no doctor able to sign a certificate (i.e. a doctor did not see the deceased after death, or within the fourteen days before death, or during their last illness).

In 2019 around 40% (210,900) of deaths in E&W were reported to a coroner; 478 of these reported deaths occurred in State detention.

Postmortems and inquests

Where no cause of death is given, a postmortem examination will usually be ordered to ascertain it.[22] If a natural cause of death is established, the investigation will usually cease, unless there is reason to suspect that it resulted from some culpable human failure. An inquest or Fatal Accident Inquiry (FAI) must be held if the criteria in the Box 17.4 are met.

> ### Box 17.4 Main grounds for an inquest or Fatal Accident Inquiry
>
> - If the death was in custody or State detention
> - If it was violent or unnatural (in Scotland, sudden or suspicious)
> - If the cause of death remains unknown despite a postmortem
> - In Scotland, after an accident at work
> - Certain deaths overseas if the body is returned[23]

Inquests and FAIs are fact-finding inquiries, to establish who the deceased person was, and when, where, and how they died. They should be held within six months of the death; some can take years to conclude, particularly if they are adjourned while separate criminal trials and/or a public inquiry take place. Approximately 30,000 inquests were opened in 2019 in

---

21 Usually by GPs, hospitals, and the police, but any person may report a death. In E&W doctors have a duty to report such deaths as soon as practicable, unless another doctor has already done so.

22 This amounts to around 20% of all deaths in E&W, or around 10% of those in Scotland and NI.

23 Service personnel only in Scotland.

E&W; approximately fifty to sixty FAIs, presided over by a Sheriff, are held in Scotland each year.

'Article 2' Inquests

Inquiries into deaths in custody or State detention (including under mental health law), or where the State allegedly has some direct responsibility for the death (including by failing to take reasonable steps to protect life where a risk of death was known or ought to have been known), may have additional obligations under article 2 of the ECHR (p.518), which protects the right to life. Such inquests or FAIs must consider the wider circumstances surrounding the death. They are often longer and more complex as, in addition to scrutinising individuals' actions, they will consider the systems and protocols put in place by State bodies to protect lives.

Inquest conclusions and Sheriff's determinations

At the end of the inquest or FAI, the coroner or jury will record a conclusion, or the Sheriff will make a determination. Sheriffs' determinations are always 'narrative': in that they set out the facts of the death in detail and explain the apparent causes in a few sentences. A coroner's 'Record of Inquest' may also adopt a narrative style to formally record a conclusion (and did so in around 20% of cases in 2019), but in the majority of cases a more traditional 'short form' conclusion will be returned such as:

• accident (or misadventure)—25% of inquests in 2019;
• suicide—15%;
• natural causes—13%;
• unlawful/lawful killing—0.5%; and
• industrial disease.

The standard of proof (p.380) for all inquest conclusions is the balance of probabilities. Although an inquest conclusion cannot be incompatible with a prior criminal finding of fact, there is no bar to an inquest returning a finding of unlawful killing following acquittal for a homicide offence because of the different standards of proof.

If the coroner finds that there is a risk of similar such deaths occurring in the future (typically because systems and protocols used by State bodies to protect life have not been sufficiently improved), they may issue a Prevention of Future Deaths report to which the body must respond.

Part V

Psychiatry within the legal system

The criminal justice system

The system

The criminal justice system (CJS) comprises a variety of State and private agencies and institutions that <u>define</u> (pp.22, 400), detect, prosecute, try, and punish crime according to <u>criminal process</u> (p.398). Other organisations with a role in crime prevention (including education, health, and social services) are not usually seen as part of the CJS.

Detection and investigation

The <u>police</u> (p.570) are the organisation with primary responsibility for identifying crime, by responding to reports of possible crime from victims and others (including police officers), investigating those reports, and gathering evidence for prosecution. Other specific bodies, some of which are part of the police service in the UK and RoI, include:

• The Royal Military Police and the Military Police Corps, each of which is responsible for policing British and Irish armed forces respectively, at home (when on duty in military facilities) and abroad.
• The UK National Crime Agency (NCA) and the National Bureau of Criminal Investigation in RoI, which co-ordinate specialist technical, cybersecurity and intelligence teams and local police forces to target serious and organised criminals.
• Specialist intelligence agencies with their own powers of investigation and sometimes arrest, including MI5 (the Security Service) and MI6 (the Secret Intelligence Service) in the UK, and G2 (Directorate of Military Intelligence) in RoI.
• The Home Office's Border Force, concerned with <u>immigration</u> (p.558) matters, and Her Majesty's Revenue and Customs also have powers of investigation and arrest. In RoI, these tasks are performed by the police.

Prosecution

In E&W the Crown Prosecution Service is a nonministerial department responsible for public prosecution of individuals charged with criminal offences. The same role is performed by the Public Prosecution Service in NI, the Office of the Director of Public Prosecutions in RoI, and the Crown Office and Procurator Fiscal Service in Scotland. These services are responsible for criminal cases beyond the police investigation, and involve giving advice to the police on bringing charges, and preparing and presenting cases for court.

Trial

Criminal charges are heard in criminal <u>trial courts</u> (p.372), comprising lower courts that hear less serious charges such as Magistrates' Courts and District Courts, and higher courts for more serious charges such as Sheriff Courts, Circuit Courts, and Crown Courts. These courts have their own <u>roles at court</u> (p.376), <u>procedures</u> (p.378), and <u>rules</u> (pp.380–383).

Offences committed by serving members of the armed forces and by prisoners of war are tried by Courts-Martial, according to military law. Their processes and personnel are similar to those of ordinary criminal courts, but in addition to ordinary offences Courts-Martial try offences relating to breaches of military discipline, and can impose military penalties (e.g. demotion to a junior rank).

The Criminal Cases Review Commissions[1] in the UK review convictions if new evidence comes to light that may render them unsafe, and can then refer a conviction back to an <u>appeal court</u> (p.372).

Sentences and punishment

Sentences imposed by criminal courts can be divided into three main types:

- Sentences of <u>imprisonment</u> (pp.448–453), carried out by the <u>prison service</u> (p.578).
- <u>Community sentences</u> (p.454), supervised by the <u>Probation</u> <u>Service</u> (p.584), which also advises the court on sentencing options.
- <u>Fines</u> (p.456) and other sentences, which are monitored by the court itself or by its agents such as bailiffs.

In addition, <u>court-imposed mental health orders</u> (p.461) are supervised by a government department if <u>restrictions</u> (p.510) are added to the order. In E&W and RoI, this is the Ministry of Justice; in Scotland, the Directorate of Criminal Justice; and in NI the Department of Health, Social Security, and Public Safety. Each department contains a unit that <u>manages restricted patients</u> (p.588), approving decisions on leave, transfer, and discharge.

---

1 The CCRC covers E&W and NI; it has been criticised in recent years for failing to investigate adequately, and for referring fewer cases to the court (down from an average of 3.3% when first set up, to less than 1% by 2018). The Scottish Criminal Cases Review Commission performs the same role in Scotland. In RoI, there is a procedure for applying to the Court of Criminal Appeal with evidence of a miscarriage of justice.

Social services

Across the UK and RoI <u>social workers</u> (p.226) are based in a variety of public and voluntary settings including schools, hospitals, community health settings, and prisons. In the voluntary sector, social workers work for fostering and adoption agencies, organisations related to substance use, domestic abuse, rape, group work programmes, and many others targeting specific service user groups.

Partnership working

Social care support requires working in close collaboration with other local services, including health, criminal justice, education, and voluntary and community organisations. There is an increasing convergence, in both policy and practice, of social care and criminal justice, which can create new opportunities to improve support for offenders with multiple needs, those at risk of offending, and their families.

Local authorities can use wider powers to create safer and stronger communities to help people with multiple needs in the CJS. Every local authority in the UK and RoI is involved in a number of overlapping partnerships, such as Community Safety, Integrated Offender Management, Troubled Families, Safeguarding Adults, and Health and Wellbeing Boards. These each offer an opportunity to co-ordinate efforts, to improve outcome for individuals and the communities in which they live.

Adult criminal justice

Social care has a key role in reducing offending through, for example, resolving problems with housing, financial welfare, or the needs of children and families. There is a considerable overlap between social care and probation, and in RoI, the Probation Service is staffed entirely by qualified, registered social workers and performs the functions that would be performed by social services in other contexts.[2] In the UK, <u>probation organisations</u> (p.584) and social services tend to share some roles in a variety of partnerships. With these, social services:

- influence local strategies to support people with multiple needs,
- work with other services to meet those needs more efficiently, and
- offer personalised social care support, including to those in prisons in their area.

Changes to sentencing laws in the UK over the past twenty-five years have led to significantly greater numbers of elderly prisoners (including some who are frail or have dementia), with far greater social care needs.

Youth justice

People who have been 'looked after' by social services are over-represented in the CJS, both as children and later as adults. They are likely to have experienced multiple disadvantages, trauma, and abuse, which can contribute to challenging behaviour and other difficulties. Around half of children in

---

2 In the case of adults. In respect of children, most social services in RoI are provided by Tusla, the Child & Family Agency.

custody in E&W have been in care at some point. Social services are involved in preventative programmes that aim to reduce the chances of children in care offending (including <u>multisystemic therapy</u> and <u>functional family therapy</u>, p.218).

Police services

Whereas there is a single national civilian police service in RoI, the Gardai,[3] in the UK police functions are divided between a patchwork of services[4]:

- Territorial police forces, such as the Metropolitan Police in London or the Yorkshire Police, which carry out the majority of policing.
- Special national forces for particular functions, such as the British Transport Police (patrolling public transport), the Civil Nuclear Constabulary (protecting nuclear installations), and the National Crime Agency (co-ordinating agencies fighting serious and organised crime).
- Small, specific police forces created by miscellaneous laws, such as local Parks Police and Port Police forces.

Personnel

All police officers are legally known as 'constables' in the UK, and 'guards' (Gardai) in RoI. More senior officers include sergeants, responsible for a team of constables or Gardai; inspectors, in charge of day-to-day policing on a given shift; superintendents, responsible for a police station; and chief superintendents ('borough commanders' in London), responsible for policing a subdivision of the police area.

Many E&W forces employ civilians (who lack police powers of arrest[5]) such as Police Community Support Officers who patrol areas alongside regular officers.

Throughout the UK and RoI, Criminal Investigation Departments are staffed by detectives whose role is to investigate reported crime and to gather evidence for prosecution.

In 2012, the College of Policing was established with the aim of ensuring future officers are qualified to degree level, and Police and Crime Commissioners were elected across E&W to provide local political oversight.

Functions of the police

The original role of the earliest police forces was to maintain public order. Police roles have diversified since then, and now include:

- maintaining public order (preventing a <u>breach of the peace</u>, p.425),
- protecting people (especially politicians and royalty) and property,
- detecting and recording crime,
- investigating reported crime and gathering evidence for prosecution,
- arresting and detaining (suspected) criminals for prosecution,
- recovering and restoring stolen property, and
- deterring crime by having a high profile.

---

3 In full, the *Garda Síochána na hÈireann* (Guardians of the Peace of Ireland).

4 This is largely because of the historical British aversion to creating a single civilian organisation that a tyrannical monarch could use to subjugate and control the population. The Gardai, by contrast, evolved from the former colonial police in Ireland: rulers in London had no compunction about controlling the Irish population, and a single force was therefore formed.

5 Though some have limited powers to detain suspects until police officers arrive, in addition to powers to issue <u>fixed penalty notices</u> (p.441), confiscate alcohol and drugs, or seize vehicles, and the power of citizen's arrest mentioned above.

Police powers

Most police officers can exercise the following powers in certain circumstances (e.g. where an officer has reasonable grounds to suspect the person has committed a serious crime):

* stop and search people,
* arrest and detain people for questioning,
* search vehicles or premises and seize property, and
* take fingerprints and bodily samples for testing.

Citizen's arrest

All citizens, not merely police officers, have limited powers to prevent a breach of the peace (p.543); to detain mentally disordered persons (p.542) if they pose a danger to themselves or others; and to make a 'citizen's arrest'. The latter limited power[6] only applies if it is not reasonable or practical to wait for a police officer, and:

* if the suspect is (or the person has reasonable suspicion that the suspect is) **in the act** of committing a serious offence or
* if a serious offence **has been committed** and the suspect is (or the person has reasonable suspicion that the suspect is) guilty of it.

Policing strategies

The techniques police services use, and the functions they prioritise, have varied as technology and social expectations have developed. Some alternative strategies include:

* reactive policing (i.e. responding rapidly to reports of crime);
* community policing (i.e. high-profile officers getting to know a local area and its inhabitants well, deterring crime, and reassuring the public);
* intelligence-led policing (i.e. actively gathering information on possible crime); and
* problem-oriented policing (i.e. analysing patterns of crime in order to prevent crime).

Roles of the psychiatrist in relation to the police

Many people who come into contact with the police have a mental disorder. Psychiatrists may be involved in assessing suspects:

* in response to the use of police powers (p.494) when a person in public appears to be suffering from mental disorder;
* advising on diversion from custody;
* attending to medical needs;
* advising on fitness to be interviewed (p.573); and
* advising on necessity for an appropriate adult (p.574) during interview.

---

6 Under s24A of the Police and Criminal Evidence Act 1984 in E&W, art26 of the Police and Criminal Evidence (NI) Order 1989, s4 of the Criminal Law Act 1997 in RoI, and under common law in Scotland. Serious offence means 'indictable offence' in E&W, and 'arrestable offence' in NI and RoI.

In the police station

Arrest

Someone reasonably suspected of an offence may be arrested for questioning. They are taken to a police station unless the police take them to hospital for psychiatric assessment using <u>mental health powers</u> (p.494).

On arresting a suspect, the police officer must caution them about their rights. In RoI, NI, and Scotland, suspects have the **right to remain silent**, but anything they say may be recorded and used in evidence against them. In E&W, the right to silence is restricted by the fact that courts are allowed to draw inferences from it[7] (e.g. that they are trying to avoid revealing information that could be used to convict them).

Initial procedure

The custody officer[8] is independent of the investigating officers, and is responsible for:

- ensuring that the detainees' rights are upheld;
- informing the detainees of the reasons for arrest and the grounds for detention;
- informing the detainees of their right to private consultation with a solicitor;
- keeping a record of detention in custody;
- deciding whether there is sufficient evidence to charge them;
- calling in a healthcare professional—
  - for assessment of possible mental or physical disorder
  - for assessment of any injuries, or after allegations of excessive force or assault
  - if medical examination is requested—; and
- requesting an <u>appropriate adult</u> (p.574) to be present during interviews for all children and vulnerable adults.

Criminal justice liaison and diversion services

These psychiatric <u>diversion schemes</u> (p.268) provide direct access to a specialist mental health professional based within the police station, and can undertake initial mental health assessments, arrange transfer to hospital, and liaise with psychiatric services in courts and prisons.

Forensic medical examiner (FME)

FMEs or police surgeons are increasingly being replaced by nonmedical professionals, sometimes with the general title, health care professional. There is similar provision in all jurisdictions. They may consider:
- need for formal assessment under <u>mental health law</u> (p.461), and
- the detainee's fitness to be interviewed.

7 This makes the assessment of fitness to be interviewed all the more important, as someone interviewed when unfit might later improperly have adverse inferences drawn from their silence.
8 In RoI, the Gard in charge of the station is the equivalent of the UK custody officer. These duties are less clearly set out than is the case in the UK.

Fitness to be interviewed

Detainees should not be interviewed if they are likely to be harmed by the interview, or if it would later be considered unreliable. Any mental disorder may or may not render a person unfit to be interviewed; it is a functional test similar to capacity assessment (p.522).[9] The assessment includes mental state assessment and how it might affect ability[10] to:

• understand the interview's nature and purpose;
• comprehend questions;
• appreciate significance of answers given;
• make rational decisions about what to say; and
• reply in a manner unaffected by their mental condition (without necessarily having to be rational and accurate).

Sample questions are shown in Box 18.1.

Box 18.1 Sample questions for assessing fitness to be interviewed

• Do you understand why you were arrested?
• What did the caution given mean?
• What will the police want to find out at interview?
• What impact might it have if you said (e.g. an incriminating statement)
• What would you do if you did not want to answer a question?

Police options for dealing with vulnerable suspects

• Charge and bail (p.398) with or without conditions until the next court hearing.
• Charge and remand into custody (p.398) until the next court hearing.
• Give bail to return to police station at later date.
• Give a caution (p.440).
• Release and take no further action ('NFA').
• Arrange admission to psychiatric hospital (i.e. diversion, p.268), instead of or in conjunction with any of the above.

9 For detailed advice see Ventress, M.A., Rix, K.J.B., and Kent, J.H. (2008), Keeping PACE: fitness to be interviewed by the police. *Advances in Psychiatric Treatment*, (14), 369–381.

10 In E&W, the Police and Criminal Evidence Act (1984), Code C (2019), Annex G contains guidance.

Vulnerable suspects

Vulnerable adults are those who, due to a mental health condition:
- have difficulty understanding processes and procedures connected with arrest, detention, voluntary attendance, or their rights;
- do not appear to understand the significance of information, questions, or their replies;
- become confused;
- provide unreliable, misleading, or incriminating information without knowing or wishing to do so; or
- are <u>suggestible</u>, <u>compliant</u>, or <u>acquiescent</u> (p.160).

Appropriate adults

These are mostly volunteers with appropriate experience and some specific training in supporting vulnerable people in police custody. In the UK, vulnerable adults can only be interviewed if an appropriate adult is present, even if they do not request a legal representative or are interviewed voluntarily. There are statutory schemes for providing appropriate adults in E&W and NI, and an informal scheme in Scotland.

Who can be an appropriate adult?

An adult who is not a police officer, but is either:
- a relative or guardian (except in Scotland), or
- a professional with experience of dealing with those with mental disorder or other vulnerabilities (e.g. a social worker or psychiatric nurse).

In Scotland, vulnerable witnesses and victims are entitled to appropriate adults as well as suspects.

An appropriate adult should

- Offer advice and assistance.
- Observe that interviews are conducted properly and fairly.
- Facilitate communication with the interviewee (to protect them, and ensure that decisions to charge are not based upon misunderstandings).
- Help stop highly <u>suggestible</u> or <u>compliant</u> (p.160) people from making unreliable or false confessions or statements.

Children

In the UK, an appropriate adult must be present for interviews of anyone younger than eighteen years old.

In RoI, children under twelve cannot be arrested or detained in a station unless the offence is murder, manslaughter, rape, or aggravated sexual assault; instead, they must be taken to their parent or guardian to be questioned. Children younger than fourteen years old can only be charged with the permission of the Director of Public Prosecutions.

Court

Children and vulnerable adults may have difficulty understanding a court's language and what is expected. Article 6 of the <u>ECHR</u> (p.518) asserts that for a fair trial, defendants must be able to understand proceedings, and also 'participate effectively' (p.602). Judges can adapt proceedings to make them easier for vulnerable defendants to understand. This might include providing sign language interpreters; giving information slowly, in writing and orally; allowing a supporter to sit or stand with the defendant and explain proceedings; or allowing more adjournments than usual. Such adjustments are dependent upon identifying and assessing vulnerable defendants.

Liaison and diversion schemes

Criminal justice liaison and diversion psychiatric teams (p.268) work with police and courts to assess defendants and provide information to courts about their needs. They can support those in early stages of the criminal justice pathway and refer vulnerable defendants for treatment and support.

Investigative psychology

Investigative psychology has expanded and evolved significantly since its inception in the mid-1990s, and it seeks to ensure that any contributions psychologists make to police investigation or legal process must have an empirical, systematic, and scientific basis.

Investigative inferences

This includes offender profiling, geographical profiling, modelling offence styles, actions-characteristics equations, and psychological correlates of offence style.

Offender profiling ◐ draws inferences from available evidence about the mind and other characteristics of a perpetrator. It is employed most often in murder and rape cases, especially high-profile serial cases where police investigation is not progressing well. Currently offender profiling provides police with supportive investigative advice through experience, statistics, and information-sharing. Many police officers appear to view profiling favourably. However, it is rarely used as a basis for an arrest, merely for further investigation.

Evidence of the effectiveness of profiling is varied at best, with the least evidence in support of the pure clinical practitioner approach.[11] A major criticism of profiling is that there is currently no standardisation in profiling techniques or even awareness of recurring offender profiles.

Geographical profiling, by contrast, is uncontroversial. It assumes that crime locations are not random, and that geographically plotting them may reveal useful patterns, such as propinquity (the proximity of crime locations to significant places in the offender's life). Analysis of geographical morphology or geo-behavioural patterns may provide new lines of enquiry or focus existing ones. Geo-profiling software is sometimes used to support decisions in investigations.

Assessment of investigative and legal information

Psychological approaches help investigators in obtaining, handling, prioritising, and evaluating the utility, validity, and reliability of information gathered throughout the investigation. Psychologists support with the trajectory of the investigation and the synthesis of large amounts of data to ensure the most relevant factors are explored (on the basis of research evidence) and limiting the influence of individual investigator heuristics. They may also assist information gathering when a suspect is taken to a crime scene, or recreate the incident with a suspect using sounds, smells, and images in a 'cognitive interview'.

---

11 Offender profiling deriving from a clinical paradigm and aimed at direct self-incrimination by a suspect can prejudice a trial. In E&W the trial of Colin Stagg for the murder of Rachel Nickell was halted by the judge on the first day, when it transpired that the defendant had been induced to make incriminating statements to an undercover police officer who asked leading questions based on the profiling psychologist's advice. Some years later, another man was convicted of the murder based upon DNA evidence.

Investigative psychologists also examine material collected during investigations and presented in court to detect deception in false crime reports or false allegations and confessions. Research continues into factors influencing the reliability of witness testimony, facial recognition, children's evidence, and whether deception can be detected.

Prison services

Prisons and jails[12] perform two main functions: detaining people before trial (on <u>remand</u>, p.398), and isolating them from the rest of society as a punishment (a <u>sentence of imprisonment</u>, pp.448, 452). They can be divided into the following major groups, although in practice a single institution will often perform functions from more than one group:

• secure or 'closed' prisons,
• resettlement or 'open' prisons with minimal security, and
• juvenile prisons and <u>Young Offender Institutions</u> (YOIs, p.580).

Women and men (and male and female young offenders) are detained separately, usually in separate prisons. Closed prisons provide varying levels of perimeter security (<u>physical security</u>, p.190) and internal security (<u>procedural</u> and <u>relational security</u>, p.190); in E&W, they, and their inmates, are described as category A (maximum security), category B (medium security[13]), and category C (low security), with open prisons being described as category D; similar high/medium/low levels are used in the other jurisdictions. See Table 18.1.

Table 18.1 Prison estates in the UK & RoI, 2020-21

Prison type	England & Wales	Scotland	Northern Ireland	Republic of Ireland
Adult category A/high	8	1	1	1
Adult category B/medium	41	7	1	9
Adult category C/low	57	3	1	2
Adult category D/open	14	2	0	2
Young offender institution[14]	23	3	1	1
TOTAL[15]	120	15	3	12
Number of prisoners	78,081	8,195	1,442	3,729

Prisons in E&W, NI, and RoI often specialise in a single function (e.g. housing remand prisoners or young offenders), whereas those in Scotland more often comprise several units with different functions. Only a small proportion are women's prisons, as many fewer women are imprisoned.

Prison is expensive, costing from around £20,000 per year per prisoner in an open prison to £50,000 per year in maximum security (though still far cheaper than a secure hospital). <u>Reoffending rates</u> (p.587) after release are high, which may in part reflect the nature of offenders who are imprisoned, not merely the failure of prison to change their behaviour.

---

12 In the UK and RoI the terms are used interchangeably; in the USA, a jail is a local remand institution and a prison houses convicts. The term *training prison* is used in E&W to indicate the latter.

13 These are not equivalent to the security levels of <u>secure hospitals</u> (p.258). A high secure hospital corresponds roughly to category B, a medium secure unit to category C, and a low secure unit falls somewhere between categories C and D.

14 Those taking under eighteens plus those taking eighteen to twenty-four year olds.

15 Totals are lower than the sum of the lines above because some prisons contain areas of more than one category.

Areas of a prison

A typical British or Irish prison comprises the following units, although not all will be found in all prisons, depending on the prison's functions:

- a reception centre, where new inmates are assessed (including a brief assessment of mental health, suicide and self-harm risk and drug dependency), and where searches and other checks take place;
- a first night centre, where new inmates undergo an induction before moving into the main prison accommodation;
- a number of wings (long open galleries of cells) or houseblocks (cells/ rooms on separate enclosed floors) providing accommodation for prisoners on 'ordinary location';
- a vulnerable prisoner unit for groups of prisoners at risk of victimisation by other prisoners (e.g. sex offenders, former police officers);
- a segregation unit for individual detention of prisoners who have seriously breached prison rules, or who are at extreme risk of victimisation by others;
- a special unit (in some prisons, a Close Supervision Centre) for prisoners at very high risk of violence and/or escape;
- a healthcare centre or wing for the assessment and treatment of physically or mentally unwell prisoners, including outpatient facilities;
- an education and training centre;
- a workshop in which prisoners can learn practical skills, and make items that can be sold by the prison;
- one or more indoor and outdoor recreation areas; and
- a visitors' centre where supervised visits can be held.

Prison GP or medical officer

Every prison has one or more doctors, usually former or part-time GPs, who provide general medical services to the prisoners, from an outpatient clinic at the healthcare centre. Prisoners can usually refer themselves or be referred by prison officers.

Those requiring treatments that cannot be provided by a GP in an outpatient setting can be referred to local NHS secondary care services; a few services will offer specialist outpatient clinics within the prison, but in most cases (and for all urgent or inpatient treatments) prison officers will need to escort the prisoner to the hospital.

Role of the psychiatrist

The prison medical officers are supported by a number of other specialist staff, including in particular drug misuse and mental health 'inreach' (outpatient) and inpatient teams, often led clinically by a psychiatrist. Prison psychiatric services are described in more detail on p.270.

Adolescent secure services

In addition to adult prisons (p.578), a variety of services exist to keep children and young people in the custody of the State (Table 18.2). Unlike prisons, youth custody services not only detain people on remand (p.398) and as a sentence (p.442), but also under civil child care law, when their behaviour cannot be managed in foster care or an ordinary children's home.

There has been a very substantial decline in the use of secure facilities for children in the past twelve to fifteen years, especially in E&W and RoI. From 2009–2019 in E&W, for instance, there was a 70% decrease in the number of ten to seventeen year olds in custody, as it became used only for more serious offences.

A significant number of young people in the secure estate have previously been in local authority care (26% in YOIs, 36% in STCs and 40% in SCHs).

Young offender institutions

These are the juvenile equivalent of a prison, run by the prison service. However, the intended ethos is care, education, and rehabilitation, rather than punishment.

In E&W, there are two groups of detainees in YOIs: juvenile offenders aged fifteen to seventeen (units that take only this group are sometimes referred to as 'juvenile units' instead of YOIs) and young offenders aged eighteen to twenty-one. In Scotland and RoI, young people up to twenty-one are held in YOIs; in NI, children aged ten to seventeen can be detained in the sole Juvenile Justice Centre; those over eighteen are held in adult prisons. The sole such institution in RoI, Wheatfield Prison, no longer takes new prisoners, and will no longer act as a YOI once the remaining few inmates are released or transferred.

Secure Training Centres (STCs) and detention schools

STCs are purpose-built centres for young offenders up to the age of seventeen years in E&W and NI. They are often run by private operators under contract. STCs house vulnerable young people who are sentenced to custody or remanded to secure accommodation. They have a higher ratio of staff to young offenders ratio than YOIs and are smaller, so that an individual's needs can be met more easily.

In RoI, the State's three children detention schools for those aged eleven to seventeen were amalgamated into the Oberstown Children Detention Campus in June 2016, which will be the only secure institution for children once Wheatfield Prison YOI closes to children.

Local Authority Secure Children's Homes (LASCHs)

These accommodate young offenders and certain other vulnerable children between the ages of twelve and sixteen in the UK. They are run by local authority social care departments, overseen by national government health and education departments.

Adolescent secure hospitals

There are five <u>medium secure forensic psychiatric hospitals</u> (p.258) and six <u>low secure units</u> in the UK that care for under eighteens suffering from mental illness associated with difficult or offending behaviour. There are an additional two medium, and three low secure neurodevelopmental disorder (NDD) units. All children in secure mental health settings are detained under the MHA.

A new framework for integrated care for children and young people in the secure estate is being developed (SECURE STAIRS) in E&W and NI. This offers a 'whole system' approach to integrated care within the Children and Young People's Secure Estate. It draws on Trauma Systems Therapy, Enabling Environments, and Psychologically Informed Environments.

Table 18.2 Adolescent secure services in the UK & RoI, 2020-21

Institution type	England & Wales	Scotland	Northern Ireland	Republic of Ireland
YOI Juvenile units[16]	5	3	1	1
Secure training centre	3	-	1	1
Secure children's home	14	5	1	-
Adolescent secure hospital	6	-	-	-
TOTAL	28	8	3	2
Number of detainees	782	692	68	61

16 That is, only those taking under eighteens (plus eighteen year olds awaiting transfer to other institutions). The figure in the table on the previous page, by contrast, includes YOIs that take eighteen to twenty-four year olds.

Parole Boards

In the UK and RoI these boards direct or recommend the release of prisoners serving long sentences. They must consider the risk to the public on release. Their membership includes judicial, mental health, probation, criminology, and community or lay members. Hearings may be oral or paper-based, and are usually held in prisons.[17]

Decisions may be challenged by judicial review (p.374). In addition, in E&W provisional Parole Board decisions are checked by a unit in the Ministry of Justice (MoJ), which may request reconsideration if it thinks the decision might be unlawful or irrational; if the Board agrees, there will be a new hearing.[18]

Psychiatry and the Parole Boards

There are three main roles for psychiatrists at parole hearings:

- **Reports on patients under a psychiatrist's care** in prison or hospital. Such reports for the Parole Board (p.696) should deal with risks associated with release into the community in the same way as for Mental Health Tribunals, not within a criminological paradigm.
- **Independent expert reports** commissioned by the prisoner or the Minister, to advise on future risk in the community related to any mental disorder, and whether the prisoner requires psychiatric or psychological treatment to reduce the risk. Psychiatrists should not comment on risk in offenders who do not have a mental disorder.
- **Sitting as a Parole Board member** is practically and ethically distinct from the above, in that the psychiatrist is contributing a mental health perspective directly to making the decisions to release or not. They are expected, with the other Board members, to weigh up *all* of the available evidence in a judicial fashion.[19]

The Parole Board is concerned almost solely with protecting the public. Other factors, including the prisoner's interests, are considered but are given much less weight than in a clinical context. Whereas attempting solely to predict harms (as opposed to assessing risk of harm; see p.163) is discouraged in psychiatric practice, parole boards may seek the advice of a psychiatrist member about the relationship between future risk and mental disorder in those terms; as well as concerning:

- the prisoner's mental health and personality function,
- the interpretation of previous and current psychiatric reports,
- the current evidence base in relation to risk assessment and outcome,
- the role of drug and alcohol abuse in offending, and
- management strategies or interventions in relation to mental disorder.

The contractual duty of the psychiatrist is to the Board, which may conflict with their ethical professional duties (p.298).

---

17 Hearings for prisoners transferred to hospital may occasionally be held at the hospital: see p.506.

18 This mechanism was created following the Worboys (p.771) judicial review.

19 This is different from sitting as the medical member of a Mental Health Tribunal (p.513) since they have also to contribute to the criminological approach of the Board.

Patients in hospital

A patient who was transferred from prison cannot be released directly by a mental health tribunal prior to their earliest date of release (p.452) from prison: instead, the tribunal[20] will deem them ready for discharge, and a parole hearing will take place automatically, often in hospital.

The Parole Board hearing will address very similar evidence in a different and more adversarial paradigm: its presumption is continued detention, whereas the tribunal focuses on release; the burden of proof (p.380) lies with the prisoner rather than the detaining authority; and it can recommend less secure or open conditions as well as release.

Women and young offenders

There may be particular difficulties in commenting on risk in life sentenced women and young offenders, partly because they are unusual, and so may be subject to additional public scrutiny. High-risk, high-profile female offenders may be categorised as 'restricted status' (RS), meaning that they cannot be released by the Parole Board until their RS status is lifted. There are also anecdotal reports of the Parole Board wrongly failing to release women because of concerns about risk to themselves.

Details of the Parole Board in each jurisdiction

See Table 18.3.

Table 18.3 Details of the Parole Board in each jurisdiction

	E&W	Scotland	NI	RoI
Primary function	Risk assessing prisoners to decide whether they can be safely released into the community	Ensuring those prisoners no longer regarded as a risk are released into the community	Conside ration of suitability for release of prisoners sentenced to life imprison ment	To advise the Minister in relation to the administ ration of long-term prison sentences
Primary legislation	Criminal Justice Act 1967 Criminal Justice and Public Order Act 1994	Prisons (Scotland) Act 1989 Prisoners and Criminal Proceedings (Scotland) Act 1993	Life Sentences (Northern Ireland) Order 2001	Non statutory
Sentences considered by the Parole Board	All life, indeterminate (p.448) and extended sentences, plus determinate sentences (p.452) for serious sexual or violent crimes, or if recalled on licence	All life sentences Imprisonment >4 years	All life sentences	All life sentences

20 In the UK; in RoI, transferred prisoners cannot appeal to the tribunal.

Probation services

Probation began in the USA as an informal system allowing <u>sentencing</u> (p.442) to be delayed while convicted offenders submitted to supervision by local volunteers. If offenders 'proved' they had reformed their behaviour, they received a lighter sentence. In the early twentieth century, the system spread across the UK and became statutory. The aims of probation are to protect the public and reduce offending, with considerable debate about how this is best achieved.

Probation may be both a sentence in its own right and a form of supervision after a prison sentence. In the mid-to late-twentieth century, probation officers in the UK and RoI were trained as specialist social workers who provided personal support to offenders to help them avoid reoffending. From 1993 onwards, successive UK governments recast probation as a punishment, particularly in E&W, and probation officers as 'offender supervisors' acting on behalf of the courts—against resistance from probation officers who asserted the <u>welfare model</u> (p.355).

Roles of probation services

- Assessing offenders before sentencing and providing presentence reports advising courts on various sentencing options.
- Monitoring progress of offenders sentenced to <u>imprisonment</u> (p.448).
- Advising <u>Parole Boards</u> (p.582) on prisoner suitability for release.
- Supervising offenders released from prison under <u>licence</u> (pp.448, 452), and recalling them to prison if they breach licence terms.
- Managing Approved Premises (APs) where some offenders released on licence must live on release.
- Supervising offenders' compliance with <u>community sentences</u> (p.454) and reporting any breach of their sentence terms to the court.
- Advising offenders on available services in their local area, to help them avoid reoffending.
- Providing support or treatment to offenders, especially <u>group psychology programmes</u> (p.214; e.g. Think First).
- Specialist work with high-risk offenders with personality disorders within the <u>OPD programme</u> (p.260); screening offenders for PD and consulting with psychologists or psychiatrists attached to the programme.

England & Wales

National Probation Service—adults[21]

In E&W, most offenders under probation supervision are on community sentences; only about 30% are on licence following release from prison. NPS's work includes <u>risk assessment</u> (p.163) using tools such as <u>OASys</u> (p.170), and risk reduction through provision of accredited offender behaviour programmes. Its primary aims are to protect the public and reduce reoffending; although many individual probation officers believe strongly in promoting the welfare of (ex-)offenders, this is not an official priority.

---

21 In 2010, NPS was reduced to a rump supervising high-risk offenders, with contracted-out Community Rehabilitation Companies managing low-risk offenders. The reform has proved ineffective, and in 2020 the government announced that the CRCs would be reabsorbed by NPS.

Youth Offending Teams (YOTs)—age ten to seventeen years
There specialist multiagency services include offender managers and supervisors, police, CAMHS professionals, social workers, and education professionals. The team identifies the needs and risks posed by each young offender using a structured assessment process (e.g. ONSET and ASSET, p.170), planning interventions according to the assessment results. The emphasis is on offender welfare, and avoiding future reoffending, with a focus on re-engaging in education and involving caregivers and family, and in the case of restorative justice (p.440) measures such as referral orders (p.458), victims and local community representatives.

Northern Ireland

The NI probation system has a stronger rehabilitation focus than in E&W but is otherwise similar, with a split between the Probation Board for adult offenders, and the Youth Justice Agency (YJA, p.586) for young offenders.

YJA local offices organise diversionary youth conferences (p.458) providing community services to help local community re-integration and reoffending avoidance. Unlike YOTs, YJA directly employs all its local staff, who liaise with other agencies as needed.

Republic of Ireland

In the RoI the Probation Service is a single agency providing supervision to both adults and to young offenders (through its Young Persons' Probation division). Its focus is on providing assessments to the courts, and supervising offenders on licence and on community sentences. It also supports a number of practical (as opposed to psychological) training and outreach programmes.

Scotland

There is no Probation Service in Scotland. Instead, local authorities employ Criminal Justice Social Workers who assess and supervise over-sixteen-year-old offenders in Community Justice Partnerships, alongside social workers who supervise young offenders through the noncriminal Children's Hearings (p.386) system.

Psychiatrists and the Probation Service

Psychiatrists commonly have contact with probation officers through joint management of MDOs, on community orders (p.488) with a condition of treatment, or patients on licence (p.448), or through contributing to the risk management (p.237) of a patient subject to Multi-Agency Public Protection Arrangements (MAPPA) (p.592). Psychiatrists may also be involved in the Offender PD Programme (p.260), especially Pathfinder services and Intensive Risk and Rehabilitation Managements Services, which support high-risk offenders with personality disorders to improve their mental health and reduce their risk of reoffending. Psychiatrists may be involved in risk assessment, formulation, and care planning, including medication reviews.

Offender management

From the late-twentieth century onwards, governments in the UK in particular have come to see sentencing less as a semi-private matter between an individual judge and an individual offender, and more as a public act of a single overarching CJS. The collection of courts, prisons (p.578), and probation services (p.584) that deal with convicted offenders came to be seen as engaged in 'offender management', and new bodies were created to ensure they served the CJS's aims coherently.

England & Wales

The main agency dealing with offender management is Her Majesty's Prison and Probation Services (**HMPPS**), an executive agency of the MoJ. HMPPS manages[22] prisons including offender treatment programmes (p.220). In the community, it oversees probation hostels, APs, and victim support services (p.234). It conducts research evaluations to improve service specification, benchmarking, and costing. It advises government departments on offender needs, providing judges with information on costs and benefits of sentencing options.

The **Youth Justice Board** is a nondepartmental public body overseeing youth justice. It works with local authorities to provide secure schools and grants for services such as Youth Offending Teams (YOTs) (p.585).

The MoJ **Mental Health Unit** (MHU) oversees treatment of patients subject to restriction orders and directions (p.510). Their primary focus is public safety, not clinical need. Their staff consider applications for transfer to hospital (p.506), and for subsequent leave (p.486), transfer, remission to prison, or discharge. They provide opinions to tribunals (p.512). The MHU can also recall (p.589) conditionally discharged patients, vary their conditions, or absolutely discharge them.

Scotland

Community Justice Scotland co-ordinates public services, third sector and other bodies to reduce offending. The **Scottish Prison Service** manages the prisons. Police Scotland has a **National Offender Management Unit** contributing to the management of high-risk offenders in the community in coordination with the Risk Management Authority.

In 2019, a **Forensic Mental Health Unit** (FMHU) was set up within the Mental Health Directorate of the Scottish Government. The FMHU includes a Restricted Patients Team that manage restricted patients in Scotland on behalf of the Scottish Ministers. Like the MHU in E&W, each caseworker takes responsibility for a group of patients on an alphabetical basis. The team is responsible for approving transfers between hospitals, returns to prison, cross-border transfers, suspension of detention (p.486), recall from conditional discharge, and variations of conditions.

Northern Ireland

The **Department of Justice** oversees prisons, youth justice, policing, and community safety. It also works with the Courts and Tribunal service,

22 It runs public sector prisons directly, and manages contracts with private sector prisons.

and the Police and Probation Services of Northern Ireland. Each prison has an Offender Management Group, responsible for oversight of the review system, supported by senior probation officers and psychologists.

The **YJA** is responsible for dealing with offending by children and young people, through the delivery of a range of community based, court-ordered, and diversionary interventions, including youth conferences (p.458) and custody (p.580) where necessary.

Staff in the DoJ's **Criminal Justice Policy Division** perform the same functions in relation to restricted patients as the MHU in E&W and the Scottish Restricted Patients Team.

Republic of Ireland

The **Department of Justice and Equality** works with the Probation Service and the Irish prison service to reduce offending. A joint Strategy on the Management of Offenders was agreed in 2016 to improve coordination between departments. Restricted patients are managed by the same unit that oversees high-risk prisoners.

Reoffending and the effectiveness of offender management

There are many methodological problems (p.22) in the comparison of offending rates between countries, including offence definitions, data collection, and the provision of services that reduce offending risk after release such as housing and occupation. Table 18.4 shows some general figures, not broken down by age, sex, or ethnicity.

Table 18.4 Reoffending statistics

Rates of reoffending after one year	E&W	Scotland	Netherlands	
Harmonised rate (2019)	39.3%	27.2%	40.0%	
Rates on different bases	E&W	Scotland	NI	RoI
Imprisonment	60%	46.7%	37.7%	27.4%
Community sentences	32.8%	27.1%	27.5%	17%
Restriction orders	5.8%	No data	No data	n/a

Managing the restricted patient

In E&W, risk management of patients subject to <u>restriction orders</u> (p.510) is co-ordinated[23] with the MHUs of national <u>offender management agencies</u> (p.586). Clinicians discuss proposed admissions, <u>transfers</u> (p.506), <u>leave</u> (p.486), and <u>conditions of discharge</u> (p.511) with the patient's allocated MHU caseworker. Developing good working relationships with MHU caseworkers is a useful skill.

In hospital

Clinical care of restricted patients detained in hospital should not differ from unrestricted, or civilly detained, patients. Like all compulsorily detained patients, their care must be supervised by a Responsible Medical Officer (<u>RMO</u>, or <u>RC</u> in E&W, p.468), usually a consultant forensic psychiatrist, except where the MHU approved admission to a PICU or general psychiatric unit.

Leave

Leave (or in Scotland, <u>suspension of detention</u>, p.486) outside the ward, unit, or hospital[24] specified on the court order or transfer warrant must first be approved by the MHU. Clinicians must apply for leave using standard forms which require details about the patient's condition, the leave purposes, assessment of potential risks, and contingency plans to manage such risk. Applications can take several weeks at busy times. Emergency approval can be given over the telephone in rare circumstances. If emergency medical treatment is required, this does not require prior MHU approval, but they must be informed as soon as possible. Permission is not required for court appearances in E&W, but is required in Scotland.

Transferred prisoners who would not be eligible for parole or release (who have not reached their <u>EDR</u>, p.452, or completed their <u>minimum term</u> or <u>tariff</u>, p.448) are usually refused leave.

Incidents

Incidents involving restricted patients that result, or could have resulted, in serious harm must be reported to the MHU, including:
- serious injury, death, or serious property damage;
- <u>hostage-taking</u> (p.244);
- public protests (e.g. following access to a rooftop);
- <u>escape</u> or <u>absconding</u> (p.250); or
- any other incident requiring a formal serious incident review.

Transfer between hospitals or wards

Restricted patients cannot be transferred between hospitals without MHU permission—even emergency transfers to a higher level of security (in such cases permission will usually be given immediately by telephone, by the on-call MHU manager). Transfers between wards may be possible without

---

23 The MHU wishes the co-ordination to be on the basis of a partnership between it and the clinician, and many clinicians accept this model. Others, however, see the relationship as one of a 'productive tension' to balance patient and public welfare.

24 If the court order or transfer warrant specifies an entire hospital, leave within the hospital grounds can legally be granted without permission from the MHU, although this may be unwise if there is no secure barrier between the grounds and the community.

permission if the court order or warrant specifies a whole unit or hospital and both wards are within that unit. A standard form is required, and the process may take some time.

After conditional discharge

The main impact of restriction orders is seen when patients are conditionally discharged. Discharge planning for restricted patients should be as thorough as for any forensic patient. Conditions for each patient are derived from individual risk assessments and are designed to manage relevant risk factors. They usually include:

• residing at a particular hostel or other address;
• compliance with medication and other aspects of the care plan;
• attending appointments or accepting visits from supervisors;
• giving samples for drug or alcohol testing (and occasionally, refraining from drug or alcohol use entirely or only with permission[25]); and
• not entering an exclusion zone (specific streets or a whole postcode near a former victim's home or place or work, for example).

The MHU accept that junior doctors and junior social workers (or other care co-ordinators, who act as social supervisors with appropriate training) in practice often manage conditionally discharged patients. There must be a supervising RC/RMO and/or senior social supervisor who countersigns their statutory reports (p.511).

The psychiatric supervisor must have contact with the patient (including home visits) at least every three months, and ideally monthly; the social supervisor must see them weekly at first, reducing to no less often than monthly.

Recall to hospital

Patients who relapse, or breach conditions such that risk of relapse is increased (e.g. drug use in a patient known to become psychotic when using drugs), may be recalled from conditional discharge. The MHU will recall patients to available beds on the advice of supervisors, but the MHU can itself direct recall if there are reports of increased risk behaviours or if restricted patients are admitted informally for over six weeks. It is crucial to discuss concerns openly with the MHU or equivalent, even if you oppose recall, so that you maintain the trust of caseworkers.

---

25 This condition is only really practical if the patient accepts the legitimacy of it (e.g. because they are trying to stop using drugs, but have poor self-control). Imposing this condition on a noncompliant patient will result in frequent, unproductive recalls to hospital.

Safeguarding

Safeguarding comprises measures to protect the health, wellbeing, and human rights of children, young people, and vulnerable adults, so that they may live free from abuse, harm and neglect. It requires people and organisations to work together to stop abuse and neglect, and to promote wellbeing. It encompasses handling complaints and incidents, as well as preventing future harm.

Whereas all under eighteens fall within the ambit of safeguarding arrangements, adults are only covered if they are 'vulnerable' through being at risk of abuse or neglect because of their particular need for care or support (e.g. arising from mental disorder).

Legal frameworks

- In England, the Children's Acts 1989 and 2004 place a duty on local authorities to assess the needs of vulnerable children and make services available to safeguard and promote welfare. Similar duties apply in relation to vulnerable adults under the Care Act 2014.
- The Social Services and Well-being (Wales) Act 2014 covers children and all other vulnerable groups in need of safeguarding and support services, and provides powers to protect adults and children at risk.
- The Children's (Scotland) Act 1995 and Children and Young People (Scotland) Act 2014 set out local authorities' responsibilities to children, including protection and supervision, and the role of Children's Hearings (p.386). More limited provisions for adults are found in the Adult Support and Protection (Scotland) Act 2007; these include a power to remove a vulnerable adult from their home for their health or safety or to protect others.[26] Safeguarding is more commonly referred to as 'Child protection' or 'Adult protection' in Scotland.
- The Children (Northern Ireland) Order 1995 establishes similar powers and duties as those in England, to which the Children's Services Cooperation Act (NI) 2015 adds provisions for services to work together effectively to promote a child's welfare.
- In addition, in all jurisdictions additional powers are available to protect those at risk because of mental incapacity, under mental capacity legislation (p.522), and guardianship provisions of mental health law where those exist (p.505).

Working together

The harm caused by failures of interagency collaboration (p.252) and information-sharing have been highlighted by numerous reviews and inquiries, including those into the high-profile deaths of Victoria Climbié, Caleb Ness, and Peter Connelly ('Baby P') in the UK. All have emphasised the importance of effective sharing of information between practitioners and local organisations and agencies for early identification of need, assessment, and service provision to keep children safe. Laws and guidance on confidentiality (p.320) explicitly allow for the proportionate sharing of information in order to protect children and vulnerable adults from serious harm.

---

26 An equivalent power was abolished in E&W by the Care Act 2014.

Administrative arrangements exist in each jurisdiction to facilitate working together, typically bringing together local authorities, police, health services, and probation services. These include regional Children's Safeguarding Boards in E&W, Child Protection Committees in Scotland, Area Child Protection Committees in NI, and Safeguarding Ireland in RoI.

Public Protection Arrangements

In the three UK jurisdictions, the process of interagency co-operation for protecting the public has been formalised under the MAPPA for E&W and Scotland, and the Public Protection Arrangements for Northern Ireland in NI. Under this statutory scheme,[27] the so-called Responsible Authorities (RA)—the police, probation, and prison services[28]—must jointly manage offenders deemed to pose a 'serious risk of harm to the public', and are entitled to co-operation from other relevant agencies, such as health, housing, education, and social services.

Identification of offenders to be supervised

This is generally determined by the offender's offence and sentence, but also by assessed level of risk. There are three formal categories, as shown in Box 18.2. Note that agencies can also co-operate in the management of offenders not covered by MAPPA, under informal arrangements (see p.252).

Box 18.2 MAPPA offender categories

Category 1: Sex Offenders
This includes all sex offenders on the Sex Offenders Register (p.457) and any other convicted or cautioned (p.440) sex offender assessed as posing a high risk to the community.

Category 2: Violent Offenders
This comprises all offenders convicted of a violent offence (one which led, or was intended or likely to lead, to death or physical injury) who are sentenced to at least twelve-months' imprisonment (p.452), or a hospital order (p.500).

Category 3: Potentially Dangerous Offenders
Offenders who have been cautioned for or convicted of an offence that indicates they are capable of causing the public serious harm.

Only the RA can definitively allocate referred offenders to a category and thereby make them subject to MAPPA. Category 3 offenders can only be managed under MAPPA for up to three months—unless they can be reallocated to category 1 or 2.

Sharing of information about offenders

Statutory procedures promote information-sharing between all the agencies, with the intention of more effective supervision and better public protection. The process of information-sharing with other agencies (p.321) can raise ethical dilemmas (p.298).

27 Brought in by the Criminal Justice and Courts Services Act 2000 and extended under the Criminal Justice Act 2003 for E&W, and brought in elsewhere in the UK by the Criminal Justice (Northern Ireland) Order 2008 and the Management of Offenders (Scotland) Act 2005.

28 Except in Scotland, where the responsible authorities are the police, prison service, social services, and health boards.

Assessment of the risks posed by offenders

<u>Risk assessment</u> (pp.163–180) should be based on a good-quality process involving both clinical and actuarial data. These statutory procedures enable resources and attention to be focused on offenders who present the highest risk to the public, who are a minority of those reviewed by MAPPA. Victims' needs are represented at discussions, and additional measures are put into place to manage the risks posed to known victims. The offender's view should also be noted, even if it is considered to be unreliable, insightless, or self-serving.

Management of the risk posed by individual offenders

MAPPA offenders are categorised at one of three levels in terms of risk and the degree of management intervention required.
- **Level 1**: Involves normal agency management by one, or sometimes two agencies. Generally, offenders managed at this level will be assessed as presenting a low or medium risk of serious harm to others. Most MAPPA offenders are managed at this level.
- **Level 2**: The risk management plans require active involvement of several agencies via regular multiagency public protection meetings.
- **Level 3**: Appropriate for those offenders who pose the highest risk of causing serious harm or whose management is so problematic that multiagency co-operation and oversight at a senior level is required with the authority to commit exceptional resources. Applies to under 1% of offenders.

The Risk Management Authority

The Risk Management Authority (RMA) was established in Scotland in 2005 to ensure effective risk assessment and risk management to reduce the risk of serious harm posed by violent and sexual offenders. It has a special responsibility for the small number of offenders sentenced to an order for lifelong restriction (OLR, p.449). There were fourteen OLRs imposed in 2019-20. It is principally concerned with the sentencing of serious offenders who pose a risk of future serious offending, and not mentally disordered offenders.

The RMA's functions are to:

- give advice and make recommendations to Scottish ministers;
- carry out research into effective practice in risk assessment and management;
- provide guidance, education, and training for those involved in the assessment and management of risk, including accrediting practitioners and monitoring risk management plans for those offenders who receive an OLR; and
- support the Level of Service/Case Management Inventory (LS/CMI), which is a risk or need assessment and case management planning tool.

OLRs and Risk Assessment Reports (RARs)

An OLR can only be imposed after the judge has considered an RAR prepared by an accredited risk assessor under a risk assessment order (p.504). There are currently thirteen accredited risk assessors (including two psychiatrists), who act solely to determine the risk to public safety of the person being at liberty. Accredited assessors come from a range of professional backgrounds, including psychiatry, psychology and social work. There is no requirement that risk be linked to mental disorder for the court to make an OLR. The RAR is prepared according to rigorous standards of risk assessment, set and reviewed by the RMA; generally based on structured professional judgement (p.167) techniques.

Ethics of the role of the accredited risk assessor

The duty of the accredited risk assessor is to support the justice process and ensure the judge has good-quality information to make decisions which are compatible with the Human Rights Act. Some may see this duty as outside the scope of medical ethics, as the risk assessment is done for the benefit of the court, not the offender, whose interests in terms of liberty may be harmed by the use of the OLR for public protection. This raises the issue of their consent to risk assessment (p.342); the individual must be informed that the risk assessment is being conducted because of a court order, that it is part of the sentencing process (p.442) and not part of a therapeutic treatment process, that any information provided might be used in the risk assessment report (i.e. there is no confidentiality, p.320), and that the outcome could be an indefinite sentence of imprisonment (p.448) or another restrictive sentence such as the OLR.

Some mental health professionals may have ethical objections to their involvement in risk assessments for the RMA (much as they may to involvement in courts' assessments of culpability or <u>dangerousness</u>, p.672).

Others may hold that the justice process has a legitimate claim on their knowledge, and that it is good for all citizens if the courts have access to the best-quality judgements about risk. Those clinicians who do work as accredited risk assessors should ensure that they have the right training and supervision for their work.

Crime prevention and PREVENT

Police, probation, and intelligence services have a duty to prevent crime, using a variety of legal measures and multiagency working. Services range from probation teams working to rehabilitate offenders so that they do not reoffend, to specialist police and intelligence agencies[29] combating foreign agents aiming to commit terrorist offences (p.430).

Disclosure for crime prevention

NHS and HSE codes of ethics permit staff to disclose patient information for the prevention, detection, and punishment of serious crime,[30] including disclosure without consent (p.321) if necessary. 'Serious' in this context refers to offences involving significant violence or other serious harm.[31] Mental health professionals, especially those in forensic services, may also attend multiagency public protection (p.592) or safeguarding (p.590) meetings in relation to patients at risk of serious offending.

UK counter-terrorism strategy

Increased concern about terrorist violence following the 9/11 terrorist attacks of September 2001 led the UK government to develop a counter-terrorism strategy (CONTEST, Box 18.3) and to pass a series of counter-terrorism and security acts. There is no equivalent strategy covering the HSE (or other bodies such as schools) in RoI; the Department of Justice & Equality co-ordinates a more limited strategy involving the Gardai.

Box 18.3 The UK government's CONTEST strategy

- PREVENT: to stop people becoming terrorists or supporting terrorism.
- PURSUE: to stop terrorist attacks.
- PROTECT: to strengthen protection against a terrorist attack.
- PREPARE: to mitigate the impact of a terrorist attack.

The PREVENT programme focuses on trying to divert individuals who may be at risk of being drawn into terrorism and nonviolent extremism. Those identified at risk of radicalisation may be referred to the Channel programme.

There are few public data on the effectiveness of the CONTEST strategy. There is considerable academic debate internationally about the effectiveness of Channel and prison deradicalisation programmes, with evidence for and against their effectiveness at reducing extremist and radical views (p.42).

---

29 Such as the Special Branch of the Metropolitan Police, and the Security Service (MI5) in the UK; or the Garda Counter-Terrorism International in RoI.

30 The wording in the HSE guidance for RoI is 'to prevent or lessen a serious and imminent threat to life or health ... [or] reasonably necessary for the enforcement of the criminal law'.

31 For example, the definition in the UK Serious Crime Act 2015 includes drug trafficking, human trafficking, child sexual exploitation, high-value financial crimes, organised crime, and cybercrime.

NHS staff and the PREVENT programme

In the UK, the NHS and other specified public authorities have duties to:
• have 'due regard' to the need to prevent people being drawn into terrorism and to
• disclose information they know or believe likely to be of material assistance to preventing an act of terrorism or securing the arrest, prosecution, or detention of those involved.

Employers are required to train all staff to recognise, in the course of their normal activities,[32] who might be at risk of radicalisation, and to have arrangements for sharing information if a risk is identified. Recognition may, where appropriate, involve the use of extremism risk assessment instruments such as the Violent Extremist Risk Assessment, version 2 (VERA-2); Extremist Risk Guidance 22+ (ERG22+); and the Vulnerability Assessment Framework. Such tools are based on structured professional judgement (p.167) and devised for use in different settings by those with specific training.

The NHS has made PREVENT part of safeguarding (p.590) arrangements; and all staff are required to undergo PREVENT training. Each Trust or Board must have a PREVENT lead, who makes decisions about information-sharing and may make referrals to the Channel programme.

Many mental health professionals express concern that the PREVENT strategy unfairly stigmatises psychiatric patients as being at risk of radicalisation, especially those of Asian heritage; and also express concern about pressure to breach patient confidentiality if the patient is perceived to be at increased risk, which may harm the therapeutic relationship and inhibit future recovery.

---

32 That is, no special or covert activity is permitted.

Homicide and suicide inquiries

Since 1994, the UK government has required various kinds of inquiries into deaths related to patients with mental disorder.[33] There is no equivalent requirement in RoI, although ad hoc inquiries may be held into certain high-profile homicides and suicides by people with mental disorder.

Suicide inquiries

Deaths by suicide of patients who are under the care of mental health services (or within six months of discharge) are investigated by the mental health Trust or Board. Investigations seek to identify system failures and potential for organisational learning. The findings of a Serious Incident Investigation may be introduced as evidence at a Coroner's inquest into how the death occurred. An independent inquiry would only be commissioned in circumstances which suggested the need for additional external scrutiny or where there were a cluster of deaths by suicide within one organisation.

Homicide inquiries

If a patient under the care of mental health services (or within six months of discharge) commits a homicide, the mental healthcare provider investigates locally. Good investigations can identify system failures without blame and opportunities for prevention in the future. Such investigations may also identify failures in care, and may be an opportunity for families and carers (of both perpetrators and victims) to feel consulted and heard. Providers' investigation findings are commonly adopted by subsequent broader inquiries, such as Domestic Homicide Reviews, Serious Case Reviews, or ad hoc independent inquiries. All such inquiries produce reports which may form the basis of negligence (p.550) claims against staff or NHS bodies, or prosecution under health and safety legislation.

Independent inquiries may be asked to comment on the internal inquiry's process and findings. It is not unusual for the internal inquiry to focus blame on frontline clinical staff, whereas the independent inquiry will often identify systemic service or organisational factors that contributed to the homicide, and which were not addressed in the internal inquiry. Having psychiatric experts as part of the independent inquiry process may be valuable here in terms providing a clinical and 'real-world' perspective.

One review of homicide inquiries found only about a quarter of homicides were deemed to have been 'predictable'. But two-thirds were thought to have been 'preventable' since they would have been prevented if there had been earlier clinical intervention, driven by patient need, which would, coincidentally, have interrupted the chain of events leading to the homicide (p.240).

33 See Part C of the *Oxford Casebook of Forensic Psychiatry*, 'Critiquing Decisions Made', which contrasts in detail a variety of both legal and other 'paradigms' applied to investigating decisions made.

Concerns about suicide and homicide inquiries

Clinicians whose patients have committed either suicide or homicide may experience high levels of stress, and report that the Serious Incident Investigation processes (both internal and external) contribute to that stress.

- Such processes are often experienced as adversarial, not inquisitorial, and as lacking ordinary legal protections such as access to relevant documentation, rules of procedure and presumption of 'innocence'. They offer witnesses few procedural or prescriptive rights or safeguards,[34] including the lack of opportunity to cross-examine other witnesses.
- Clinicians may not be legally represented, and may be advised early that their interests conflict with those of their employer's, and they may need to seek their own legal advice. Not all clinicians may be able to access support from their medical defence organisation.
- Inquiries usually deliberate in private, and may not have time to examine in detail the 'fine-grained' processes that lay behind clinical decisions.[35]
- Inquiries may not address <u>causation</u> (p.549) in a legally coherent way. It is possible for an inquiry to conclude that a single clinician was responsible for a negative outcome not directly related to their own actions, or where other factors were necessary and contributory.
- There is no 'right of appeal' to any court to challenge the inquiry's findings unless the inquiry procedure was so deeply flawed as to be found unreasonable after <u>judicial review</u> (p.374).

National Confidential Inquiry into Suicide and Safety

Until 2019, details of serious incident reviews of suicides and homicides by mentally ill people, as well as sudden unexpected deaths, were collected and studied by the National Confidential Inquiry into Suicide and Safety in Mental Health. The Inquiry no longer addresses homicides, and seeks to use aggregate data to make recommendations to services on reducing the risk of further incidents. Key findings from the NCISS include:

- The numbers of suicides have fallen steadily, including in the general population, amongst patients, and amongst inpatients.
- The commonest methods of completed suicide were hanging, followed by self-poisoning; the highest risk of suicide after hospital discharge came in the first one to two weeks, and especially the first forty-eight to seventy-two hours.
- Suicides preceded by noncompliance with treatment are less common.
- Changing patterns of ligatures and ligature points continue to be found: recognised types of points, for example, are eliminated when wards are redesigned, but those designs introduce new, unrecognised, points.
- The numbers of homicides by people receiving mental healthcare are also failing; where they do occur, it is more commonly on weekdays.

---

34 Other than via a 'Salmon letter', which warns a witness in advance of them giving evidence (or publication of the final report) that they may be subject to criticism.

35 See Parts A and C of the *Oxford Casebook of Forensic Psychiatry*.

Chapter 19

Legal tests relevant to psychiatry

Fitness to plead

A criminal trial can proceed only if the defendants are 'fit to plead', in terms of their mental ability to participate. Fitness to plead is determined by the court, based upon expert psychiatric (or sometimes psychological) evidence, taking into account the complexity of the trial issues and trial context[1] Physical conditions may be relevant (e.g. deafness). Fitness to plead is different from <u>fitness to attend court</u> (p.606).

All defendants are presumed fit until evidence demonstrates otherwise. The relevant legal tests are therefore of *unfitness*. Tests vary between jurisdictions, but are all tests of cognitive ability, considering the degree to which this is affected by psychotic or other symptoms, or disabilities.

Tests of unfitness

E&W and NI R v Pritchard (p.765)

The precise wording of the test has changed as it has been restated by judges in various cases, the most recent leading case being <u>R v M (John)</u> (p.761). A finding of unfitness to plead involves the defence demonstrating to the judge, on <u>balance of probabilities</u> (p.380), that the defendant is incapable, during any part of the trial,[2] of one or more of:

- understanding the charge(s);
- deciding whether to plead guilty or not;
- exercising their right to challenge jurors (even for irrational reasons);
- instructing solicitors and counsel;
- following proceedings; and
- giving evidence in their defence and being cross-examined (<u>R v Orr</u>, p.763).

Inability to remember events related to the alleged offence is insufficient for unfitness (<u>R v Podola</u>, p.764). Muteness rarely reflects unfitness.

A mental disorder is not necessary for an unfitness finding.

Criminal Justice and Licensing (Scotland) Act 2010

The test is whether the defendant is incapable, by reason of a mental or physical condition, of participating effectively in a trial. Being unable to remember the alleged offence is insufficient; the court must consider the defendant's ability to understand the:

- nature of the charge;
- requirement to tender a plea to the charge and the effect of such;
- purpose, and follow the course, of the trial;
- evidence that may be given against them; and
- instruct and communicate with their legal representative.

RoI Criminal Law (Insanity) Act 2006

Accused persons shall be deemed unfit to be tried if they are unable by reason of mental disorder to understand the nature or course of proceedings so as to:

---

1 <u>R v Marcantonio</u> (p.VI.12)) and *R v Thomas (Dean)* [2020] 4 WLR66 respectively.

2 <u>R v Mercantonio</u> (p.762).

- plead,
- instruct legal representatives,
- make a choice (where available) on trial summarily or by jury,
- make a proper defence,
- understand the evidence, or
- challenge a juror.

Problems with tests of unfitness

The definitions and applications in practice of unfitness tests have been widely criticised for disproportionately emphasising cognition, ignoring other mental symptoms influencing decision-making capacity, and ignoring suggestibility and compliance (p.160). For example, in _R v Robertson_ (p.766), a defendant who had delusions relating directly to the alleged offence and low intelligence was held capable of meeting the _Pritchard_ tests, by merely 'failing to act in his own best interests'.

Human rights law (p.516) implies that defendants should be able to offer 'effective participation', and be able to 'plead with understanding'. If a defendant is deluded about the consequences of a plea (as in _R v Erskine_, p.755, where he believed that if he acknowledged his multiple killings he would be deported to the USA and executed), then they cannot plead with understanding; yet they might be held fit to plead.

A mentally disordered defendant who has killed might meet criteria for diminished responsibility (p.624), but still be fit to plead if their 'abnormality of mind', or in E&W or NI, 'abnormality of mental functioning', does not affect those cognitive abilities. If they lacked insight into their mental disorder, they might be allowed to refuse to plead diminished responsibility, resulting in an unfair conviction for murder.[3] The disorder which would _allow_ a successful plea of diminished responsibility might be the reason they _refuse to plead it_, and yet they may well be found fit to do so.

Psychiatrists are commonly encouraged to give evidence directly addressing whether the defendant is fit to plead (i.e. the ultimate issue, p.664). This can mean that they interpret the legal test for themselves, rather than describing relevant mental disabilities and leaving the court to determine whether they infer unfitness. Apparent disagreements between psychiatrists may not be about the defendants' medical disabilities, but their legal interpretation.

These criticisms may explain why findings of unfitness to plead are rare.[4] The E&W Law Commission published proposals in 2016 to replace the Pritchard test with a broader one based upon decision-making capacity, similar to mental capacity within the Mental Capacity Act (p.522) of civil law. It is a point of debate whether a new legal unfitness test should allow 'proportionality' of threshold of unfitness, to be commensurate with the gravity of potential outcomes and proportionate to the anticipated complexity of the case. Given the predictability difficulties of 'proportionality',

---

3 The issue of diminished responsibility can only be raised by the defence, not the prosecution or the judge.

4 Numbering in the tens or hundreds in a typical year in E&W, compared with around 12,000 in the USA.

the Commission recommended a decision-making capacity test which is informed by the spectrum of potential trial decisions and incorporates measures to support effective participation into a legal framework.

Procedures

The issue of fitness to plead can be raised by the defence, prosecution or judge.

E&W Criminal Procedure (Insanity) Act 1964 (amended 1991, 2004)
- Two medical practitioners must give evidence on fitness
- For the prosecution, it must be proved <u>beyond reasonable doubt</u>; for the defence, on <u>balance of probabilities</u> (p.380)
- Determined by the judge, not jury,[5] in the <u>Crown Court</u> (p.384)

Scotland Criminal Procedure (Scotland) Act 1995 (amended 2010)
- Called unfitness for trial[6]
- No medical evidence requirement
- Case may be adjourned for investigation of mental condition

NI Mental Health (NI) Order 1986 / Mental Capacity Act NI 2016[7]
- Called the question of fitness to be tried
- Two medical practitioners must give evidence (one oral)
- Determined by judge

RoI Criminal Law (Insanity) Act 2006
- Determined by court
- Evidence of approved medical officer required

Delaying trial

Where unfitness to plead is likely but the relevant mental condition is likely to respond to treatment within a reasonable period of time, it is sensible to advise the court to delay trial, rather than proceed to an unfitness hearing.

If a defendant is fit to plead but seriously mentally unwell with a condition where treatment would be likely to improve their ability to participate it is sensible to advise the court of this and suggest delay, in 'natural justice'.

Outcome following unfitness to plead

After a finding of unfitness to plead, a 'trial of the facts' determines whether, on the balance of probabilities,[8] the defendant did the acts or omissions (i.e. the <u>conduct element</u>, p.400) of the offence[9] to avoid long-term detention

---

5 There is no procedure for testing unfitness to plead in the magistrates' court. Under s37(3) of the MHA, magistrates can make a <u>hospital order</u> (p.500) or <u>guardianship</u> (p.505) if the offence is punishable with imprisonment and they are satisfied that the defendant did the acts or made the omissions charged.

6 Previously 'insanity in bar of trial'

7 This part of the MCANI has not yet been brought into force at the time of writing, but it does not significantly change this area of law.

8 Beyond reasonable doubt in RoI.

9 In E&W, the Law Commission has proposed allowing consideration of the <u>mental element</u> (p.402), such that if there is clear evidence (unrelated to the cause of the unfitness to plead) that defendants lacked the relevant *mens rea*, they can be acquitted rather than found unfit to plead.

of a defendant who might not have done what is alleged. If proved, the
court may make the following orders:

E&W, NI, and Scotland
- <u>Hospital order</u> (<u>compulsion order</u> in Scotland) (p.500)
- Hospital/compulsion order with <u>restrictions</u> (p.510)[10]
- Interim compulsion order (Scotland)
- <u>Guardianship order</u> (p.505) (Scotland and NI)
- <u>Supervision & treatment order</u> (Supervision order in E&W) (p.504)
- Absolute discharge

In E&W, even if there has been a disposal as above, the patient can be re-
tried if they become fit to plead.

RoI
- <u>Committal for treatment</u> (p.500) to a designated centre for days for
  inpatient/outpatient care/treatment

Return to court
A trial of facts finding that the defendant did the acts or omissions alleged is
not a conviction. If later found fit to plead, a defendant may wish to be tried.
In practice, subsequent trial is unusual, and government policy opposes it
(because, for instance, witness memories and important documents may
be lost over time).

10 In E&W, this is mandatory if the charge was murder.

Fitness to give evidence

Whereas <u>fitness to plead</u> and stand trial (p.602) applies only to defendants, all witnesses, not only defendants, must be fit to give evidence. Whether they are fit to do so is an issue for the judge, aided where necessary by psychiatric or psychological evidence.[11]

There is a history of trials not proceeding due to assumptions that witnesses were unfit, or their evidence was likely to be unreliable; most often with prosecution witnesses, particularly victims (e.g. of <u>rape</u>, p.418, where their evidence may be the sole evidence).

Fitness to give evidence must be distinguished from concerns about:

- evidence <u>reliability</u> (p.156), which might lead to it being <u>excluded</u> (p.383), or admitted with caution, and
- witness <u>vulnerability</u> (p.157), which might lead to 'special measures' to protect them, such as the court concealing their identity (e.g. the young, elderly or intellectually disabled).

Test of fitness to give evidence

Specific tests have not evolved in each jurisdiction. One model is that provided in E&W by <u>R v M</u> (John) (p.761), in which the judge ruled that the defendant giving evidence—and by extension other witnesses—must be able to:

- understand questions;
- apply their mind to answering them; and
- convey intelligibly to the jury answers they wish to give.

These principles apply to child as well as adult witnesses.

It is not necessary for fitness that a witness' answers be plausible, believable, reliable, or seen as such by the witness.

Problems with the test

The test may not allow for some subtleties of disability or vulnerability. In police interviews, where <u>suggestibility</u> or <u>compliance</u> (p.160) must be considered, there is arguably greater protection for vulnerable individuals than when they are hostilely cross-examined in court—albeit the judge is present to ensure fair questioning. Conditions such as dysexecutive syndrome or autistic spectrum disorder, for example, may result in a witness meeting the test, despite reduced ability to deal with rapid, subtle, and pointed cross-examination.

The impact of defendants' relative vulnerability can sometimes be counterbalanced by allowing expert evidence to describe the nature of the defendants' mental disorder and how this may influence their answers to questions and their body language (evidence which may be allowed under current <u>rules on expert evidence</u>, p.651). Special measures, such as allowing frequent breaks for the witness to regain composure, may also assist.

---

11 It is of particular relevance to defendants in E&W, because s35 of the Criminal Justice and Public Order Act 1994 allows courts or juries to regard a defendant's 'failure' to give evidence as a factor supporting the prosecution case (the so-called adverse inference (p.378) from the defendant's silence)—unless the judge accepts that it would be 'undesirable' for them to do so.

Fitness to attend court

A witness unfit to give evidence will not be required to attend court, but a defendant may still be expected to attend. For some mentally disordered defendants, therefore, it may be necessary for a psychiatrist to consider whether they are fit to attend. This is more likely to be an issue with in-patients, where severe psychotic or other symptoms, or attempts at self-harm, would make it unsafe for them to leave hospital, even with staff escorts.

If you consider that this applies to one of your patients, it is important to communicate this to the clerk of the court in good time, as some hearings will have to be adjourned if the defendant cannot be present. It is helpful to indicate how soon the defendant may become fit.

Confessions

A confession can be a direct admission of guilt or effectively any statement that harms the suspect's criminal legal interest. In E&W, NI, and RoI a defendant may be convicted on the basis of confession alone; in Scotland, confessions, like all evidence, must be corroborated.

- A genuine confession is one in which the suspect confesses truthfully.
- A false confession is one in which the suspect confesses to a crime they did not commit.
- A retracted confession is one in which the suspect, after having made a confession, later claims that their original confession is untrue. Retracted confessions are common in criminal proceedings, and may be genuine or false.

Any confession is legally problematic if obtained by threats or coercion; a false confession may also lead to unjust conviction and failure to apprehend the actual offender.

Types of false confessions

- A **voluntary** false confession occurs in the absence of obvious external pressure, and may result from ulterior motives for being prosecuted (e.g. to protect another or for notoriety).
- A **coerced-compliant** confession occurs with awareness that the confession is false, but where the suspect <u>complies</u> (p.160) because of objective or perceived coercion. It can arise from eagerness to please, seeking self-esteem in the company of others, or a desire to avoid conflict.
- A **coerced-internalised** confession occurs when suspects come to believe (wrongly) that the confession they are making is true; usually related to <u>suggestibility</u> (p.160) affecting responses during high-pressure interrogation.

Factors encouraging false confession

Situational and individual factors, and the interaction between them, can lead to an interviewee making a false confession. The conditions in which the interrogation takes place can therefore be crucial. **Situational factors** include the effects of custody and isolation prior to interview, the process of interrogation, coercion by the interrogator, interrogators' prior belief that the suspect is guilty, plus 'case building' (which may lead to giving information about the offence, which is then taken as proving guilt when repeated by the interviewee).

A degree of situational pressure may be desirable in interviews where the suspect might lie; a balance must be struck between this and risking false or unreliable confessions.

Individual factors (individually or in combination) include mental disorder, intellectual disability, distress, guilty feelings, a desire for publicity or notoriety, and a desire to protect the true perpetrator.

Individual factors may be mitigated by the presence of an <u>appropriate adult</u> (p.574) or an effective solicitor.

Demonstrating traits of suggestibility or compliance is insufficient to render a confession unreliable and potentially <u>inadmissible</u> (p.382). It must also be demonstrated that such traits were in operation in making the confession.

Admissibility of confessions

In **E&W** and **NI**, confessions must be excluded if they were obtained by 'oppression' (e.g. torture, coercion, or threats) or anything else likely to render them unreliable.[12] Any evidence, including confessions, may be excluded at the court's discretion if it would have too great an adverse effect on fairness. Confessions made by 'mentally handicapped' persons may still be admitted, but the jury or magistrates must be warned that there is a 'special need for caution' before convicting on the basis of it.

In **Scotland**, there are no special rules on the admissibility of confessions and fewer <u>rules of evidence</u> generally (p.382); the main protection against conviction based on false confessions is the requirement of corroborating evidence.

In **RoI** there are no special rules on admissibility of confessions. The jury or court must be warned about any absence of corroboration before convicting.

Even if a confession is admitted, there may still be expert evidence in regard to its 'evidential weight'.

Expert assessment of confessions

An expert psychologist might be required when there are concerns about the reliability of a confession. A psychiatrist may also be required if there is evidence of relevant mental disorder. In addition to following the usual <u>principles of assessment</u> (p.122) and rules for <u>criminal court reports</u> (p.694), experts should:

- assess for mental disorder, especially psychosis or personality disorder, or any condition known to be associated with confession unreliability;
- assess individual characteristics that may make the suspect more vulnerable to confessing, using where appropriate <u>psychometric tests</u> (p.136) of intelligence, memory, suggestibility, and compliance;
- read, listen to, or watch transcripts and video tapes of police interviews—with particular attention paid to leading or closed questions, undue pressure by the interrogator, evidence of the possible operation of suggestibility or compliance, and the possible effects of the absence of an appropriate adult or solicitor; and
- only state whether these factors *may* have affected the reliability of the confession, never that they *did* (<u>Pora</u>, p.765).

12 ss76–78 PACE in E&W, aa74–76 PACE(NI)O1989, and s10 Criminal Procedure Act 1993 in RoI.

Capacity to form intent

Psychiatrists and psychologists are often asked to assess whether a defendant could have formed the relevant <u>mental element</u> (p.402) of the alleged offence: most often, whether they would have had the capacity to have formed a particular <u>intent</u> (p.402). They should not comment on what the defendant actually intended.

The legal test

The required mental element is specific to the offence: often <u>specific intent</u>[13] or <u>recklessness</u> (p.403). Generally, E&W has very detailed definitions of different mental elements, and Scotland leaves great discretion to the judge, with NI and RoI in between.

Some mental element examples are shown in Box 19.1. What legal test will apply in a given case should be specified in the <u>written instructions</u> (p.680).

> ### Box 19.1 Examples of questions regarding capacity to form the mental element
>
> Did the defendant have the capacity to:
> - Intend to kill or cause serious injury? (murder, E&W, NI, or RoI)
> - Kill with wicked recklessness or intent? (murder, Scotland)
> - Foresee the risk of death a reasonable person would have foreseen? (manslaughter or culpable homicide)
> - Foresee a co-defendant's actions and intend to assist them? (joint enterprise)
> - Intend the bodily contact that they made? (e.g. battery, ABH)
> - Reasonably believe the victim consented? (defence to rape, E&W)
> - Intend life to be endangered? (arson with intent, E&W or NI)
> - Intend permanently to deprive the owner of property? (theft)

The role of the psychiatrist

As with all expert evidence, it is important only to answer questions within your <u>professional expertise</u> (p.654), and not to attempt to answer <u>ultimate questions</u> (p.664) that are for the court. A valid question is, 'would the defendant's mental condition at the time have been likely to prevent them forming the relevant mental element?'

Symptoms and conditions that might prevent formation of a particular mental element include:
- **specific delusions** relating to the knowledge in question, or another relevant aspect;
- an **abnormal mood state** (e.g. severe depression or mania), associated psychomotor agitation or retardation, or impaired concentration that would have prevented consideration of risks or facts a reasonable person would have considered; and

---

13 There is a rule of law, at least in E&W, that psychiatric evidence of incapacity to form intent is usually <u>inadmissible</u> (p.382) in crimes of <u>basic intent</u> (p.403).

- severe **cognitive impairment** (e.g. in dementia),
- an **acute confusional state**, or
- **acute intoxication**.[14]

Incapacity and public policy

The result of a finding of incapacity is outright acquittal, which legislatures and courts see as unacceptable in the case of defendants with mental disorders who cause serious harm to others, which may be repeated. The bar is therefore set very high. Scottish law allows order for the <u>urgent detention of acquitted persons</u> (p.504).

---

14 Public policy profoundly limits the relevance of self-induced intoxication to removing the capacity to form intent, and then only 'specific intent', setting the bar extremely high (*DPP v Majewski*, p.761).

Automatism

An action which the mind of the defendant did not will is an automatism: the body is said to have moved involuntarily. Automatism is a full defence (p.412) to any offence, provided there is total lack of control: partial
control rules it out (A-G's ref, p.746). Automatism can be caused by physical
or mental disorder, but not voluntary intoxication (p.616) in crimes of basic
intent (R v Coley, p.752).

Insane versus noninsane automatisms

Automatisms can be **insane**,[15] resulting in a finding of not guilty by reason
of insanity (p.620), or **noninsane**, resulting in acquittal (Table 19.1). The
distinction is legal, not medical. An automatism is insane if its *cause* is a legal
'disease of the mind', meaning:

- it was intrinsic to the mind (R v Quick, p.765); in other words where
  there was no 'external blow', physical or mental; or
- it resulted in violence and is prone to recur (Bratty v A-G NI, p.749).

Table 19.1 Insane and noninsane automatisms

Insane automatisms	Noninsane automatisms
Epileptic fits (R v Sullivan, p.768)	Concussion after head injury
Arteriosclerosis causing transient ischaemia (R v Kemp, p.759)	Hypoglycaemia after taking insulin (R v Quick, p.765)
Parasomnias (p.115) e.g. sleepwalking (R v Burgess, p.750)	Dissociation precipitated by unusual external stressors e.g. rape (R v T, p.769)
Dissociation caused by 'ordinary stresses' (R v Rabey, p.765)	

Medico-legal incongruence

The distinction between intrinsic and extrinsic causes is incoherent medically.[16] For example, if a man with BPD (p.84) impulsively takes insulin,
becomes hypoglycaemic, and assaults someone, does the insulin make
the automatism noninsane, or the BPD make it insane? Is an epileptic fit
triggered by high-dose clozapine an insane automatism because of the fit,
or noninsane because of the drug? Is hypoglycaemia caused by an insulin-
secreting pancreatic tumour an insane automatism because the source is
intrinsic to the body, or noninsane because it is extrinsic to the brain?

---

15 This raises the question, what is the legal difference between an insane automatism and insanity?
   The legal test for insanity (e.g. the McNaughten rules) applies in both cases, but only those
   cases of insanity in which the defendant's actions are involuntary will also be cases of (insane)
   automatism.

16 The incompatibility of the legal concepts of automatism and insanity with modern medical understanding led to the Law Commission's 2013 recommendations for legal reform.

Epilepsy

To doctors epilepsy as not a 'disease of the mind'; and it is not a ground for detention under mental health law. Someone with epilepsy who kills during a fit would be deemed to have been in an insane automatism and yet might not be detainable under mental health legislation, whilst the alternative supervision order (p.504) might not be adequate for public protection.

Dissociation

Dissociation is deemed 'intrinsic' and thus (if the threshold for automatism is reached) an insane automatism; but if it is triggered by a severe external blow, a noninsane automatism (R v T, p.769).

Scotland and RoI

Scottish law does not recognise insane automatism as such; defendants must raise the insanity defence instead. In Scotland the defence of (noninsane) automatism requires:
- an external factor causing loss of reason that must not be self-induced and could not be foreseen, and
- a resulting 'total alienation of reason' amounting to complete loss of self-control, demonstrated by expert medical evidence.

Courts in RoI have recognised the distinction but have generally only accepted noninsane automatisms.

Resolving medico-legally contentious issues

Confusion at the medico-legal interface (p.358) is for the court to unravel, not the expert, who should remain within the limits of psychiatric opinion; describing only the medical condition and its causes and effects, leaving the court to determine whether it amounted to an automatism, and if so, whether insane or not.

Involuntary intoxication

Intoxication with drugs or alcohol alters a person's mental state, and may well have an impact on their decision to commit an unlawful act. However, under the **prior fault** rule, it can only contribute to acquittal or a partial defence if it is involuntary.

When is intoxication 'involuntary'?

Intoxication is presumed to be voluntary (i.e. intentional or reckless) unless there is clear evidence that the defendant was unaware of the risk of becoming intoxicated. For example:

- Someone putting alcohol in a soft drink unbeknownst to the defendant, or drugging their mild alcoholic drink with flunitrazepam (Rohypnol).
- Taking a prescribed drug on the professional advice of the prescriber.
- Using a substance that is not dangerous[17] and does not normally cause intoxication, unless the use was itself somehow reckless.
- Using a substance on which one is sufficiently dependent.

A drink or drug being much stronger or more potent than expected does not make the intoxication involuntary: the prior fault was in taking the substance at all.

Dependence and involuntary intoxication

Intoxication was previously deemed involuntary in dependent users only if they had an 'irresistible impulse' to use the substance (_R v Tandy_, p.769). This strict approach was modified by _Wood_ and _Stewart_ (pp.768, 771), which require the jury to consider:

- the extent and seriousness of the defendant's dependence (p.76);
- the extent to which the ability to control drinking, or to choose whether to drink, was reduced; and
- whether the defendant was capable of abstinence and, if so, for how long, and whether they had a particular reason (other than dependence) to drink.

Voluntariness is a legal construct (p.354): an expert should only give an opinion on dependence, not on voluntariness.

When is involuntary intoxication a defence?

If the degree of involuntary intoxication prevents the defendant forming the mental element (p.402) of the offence, they will be acquitted.[18]

Evidence of involuntary intoxication may be taken as evidence suggestive that the necessary state of mind was absent, but it does not prove it: it must be weighed alongside other evidence, which might show that the defendant did in fact have the necessary *mens rea* (as in _R v Kingston_, p.760, where it

---

17 A 'dangerous' drug is one where it is 'common knowledge' that the user 'may become aggressive or do dangerous or unpredictable things' or become incapable of appreciating risks. Amphetamines and LSD have been held to be dangerous; diazepam to be 'nondangerous' (_R v Hardie_, p.757).

18 In contrast to the rules on voluntary intoxication (p.616), this includes offences of basic as well as specific intent (p.403).

was accepted that the defendant was involuntarily intoxicated, but the jury convicted on the basis of photographic and audio evidence that he had formed the intent to commit indecent assault).

Where involuntary intoxication is insufficient for acquittal, it may still be a <u>mitigating factor</u> (p.638) sufficient to reduce the sentence.

Voluntary intoxication

Generally, courts hold defendants responsible for their behaviour whilst intoxicated, unless they can prove their intoxication was <u>involuntary</u> (p.614). However, it is often difficult to determine a defendant's state of mind whilst intoxicated, and the courts have therefore devised a set of somewhat arbitrary rules governing such situations. These are followed strictly in E&W and NI, and more flexibly in Scotland and RoI.

Exceptions to the need to prove *mens rea*

As a general rule, the <u>mental element</u> of the offence (p.402) must still be proved; if it cannot be shown that the defendant possessed the relevant *mens rea*, then they cannot be convicted. However, the courts have established two major exceptions to this rule:

- If there is evidence that the defendant formed the *mens rea* for the offence beforehand, then became voluntarily intoxicated (e.g. in order to overcome their inhibitions) by the time they committed the offence, they can be convicted on the basis of their earlier *mens rea*.[19]
- If the criminal behaviour can be seen as a 'natural and probable' consequence of becoming voluntarily intoxicated, the defendant can be presumed to have intended or foreseen[20] that behaviour: as in <u>DPP v Majewski</u> (p.761), where the defendant drank heavily and then assaulted police officers.

Mistake and specific intent

If, **and only if,** neither of the exceptions above applies, then a lack of evidence of the required *mens rea* leads to acquittal, even if it is clear that the lack was due to voluntary intoxication. This means, for example, that:

- If voluntary intoxication causes the defendant to form a <u>mistaken belief</u> (p.404) that negates an element of the offence, they will be acquitted. For example, a person who genuinely believes (because of the influence of drink or drugs) that they own the property they are smashing cannot be convicted of <u>criminal damage</u> (p.422).
- If the offence is one of <u>specific intent</u> (p.403), and there is evidence that the defendant was not <u>capable of forming that intent</u> (p.610) because they were intoxicated, they will be acquitted. For example, a grossly drunken man who clearly cannot control his behaviour and who drops a lit cigarette into a pool of brandy he spilt earlier, causing a major fire, would be acquitted of <u>arson with intent</u> (p.422), although he might still be convicted of simple arson.

In very few cases, however, will voluntary intoxication be accepted as a defence to a crime of specific intent: a very high degree of intoxication is required. The courts have held that:

---

19 This is also an exception to the rule that the defendant must be shown to have *mens rea* at the time of the <u>*actus reus*</u> (p.400). Lord Denning notoriously described it as seeking 'Dutch courage'.
20 That is, been <u>reckless</u> (p.403).

- The degree of intoxication required is not defined by any particular blood alcohol level (because tolerance can vary between individuals due to varying metabolic rates and varying cerebral susceptibility).
- Ordinary evidence showing the defendant exercised a degree of control over their actions will neutralise the defence.

Scotland and RoI

The same rules exist in Scotland and RoI but are often interpreted more leniently: even recklessly voluntarily intoxicated defendants have been convicted of lesser offences (e.g. manslaughter instead of murder).

Expert evidence

A medical expert should comment only upon the capacity to form intent (p.610), not upon whether the defendant actually formed a particular intent, which is for the court to determine. There may be ordinary evidence showing that intention was in fact formed, negating any expert opinion favouring lack of capacity to form intent.

Intoxication and specific defences

Intoxication must be distinguished from mental disorder caused by substance use (e.g. dependence or a drug-induced psychotic episode), and from the effects of chronic substance-induced brain damage. Such mental disorder or brain damage may be relevant to <u>specific defences</u> (p.412), but the intoxication itself is usually not, even if it is involuntary.[21]

Diminished responsibility

Mental disorder or brain damage resulting from substance use
Substance-related mental disorder or chronic brain damage can amount to a 'recognised mental disorder', giving rise to an 'abnormality of mental functioning' (E&W, NI), to an 'abnormality of mind' (Scotland), and to a 'mental disorder' in RoI, for the purposes of <u>diminished responsibility</u> (p.624).

Intoxication in addition to a recognised medical condition
If the conditions of the defence are otherwise met (e.g. because of schizophrenia), the fact that the defendant was also intoxicated does not negate the defence (<u>R v Dietschmann</u>, p.753). Moreover, a combination of recognised medical conditions (e.g. bipolar disorder and alcohol dependence) can suffice for the defence. But if there would have been no 'substantial impairment' of the relevant capacity without the voluntary intoxication, the defence will fail (<u>R v Joyce</u>, p.759).

Intoxication as a recognised medical condition
In Scotland and RoI, the position is clear: intoxication is excluded from the definitions of diminished responsibility[22] and mental disorder for diminished responsibility,[23] respectively.

The definitions in NI and E&W[24] include the concept of a 'recognised medical condition', which acute intoxication is (and it is present in both ICD11 and DSM-5). However, the courts have ruled that intoxication is not *legally* a recognised medical condition (<u>R v Lindo</u> (p.760); <u>R v Dowds</u> (p.753)).

Automatism

If an <u>automatism</u> (p.612) is induced solely by involuntary intoxication, it is a noninsane automatism, and the defendant will therefore be acquitted (assuming the criteria for automatism are met). If, however, the automatism was induced solely by voluntary intoxication, the defence is unavailable (<u>R v Coley</u>, p.752).

---

21 However, involuntary intoxication (p.614) may act as a *general* defence in the same case, if it prevented the defendant forming the relevant mental element (p.402).

22 Criminal Procedure (Scotland) Act 1995 s51B(3).

23 Criminal Law (Insanity) Act 2006 s1.

24 Under the new tests. Appeals relating to the old tests for diminished responsibility (p.624) could not succeed on the basis of acute intoxication, as that is not a condition of arrested or retarded development of mind, an inherent cause, or induced by disease or injury.

An automatism induced by substance-related mental disorder or chronic brain damage will be an <u>insane automatism</u> (p.612).

Insanity

Intoxication, no matter how severe, cannot on its own cause <u>insanity</u> (p.620), because it is not *legally* a 'disease of the mind' (<u>*R v Quick*</u>, p.765). However, substance-related mental disorder or brain damage may form the basis of a defence of insanity.

Temporary insanity arising from voluntary intoxication

In NI, a statutory provision[25] provides an exception to the rule above. It concerns defendants who, at the time of an alleged murder, were 'labouring under such a defect of reason ... as not to know the nature and quality of [their] act [or, that it] was wrong' because of voluntary intoxication. If before becoming intoxicated, they had the intention of killing or causing serious harm, they will be convicted of murder, otherwise they will be convicted of manslaughter. In other jurisdictions, such defendants could still be convicted of murder.

25 Criminal Justice Act (Northern Ireland) 1966, s6.

Insanity

Insanity is a defence to any crime and is available in all criminal cases (*R v Loake*, p.761). If successful, the verdict is 'not guilty by reason of insanity'. Criticisms of it include:

- The purely cognitive nature of the test, and very high threshold excluding even some severely psychotic defendants.[26]
- Inconsistency with modern psychiatric understanding.
- *Insane* is an outdated word for describing those with mental illness, and is wrong in describing intellectual disability or epilepsy.

The McNaughten rules

These common law rules still form the insanity test in E&W.

> At the time of the committing of the act, the party accused was labouring under such a **defect of reason**, from **disease of the mind**, as not **to know the nature and quality of the act** he was doing; or, if he did know it, that he did not know what he was doing **was wrong.**
> **McNaughten rules, 1843**

Defect of reason excludes all mental functioning other than reasoning. Unlike diminished responsibility (p.624), it does not represent 'the mind in all its aspects' (*R v Byrne*, p.750). Uncontrollable urges do not amount to defect of reason.

Disease of the mind includes:
- brain arteriosclerosis (*R v Kemp*, p.759),
- epilepsy (*R v Sullivan*, p.768),
- hyperglycaemia in untreated diabetes (*R v Hennessy*, p.757),
- sleepwalking (*R v Burgess*; p.750, cf. automatism, p.612), and

States induced by external factors are not included, such as insulin-induced hypoglycaemia (*R v Quick*, p.765) or cannabis intoxication (*R v Coley* p.752).

Not knowing the nature of quality of the act suggests, for example, being delusional about the act itself or its object.[27]

Wrong means legally, not morally wrong (*R v Windle*, p.771).
- Psychosis or other mental states may explain the behaviour but not prevent the defendant knowing[28] their actions were legally wrong.
- Evidence of stopping when the police arrive might suggest knowing that the act was illegal.

26 The Law Commission reported in 2013 that in E&W there were fewer than thirty successful insanity pleas each year.

27 Arguably this should result in acquittal, as it means the defendant lacks the required mental element; but public policy dictates that there should be a mechanism for protecting society from people who commit serious offences in such states, hence their inclusion within the insanity defence.

28 The narrow legal interpretation of 'knowing' is straightforward, but someone psychotically driven to offend by command auditory hallucinations or passivity phenomena, for instance, might be unable to *appreciate*, or *pay attention*, to the knowledge they might otherwise have that their acts were legally wrong.

Statutory forms of the insanity defence

Scotland s51A Criminal Procedure (Scotland) Act 1995[29]

This statutory test is referred to as the 'special defence'; the term *insanity* is not used. It excludes personality disorder characterised solely or principally by abnormally aggressive or seriously irresponsible conduct.

> A person is not criminally responsible for conduct constituting an offence, and is to be acquitted of the offence, if the person was at the time of the conduct unable by reason of mental disorder to appreciate the nature or wrongfulness of the conduct.
> **Section 51A CPSA**

The word *appreciates* is looser than '*knows*' in the McNaughten rules.

NI s1 Criminal Justice Act (NI) 1966

Defendants suffer from a mental abnormality which prevents them:
- appreciating what they are doing or
- appreciating that it is wrong or contrary to law or
- from controlling their own conduct.

RoI s5 Criminal law (Insanity) Act 2006

- The accused was suffering at the time from a mental disorder, and
- The mental disorder was such that the accused ought not to be held responsible for the act alleged by reason of the fact that the person—
  - did not know the nature and quality of the act or
  - did not know that what he or she was doing was wrong or
  - was unable to refrain from committing the act.

Procedures

E&W Criminal Procedure (Insanity) Act 1964 (as amended)

- Applies in both Crown and Magistrates Courts
- Raised by defence, prosecution or judge
- Jury may disagree with unanimous medical evidence
- Burden of proof on defence (on balance of probabilities)

Scotland Criminal Procedure (Scotland) Act 1995

- Written/oral evidence of two or more registered medical practitioners
- Jury decision

NI Mental Health (Northern Ireland) Order 1986[30]

- Oral evidence of one and written or oral evidence of another doctor
- Jury decision

RoI Criminal law (Insanity) Act 2006

- Oral evidence of one consultant psychiatrist
- Jury decision

---

29 As inserted by the Criminal Justice and Licensing (Scotland) Act 2010.

30 The MCANI contains identical provisions.

Outcome of successful insanity defence

E&W, NI, and Scotland
- Hospital order (compulsion order in Scotland)
- Hospital or compulsion order with restrictions (in E&W these are mandatory if the charge was murder, and a hospital order is appropriate)
- Interim hospital or compulsion order
- Guardianship
- Supervision order (supervision and treatment order in Scotland)
- Absolute discharge

RoI
- Initial committal to a designated centre for not more than fourteen days for inpatient or outpatient care or treatment

Reform

The Law Commission for E&W has proposed changes to:
- improve compatibility with modern medicine;
- rename the defence;
- incorporate mental capacity into the test, in line with constructs used in s52 Coroners and Justice Act 2009, amending s2 Homicide Act 1957, but requiring total incapacity rather than substantially impaired capacity; and
- clarify when an insanity defence should be chosen over other defences.

Diminished responsibility

Tests of diminished responsibility

Diminished responsibility

Diminished responsibility is a <u>partial defence</u> (p.412) to <u>murder</u> (p.414) only. If successful, the defendant is convicted of manslaughter (culpable homicide in Scotland) and avoids the <u>mandatory life sentence</u> (p.448).

Diminished responsibility can only be raised by the defence (unlike <u>insanity</u>, p.620, and <u>unfitness to</u> plead, p.602). It is determined on the <u>balance of probabilities</u> (p.380). And, since an insightless defendant may refuse to plead diminished responsibility, you should always assess <u>fitness to plead</u> (p.602).

Tests of diminished responsibility

E&W and NI s2 Homicide Act 1957; s5 Criminal Justice Act (NI) 1966[31]

A defendant, D, is not to be convicted of murder, but only manslaughter, if D was suffering from an

- **abnormality of mental functioning** which:
- arose from a **recognised medical condition** and
- **substantially impaired** D's ability to—
  - understand the nature of D's conduct or
  - form a rational judgment or
  - exercise self-control;
- and which **provides an explanation** for D's acts and omissions in doing or being a party to the killing; (meaning that it caused, or was a significant contributory factor in causing, D to carry out the killing).

Scotland <u>Galbraith v HM Advocate</u> (p.756)

Diminished responsibility requires:

- an abnormality of mind (including psychopathy),
- which need not 'border on insanity', and
- which had the effect that the accused's ability to determine or control their actions was **substantially impaired**.

RoI s6 Criminal Law (Insanity) Act 2006

If the jury or court finds that a defendant charged with murder:

---

31 As amended by the Coroners and Justice Act 2009. An older version applied to offences in E&W before 4.10.10 and in NI before 1.6.11, and can therefore still be relevant to appeals against such offences. Instead of the four limbs above, the older test had two: 'abnormality of mind (whether arising from a condition of arrested or retarded development of mind or any inherent cause or induced by disease or injury)' and 'substantially impaired his mental responsibility for his acts'.

- did the act alleged,
- was at the time suffering from a **mental disorder**, and
- that disorder did not amount to <u>insanity</u> (p.620), but
- it **diminished substantially** his **responsibility** for the act,

the jury or court shall find them not guilty of murder, but guilty of manslaughter on the ground of diminished responsibility.

Which mental disorders qualify?

Abnormality of mind[32] has been defined (p.753) as 'a state of mind so different from that of ordinary human beings that the reasonable man would term it abnormal', and as covering 'the mind in all its aspects' (<u>R v Byrne</u>, p.750). This is not a medical test, but requires medical evidence in support of it (R v Dix, p.VI.12). It includes abnormalities of consciousness, perception, cognition, mood and volition; and is therefore effectively much broader than is required by the amended defence in E&W and NI. Courts have allowed the following examples:

- schizophrenia and paranoid psychosis (<u>R v Sanderson</u>, p.767);
- paranoid personality disorder (<u>R v Martin (Anthony)</u>, p.762);
- premenstrual stress & postnatal depression (<u>R v Reynolds</u>);
- chronic alcoholism causing brain damage (<u>R v Tandy</u>, p.769);
- irresistible perverted sexual desires (<u>R v Byrne</u>, p.750); and
- 'battered woman syndrome' (<u>R v Ahluwalia</u>, p.746).[33]

In E&W and NI, despite its name, whether a condition is a **recognised medical condition** is a legal test. Doctors and international classification systems defining a medical condition is necessary but not sufficient (<u>R v Dowds</u>, p.753). Hence intoxication is not legally a 'recognised medical condition', and cannot add to a condition so as to result in diminished responsibility if that other condition alone would have been insufficient (see pp.614, 616 for details)—although it cannot invalidate an otherwise valid responsibility defence (<u>R v Dietschmann</u>, p.753). Psychosis brought on by drug intoxication is not a 'recognised medical condition'[34]. However, a defendant who chronically abuses substances for years and has alcohol dependence syndrome, and then is intoxicated at the time of the offence, may be able to rely on the defence (<u>R v Tandy</u>, p.769; <u>R v Stewart</u>, p.768; <u>R v Wood</u> p.771).

In RoI the legal definition of **mental disorder** for the purpose of diminished responsibility excludes intoxication.

Substantial impairment

The UK Supreme Court has defined 'substantial'[35] (in the context of impairment of mental responsibility or of a qualifying ability), as having its ordinary

---

32 Part of the test in Scotland, and the old test in E&W and NI; the courts in E&W and NI have generally applied similar criteria to the new term, 'abnormality of mental functioning'.

33 However, it would not now be a 'recognised medical condition', unless the D had another disorder (e.g. PTSD); since it lacks symptom validity; arises more clearly from social theory and psychology than from psychiatry, and is defined not only in terms of the 'symptoms' of the abused woman but also of the abuser's behaviour and the characteristic interaction pattern of the couple.

34 R v Foy [2020] EWCA Crim 270.

35 Caselaw in E&W previously defined 'substantial' as 'having substance' and as 'less than total and more than trivial' (<u>R v Lloyd</u>, 760).

meaning; and that, if the jury asks for direction, they should be advised that it means 'weighty', not just 'more than trivial' (*R v Golds*, p.757).

Causation

The final limb of the amended test in E&W and NI requires the abnormality of mental functioning to **provide an explanation** for the killing, meaning that it caused it or contributed significantly to it.

Psychiatry cannot address causation with scientific rigour; instead, any expert comment must be expressed as a formulation (p.146) of the role of the 'abnormality' within the narrative of the killing. Where relevant facts have not yet been determined by the court, this may need to be a conditional opinion ('if X is found, then my opinion would be A; if Y then B').

Expert psychiatric evidence concerning causation is allowed; and there was, prior to amendment in E&W, emphasis on jury decision-making (*R v Khan*, p.759). However now if there is uncontested expert evidence it cannot be ignored 'irrationally' by a jury; so that the judge should remove the charge of murder from consideration by the jury if there is unchallenged expert evidence of diminished responsibility (*R v Brennan*, p.749).[36]

Scotland, and the old test in E&W and NI

The Scottish test, as with the old test in E&W and NI, leaves it open to juries to weigh medical evidence about the killing against competing explanations. It is not necessary that the abnormality of mind is the only explanation for the killing (*R v Dietschmann*, p.VI.12); only that it itself substantially impaired responsibility.

Is it a medical or moral test?

This question becomes enmeshed with the right, or not, of juries to ignore unanimous expert evidence supportive of the defence (see above).

Diminished responsibility is a legal test based on moral foundations, but for which expert evidence is required.

Notably the term 'diminished responsibility' in E&W does not occur in the body of s52; since there is a presumption that if all the limbs of the defence are satisfied, based upon expert evidence, then responsibility is indeed diminished. This reflects the wish of the Law Commission to ground what is a moral defence in medical constructs and reasoning.

The case of a soldier convicted of the murder of an Afghan insurgent, reduced by the Court of Appeal to manslaughter based upon unanimous expert evidence of only 'adjustment reaction' (a diagnosis lacking pathognomonic symptoms and based upon clinically differentiating 'normal' from

---

36 Assuming the prosecution has not by this stage accepted the plea of diminished responsibility.

'abnormal' reactions), in the face of head camera and audio evidence clearly indicative of a revenge killing, suggests that the essentially moral interpretation of diminished responsibility continues to assert itself (_R v Blackman_, p.748).

Effect of a finding of diminished responsibility

The sentencing options for manslaughter and culpable homicide range from <u>absolute discharge</u> (p.456) to discretionary <u>life imprisonment</u> (p.448), or <u>treatment in hospital</u> (p.500). It is not uncommon for a plea of diminished responsibility to be accepted and for the defendant still be to be sentenced to imprisonment—for instance, because the mental condition was a temporary one, or other criteria of mental health law are not met.

In E&W, the decisions in _Vowles_ and _Edwards_ (pp.754, 770) have emphasised that discretionary life imprisonment may be appropriate despite diminished responsibility, for reasons of required punishment and/or public protection.

Controversies

Developmental immaturity

None of the tests allow a plea of diminished responsibility based upon non-pathological developmental immaturity in a child defendant, as this is not a recognised medical condition. (E&W and NI), abnormality of mind (Scotland) or mental disorder (RoI)[37] This means that a ten year old (without mental disorder) who, when emotionally overwhelmed, was substantially impaired in their ability to exercise self-control, for example, is not able to plead the defence; whereas an 'immature' adult with personality disorder may be able to do so.

In Scotland and RoI

The defence has generally been used very flexibly in these jurisdictions, with responsibility resting on juries to follow, or reject medical evidence as they see fit. In Scotland, there has been some limited debate over the exclusion of psychopathy (or effectively ASPD more widely). In RoI, there has been some disquiet over sentencing after a finding of diminished responsibility, where there is no option to send the defendant to hospital (although they may be <u>transferred from prison</u>, p.506), and sentencing guidelines do not take the mental element of the crime into account in determining the length of imprisonment.

---

37 The Law Commission recommended including this in the new test in E&W and NI, but its proposal was not accepted.

Frequency of the finding

The number of cases successfully pleaded in E&W, either with the agreement of the Crown or at trial, steadily diminished under the old test. There is no clear explanation for this. It may have related to:
- changing social attitudes, and a reduced willingness for juries to accept what appear to be excuses for killing, and
- 'targets' set for the CPS which value conviction more highly than accepting a plea of diminished responsibility.

There is little evidence that this decline has been reversed by introduction of the reformed test in E&W, as might have been expected. Decisions of the Court of Appeal and Supreme Court in pulling the role of the jury again into prominence (see above) may continue to be influential in this.

Variability of findings

Apparent limitation, on the face of the statute, of the freedom of juries now to balance competing explanations for the killing, plus emphasis of the role of experts, might have been expected to reduce the variability in outcomes between defendants in similar cases in E&W and NI, by comparison with Scotland, or E&W pre amendment. There is as yet no evidence of this.

Expert interview and reporting

You should interview the defendant at the earliest opportunity, albeit usually once the relevant medical and legal papers are available. It is common for psychiatrists instructed by the prosecution to wait until they have received a defence expert report before instructing assessment of the defendant (because legally the defence must raise the issue); however, this practice may invite a wrong expert approach, driven by the question of whether there is a basis upon which to rebut the defence report—rather than production of an independent opinion. This risk can be managed by:
- if instructed by the Crown, carrying out your assessment before reading any other expert's report and,
- if instructed by the defence, submitting an interim report containing only a summary of your opinion (thus allowing the defendant to enter a plea and the prosecution to know whether it needs its own expert report), whilst reserving your full report, with data and reasoning, to be produced in parallel with that of the prosecution expert.

Discussing the alleged offence

Experts may be cautious when asking the defendant about the alleged offence in case it prejudices the case. However, it is proper to do so because:
- The defendant's account of the alleged offence may itself reveal symptoms of mental disorder at the time.
- It will be necessary to develop a formulation of the killing (including through the defendant's own description) in terms of the potential relationship between the killing and any mental abnormality.

Considering disposal

Instructions from solicitors in a murder trial will usually focus upon the question of diminished responsibility (or some other trial related issue) rather than on sentencing. However, if an expert's findings are supportive of diminished responsibility it may seem natural then also to offer an opinion on disposal (p.456) in the event that defence were to be successful. If the recommendation is not for hospital admission (p.500), then, even though this cannot be disclosed in front of the jury, this may give the false impression that the defendant was seriously mentally disordered at the time at the time of the killing. It may therefore be wise to exclude any recommendation from the report, unless there has been a specific instruction to address it.

Loss of control & provocation

The common law developed the concept of provocation in the seventeenth century as a 'concession to human frailty', when murder carried the death penalty: it partially excused 'loss of mastery over the mind in response to things said or done' by resulting in a <u>manslaughter</u> (p.414) conviction.[38] Over time, the defence became viewed first as too restrictive, and then as too subjective[39]; and it has been replaced in statute in E&W and NI by 'loss of control' but has evolved more gradually in Scotland and RoI.

Tests of provocation and loss of control

Scotland <u>Robertson v HM Advocate</u> (p.766)
- Provocation requires a **loss of self-control**, and
- a reasonably **proportionate** (i.e. not grossly disproportionate) **relationship** between the provocation and the reaction to it.
- It can only apply where the defendant 'has been assaulted and there has been substantial provocation ... no mere verbal provocation can palliate killing. ...To this [there is] one exception ... when an accused discovers that their partner ... has been unfaithful' (<u>Drury</u>, p.754).
- There is no requirement to show that an ordinary person might have acted in the same way (<u>Gillon</u> p.757).
- A finding of provocation usually results in conviction for culpable homicide, but could sometimes still be for murder (<u>Drury</u>, p.754).

RoI <u>R v Duffy</u> (p.754)
- Provocation is one or more acts by the victim which cause a **sudden and temporary loss of self-control** and which
- would cause such loss of self-control **in any reasonable person**;
- 'temporary' means that the defendant must act before having had an opportunity to regain composure (<u>Masciantonio v The Queen</u>[40]).

E&W and **NI**: s54 Coroners and Justice Act 2009
A defendant, D, is not to be convicted of murder (but only manslaughter) if:
- D's acts and omissions resulted from D's **loss of control** (**which need not be sudden**);
- the loss of self-control had a **qualifying trigger** (fear of serious violence and/or acts or words that constitute circumstances of an extremely grave character and give a justifiable sense of being seriously wronged[41]);

---

38 <u>R v Duffy</u> (p.VI.12). In other jurisdictions, including some US and Australian states, provocation can be a defence to any <u>offence against the person</u> (p.416). In Scotland and elsewhere, the term is also used to refer to circumstances that <u>mitigate</u> (p.638) offence seriousness, and therefore can reduce the sentence.

39 The peak of subjectivity was represented by the decision in <u>Morgan Smith</u> (p.763), where the defendant's depression was taken into account in deciding not just his sensitivity to things said or done, but whether his violent response to the provocation was reasonable.

40 The English case of <u>Duffy</u> and this Australian case have been accepted as authoritative in RoI.

41 The feared violence must be from the victim to the defendant or another person. Feared violence does not count insofar as it was caused by anything D 'incited to be done or said for the purpose of providing an excuse to use violence'. Similarly, a sense of being seriously wronged is not a qualifying trigger if it was caused by something D incited for the purpose of gaining such an excuse.

- a person of D's sex and age, with a **normal degree of tolerance and self-restraint**, and **in the circumstances of D**, might have reacted in the same or a similar way to D; and
- D did not act in a considered desire for revenge.

Sexual infidelity is explicitly excluded as a ground for feeling 'seriously wronged', although it may be taken into account alongside other grounds if it is integral to the facts as a whole (*R v Clinton*, p.751).

Once sufficient evidence has been adduced for a jury reasonably to conclude that provocation or loss of control might apply, the burden of proof (p.380) is then on the prosecution to prove beyond reasonable doubt that it does not.

Problems with the reasonable person test

This test, which is inherent to the defence in E&W, NI, and RoI, has caused problems in many jurisdictions because of dispute about the extent to which the reasonable person should be imbued with the specific characteristics, including mental characteristics, of the defendant (ranging from youthfulness to learning disability to particular personality traits).[42] The statutory rules in E&W and NI for 'loss of control' are an awkward compromise between a purely objective, and an excessively subjective test. It is already clear that mental disorder cannot be taken into account insofar as it bears on the defendant's general capacity for tolerance and self-restraint (*Rejmanski*, p.766), making this element of the test purely objective. There does remain, however, scope for subjectivity in how broadly judges interpret 'in the circumstances of D' in regard to the defendant's sensitivity to, or 'woundability' by, any alleged qualifying trigger.

Scotland avoids these difficulties, with its simpler proportionality rule.

Role of psychiatric evidence

Psychiatric evidence may be relevant where a mental disorder or characteristic might have affected a defendant's woundability (part of their circumstances) in response to qualifying triggers in the defence. For example,
- A history of childhood sexual abuse might be relevant to a sexual assault in adulthood acting as a trigger or provocation.

---

42 The courts have adopted varying views: see *Camplin*, *Morgan Smith*, and *Holley* (pp.750, 763, 758). This is the same tension as is found between subjective and objective approaches to intention (p.402).

- Evidence of a mental characteristic such as depressed mood, or a depressive illness, might make the defendant more 'woundable' by taunts (e.g. about inadequacy).
- Chronic spousal abuse might affect the abused victims mentally such that they are the more easily wounded by things said or done by their abuser, such as further taunts or violence.

Controversies

- Men tend more to react immediately to provocation, including in response to sexual infidelity or relationship loss; whereas many women react after delay, or what has been called a 'slow burn'.[43] This is particularly the case in 'battered woman syndrome' (which can include PTSD, p.96). The provocation defence was thought to discriminate against women because of the requirement for the response to be sudden; the loss of control defence is intended to remedy this.[44]
- The rules on the 'qualifying trigger' in E&W and NI may greatly restrict the scope of the defence, as may the policy-driven exclusion of sexual infidelity (which is difficult to define).
- Some authors suggest that provocation should either be available as a general defence, or be abolished (alongside abolition of the mandatory life sentence for murder, so that provoked killers could potentially be given a more lenient sentence).

Relationship with diminished responsibility

Pleading the defences in tandem

It is possible to plead loss of control or provocation, and diminished responsibility (p.624) simultaneously, even adding self-defence (p.410). Juries are usually instructed to consider self-defence, which is highly restricted, first, then diminished responsibility, and finally loss of control or provocation.

Legal polarising of a psychological spectrum

Provocation or loss of control and diminished responsibility represent two poles of a psychological spectrum: in the purest form of the latter, the cause of killing is entirely internal (i.e. solely the product of mental disorder); whereas in 'pure' loss of control or provocation, the cause is entirely external. In between lie degrees of mixed causation, such as where the other's words or actions play upon an abnormality of mental functioning (e.g. in delusional misidentification or severe depression), or where the provocation is slight and, although someone else might not be particularly woundable by such provocation and retaliate, someone with the characteristics (or in the circumstances) of the defendant might do so. There remains a large gap in the middle where neither defence is available.

---

43 *R v Ahluwalia* (p.746).

44 However, the requirement might actually disadvantage abused women, who typically kill in a very considered fashion, often having developed learned helplessness: the consideration might mean they are not found to have lost control, whereas it has in the past met the old common law test of 'loss of mastery over the mind'. Only if the test is interpreted to include distorted and restricted reasoning on a defendant's options will the defence afford itself to most abused women who kill.

Duress, coercion, and necessity

Duress is a complete defence to an offence as a result of specific **threats** or **circumstances**. In Scotland, duress by threats is known as *coercion*; duress of circumstances is known as *necessity* in Scotland and RoI.

Once evidence suggesting duress has been raised, the <u>burden of proof</u> (p.380) is on the prosecution to show that the defendant did not act under duress. The defence does not apply to murder,[45] attempted murder or treason: the law protects the 'sanctity of life' (<u>R v Gotts</u>, p.757).

Duress by threats (coercion)

The basis of the defence is that another person's threats overwhelmed the defendant's will (a **subjective** test), and would have overwhelmed the will of a person of ordinary courage or fortitude (an **objective** test).

E&W and NI <u>R v Hasan</u> (p.757)

Threats can amount to duress if:
- they concern serious bodily harm or death to the defendant, their family, or someone close to them;
- a reasonable person of their age and background[46] would have been forced to act in the same way;
- the threats directly caused the criminal conduct;
- the criminal conduct could not have been avoided without the threatened harm; and
- the defendant did not voluntarily run the risk of such threats (associating with the threatener, e.g. another gang member).

Scotland <u>Thomson v HM Advocate</u>

'It is only where, following threats, there is an immediate danger of violence ... that the defence of coercion can be entertained; and even then only if there is an inability to resist or avoid that immediate danger ... It is the danger which has to be "immediate", not just the threat.'

RoI <u>A-G v Whelan</u> (p.746)

Duress requires:
- 'threats of immediate death or personal violence ... so great as to overbear the ordinary power of human resistance';
- the defendant's will must actually have been overborne;
- the duress must have been operating when the offence was committed; and
- there must have been no opportunity for the defendant to escape.

Duress of circumstances (necessity)

This defence concerns situations in which an offence is committed in order to avert death or serious physical injury.

---

45 Including aiding and abetting, counselling or procuring murder; but it is available on a charge of conspiracy to murder.

46 This can include pregnancy, serious physical disability, or mental disorder, but no other 'woundability' characteristics such as traits of emotional instability (<u>R v Bowen</u>, p.749). It no longer includes simply being a married woman: the E&W defence of marital coercion was abolished in 2014.

E&W, NI, and RoI <u>R v Martin</u> *(p.761)*
- The defendant had good cause to fear death or serious injury
- and was therefore impelled to commit the offence to avert this
- because of what they reasonably believed to be the situation.
- From an objective standpoint, the defendant acted reasonably and proportionately to the danger.
- A sober person of reasonable firmness, sharing their characteristics, would have responded to the situation in the same way.
- The danger was not brought about by the defendant themselves.

Scotland <u>Moss v Howdle</u> *(p.763)*
- The defendant acted under an immediate threat of death or great bodily harm to themselves or another person.
- The criminal conduct was an endeavour to escape the danger.
- There was no reasonable, alternative course of action.

In addition, the common law doctrine of <u>medical necessity</u> (p.542) provides a defence to offences such as <u>battery</u> (p.416) which would have been committed by giving treatment.

Duress and undue influence in civil law

Duress applies if force or violence is used to compel a person to enter into (or discharge) a contract. If the defence succeeds, the contract is invalidated and may be rescinded. There are two broad categories:
- Physical duress (the use or threat of physical force or violence)
- Economic duress (the use or threat of financial inducements or penalties).

There is a related civil law <u>equitable doctrine</u> (p.366) of **undue influence** in making a contract or will. This arises if the claimant and defendant have a 'special relationship' and the contract is made on unfairly advantageous terms, or the bequest is over-generous. If the relationship is a recognised one (e.g. parent-child or doctor-patient) there need be no proof of actually placing special trust in the defendant.

Relevance of psychiatric evidence

Psychiatric evidence may be relevant in criminal proceedings where the defendant had a recognised mental disorder which can be held to have reduced the defendant's fortitude to below 'reasonable fortitude' (see above). For example, an abused woman with PTSD whose children are threatened with harm if she does not smuggle drugs may not have the 'reasonable fortitude' to resist the threats. Expert comment should not address whether or not they were 'coerced', or acted out of 'necessity', per se.

Amnesia

Amnesia for an alleged offence is potentially legally relevant because it can be (though usually is not) suggestive of an abnormal state at the time of the offence or because the defence may call expert evidence to give credibility to the defendant's claimed amnesia.

Law

Amnesia for events surrounding an alleged offence cannot be a defence or render a defendant unfit to plead (R v Podola, p.764). Even if the defendant truly cannot recall the relevant events, they can respond to evidence in the trial, and it would be simple to claim 'I can't remember' to avoid trial. However the rule may put a defendant at a disadvantage, particularly if only they and the victim were present and the issue is whether the victim is telling the truth, or if the victim is dead. If the amnesia is due to a generalised memory disorder, or other cognitive impairment, that disorder or impairment can be relevant to fitness to plead (p.602).

If amnesia for an offence is genuine, this can bear upon the reliability of a defendant or witness (p.156), especially if they attempt to 'do their best' to remember ('I must have done ...' rather than 'I remember ...'). A generalised memory disorder will also be relevant to reliability, most obviously where there is amnestic syndrome and confabulation.

Questions put to experts

- Is the defendant's amnesia for relevant events genuine?
- Does the amnesia suggest an underlying condition which could be a basis for a mental condition defence (p.412)?
- Does the amnesia suggest the defendant lacked the capacity to form the mental element (p.402) for the offence?
- Does the defendant have a generalised memory disorder relevant to fitness to plead (p.602) or to reliability (p.156) in police interviews or to the ability to give evidence (p.606)?

Clinical assessment

Assessment includes reading all medical and legal documents for evidence of the consistency and extent of the claimed amnesia. Police interviews and witness statements should be read carefully: it is embarrassing to suggest amnesia at the time of the alleged offence and then to be cross-examined with evidence which clearly suggests relevant memories.

Relevant clinical issues include whether there have been multiple episodes of amnesia, or whether the amnesia is solely for events surrounding the offence: if the latter, then it is most likely to have arisen either from a disorder of consciousness at the relevant time (preventing the laying down of memory) or from 'psychogenic amnesia' (dissociation preventing the recall of memory[47]).

---

47 Some authors, confusingly, use the term *dissociative amnesia* to include amnesia resulting from dissociation at the time when memory would otherwise have been formed.

Dissociative disorders and dissociative amnesia

Clinically it is difficult to distinguish between psychogenic **dissociative amnesia**, and the effects on memory formation of a **dissociative state** at the time of the offence. Dissociative amnesia (p.101) has a number of characteristics: it is often patchy; it is associated with emotionally significant, arousing events (e.g. the offence); and it can resolve gradually.

Other evidence is required to demonstrate that there was dissociation at the time of the offence, such as:

• depersonalisation and/or derealisation recalled as occurring prior to the time of the offence;
• dense amnesia for the offence, with clear previous and next memories;
• acts out of character with apparently purposeful behaviours despite lack of memory;
• observed confusion after the offence;
• presence of other factors predisposing to dissociation (e.g. head injury or traumatic brain injury), previous episodes of dissociation, depersonalisation, or derealisation;
• precipitation by a psychologically significant event (e.g. being sexually assaulted when there is a personal history of sexual abuse).

Dissociative amnesia is the most likely explanation of amnesia for an offence; amnesia resulting from dissociation at the time of the offence is uncommon. There is often suspicion that such amnesia may be at least partly feigned (see malingering p.118), and cross-examination of the expert is therefore often robust.

Alcohol-induced amnesia

Alcohol-induced amnesia can occur in the context of chronic alcohol abuse and can reflect **alcohol blackout** syndrome, in which the individual wakes with no recollection of the events of the previous day or evening. Since violent offending is also often associated with intoxication the two commonly occur together.

Other organic causes

Head injury occurring at the time of the offence can cause a transient organic amnesia. A history of any other neurological condition that might explain claimed amnesia for the offence, for example 'transient epileptic amnesia', requires thorough assessment and investigation, especially if there are no records of previous diagnosis.

Aggravating and mitigating factors

These factors, taken into account by judges when sentencing offenders, (p.IV,91) are distinct from risk factors or dangerousness (p.672), although some risk factors may be relevant to aggravation. In E&W, and to a lesser extent NI, judges are constrained by sentencing guidelines (p.443) which define such factors, how they should affect the sentence, and how this should be explained to the defendant (see Box 19.2). In Scotland and RoI, judges have wider discretion in taking such factors into account.

Aggravating factors

These are features of an offence that indicate either that particularly grave harm was caused, or that the offender was particularly culpable for it.

Factors indicating greater degree of **harm** include:
- victimising someone vulnerable;
- offending against a public servant (e.g. police officer, nurse);
- harming multiple victims;
- causing particularly serious injury, mental trauma or other harm; and
- committing the offence against, or in the presence of children.

Examples of greater **culpability** include:
- offending while on bail awaiting trial for another offence;
- being motivated by the victim's religion, sexuality or race (hate crimes);
- planning the offence in advance, or as part of an organised crime group;
- concurrent use of drugs or alcohol;
- using a weapon; and
- abusing a position of power or trust.

Mitigating factors

Some factors may indicate lesser culpability, or that the harm caused by an offence is less serious than usual. Examples include:
- being provoked (p.630) into committing an offence other than murder,
- suffering from a relevant disability or mental disorder,
- being young or otherwise vulnerable or immature,
- playing only a very limited role in the offence,
- showing remorse or trying to make amends,
- reporting oneself to the police, and
- pleading guilty at the first opportunity.

Weighing up the factors

Even within the guideline of E&W, there is no formula to decide what weight should be given individual factors, although there are suggested thresholds above which community or custodial sentences may be appropriate.

Relevance of psychiatric evidence

A psychiatrist should not comment upon mitigation or aggravation. However, any presentence report they provide on a defendant's mental disorder may then be used in mitigation, but also for determining dangerousness (which may pose an ethical dilemma, p.318).

Expert reports may also inadvertently raise or imply other aggravating or mitigating factors even though written for other purposes:

- Psychological or psychiatric formulations may suggest a motivation for offending, including arising out of mental pathology.
- A psychiatric history may contain evidence of aggravating or mitigating factors (e.g. being abused or hating people from a certain minority group).
- The report may recount the defendant's attitudes towards, or remorse for, an offence.
- Some diagnoses may themselves be seen as aggravating factors, especially certain personality disorders such as <u>narcissistic</u> (p.86) or <u>antisocial</u> (p.82) personality disorder.

Box 19.2 Example from E&W sentencing guidelines for magistrates

Sentencing and mitigation in **common assault**
- Starting point: fine
- One aggravating factor indicating greater culpability: usually community sentence
- Two factors: usually custodial sentence

Common aggravating factors indicating **greater culpability**
- Weapon use
- Planned or sustained offence
- Head-butting, kicking, biting, or attempted strangulation
- Motivated by sexual orientation or disability
- Motivated by hostility towards a minority group
- Abuse of position of trust
- Offence as part of a group

Common aggravating factors indicating **greater harm**
- Serious injury
- Victim providing a public service, or was highly vulnerable
- Additional degradation of victim
- Offence committed in the presence of a child
- Forced entry into victim's home
- Offender prevented victim seeking or obtaining help
- Previous threats or violence to the same victim

Common **mitigating factors** for common assault
- Provocation
- Single push, shove or blow

Legal tests in personal injury cases

Personal injury claims alleging <u>negligence</u> (p.548) in allowing an injury to occur represent a lucrative industry. Psychiatric injury is often the claimed harm (Box 19.3).

> **Box 19.3 Basis for a claim for compensation for psychiatric injury**
>
> Compensation for psychiatric injury requires:
> - a recognisable psychiatric illness is present (not just 'mental distress')
> - the disorder was caused or aggravated by the acts or omissions of a negligent defendant

Specific legal rules in psychiatric injury cases

- Both primary and secondary victims may be entitled to compensation but the distinction, and implications, can be complex. 'Innocent bystanders' are not entitled to compensation, as harm to them is deemed too <u>remote</u> (p.549).
  - A **primary victim** suffers psychiatric illness as a result of being directly (physically) injured, or put in fear of injury.[48]
  - A **secondary victim** suffers psychiatric illness ('nervous shock'), as a result of being in a 'close tie of love and affection' with a primary victim, and being present at, and directly perceiving, an incident that caused them direct injury (or its immediate aftermath).
- The danger arising from a situation must have been **reasonably foreseeable**. If harm was reasonably foreseeable, and the fear of this caused psychiatric illness, there need not be proof of actual harm.
- People who act as **rescuers** (private individuals or professionals e.g. police and fire officers) may claim compensation for psychiatric injury on the ground that it is reasonably foreseeable that people will attempt to rescue victims of a dangerous situation.
- People who are **involuntary participants**[49] in the creation of a dangerous situation that results (or could reasonably foreseeably have resulted) in injury may be entitled to compensation if they suffer psychiatric illness.
- Psychiatric illness caused by **workplace stress** can be a ground for compensation, again if the psychiatric illness was reasonably foreseeable.
- Both ill-treatment by prison officers and insensitively breaking bad news have also been held to be grounds for compensation when reasonably foreseeable psychiatric illness has resulted.

The shock requirement for secondary victims

The psychiatric illness must have been induced by 'a sudden assault on the nervous system'. For example, the courts have ruled that psychiatric illness resulting from years spent caring for a negligently injured spouse, or dealing

---

48 They must be 'directly involved in the accident … and well within the range of foreseeable physical injury': _Page v Smith_ (p.764).

49 For example, the crane driver in _Dooley v Cammell Laird_ (p.753) was an involuntary participant in feared injury caused by his employer's negligence.

with a negligently brain-damaged child's challenging behaviour, did not warrant compensation, because there was no 'shock' nor, for the same reason, did viewing a disaster involving loved ones on live television.

The shock requirement is deliberately restrictive: the courts fear opening the 'floodgates' to a large number of claims, which might lead to general increases in insurance premiums.

What is a recognisable psychiatric illness?

The mental disorder most clearly related to injury or trauma is <u>PTSD</u> (p.96). <u>Depression</u> (p.94), <u>anxiety disorders,</u> and <u>adjustment disorders</u> (p.98) are also common bases of claims. Other conditions that the courts have accepted as 'recognisable psychiatric illness' include <u>hysterical (histrionic) personality disorder</u> (p.78), <u>pathological grief</u> (p.98), and <u>chronic fatigue syndrome</u> (p.101).

The 'eggshell skull' rule

There is a general legal rule that you take your victim as you find them: any vulnerability the victim may have (meaning that they suffer more serious injury than you could have foreseen, or suffer injury when another person would not have done) does not reduce liability either in <u>criminal law</u> (p.397) or in <u>tort law</u> (p.548), provided in the latter case that some degree of injury was reasonably foreseeable.

This is known as the 'eggshell skull' rule in the context of head injury. If you are negligent (or act criminally), the fact that the victim suffered serious brain injury instead of mere bruising only because they have an abnormally thin cranium does not reduce your liability for the damage suffered. This generalises to vulnerable mental states, to 'eggshell' personalities and to previously traumatised individuals who are more likely to be traumatised by subsequent events.

Compensation under other arrangements

Victims of injury, including psychiatric illness, that resulted from a **violent criminal offence** can also claim compensation under statutory schemes.[50] Close relatives who are **bereaved** may also sue those who caused the death, particularly if they were financially dependent on the person who was killed.

---

50 From the Criminal Injuries Compensation Authority in E&W and Scotland; the Compensation Agency in NI; and the Criminal Injuries Compensation Tribunal in RoI.

Fitness to practise professionally

The grounds for raising fitness to practise proceedings in the UK and RoI are:
• professional misconduct;
• poor professional performance;
• a relevant criminal conviction;
• relevant physical or mental ill-health;
• a breach of a relevant condition of registration, rule, or undertaking; and
• a finding by a regulatory body elsewhere of impaired fitness to practise.

A complaint that appears to show one or more of these grounds will result in a preliminary <u>investigation</u> and possible <u>sanction</u> (p.393) if the relevant professional <u>standards</u> (p.552) have been breached.

What are the relevant tests?

Unfitness to practise is defined as a **serious or persistent failure to follow the relevant professional standards**. This must be proved by the regulator on the <u>balance of probabilities</u> (p.380)[51] in the UK, but <u>beyond reasonable doubt</u> (p.380) in RoI. More specifically, that can mean:
• persistent technical failings or other repeated departures from good practice which cannot safely be managed by the employer;
• a deliberate or reckless disregard for clinical responsibilities to patients;
• working despite a health problem that compromises patient safety;
• abusing a patient's trust, autonomy, or other fundamental rights; or
• behaving dishonestly, fraudulently, or otherwise so as to harm public trust in the profession.

Complexity and causation

A key issue may be distinguishing between individual clinical responsibility, the responsibility of other clinicians, and the failings of a system as a whole. This is very frequently the case because of the complexity of modern healthcare, with multiple teams involved in many patients' care, each involving a range of professionals, sometimes spanning several organisations. The actions of several of those professionals may have contributed to the harm suffered, as may the rules they were required to operate within. This is the context within which the actions and omissions of the practitioner under investigation must be assessed.

Unlike in <u>clinical negligence</u> (p.550) proceedings, the degree to which the practitioner's failure to meet the relevant standards caused or contributed to the eventual harm is not relevant, only the failure itself. Thus a serious failing can result in sanction even though others may have succeeded in saving the patient's life, and conversely, a minor oversight that led to very great harm would result in only a minor sanction.

---

51 This standard of proof in this setting has caused controversy: see the discussion on p.393.

Legal tests in family law

In very general terms, <u>family law</u> (p.554) aims to protect members of families from harm, assist in the adjustment to separation of family members, and support family life. In family courts, <u>public law cases</u> (p.554) are usually brought by local authorities, whereas private law cases are brought by individuals. The emphasis in all family law is on protecting children and vulnerable adults.

Rights and responsibilities in family law

A person's life in law begins at birth. Like all natural persons,[52] children have rights under the law; parents are no longer regarded as having rights in relation to their children that they would not have if they were not parents. Instead, the law assigns **parental responsibilities**, from which additional rights may flow (e.g. you must have the right to feed your child if it is your responsibility to care for them). The welfare of parents is only taken into account insofar as it might impact the welfare of the child.

Proof of facts in family courts

The judge decides disputed facts, such as whether an adult has harmed a child. Expert evidence may be called as part of the fact-finding process, for consideration alongside other evidence. Family courts hear evidence about, and test disputed facts, using the <u>standard of proof</u> (p.380) of the balance of probabilities, and may therefore come to different conclusions from criminal courts on similar issues.

Role of psychiatric evidence

Divorce

Most divorce cases do not have to address issues of parental contact, or residence, because these are settled amicably between the parties. The court will only be involved where there is disagreement (about 30% of cases). <u>Psychiatric evidence</u> (p.698) may be called where one party claims to have been abused by the other, usually in cases of domestic violence, and in other cases where one parent seeks to restrict access to the children by the other parent. There may be misguided attempts to 'prove' that domestic violence has taken place because one parent suffers from <u>posttraumatic stress disorder</u> (p.96).

Annulment

Rarely, psychiatric evidence may be introduced to support the annulment of a marriage on the grounds that one or other party lacked the <u>mental capacity to marry</u> (p.540) at the time; but this is unusual.[53]

Parenting and child protection

The questions that require psychiatric advice include:
• Does this parent have a mental disorder that impacts their capacity to parent (i.e. to care safely for their child)?

---

52 As opposed to other categories of legal person, such as corporations.
53 This may be more relevant to Catholic couples who cannot remarry in church if they divorce and therefore seek annulment instead.

- Does this parent pose a risk of harm to their child because of mental disorder? (It is important not to consider risk of harm arising from causes other than mental disorder.)
- Can any mental disorder be treated, and if so what is the time scale?
- Does this child have a mental disorder?
- If so, to what extent is it caused or exacerbated by the home environment or by the actions of one or other parent?
- What attachment relationship is there between parent and child?

This list is not exhaustive. The family courts use such testimony to make decisions about where children will live and whether they will have access to their parents.

Fitness for work and dismissal

Legal tests

The specific tests applied by the court or <u>employment tribunal</u> (p.557) will depend upon the employer's rules, policies, and procedures, but in general terms, the legal test applied is a serious or persistent failure to follow those rules. In addition, the tribunal will require the employer to demonstrate that it has applied its rules consistently and fairly, and only applied a sanction (e.g. demotion, change of duties, or dismissal) after a proper investigation.

The role of psychiatric evidence

There may be scope for a psychiatric opinion in disciplinary proceedings:
• If there is evidence of mental disorder which might provide some explanation, for example, of inappropriate conduct in the workplace (e.g. hypomania causing sexual disinhibition). Here the employer or regulatory body might agree to withhold or suspend disciplinary sanctions to allow treatment of mental disorder.
• Where proceedings relate to alleged clinical malpractice or incapability on the part of a fellow psychiatrist.

Before accepting instructions in either of these cases, the experts should ensure they are aware what legal <u>standard of proof</u> (p.380) applies, and what definitions of key concepts (e.g. 'breach of duty of care') are adopted within the relevant employment contract or <u>professional guidelines</u> (p.294).

Legal issues commonly encountered by psychiatric experts

• **Work-related stress**: this issue may arise with respect to the link between work, stress, and mental disorder, particularly conditions such as <u>depression</u> (p.94), <u>adjustment disorder</u> (p.98) and <u>PTSD</u> (p.96).
• **Fitness to work** in relation to psychiatric disorder may have many implications for employee and employer. Psychiatric opinion is unlikely to be sought unless there is a complex or highly contentious issue. General practitioners and occupational health departments are more likely to be involved in writing such reports.
• **Unfair or wrongful dismissal**: if employees contend that they were unfairly or wrongfully dismissed[54] because of their mental disorder or its consequences (which might also amount to a breach of <u>equality law</u>, p.556), psychiatrists may be instructed to give an opinion on the nature and symptoms of the mental disorder, its cause(s), its impact on work, and the patient's response to work.

As in <u>professional regulatory proceedings</u> (p.552) (where the issue is one of conduct or competence in relation to clinical practice), it may be necessary to take into consideration the complexity of modern healthcare and the involvement of other professionals, but whether the employee's failure was the cause of any harm or not is irrelevant to the employment tribunal.

---

54 Wrongful dismissal is any kind of sacking that is in breach of the contract of employment (e.g. because the required notice period was not given or because there was no adequate reason for it). Unfair dismissal is a subcategory of wrongful dismissal, where the dismissal did not follow a procedure required by statute or was for a prohibited reason (e.g. because a female employee has become pregnant).

Fitness for extradition & deportation

Common psychiatric issues

- The presence of any severe mental disorder.
- PTSD (p.96) and adjustment or other disorders relating to trauma.
- Prognosis in relation to deportation or extradition.
- The availability of treatment and support in the proposed destination, and the impact of not receiving necessary treatment.

Fitness for deportation

Psychiatric evidence concerning persons at high risk of suicide if deported may, exceptionally, lead to court ruling that this would breach their ECHR article 2 or 3 rights (p.516), particularly if the persons were tortured in that country before.[55] The test is now 'a real risk, on account of the absence of appropriate treatment in the receiving country or the lack of access to such treatment, of being exposed to a serious, rapid and irreversible decline in his or her state of health resulting in intense suffering or to a significant reduction in life expectancy.'[56] An article 2 or 3 breach is an absolute bar to deportation or removal.

Mental health is part of the 'moral and physical integrity' of a person that article 8 (the right to private and family life) seeks to protect. Mental disorder and/or a risk of suicide on return or a high risk of relapse preventing reintegration into the new society,[57] may all therefore be relevant to a claim to resist removal under article 8. As this is a qualified rather than an absolute right, this is subject to a proportionality assessment (p.559) and to additional restrictions in the case of 'serious foreign criminals'.

Detention of mentally disordered people

- Detention in removal centres of those suffering from **serious medical conditions** or **mental illness** should be avoided pending deportation or removal.
- A medical report stating that a period of detention would be likely to lead to a risk of harm creates a very strong presumption against detention in the absence of exceptional circumstances relating to immediate removal or significant public protection concerns.[58]
- Mental healthcare in detention centres and access to appeals is limited and has been criticised in inspection reports.
- Under equality law (p.556), the State must ensure mentally ill or incapacitated detainees receive help challenging detention or its conditions.
- Detainees may be transferred to hospital (p.506) under mental health law if necessary. Failure to make such a transfer after it has been recommended by a psychiatrist may breach the detainee's human rights.[59]

55 *Y and Z (Sri Lanka) v Secretary of State for the Home Department* [2009] EWCA Civ 362.
56 *AM (Zimbabwe) v Secretary of State for the Home Department* [2020] UKSC 17.
57 *Secretary of State for the Home Department v KE (Nigeria)* [2017] EWCA Civ 1382.
58 In the UK, Immigration and Asylum Act 2016 S59 and associated guidance (Adults at Risk in Immigration Detention Statutory Guidance and Policy, Version 5).
59 *Rooman v Belgium* [2019] ECHR 105.

Fitness for extradition

In addition to being barred for breach of article 2, 3,[60] or 8 as with deportation, extradition from the UK (but not RoI) may be prevented if it would be **unjust or oppressive**, given the person's physical or mental health. If this test is met, extradition must be denied, or suspended until it would no longer be unjust or oppressive. Courts address the test case-by-case,[61] on the basis of medical assessment, and data on likely treatment in the receiving country.

- The test has a high threshold, requiring for example a 'substantial risk of suicide ... whatever steps are taken ... with no capacity to resist the impulse to commit suicide', or a serious mental disorder that is unlikely to improve, because of the public interest in meeting obligations under the relevant extradition treaty.[62]
- Recency of suicidal acts and concertedness of effort have been decisive factors in some extradition cases.[63]
- Judgements have also considered the impact of the extradition proceedings as a source of uncertainty that could precipitate or potentiate the mental disorder or suicide risk,[64] as well as likely conditions in the receiving country and the loss of protective factors (e.g. family) in the UK or RoI.
- Being unfit to plead (p.602),[65] though relevant, does not automatically meet the test: assurances of adequate safeguarding and treatment while awaiting recovery before trial can allow extradition to go ahead.[66]

In cases involving unfitness to plead, the court may also have to consider whether persons would face a 'flagrantly unfair' trial that would breach their article 6 right to a fair trial.[67]

---

60 For example, in *Aswat v United Kingdom* (2013) 56 EHRR 1, the court ruled there was a real risk that extradition to the USA and to a potentially more hostile prison environment (ADX Florence) would result in a significant deterioration in mental and physical health that could breach article 3.

61 *United States v Tollman* [2008] 3 AllER 150.

62 *Turner v USA* [2012] EWHC 2426.

63 For example *USA v Dunham & Anor* [2014] EWHC 334; *Poland v Wolkowicz* [2013] 1 WLR 2402.

64 For example in *South Africa v Dewani* (p.752).

65 Using the E&W fitness criteria (though those of the receiving country would be more relevant).

66 *South Africa v Dewani* (p.752).

67 For example, in *Meadows v Spain* [2019] EWHC 2084 (Admin), the court was satisfied that despite the defendant being deaf, mentally disordered, and unable to read or write, arrangements would be in place to enable him to have a fair trial, and his treatment would not be unjust or oppressive.

Chapter 20

The psychiatrist in court

Witnesses, experts, & expert evidence

Types of witness

There are three main types of witness to the court:
- an ordinary witness,
- a professional witness, and
- an expert witness.

Ordinary and professional witnesses may describe only factual matters (ordinary or professional fact); expert witnesses may give their professional opinion. Ultimately, the court makes the <u>distinction between fact and opinion</u> (p.654).[1]

Professional and expert witnesses in the UK

Factual, including professional, witnesses most commonly write, often with assistance from the police or a solicitor, **statements** that will become part of the case papers. Experts write **reports** to the court (although a report can sometimes be transformed into a statement). All types of witness may then be required to give oral evidence.

Professional and expert witnesses in RoI

In RoI, no rigid distinction is maintained between expert and professional witness, at least where consultants giving evidence in their speciality are concerned. If a patient is under the care of a psychiatrist then that treating doctor becomes the expert witness in any relevant proceedings.

Roles of an expert witness

There are various potential roles of an expert witness, including:
- **Clinical**—This requires direct contact with a defendant/witness and involves making an <u>assessment</u> (p.122) of mental condition, perhaps including the use of <u>psychometric tests</u> (p.130) of mental functioning.
- **Experimental**—This impersonal role does not require direct contact with the patient/defendant/witness. It is useful for obtaining facts and extracting them in situations relevant for a jury (e.g. the reliability of eyewitness testimony).
- **Actuarial**—Here the expert presents evidence of the probability of some event, or of the prevalence of some condition. It is based upon probabilistic reasoning, and the use of statistics, and is increasingly applied in judicial proceedings. It can be achieved through literature searches or by fieldwork.
- **Advisory**—A contrasting role in which the expert may be asked to examine and critique the evidence of another expert, and perhaps write <u>advice to counsel</u> (p.666). This is not an 'expert report', and the experts are not an 'independent expert witness', since they are effectively partisan, and will not give evidence to the court. This role has had greater prominence in recent times, and expert reports are increasingly subjected to peer review by experts appointed by the other side.

---

1 Some civil legal situations blur the distinction between factual evidence and expert opinion, such as when a treating psychiatrist (in theory a professional witness) is asked by a tribunal whether the patient's disorder is of a nature warranting detention (a matter of opinion).

Criteria for allowing expert evidence

For expert evidence to be allowed in legal proceedings, it must be:
- **relevant** to a matter in the proceedings,
- legally **admissible** (p.382),
- **necessary** (i.e. outside the court's knowledge and experience),
- from a witness **competent** to give that evidence, and
- sufficiently **probative**.

The 'probative value' of evidence depends on how much it tends to prove or disprove a relevant fact, or state of mind. There are several specific legal rules (p.656) governing what psychiatric evidence is allowed in certain types of cases.

The judge determines the competence of a witness to give expert evidence and whether what the expert intends to assert is relevant, necessary and admissible. The judge may accept the expert's qualifications, but exclude part or all of their evidence.

The single joint expert

In civil and family proceedings there may be a request for a psychiatrist to act as a joint expert. One solicitor will be appointed as the lead solicitor to instruct them. In cases where a party then wants to instruct another expert, this will need to be agreed separately by the judge with a clear rationale given. At the time of writing, criminal proceedings do not use joint experts.

Principles & law of expert evidence

Who is an 'expert'?

Expert witnesses come from a range of disciplines and fields. Expertise is based upon possessing **knowledge** and **experience** rather than professional status or registration, and on:

- whether the **subject matter** of the opinion forms part of an organised and recognised body of knowledge or experience, and
- whether the witness has acquired by **study or experience** sufficient knowledge of the subject.[2]

Hence trainees may provide expert evidence under supervision.[3]

If detailed testing of the admissibility of expert evidence is not practical, then the court may consider:

- whether the expert's methodology accords with established practices in the profession or field, and
- the extent to which the basis of the expert's opinion can be properly explained and shown to be sound.

Fact and opinion

The judge distinguishes fact from opinion. Fact can include 'medical fact' which is attested to by doctors, but distinguished from medical expert opinion (Box 20.1). For instance:

- 'He was unsteady on his feet' is fact, albeit with some element of judgment contained within it, whereas 'His gait was consistent with his diagnosis of multiple sclerosis' is expert opinion.
- 'He was suffering grief at the loss of his wife' might be an inference drawn by an ordinary witness, whereas 'he was suffering from an arrested grief reaction' would require expert knowledge.

> ### Box 20.1 Fact and opinion
> - A junior A&E doctor called to give evidence of what she found when she examined a victim of a knife attack might give factual medical information such as, 'He had a single clean wound extending 6 cm across the left side of the face, which had penetrated the muscle.'
> - If she then answered the question, 'Is it likely that the wound was made by a knife such as the one I am now holding up?', this would amount to an expert medical opinion.

Expert evidence and hearsay

Evidence by a psychiatric expert will often include things said to the expert by the defendant/claimant and others. If presented to court by the expert, such evidence is essentially <u>hearsay</u> (p.383) in character. It is admissible because it forms part of the <u>information</u> (p.356) upon which the expert

---

2 <u>Kennedy v Cordia</u> (p.759); *Pool v General Medical Council* [2014] EWHC 3791.

3 For example as set out in the Royal College of Psychiatrists' *Council Report CR193* on psychiatric experts (p.774).

formed their expert opinion—it is not presented as true per se. This distinction is fine and can be problematic since the court (or a jury) is required to accept that the information is relevant to the view the expert formed, but to ignore it as regards proof of other matters.

Disagreement and joint statements

In the UK and RoI, in civil and (increasingly) criminal proceedings, experts are often asked to attend a legally privileged experts' meeting and to issue a 'joint statement' summarising the areas of agreement and disagreement, and making clear the reasons for any disagreement.

Joint statements should be brief and focused on describing disagreements and the reasons for them. In some civil cases, the court may instead appoint a single joint expert (p.653).

Other principles

Experts should:
- know the legal questions to which their evidence is relevant,
- understand the potential relevance of their medical findings,
- give reasons for their opinion,
- cite evidence both for and against their opinion,
- cite other potential opinions and give reasons for rejecting them,
- give 'conditional' opinions where their opinion would vary depending upon what findings of fact the court makes,
- be prepared to change their opinion in response to new information,
- acknowledge the limits of their expertise (and point out where the opinion of an expert from another profession would be useful),
- provide impartial, unbiased evidence, and
- refrain from being an advocate.

Beyond various legal duties (p.656), and duties laid down in codes of practice (p.658), experts have an ethical duty (p.776) to the court and to their profession. Expert work is subject to scrutiny by professional bodies, and poor or unethical performance may lead to professional liability proceedings.[4]

---

4 Such as in _Kumar v GMC_ (p.760).

Specific legal rules of expert evidence

Beyond the general <u>principles of expert evidence</u> (p.654), higher courts across the UK and RoI have issued a number of specific legal rules for experts. These have not always been consistent.

Most of the rules on this page come from courts in E&W, many of which apply in NI and some in Scotland. Similar principles are followed in all jurisdictions, but courts in Scotland and RoI tend to allow greater discretion in the <u>admissibility of evidence</u> (p.382).

Mandatory evidence

In certain circumstances, psychiatric evidence may be required before a court can make certain decisions:
- All jurisdictions require psychiatric evidence from one or more registered medical practitioners to support a finding of <u>insanity</u> (p.620), and E&W, NI, and RoI require it for <u>unfitness to plead</u> (p.602).
- Psychiatric evidence is mandatory before an order for <u>compulsory treatment</u> (p.500), such as a hospital order, is made.
- Oral expert evidence is required from at least one suitably approved psychiatrist before a court can make any <u>restriction order</u> (p.510).
- Psychiatric evidence may be practically essential but not required by statute, such as when considering a <u>risk assessment order</u> (p.504) in Scotland, before imposing an <u>extended sentence of imprisonment</u> (p.453) in some cases, or before making a <u>community order</u> (p.454) with a mental health treatment requirement, or where partial defences such as of <u>diminished responsibility</u> (p.624) are pleaded.

How mentally disordered?

Courts refuse expert evidence on issues they consider within the experience of ordinary people (<u>R v Turner</u>, p.770):
- There cannot be evidence from a psychiatrist on psychological functioning of someone who is not mentally abnormal.
- Evidence of psychiatric abnormality (e.g. relating to a propensity to violence) is not admissible for the purpose of determining whether a defendant committed an offence, or which of two defendants committed the offence (<u>R v Kemp,</u> p.759).
- Diagnostic evidence is usually allowed as it is founded on scientific principles.
- Evidence relating to intellectual disability has tended to be allowed if a formal assessment shows or suggests an IQ of less than 70.
- Psychiatric evidence is inadmissible when the issue concerns how an ordinary person reacts to stress (<u>R v Weightman</u>, p.770); however,
- Expert evidence on complex psychological phenomena such as 'learned helplessness' as a basis for a defence of <u>duress by threats</u> (p.634) may be admissible (<u>R v Emery</u>, p.755).
- Psychiatric evidence relating to complex reactions to trauma is often allowed.

Specific issues

Reliability

- Psychiatric evidence must be relevant and reliable (_R v Mohan_, p.762).
- An expert may comment on the reliability of a witness if there is a mental disorder that makes a witness incapable of giving, or less likely to give, reliable evidence (_R v O'Brien_, p.763). This may include personality disorder.
- Expert evidence concerning the reliability of <u>confessions</u> (p.608) when related to mental disorder, or related personality features such as unusual <u>suggestibility</u> or <u>compliance</u> (p.160), is usually allowed.
- Where interviews have been conducted with a defendant who was mentally disordered, expert evidence is allowed on the reliability of the content of the interview.
- Evidence from psychiatrists or psychologists as to which of two defendants is the more likely to be violent is not usually allowed.

Veracity

- An expert may not bolster a witness's credibility (_R v Robinson_, p.767); however, evidence is admissible of 'disabilities' which the jury, or court, should know about in properly interpreting the witness's evidence.
- Child psychiatrists have been allowed to give evidence on whether children's evidence that they have been abused is likely to be reliable (_In Re M & R_, p.761).

Mens rea, intent, and recklessness

- Experts must distinguish <u>intent</u> (p.402) from <u>capacity to form intent</u> (p.610) as follows:
- They may give evidence relevant to the capacity to form intent if there is mental disorder;
- They may give evidence relevant to jury consideration of whether the defendant formed the relevant _mens rea_ if there was mental disorder.
- An expert may not give evidence on the intent of an ordinary person, unless there is a medical condition that may affect it, such as hypoglycaemia (_R v Toner_, p.769).

Capacity to consent

- In <u>sexual offences</u> (p.418) an expert may consider the defendant's capacity to assess another person's ability to consent.

Criminal convictions

- There is a general rule that no criminal conviction can be based on expert evidence alone.

Codes of practice for experts

Some jurisdictions have specific codes of practice for experts.[5] In E&W they are detailed and specific. The box contains an abridged version of the Criminal Procedure Rules for expert witnesses (CPR19)[6] and associated Practice Directions; the sections of the Civil Procedure Rules and Family Procedure Rules referring to expert witnesses (CivPR35, FPR25); and other jurisdictions' codes, embody similar principles.

19.1 A reference to an 'expert' in this Part is a reference to a person who is required to give or prepare expert evidence for the purpose of criminal proceedings, including evidence required to determine fitness to plead or for the purpose of sentencing.

19.2 1) An expert must help the court achieve the overriding objective by giving opinion which is:
(i) objective and unbiased, and
(ii) within the expert's area or areas of expertise.
2) This duty overrides any obligation to the person from whom the expert receives instructions or by whom the expert is paid.
3) This duty includes obligations:
a) to define the expert's area or areas of expertise—
(i) in the expert's report, and
(ii) when giving evidence in person;
b) when giving evidence in person, to draw the court's attention to any question outside the expert's area of expertise;
c) to inform all parties and the court if the expert's opinion changes from that contained in a report served as evidence or given in a statement; and
d) to disclose to those instructing them anything which might undermine the reliability of their opinion or their credibility or impartiality.

19.3 A party who wants to introduce expert evidence must serve it on the court and the other parties as soon as practicable; and if required, give copies of (or a reasonable opportunity to inspect) any relevant records etc.

19.4 An expert's report must
• give details of qualifications, relevant experience, and accreditation;
• give details of any literature or other information relied on;
• contain a statement setting out the substance of all facts which are material to (or the basis of) the opinions in the report;
• make clear which facts stated in the report are within the expert's own knowledge;
• where the expert has based an opinion on evidence from another person (for example a test or examination) they should
  • identify the person,
  • give their qualifications, and
  • certify that they had personal knowledge of the relevant matters;
• where there is a range of opinion on the matters:

---

5 Distinguished from <u>ethical codes</u> for experts (p.776), and from <u>professional guidance</u> (p.294).
6 Part 19 of the Criminal Procedure Rules 2015 as amended 2016–2020, and Practice Directions.

- summarise the range of opinion, and
- give reasons for the expert's own opinion;
- if the opinion requires qualification, state the qualification;
- contain a summary of the conclusions reached;
- state that the expert understands their duty to the court, has complied and will continue to comply with that duty; and
- contain the same declaration of truth as a witness statement.

[PD19A.5-7: Courts will consider **Daubert principles:** data quality and completeness, logic, precision of methods, peer review, range of opinions, honesty, and conflict of interest etc. in assessing the reliability of expert evidence.]

19.5 A party who serves an expert's report on another party or the court must inform that expert at once.

19.6 The court may direct the experts to:
- discuss the expert issues in the proceedings; and
- prepare a statement for the court of the matters on which they agree and disagree, giving their reasons.

Except for that statement, the content of that discussion must not be referred to without the court's permission. If an expert fails to take part in such a discussion, their evidence may not be admitted in court.

19.7 Where more than one defendant wants to introduce expert evidence on an issue at trial, the court may direct that the evidence on that issue is to be given by a single joint expert. Where the co-defendants cannot agree who should be the expert, the court may:
- select the expert from a list prepared or identified by them, or
- direct that the expert be selected in another way.

19.8 Where the court gives a direction for a single joint expert to be used, each of the co-defendants may give the expert instructions. Such instructions must, at the same time, be copied to the other co-defendant(s). The court may give directions about:
- the payment of the expert's fees and expenses; and
- any examination, measurement, test, or experiment which the expert wishes to carry out.

The court may, before an expert is instructed, limit the amount that can be paid by way of fees and expenses to the expert. Unless the court otherwise directs, the instructing co-defendants are jointly and severally liable for payment.

Consent & confidentiality in court

While the general duty of <u>confidentiality</u> (p.320) applies to professionals giving expert witness evidence, certain legal rules may override that duty.

Consent

When undertaking assessments for court proceedings, the expert should be mindful of explicit or implicit <u>coercion</u> (p.324) of participants, especially if they have been instructed to engage by the court. This is particularly important in assessment for criminal proceedings where the defendant may, for example, receive an <u>indeterminate sentence</u> (p.448) and where <u>consent to risk assessment</u> (p.342) is an issue. Proper care in obtaining consent is paramount. It is important to obtain consent (ideally written) from the defendant, also to speak to other informants, <u>before writing the report</u> (p.682). Consent forms may be helpful.

Confidentiality and related issues

- An expert witness's duty to the court requires them to disclose their report and any relevant information to the court and/or instructing solicitor; you must warn the evaluee of these exceptions to normal medical confidentiality.
- If the assessment reveals a serious and immediate risk of harm, a limited disclosure of this to others can also be made (e.g. telling prison inreach staff of a prisoner's suicidal intent).
- The expert witness has a duty to disclose all the evidence they have used to form their opinion.
- When citing references it is vital to have read the original source, to cite it correctly, and to be able to make it available.
- If you seek <u>supervision</u> (p.308), or specialist advice from a colleague, this must be documented in your report.
- You should ensure that your instructing party understands that you may make limited disclosures to colleagues for the purposes of supervision or advice. Prior to discussing the specifics of a case with other experts, permission should be obtained from the instructing party.
- In court, when under oath as a witness, you must answer the questions posed despite any duty of confidentiality you may be under, unless the judge orders that you do not need to answer. If your report was based upon information that you would not wish disclosed in this way, such as specific questions and scoring criteria in certain <u>psychometric tests</u> (p.136), you should discuss this in advance with your instructing solicitor, and if necessary with the judge.
- When giving evidence in a Magistrate's Court it is important to remember that the magistrates will not have been provided with a copy of your report and will not have access to information that could prejudice the outcome of a case (e.g. prior convictions of a defendant). It is important that you do not give this information in oral evidence, even though it was written in your report. In higher courts, the same applies to evidence given when the jury is present.

Chapter 21

Applied ethics and testimony

Judicial ethics and legal philosophy

Judicial ethics is a specific area of ethics, concerning the values held important by judges, which differ from those of psychiatrists (p.352).

The relevance of jurisprudence

The moral value at the heart of the law is justice. What justice means in practice, and how it relates to competing values such as fairness, duty, and rightfulness, is the subject-matter of jurisprudence (p.364), which is the theory and philosophy of law and legal decision-making, and the source of judicial ethics. *Descriptive* jurisprudence analyses how these values shape what the law is in a society; *normative* jurisprudence extrapolates what the law should be from its values.

There are three main schools of descriptive jurisprudence:

- **Natural law**—Theorists hold that there are natural, absolute foundations to law (which might be considered laws of nature) which can be deduced by the power of reason. Hobbes and John Finnis are two of the most significant natural law theorists.
- **Legal positivists**—Argue that law is wholly distinct from morality, and that societies adopt laws to reflect their social and political structures and power relationships. Positivism is, in essence, the view that law is derived from the acts of legislators, judges, and citizens, rather than from abstract moral principles.[1] There is disagreement about *how* the relationship between law and society should be analysed:
  - 'hard' positivists such as Joseph Raz maintain that the law is the sole substrate for analysis, whereas
  - 'soft' positivists such as HLA Hart argue that objective moral facts exist outside the law and must be taken into account.
- **Legal realism** is a related sociological view of law, which agrees with positivism that law is defined by what legal actors (judges, lawyers, clients, juries, and legislators) do—but differs in arguing that it should be analysed only with value-free, empirical scientific methods, not philosophical ones.[2]
  - **Legal pragmatists** follow this approach and argue that the law should be interpreted (p.364) so as to achieve desired social outcomes, rather than in order to promote coherence in the body of law as a whole, or fidelity to the law's literal meaning.
  - **Critical legal studies** is a more radical derivative of legal realism that argues that the law is a codification of power structures that exist to maintain the oppression of marginalised groups in society.

Judicial ethics

Judicial ethics comprises the norms and standards that impact judges in exercising that power.

---

1 Ironically, one of the strongest arguments against it is that it cannot explain what judges, legislators, and citizens actually do, or think they are doing.

2 Philosophers counter that empiricism and science are not remotely 'value-free', but that is a debate for another book.

There is considerable debate about how justice should be reflected in the application of the law. One view sees it as arising in judicial decisions and, therefore, in the ethical mindset of individual judges. However, different judges favour different ethical theories (286): some may be more communitarian, for example, whilst others favour liberal individualism. The importance of these schools of thought can be seen in judicial appointments, especially to each country's Supreme Court (p.372).

Codes of judicial ethics

- The European Court of Human Rights (p.390) has set out principles by which judges need to abide.
- The United Nations has adopted the six 'Bangalore Principles' of judicial ethics, which have been endorsed and elaborated in detail by the Scottish judiciary and others (Box 21.1).

Box 21.1 The Bangalore Principles of judicial ethics

All judges must:
- be independent of all outside influences
- be impartial between the different parties, cases, and views
- maintain personal and professional integrity at all times
- behave properly, and be seen to behave with propriety
- ensure all are treated equally by the courts
- exercise their duties competently and diligently

Avoiding addressing the ultimate issue

The *ultimate issue* means the final decision before a court. For example, in a murder trial, the ultimate issue is whether the defendant committed the <u>actus reus</u> (p.400) with the requisite <u>mens rea</u> (p.402). Possible mental disorder present at the time of the killing is an intermediate issue, subject to expert evidence.

Experts must limit themselves to matters within their expertise that are beyond the experience of the jury or judge, and not directly address the ultimate issue. Deciding the ultimate issue inevitably requires choosing between disputed facts, interpretations, or inferences, and might involve making assumptions. It is a fundamental principle in <u>common-law jurisdictions</u> (p.368) that such decisions are matters for ordinary people or those representing them, not for experts.[3]

In the USA, addressing the ultimate issue is prohibited by federal rules of evidence; in the UK and RoI, there is no explicit rule, but such conduct may be censured by the judge.[4]

Experts and the ultimate issue

Forensic psychiatric experts are likely to be drawn into discussing the ultimate issue in the following:

- **Insanity** (p.620)—the expert is commonly allowed to state whether defendants suffered from a 'disease of the mind', although this is legally defined, as well as its effects, but should be cautious regarding whether this rendered them 'unable to know the nature and quality of their actions', or 'whether they were wrong'.
- **Diminished responsibility** (p.624)—The expert may offer an opinion on all 'limbs' of diminished responsibility, and the courts have allowed this (e.g. *R v Brennan*, p.749), although the jury may reject these opinions.
- **Child protection** cases (p.644)—If questions are asked of the expert that assume that disputed facts have been proved (e.g. that a child has been harmed in a particular way) the expert should either not accept such instructions, until the relevant facts have been determined by the court, or give a conditional opinion ('if X is proved, then my opinion would be …, if Y, then …').

Guidelines

The following may help in avoiding addressing the ultimate issue:

- Obtain detailed instructions and request clarification concerning legal questions if necessary: reject 'Did Mr P have diminished responsibility?', but accept 'Was Mr P suffering from "substantial impairment of the ability to exercise self-control"?'
- Ensure every statement you make is based on the evidence cited in your report.

3 See, for example, *Pora v The Queen* [2015] UKPC 9.

4 Or, inconsistently, encouraged—it is normal practice for tribunal judges asking psychiatric witnesses to give an opinion on whether the legal criteria for detention are met, and even Court of Appeal judges may invite an expert to opine on whether the defendant's responsibility for killing was indeed diminished.

- Do not make assumptions or value judgments.
- Avoid giving opinions inappropriately using legal terminology.
- Distinguish between psychiatric opinion and the legal implications of that opinion.
- Express opinions in a way that can assist the court in 'mapping' (p.358) the mental state onto the legal test(s), rather than expressing a view per se on whether those tests are met.

Giving expert advice to one side

Advice instead of giving a report to the court

A distinction must be drawn between submitting an expert report to the court (irrespective of the source of instructions) and giving advice to lawyers for one side. The former requires independence and an acknowledgement of the duty of the expert to the court. The latter is likely to involve reading and critiquing of another expert's report, clinical notes, and process (without direct clinical assessment), and represents assistance to one side within an <u>adversarial</u> process (p.369).

Often the advice will be given in writing. This should be headed 'Advice to Counsel' and constructed so as to make plain:
- the nature of the instructions,
- the nature of what you are providing, and
- the distinction between such advice and a report which might be used directly within the legal proceedings.

Advice after completing a report

Where psychiatrists have already provided a report, usually based upon their own clinical assessment, they have a duty of impartiality to the court.

If they then also give advice to the lawyers that instructed them, knowing it will be used in an adversarial fashion, this creates an ethical tension with that duty. The advice offered might be in conference with counsel or the instructing solicitor, or for example, by passing notes to counsel when they are cross-examining another expert, advising them of particular lines of questioning, or of particular detailed questions to ask.

This ethical tension is unavoidable in that lawyers may not be able to understand the strengths and weaknesses opposing expert evidence without advice. Assisting the lawyers on one side of a case by explaining your own report to them, as well as its strengths and weakness, is acceptable, as is explaining the strengths and weaknesses of other experts' reports. However, you must still continue to strive for impartiality, and give honest and unbiased assessments of your own and others' evidence.

Record-keeping when giving advice

As always, you must make clinical notes, and deal with all communications, on the assumption that they may be used or tested legally, whatever your role. It is good practice to keep notes of discussions, and of the participants. Documents should be checked, dated, and either signed or electronically secured. Also keep a record of the oral information received and advice given, any documentation one has seen, and (if known) what one has not seen. If it is known that facts are in legal dispute, then it is essential to make clear that this is also known by you, and that you have not advised in advance of legal determination of the relevant facts.

Controversial clinical concepts in court

New or controversial clinical concepts or diagnoses can pose a challenge for the legal system and experts.

So:

- Present scientific information in simple terms.
- Identify any value judgments inherent in a particular concept or diagnosis.
- Acknowledge any specific inherent limitations.
- Ensure that you clearly cite, and explain, the relevant scientific evidence.
- Observe the <u>rules on expert opinions</u> (p.656) by giving the range of possible opinions on the concept, and state why you prefer yours.
- Be prepared to explain and educate, rather than argue a particular side of any debate.

Neuroscience

Knowledge about the relationship between <u>violence and neurobiology</u> (p.30) is rapidly expanding. The main issues are whether biological correlates of violence exist in particular populations, and whether they can be used to inform the assessment of culpability or risk of violence in the individual defendant. The answer to the first question is evolving into a more certain 'yes', despite methodological complexity. An answer to the second is still elusive. Extreme caution should therefore be exercised in drawing conclusions about any mental disorder, risk, or prognosis directly from the results of biological investigations—unless that investigation has been established as diagnostically relevant, such as an EEG in sleep disorders or in specific kinds of epilepsy.

Recovered or false memories

The main debate is whether such memories (usually of sexual abuse) are a product of suggestions that have been made to the individual in the course of therapy (**false memories**), or whether they reflect an uncovering of true childhood memories of repressed, stressful events (**recovered memories**). Whilst an opinion about the nature of recalled events may be necessary, any court should be informed of the controversial nature of the concepts, and that:

- memory is rarely an exact replication of true events;
- memory is likely to incorporate some distortion of events;
- recall of events can be influenced by <u>suggestion</u> (p.160); and
- repression is a psychological theory with limited scientific evidence for its existence.

Controversial diagnoses

Many of the most controversial diagnoses relate to responses to stress and trauma.

- **Complex PTSD** has some clinical validity but is only just emerging in diagnostic manuals (see ICD11). There is overlap with the features of <u>borderline personality disorder</u> (p.84). There may be potential legal significance in making one or other of these diagnoses: for example, in <u>mitigation</u> (p.638), the diagnosis of <u>complex PTSD</u> (p.96) might be less likely to be accepted by the court, but that of personality disorder might be more stigmatising.
- **Adjustment disorders** are recognised medical diagnoses but can be subject to criticism if relied on in expert evidence; because they contain no pathognomonic symptoms and incorporate judgment about what represents a culturally normal reaction to a given stressor (see *R v Blackman*, p.748).
- **Dissociative identity disorder** (or <u>multiple personality disorder</u>, p.100) is subject to continuing controversy regarding its validity as a diagnosis.
- **Sex addiction** is not included in DSM-5, but it was proposed as 'hypersexual disorder'.
- **Intermittent explosive disorder**—There is some evidence for the existence of this <u>syndrome</u> (p.114) of explosive and apparently uncontrollable violence related to abnormalities of the temporal lobes and/or other brain regions, but it is not generally accepted.

Crime-related amnesia

Although less controversial, with support from published studies, there are multiple possible psychological and biological reasons for <u>amnesia</u> (p.636), which may have legal consequences if the amnesia is accepted as being due to an underlying mental disorder or abnormal mental state present at the time of the offence such as dissociation (psychogenic amnesia).

Opinions in sentencing

Sentencing (p.442) has become progressively more concerned with public protection (p.352) from mentally disordered (and other) offenders and with 'culpability' (p.354). Hence the courts increasingly expect psychiatrists to make and interpret risk assessments for sentencing purposes in those terms, including giving opinions on the distinct legal concept of dangerousness (p.672)—as well as to consider treatment in the context of punitive sentences.

Relevant psychiatric factors

An expert witness may assist the court by commenting not on culpability but on causation, via the following[5]:
- At the time of the offence did the offender's disorder or disability impair their ability to exercise appropriate judgement, to make rational choices, or to understand the nature and consequences of their actions?
- At the time, did it cause them to behave in a disinhibited way?
- What was their degree of insight into their condition?
- Did they adhere to prescribed medication, and/or self-medicate?

Recommending inpatient treatment

Make a recommendation for court-ordered treatment (p.500) such as a hospital order only if the defendant is likely to benefit from treatment. Recommending treatment when there is evidence that benefit is unlikely would be unethical (p.340).[6] This is relevant to psychopathy (p.90) and paedophilia (p.102) in particular.

Penal sentences

No medical expert should recommend a penal disposal or punishment. Where no psychiatric disposal is indicated, you should make no recommendation.

With increasing consideration of extended sentences (p.453), mental health professionals are frequently asked for opinions on risk of harm. Even if you normally refuse such requests, if you have given a report for trial, you may still be drawn into sentencing issues per se. This raises the ethical issue (p.322) of your clinical assessment being used towards a solely punitive objective (even if it does not support an extended sentence).

Hybrid orders and hospital directions

The hybrid order in E&W and the hospital direction (p.504) in Scotland combine elements of treatment and punishment, and were created by the UK and Scottish governments because they believed that hospital orders 'did not always properly reflect an element of appropriate punishment', combined with concerns about 'dangerous' patients being released 'early' when treatment has failed or the patients no longer met criteria for detention. In E&W, judges are required to consider them[7] even if the medical recommendation is only for a hospital order, based upon considerations

---

5 These, and other, factors are endorsed by sentencing guidelines in E&W.

6 And potentially unlawful: SLL v Priory (p.768).

7 See Vowles and Edwards (pp.754, 770).

including the culpability of the defendant and the harm caused by the offence, as well as the regime that would be available for supervising the offender on release.

It is important to remain within your professional role (p.300) in giving
opinions for sentencing. It is acceptable to state that treatment, though
legally possible, has a low probability of achieving significant risk reduction, and to point out the advantages and disadvantages of long-term risk
management under different types of disposal, but it is not acceptable to
recommend the hybrid order specifically, which implies punishment. If it is
uncertain whether treatment is possible, an interim order can be recommended (though the judge may still impose a hybrid order).

Community orders with a condition of treatment

A community order (p.454) is a punitive sentence but may have a condition
of mental health or drug treatment attached to it. If the offender fails to
comply with the requirements of the treating psychiatric team, they may
be 'breached' by her supervising probation officer and returned to court.

Your report should state what treatment you think necessary, if any, and
where it may be offered (as an inpatient, or in the community). If you think
that treatment is more likely to succeed if there is an element of supervision attached to it, it is acceptable to recommend a condition of treatment,
but taking care not to recommend the community order itself, as this is
essentially a punitive sentence. A **conditional recommendation** is the
easiest way of achieving this: 'Should the court be minded to impose a community order, I would recommend a mental health treatment requirement
specifying ...'.

Before making a recommendation, you should obtain the agreement of
the probation officer (or in Scotland, criminal justice social worker) who
would supervise the order. It is important to consider the potential functions of the treating psychiatrist and supervising officer; if either appears to
have no obvious role, then the order is inappropriate.

It is also wise to consider the possibility that, as the treating psychiatrist,
you may come to have evidence that your patient is in breach of the order,
such as refusing to comply with an aspect of treatment. Consider what the
supervising officer will expect you to disclose, and what you will agree to
disclose, based on the threshold for breach.

Mitigating and aggravating factors

You should not explicitly give mitigating evidence (p.638) on behalf of a
defendant, even if they are your patient. If instructed, you may give medical
information in response to specific relevant questions (e.g. 'What impact
would the mental disorder have had on the defendant's understanding of
the seriousness of their actions?').

You should not raise aggravating factors (p.638) or accept instructions to
produce a report on them. You should always be aware of the possibility
that a report you write for some other purpose may later be used by the
court as evidence of aggravating factors.

Courts' assessments of dangerousness

One of the <u>aims of sentencing</u> (p.442) is protecting the public from 'dangerous' offenders. In determining dangerousness, courts may request expert psychiatric evidence. This can be ethically controversial for psychiatrists or psychologists, particularly where treatment is not an option, or they are asked about the defendant's <u>culpability</u> (p.354).

Dangerousness versus risk

'Dangerousness' is a purely legal concept referring to the perceived likelihood of harm to the public. As with many other <u>legal concepts</u> (p.354), it is superficially similar to the psychiatric concept of <u>risk of harm</u> (p.164), but differs in important ways. Dangerousness is conceived as a simple, static, global characteristic of an individual, whereas <u>risk assessment</u> (p.166), albeit related to the individual, is specific in regard to a given time frame and in a given set of potential circumstances.

Should clinicians assist courts in considering dangerousness?

Clinicians may be called upon to assist a court with its assessment of dangerousness where:
- they have previously written a report on a defendant with mental disorder, and the court is now considering sentencing, or
- they have not previously been involved in the case, but are asked to assess dangerousness at the sentencing stage (e.g. under a <u>risk-assessment order</u> (p.504) in Scotland).

Arguments against assisting

Some psychiatrists refuse to offer such evidence because in their view:
- It amounts to misusing medical techniques solely for a nonmedical purpose carrying a risk of doing harm to the defendant/patient.
- The courts may confuse 'risk assessment' with 'dangerousness'.
- Risk assessment is arguably too unreliable for court decisions, especially when attempted by a single clinician who has not had the benefit of substantial data collection and investigation whilst the patient has been in hospital.
- It may be invalid to use risk-assessment techniques for a 'snapshot' of dangerousness for a court, instead of as part of a continuous process of reassessment and risk management within a therapeutic relationship.
- Many risk-assessment tools, or parts of them, utilise actuarial data based upon groups, whereas evidence within justice towards sentencing requires an individual approach.
- Courts may fail to understand the distinction between stating that a group to which the defendant belongs has an average risk of committing a particular offence within a certain time period, and stating that the defendant personally has such a risk.

Arguments in favour of assisting
- The court will make an assessment of dangerousness regardless of whether a clinician assists, and, if the defendant has a mental disorder, better that the assessment is informed by expert psychiatric or psychological evidence than carried out solely by those without such training.

- Where a psychiatrist has compiled a report earlier during the trial, and then finds that the data they have presented in the report[8] will be used to consider dangerousness, better that it is interpreted by an expert rather than 'used blind' by the court.

Practical considerations

If an expert decides to assist (or not to frustrate) a court's assessment of dangerousness, the following should be considered.

- When seeking the patient's consent (p.342) to assessment, and to the completion of a report, you should explain the uses to which the report could be put by the court, beyond the requested purpose.
- The risk assessment must be of the highest quality achievable, and should set out its assumptions and limitations.
- The report or evidence must be framed in medical terminology concerning risk, leaving the court to make inferences about dangerousness: you should not cross the divide (p.358) and address any legal concept directly.
- The report must not make recommendations about management of the risk by way of a particular sentence, unless you are recommending treatment (p.500).

---

8 This is an unavoidable risk: rules of expert evidence (p.656) require experts to include relevant data in the report.

Bias influencing opinion

Impartiality and bias

Assisting justice is the proper role of the expert. Seeking to **affect** it is not. With acceptance that, even in regard to aspects of medical evidence, the law of approaches '*a* truth' and not '*the* truth' (constrained by rules of evidence and legal process, including defined burdens and standards of proof), and that the particular 'truth' found depends not only upon the clinically relevant data collected but also then upon the subset of such data that is legally admissible. Accepting also that the adversarial process itself can variously encourage bias

Clearly experts should have no personal interest in the outcome of a case and should not be drawn into the adversarial process by <u>taking sides</u> (p.666), or otherwise compromising their impartiality. But bias is more subtle than this[9]

Impartiality should be consciously pursued, but **avoidance of bias is impossible** since much bias arises unconsciously, often expressed via unconscious cognitive heuristics. For example, psychiatrists may meet patients who engage their personal values and beliefs, and as doctors, they are trained to be both sympathetic and empathetic with people's stories. Their professional identities also encourage them to do good for people and to establish a therapeutic alliance. The *clinical* ethical imperatives to 'first do no harm' and of favouring <u>beneficence</u> (p.287) may also make it difficult for a doctor to be objective about a person whom they are evaluating for *litigation* purposes.

Some situations tend particularly to bring doctors' natural inclination to care into play, most obviously where they write reports on patients whom they are, or have been, caring for (e.g. in civil litigation for cases of <u>PTSD</u>, p.96, or inpatients coincidentally involved in criminal proceedings), and especially where the therapeutic relationship is longstanding. Hence it is recommended that treating doctors do not give expert testimony (as opposed to <u>professional testimony</u>, p.652) in cases involving their patients whenever possible.[10]

However, although it may be less difficult to pursue objectivity when assessing a client who is a stranger, or whom one will never see again, there are then risks that one may fail to recognise a medical duty to them, and, by contrast, may be more open to the influence of those giving

---

9 See Part A *Oxford Casebook of Forensic Psychiatry* for a detailed description of decision-making and bias, including in regard to the sources and routes to expression of bias in expert witness practice.

10 There is no obvious way to resolve the tension between doctors' duties to the court and those to patients: if doctors only give evidence that benefits patients (whether defendants or plaintiffs) then the court will not have access to relevant evidence, and the justice process will be unbalanced.

instructions: for example, in a criminal case when acting for the prosecution, one may unconsciously emphasise evidence that the defendant was or is mentally well, or in <u>civil compensation</u> (p.548) cases, one may look for evidence that the client is <u>malingering</u> (p.118) and dismiss signs of distress that go against this.

Judicial detection of bias

Judges tend to be particularly alert to 'the dogmatic expert'; 'the expert with a scientific prejudice'; 'the expert with strongly held views even falling short of being dogmatic or prejudicial'; 'the expert expressing disapproval of a contradictory view'; and 'the expert with a preference to act for one side or the other'. Some such experts, often with limited insight, may make names for themselves, always seeking to put a particular point of view irrespective of the facts of the particular case, and appearing only for one side.

Can opinion *be* value-free?

There are reasons to think that it is impossible for doctors to be completely, or even highly objective[11]:

- the argument from sociology that a speaker always speaks from their position, and tends to assume that their perspective is the most real, and thus the most true; and
- the psychological argument that all individual personal memory and experience affects later cognitive appraisal and interpretation of facts

It is also important to be aware of one's own **personal value systems** and prejudices, and to reflect upon how they may influence opinion. Since these may influence how you give expert testimony: for example, some religious or political beliefs emphasise free will and tend towards rejecting the influence of mental illness on offending choices, except in extreme circumstances. Such beliefs may indicate potential blind spots.

   Unconscious values may be harder to access. Colleagues, however, may be able to tell one about the apparent impact of less consciously held beliefs and values, this being one of the benefits of attending professional development, peer review, and <u>reflective groups</u> (p.308).

   Finally, always ask oneself What are the arguments against my position? and carefully consider the evidence against your arguments, even if they initially seem repugnant or foolish.

Honesty versus objectivity

The risk of bias, including the application of personal values, makes it essential that the doctor should consciously attempt objectivity, but with understanding of the potential cognitive heuristic and values routes to bias. However, although objectivity is an impossible goal, **honesty** in attempting to **minimise bias** is not.

11 See also Part A *Oxford Casebook of Forensic Psychiatry* on the influence of values.

Providing reports

Aims and methods of report-writing

The main aim of a medico-legal report is to provide the court with an opinion concerning any mental disorder that may be (or have been) present, its potential legal implications, plus any recommendations for further investigation or for any disposal. The report-writer must comply with the various duties of an expert witness (p.656), which include a number of specific requirements concerning the content of reports (e.g. those in the various Practice Directions, p.658), in order to enable to court to assess the report's veracity, reliability, and validity. There should be a coherent structure to the report, so that its data (including sources) and reasoning are easy to see.

What providing a report involves

Assessment prior to writing the report involves gaining and/or interpreting clinical information, plus any legal information of clinical relevance. The task for the expert is to present clinical findings in a way that can be understood by the court, including assisting in 'mapping onto' the relevant legal constructs (p.354).

There is nothing intrinsically different between assessment for court proceedings and for clinical purposes; indeed, it is important not to distort normal clinical practice because there is a legal purpose to the assessment. However, the content and format (p.684) of the report is likely to vary from clinical reports. Also, whereas data that are considered irrelevant for clinical purposes may be excluded from clinical reports, court reports should be written so as not to be open to the accusation of being 'selective' in the data used. No presumptions should be made about the veracity of particular information, and the report should usually include a section dealing with the likely validity of any conclusions reached. Finally, reports for court should be written so that the clinical findings can easily be read in terms of their potential legal implications, with a section included which deals with those implications (though often not definitively, given the ultimate issue rule, p.664).

Most reports are based upon clinical assessment and investigation, plus consideration of medical records and legal papers, and sometimes also other medical reports, either for the current or previous proceedings. Anything potentially of relevance, either to your clinical opinion or its legal implications, should be included in the report. Where appropriate, reports may offer opinions based solely upon medical records, and/or legal papers (e.g. in retrospective assessment of others' clinical practice within clinical negligence litigation, p.550).

Why there is expertise in being an expert

Most jurisdictions increasingly recognise the importance of expertise of presenting medical and psychological evidence into legal proceedings, and the need for accreditation of experts. Experts need to understand the relationship between medical and legal constructs (p.354) and their interface (p.358), and to be adept in interpreting and using evidence that may not be solely medical, and in integrating that evidence into their opinion. For example, in a criminal trial it is necessary not only to assess the defendant with the usual medical techniques and tools available but also to consider ordinary evidence (e.g. witness statements) that may bear upon whether, at the time of the alleged offence, the defendant was mentally disordered.

Consideration of the relevance of any disorder for strictly legal issues also requires an understanding of how courts will test medical evidence, adversarially rather than investigatively. Merely making a diagnosis is inadequate: the expert must interpret its relevance to the legal questions concerned.

Such skills also include the ability to validate the diagnosis in the first place, in the special circumstance of a legal case where there may properly be a measure of scepticism about the veracity of the subject's presentation.

Expertise in being an expert does not infer being a 'courtroom hack' or 'hired gun'. In fact the reverse, since knowledge of the interface between legal and medical constructs and processes makes policing the boundary for oneself much easier, so as to inhibit the influence of one's own values on professional opinion (p.675), or of bias (p.674).

Preparation and taking instructions

Preparation for a medico-legal report should be comprehensive. You should be confident that you have understood the relevant legal questions, and that you have access to all information relevant to your potential clinical opinion and its legal implications. Often the referring solicitor will not know, without your advice, what information may be relevant.

The source of the request

'Receiving instructions' is the usual term for a formal request for assistance in a case, which should be set out in a 'letter of instruction'. Requests for medico-legal reports may come from a variety of sources:

- For criminal reports, this could be the defence solicitors, the prosecution, the court or a body such as the Criminal Cases Review Commission (p.567).
- For civil proceedings, instructions may come from the court, claimant, or defendant. Sometimes both sides may agree to appoint the same expert, or the court may require that there should be a joint expert (p.653); when one solicitor will be appointed as lead solicitor. There will be a joint letter of instruction with questions from all parties.
- For mental health tribunals requests can arise from any party with an interest, plus the tribunal itself.

Taking and refusing legal instructions

- Before accepting instructions, you should confirm that you are not only adequate as an expert for the case but also likely to be the best type of expert, both in clinical terms and in respect of the legal domain and questions involved.
- There are sometimes ethical considerations in a case; for example, you may not wish to take on a request for an independent psychiatric assessment of a patient under your care, or in any other situation that would give rise to a conflict of interest (p.298).
- You should make sure that you can complete the report by the deadline.
- It is usually necessary to provide the instructing body with an itemised estimate of the time and costs for your report. This should include time for discussing the referral in detail, reading all medical and legal papers, clinical assessment, investigations, drafting the report, and discussion with the referring solicitor. Attending a conference with counsel (a 'con') will usually be funded separately after there has been consideration of the relevance and use of your report. The likely costs associated with appearing in court are often dealt with and funded separately.
- You should alert the instructing body to any days you would be unavailable to attend court.
- You should ensure that you receive clear instructions concerning the legal questions to which the assessment and report will be directed. Do not become drawn into dealing with anything that subsequently arises that is outside your area of expertise (this is an easier error to make than initially taking on a case that is wholly outside your expertise).

- Make sure you understand the legal issues in the case and that you are familiar with the relevant legal constructs and terminology, even case law.
- Trainees should ensure that they will receive adequate supervision (p.308).

Letter of instruction

This is in effect part of a contract between you and the solicitor, listing the questions you will address. Questions may be modified after discussion. It is advisable (and required in some cases) for the letter, or your formal acceptance, to include terms and conditions. It should set out clearly your instructions, and you should ensure that you address all the questions in the letter, and usually, do not deviate from these (unless by agreement the terms are varied at a later stage).

If you become aware of an issue that the solicitors quite deliberately do not wish you to consider, you will have to decide what is an ethically justifiable response. If you identify issues that are relevant to the case, but which you have not been instructed to address, it will be necessary for you to contact the instructing body and to discuss this. If, by agreement, the instructions alter, then you should obtain amended instructions in writing.

Sources of information

- Consider whether you should receive each of the source documents shown on p.142.
- Before seeing the defendant or litigant, you should ensure you have obtained copies of all relevant documents, whether from the instructing agents or from other sources (with the client's consent).
- You will need to check that you have been sent everything listed in the index of the bundle that has been sent to you, and that the bundle contains everything that you might need to see.
- Read all the background information prior to seeing the client as questions may arise from this.

Before writing the report

The assessment

Your assessment of the subject should have been conducted with writing the report in mind (see <u>assessment</u>, p.122 onwards). If it was not, you might need to see them again; for example, to obtain specific <u>consent</u> (pp.148, 342) and to address issues not usually covered in a routine clinical assessment. Such interviews can often be a lengthy process. The quality of your report will depend upon the care with which you performed this assessment (and read the relevant medical and legal paperwork); any inadequacies are likely to be exposed during <u>cross-examination</u> (p.714).

The circumstances of the assessment are also important, particularly in criminal proceedings in prison. Psychiatric assessment often touches upon profoundly personal issues, and adequate assessment is therefore dependent upon the use of a quiet, confidential, and emotionally safe environment. A defendant who, for example, was subjected to serious sexual abuse as a child is unlikely fully to divulge such information, or the effects upon their emotional or sexual functioning, unless they are approached with care in such an environment. It follows that it is wholly unacceptable to assess a defendant facing a serious charge, other than in relation to a simple issue, in the cells just before or during trial.

What makes assessment for a court report different

Although the essence of the assessment is the same as one conducted in a clinical context, there are several important matters you must address.

- Explain very clearly to the defendant your role, including who you are, who has instructed you, and the limits of <u>confidentiality</u> (p.148).
- Explain that they can decide whether to co-operate with the assessment—and what will happen if they do not.
- At the end of your assessment, ask the defendant whether there are any matters that you have not asked about that they consider important.
- On completion of the assessment, it is usually not appropriate to give any feedback about the results, since your conclusions will be placed into the context of all of the other information in the case, and so conveyed by the lawyer.
- Inform the defendant what will happen next, including repeating your description of who will receive the report.
- At prison, ask staff, including medical staff if possible, about their observations of the prisoner, as well as viewing their <u>inmate medical records</u> (p.151).

After assessing the defendant

- If the defendant is in prison or hospital, make an entry in their <u>inmate medical record</u> (p.151) or medical notes. However, you should be cautious about entering the conclusions of your report without the consent of the <u>instructing body</u> (p.680)—although you may have to breach such confidentiality if the defendant discloses evidence of, say, significant risk of death or serious harm to self or others.

- Obtain consent from the defendant to speak to other informants (e.g. family, other professionals involved); remember that if they refuse then you are still at liberty to approach them and to listen to what they tell you, since breaching confidence refers to giving away confidential information proffered to you by the defendant. However, if you are instructed by the defence in a criminal case, check that none of these is a prosecution witness (as permission would have to be sought by defence lawyers for you to have access to them).
- If it is necessary to collect other further information following your assessment ask the instructing body to do this, or do it yourself if that is easier and appropriate.

The importance of good record-keeping

You need to treat every legal communication, and relevant clinical communication, on the basis that it may be used or tested legally (whatever your role). It is good practice to keep contemporaneous notes of discussions, including with whom they were had. Also, keep a careful record of any information given orally, any documentation you have seen, and (if known) what you have *not* seen. If it is known that facts are in legal dispute, then it is essential to make clear that this is also known by you (and that you have not taken a position in advance of legal determination). Formal documents need to be checked, signed, and dated.

General aspects of report-writing

Psychiatric disorder

The psychiatric report to court arising from the assessment and tests will describe any disorder likely to have been present at the time of the alleged offence, or relevant to any legal issue of current importance.

Legal implications

It should also describe how the disorder is, or is not, relevant to particular legal tests or issues. This may be couched in conditional terms, dependent for example on which disputed facts about the alleged offence (or event in civil proceedings) are established. You should not address the legal issues directly: instead, describe how they might be informed by diagnosis, mental state, or formulation.

Expert evidence cannot say that a mental state or diagnosis caused certain acts or omissions, in a scientific sense[1]; it can only offer an understanding of how mental disorder might have contributed to the narrative of the alleged offence or event.

Rules

Reports intended to be used in court are subject to a variety of <u>rules for expert witnesses</u> (pp.654, 656); your report must comply with them. Regulatory bodies have impugned the <u>fitness to practise</u> (p.642) of psychiatrists and other professionals, because of failings in expert evidence they have given.[2]

Context

The report should be written with the relevant legal context in mind. Reports for different legal purposes (e.g. <u>criminal proceedings</u>, p.694; <u>mental health tribunals</u>, p.692; and <u>family proceedings</u>, p.698) will demand different approaches, all of which are different from a standard clinical report such as a discharge summary or referral letter. Also remember that, once released, the report might be used in other settings—for example, a report in a criminal trial might be passed on to the prison service if the defendant is imprisoned, or used in family proceedings.

Structure

The report should separate out the following:
* *Instructions.*
* *Sources of information.*
* *Factual information* relevant to your opinion, identified by source.
* *Opinion*, distinguished into *psychiatric opinion* and *potential legal implications* (not directly addressing the <u>ultimate legal</u> issues, p.664).
* *Recommendations* in relation to disposal (if relevant and required).

A detailed list of report sections is shown on p.688.

---

1 As opposed to the legal sense of causation, for which being a significant contributory factor is often sufficient.
2 For example <u>*Kumar v GMC*</u> (p.760); *Pool v General Medical Council* [2014] EWHC 3791.

How long should the report be?

This will depend on the quantity of data, and the clinical and legal complexity of the case. Bear the following factors in mind:

- The report structure must be easy to follow, and show how the opinion flows from the data and your reasoning.
- Sufficient detail can save court time by obviating the need for follow-up questions, and may allow a hearing to be avoided. It can also avoid any appearance of not having been balanced in approach.
- If a long time will pass between preparing the report and giving oral evidence, a detailed report will aid you in recalling information later.
- However, extraneous data wastes the court's time, and may make it harder for the reader to understand what you are saying and why.

A summary enables the reader to grasp the nub of your opinion rapidly, with which therefore some authors begin their report.

Data by source

Ensure that your report indicates the sources for all the data you describe.[3] If your opinion rests on a particular fact, or set of facts, the court can <u>weigh the evidence</u> (p.383) according to its perception of its reliability and validity. For example, patients' self-report might be readily accepted in clinical settings, but might not be by the court if the defendant is shown to have lied, unless there is corroborating evidence. A clear chain of reasoning to link your opinion to important factual evidence. Evidence which does not support your opinion, including that in other experts' reports, should be included or referred to, with an explanation for the discrepancy.

Opinion

Responsible opinion

In giving an opinion, you should be confident that it would be shared by a responsible body of practitioners,[4] especially where your opinion is based on novel areas of practice.

Using diagnostic systems

Adopting accepted systems such as the DSM-5 or ICD11 ensures rigour, improves communication, and adds weight to your opinion. However, this can open the expert up to cross-examination which misunderstands the nature of diagnosis and the proper use of diagnostic classification systems. This is particularly the case with the DSM-5, which lists criteria required for a diagnosis that can easily be misunderstood as strict 'checklists', as opposed to a guide to clinical judgment.

Diagnostic validation

Legal contexts increase the possibility of <u>feigning</u> and <u>malingering</u> (p.118). That should not divert the clinician from ordinary and proper practice (it is impossible in medicine to avoid asking 'leading questions'). However, the

---

3 The era is long past when the courts wished only to know the expert's opinion, and experts in the witness box might be somewhat affronted if their opinion was questioned. An expert report today must display balanced, cogent reasoning, supported by sufficient data.

4 The *Bolam* test (p.748), which also applies to expert opinion on clinical matters.

possibility of feigning or exaggeration should be borne in mind, and mentioned in the report where relevant.

Keeping within the medical boundary

You must remain in the medical expert role. For example, a doctor could reasonably give evidence suggestive of an 'abnormality of mental functioning' at the time of an alleged murder,[5] and could describe any abnormalities of perception, emotion, thinking, volition, or consciousness, and whether these 'were a significant contributory factor' in causing the killing. However, this should fall short of addressing the <u>ultimate issue</u> (p.664) of whether the legal criteria for the defence are met.

Dealing with potential legal implications

It is important to distinguish <u>mental state</u>, <u>diagnosis</u> (p.144), <u>formulation</u> (p.146), and any other description of psychiatric or psychological status, *from* their legal implications; albeit you can offer the court an understanding of the relevance of your opinion to the legal questions under consideration.

Stick to your area of expertise

Forensic psychiatrists, like all expert witnesses, should ensure that they only express opinions that are firmly based on the evidence available to them, and that reflect the application of their specialist expertise—opinions that the court, without that expertise, could not otherwise reach. The consequences of giving evidence often go beyond medical benefit to the subject, and the psychiatrist giving evidence should be aware of the numerous <u>ethical dilemmas</u> that may result (pp.293, 311, 327).

Style

A style of writing, format, and presentation should be adopted which acknowledges that the reader will not be an expert. Technical language should be kept to the minimum necessary to allow another expert to assess the details of your assessment and opinion, and all technical terms should be explained.

---

5 In relation to a plea of <u>diminished responsibility</u> (p.624).

Suggested report structure

Suggested report structure

This structure will aid you in meeting the <u>procedural rules</u> (p.658), with which you should familiarise yourself.
- Cover page
- Basic details, such as name of client, date of birth, where seen, date of appointments, and total amount of time seen
- Name and address of instructing body
- Purpose of assessment as per letter of instruction
- Sources of information
- Information obtained from interview(s) with the defendant/litigant
- Mental state examination
- Relevant information from other sources, including other interviews; medical records; other records (e.g. school, social services); legal papers (e.g. witness statements, police interviews, and proofs of evidence)[6]
- Brief descriptions of tests applied by you and others, both medical and psychometric[7]
- Information from other reports (including for 'the other side')
- Psychiatric or psychological opinion, expressed in clinical terms
- Legal implications: explaining the relevance of the psychiatric opinion to the legal issues raised in the instructions, while avoiding addressing the <u>ultimate issue</u> (p.664)
- Recommendations: these should address clinical issues within the legal context, such as mental health disposal in a criminal trial, or treatment aimed at improving prognosis in personal injury civil litigation
- Summary (of clinical opinion and potential legal implications)
- Appendices—for example, raw data from psychometric tests
- A brief, relevant descriptive CV, giving name, professional status, professional address, qualifications, and affiliation of author, plus details of clinical and medico-legal experience
- Declaration—this is likely to be required in a specific form, so check the wording required, which may vary between courts and jurisdictions

6 Deciding which legal papers to rehearse, and how much to extract or to cite, may not be straightforward. Over-inclusion can make a report excessively long; omission of important information may result in accusations of being selective.

7 Avoid describing copyrighted psychometric tests in such detail that copyright is breached.

After writing the report

After writing the report

Failing to submit a report on time can result in a formal complaint. If you cannot comply with the timetable, then you have a responsibility to inform those instructing you at the earliest opportunity. A late report can result in proceedings being delayed at expense and inconvenience to the legal system, and even legal liability in civil proceedings.

Disclosure

- When you have completed the report, do not forget its origin. If it was requested by a third party such as a solicitor, it is likely to be the property of that third party, and you will not be at liberty to disclose it without their permission, or where <u>confidentiality</u> can lawfully be breached (p.320).
- Confidentiality can be breached where there is a significant risk of death or serious harm to others arising from nondisclosure (<u>W v Egdell</u>, p.754) or where it is in the public interest that it be disclosed for the proper administration of justice. This includes disclosing it to the court itself, for example, if the defence has decided to withhold it because it is not seen as helpful to their case (<u>R v Crozier</u>, p.752).

Changing and adding to reports

- Experts should not be asked to, and must not, amend, expand, or alter any part of a report in a manner that distorts the expert's true opinion or withholds information that it is not acceptable to withhold from the court (see p.306).
- It may be appropriate to agree to exclude information that is covered by legal privilege, or which is not relevant to the medical opinion, and which is not relevant to the court's consideration of the case.
- The opinion may be altered by newly acquired information or newly submitted evidence.
- Sometimes experts are asked to provide addendum reports addressing additional issues, and/or new information. Commonly this arises where the 'other side' have filed a report, and it is helpful to the court that your position is clarified or explained on particular points as they have emerged through the other expert's report. Care should be taken to link the two reports, for ease of reading them together.
- What is not helpful is a long sequence of addenda amounting to an argument between the experts. To prevent this, after seeing the initial reports, courts often require experts to meet and produce a 'joint statement' covering areas of agreement and disagreement.

Subsequent meetings

- Joint statements, and meetings, should be based upon an agenda agreed between the lawyers for all parties, and not made up by the experts (unless the lawyers specifically ask the experts to draft an agenda for their consideration). Also, the purpose of the meeting and statement is to clarify the areas of agreement and disagreement, and the key underlying issues. It is not an appropriate forum for experts to argue their case by rehearsing the reasons for their opinion beyond the minimum necessary to establish the areas of disagreement. The latter should be evident from the experts' detailed reports.

Reports for mental health tribunals

Mental health tribunals require you to justify the diagnosis, current treatment, or future management of a patient, usually in their presence.[8]

The report should contain a comprehensive summary of the patient's history and current condition—but without extensive pasting of voluminous computerised clinical records. It should outline their mental disorder and explain relevant risk assessments (p.163). There may be templates provided by your employer which you are expected to use. Essential elements are shown in Box 22.1.

> **Box 22.1 Essential elements of a report for a mental health tribunal**
>
> - Patient's name, address, date of birth, and reference number
> - Legal powers under which they are detained or treatment
> - Date compulsory detention and/or treatment started
> - Name of the RC/RMO and, if different, author's name[9]
> - Names of care co-ordinator and any other key staff members
> - Date of the report
> - Duration of illness and other important details of history
> - Why admission or outpatient treatment was needed
> - Why informal treatment was not possible
> - The grounds for compulsory detention and/or treatment
> - Progress during the use of compulsory powers
> - Current mental state, insight, and attitude to treatment
> - Diagnosis, using standard (ICD or DSM) terminology and codes
> - Risk assessment
> - Current treatment and risk management plan
> - Community care plan in the event of discharge
> - Opinion (psychiatric) and recommendations (psychiatric and legal)

Summary and recommendations

The information in the body of the report is summarised and synthesised into recommendations to the tribunal on the use of compulsory powers.

Opinions should be expressed on the issues that the tribunal will have to address, such as absolute or conditional (or deferred) discharge, continued detention, or transfer to a different level of care (though the tribunal can only recommend this). Whatever the recommendation, explain your reasons clearly, including citing the legal criteria (p.461) for detention that you believe are fulfilled, or not.[10] Where a recommendation is made for continued detention to allow safe arrangements for discharge to be made, the report must explain what further arrangements need to be made (e.g.

---

8 And potentially also in public: although the vast majority of tribunals are held in private, it is possible for the parties to agree to make the hearing, or part of it, public.

9 If the RC/RMO is not the author of the report, it is good practice for them to countersign it.

10 Arguably this amounts to addressing the ultimate legal issue (p.664) since they are legal and not clinical criteria. But this is glossed over in all tribunals.

obtaining funding for a hostel place, or identifying a community care co-ordinator) and how long this is likely to take.

Even where the clinical team is strongly opposed to discharge now or in the near future, the report must contain an <u>after-care</u> (p.492) plan at least in outline form, to indicate what would be done if the tribunal made a decision to discharge the patient.

In writing the report you will act as a <u>professional witness</u> (p.652) in relation to the history and examination findings, and an <u>expert witness</u> (p.652) in relation to the legal criteria for detention (which you are permitted to address directly, despite them amounting to the <u>ultimate issue</u>, p.664).

Dilemmas

There are several dilemmas you may face in making recommendations:
- **The incompletely treated patient** (including nonmedical treatment)—it may not be possible to make recommendations for discharge, but it will be necessary to explain what further treatment is required.
- **The patient recently in remission**—without overt symptoms of mental illness, it may be difficult to justify why the patient should not be discharged. It may not have been possible to test out the improvements through degrees of individual responsibility and freedom.[11]
- **Restricted patients for whom the RC/RMO recommends discharge contrary to the recommendations of the relevant minister**[12]—in these cases it is necessary to pay particular attention to the risk of relapse of mental disorder, or harm to self or others, and of subsequent offending.
- **Patients suffering from primary personality disorder**—the dilemma here is when a patient is suffering from personality disorder that does not appear to be amendable to treatment because of either a lack of ability or motivation to co-operate with therapy. The psychiatrist will need to explain what has been offered, the reasons why it was not successful and why discharge is (or is not) appropriate.[13]

It is also important to be mindful of the issue of power in the therapeutic relationship and the potential impact and effects of the outcome of the tribunal on the individual patient.

---

11 In E&W, for example, this might involve arguing that the nature but not degree of mental disorder indicates the need for detention.

12 The Secretary of State for Justice in E&W; the Secretary of State for Health, Social Security, and Public Safety in NI, the Scottish Ministers; or the Minister of Justice in RoI

13 Mental health legislation varies in the extent to which it invokes a 'treatability' test, and if it does, how closely it comes to what a doctor would consider treatability to be.

Reports for criminal cases

Reports for criminal proceedings—for example, addressing issues such as criminal responsibility (p.406), a defendant's suggestibility (p.160) affecting the admissibility of police interviews (p.383), or the relevance of a risk assessment to sentencing (p.442)—present the most focussed form of the general problem of translation (p.358) between psychiatry and law. The general advice on legal report-writing (p.684) is therefore highly relevant.

The core disparity between the natures of law and medicine should be borne in mind throughout assessing, writing reports for, and giving evidence in, criminal courts.

Pitfalls

There are several pitfalls that you should be aware of when writing a report to be used in a criminal context:

- The law uses different concepts of mental disorder in different criminal contexts, and they are always distinct from medical concepts—for example, 'abnormality of mental functioning' in diminished responsibility (p.624) or 'defect of reason', compared with much broader notions of disability or incapacity, in relation to insanity (p.620).
- Legal concepts of mental disorder used within trials are often different from those applied at sentencing.
- Psychiatrists are asked to give evidence on a defendant's dangerousness (p.672) when the court is considering extended or indeterminate periods of imprisonment, such as a discretionary life sentence. This poses ethical dilemmas (p.322).
- Advice on risk for punitive sentencing may include requests where there is no diagnosable mental disorder but where the court considers that there are mental factors which would benefit from expert comment. This raises ethical dilemmas at a further level (p.670), and most forensic psychiatrists would not provide an opinion in this situation.
- It is important not to give recommendations, explicitly or implicitly, on punishment or other nonmedical matters, other than in the context of a response to a request concerning risk (assuming you take the position of responding to such requests), or causation of the index offence, if considered relevant to culpability and sentence.
- There may be a temptation to be helpful by giving recommendations that go beyond your instructions—for example, to give advice on mental health sentencing options in a report on diminished responsibility. This should only be with prior discussion with your instructing lawyer.
- There can be circumstances where the doctor considers they have an ethical duty, as a doctor or an expert witness, to disclose additional information to the court voluntarily; this may occur in the context of having been asked for a report; or through deciding to provide a voluntary report to the court, for example on a patient the doctor is treating without being asked for it.

Keeping your eye on a next stage

From the moment that you start work on a case, even before assessing the defendant clinically, have in mind that everything you do or advise is potentially subject to subsequent scrutiny, including during cross-examination. Also when writing the report, have in mind that the particular words you use will be the words that you may have to defend in oral evidence: **words matter**.

Reports for the Parole Boards

Situations when reports are needed

There are different situations in which a psychiatrist may write a report for the Parole Board.[14]

- A prison psychiatrist may write a report for a hearing in relation to a prisoner who has not had psychiatric treatment outside prison.
- A hospital psychiatrist may write a report for a hearing where a prisoner has been transferred to hospital and has received a recommendation for discharge by a <u>mental health tribunal</u> (p.515).
- An independent psychiatrist may write a report following instruction by a solicitor, or the relevant government ministry.

Psychiatrists also sit on the Board, either as a regular assessor or as a Board member, but their role is quite distinct from that of a psychiatrist providing a report to the Board.

Instructions

The Parole Board or prisoner's solicitor may issue instructions prior to a hearing, and if they do not, ask for these. If instructions posed as questions are unanswerable then they should be declined. Where the report is prepared for a prisoner, sometimes with no history of psychiatric treatment in the health service, caution needs to be taken to avoid straying beyond one's areas of <u>expertise</u> as a psychiatrist (p.298).

Most parole reports by psychiatrists relate to prisoners under some form of indeterminate imprisonment, where a <u>tariff</u> (p.448) has passed and where the focus is on risk of harm to others, and management of that risk if released.

Where the doctor is the supervising psychiatrist for a transferred patient, it will be automatic that they will provide a report to the Board, triggered by the previous tribunal finding.

Assessment

Clinical assessment is similar to that for a tribunal report if the prisoner is currently transferred to hospital; however, notice will have to be taken of the additional model of risk assessment adopted by the Board, which is criminological and not psychiatric.

In preparing the Parole Board report you will need to read the parole file and be acquainted with the prisoner's prison history, beyond knowing their health records. You will need to have read psychology reports, usually prepared by prison-based forensic psychologists. You should consult the relevant probation officer, who will also prepare a report. Consider the nature and extent of postrelease liaison between health and probation, including monitoring and arrangements for recall.

Report content

General aspects of report-writing apply when considering reports for the Parole Board (see also <u>reports for tribunals</u>, p.692).

---

14 There is a separate Parole Board for each of the three UK jurisdictions and for RoI. In NI, the reference is usually to the 'Parole Commissioners' rather than to a Board.

The role of the psychiatrist is limited to those hearings where there is a psychiatric issue. The psychiatric or psychology member of the Board (if there is one) will have a role in interpreting these reports.

The report should cover:
• Prisoner's psychiatric history;
• Psychiatric factors associated with offending, within a comprehensive risk assessment;
• History of psychiatric treatment;
• Mental health during imprisonment (and any hospital admission); and
• Impact of changes in mental health on risk of future offending.

There may be specific questions asked by the Parole Board:
• Is the inmate's condition treatable?
• Can the mental disorder be treated postrelease?
• Can advice be given about appropriate services?
• Are there specific hospitals or psychiatrists that can be recommended?
• Is the prisoner likely to co-operate with any treatment?
• Should any mental health care input be required if released?
• Proposed conditions of release relevant to mental health care

There may also be reference to arrangements for recall if necessary, including for deterioration of mental health associated with increased risk of harm to others (since the prisoner may not be subject to mental health law once discharged and released, recall might only be possible via the probation and prison system, and this can cause difficulties if the person needs hospital care).

Rules for the Lifer Panel in E&W
• Reports for the review can be withheld from the prisoner on the grounds that its disclosure would adversely affect:
  • national security or
  • the prevention of disorder or crime or
  • the health or welfare of the prisoner or others.
• A report from a forensic psychologist will only be required in tariff-expired cases where there has been substantive psychological input to the case or where the Parole Board have particularly requested that such a report is made available for the review.
• Psychiatric reports are only required if there are mental health issues.

Reports for the family courts

Much family court work is properly conducted by experts in **child and adolescent psychiatry** and psychology, and involves assessment not just of the individual parents and children but of interactions between the parents, and between the parents and children. Social work evidence may sit alongside expert psychiatric and psychological evidence.

Where an adult involved in the case appears to suffer from a mental disorder, it may be appropriate for a **general adult psychiatrist** to be appointed to assess them, or a **forensic psychiatrist** if they are thought to pose a significant risk of violence or sexual offending.

In addition to the usual information required to prepare an assessment in a family court, you will also need any criminal, social services, and other records. You will need to interview the parent and possibly relatives and professionals.

Principles relevant to mental health expert evidence

- Expert reports must be necessary rather than just useful or desirable.
- The court is advised by the expert. The judge may not accept the advice; if judges disagree they must explain why.
- Paper-based assessments of parents are mostly unacceptable.
- The clinical need of the parent is not the focus; though any mental disorder, and its potential for treatment, may relate to child welfare.
- Single joint experts are common. Where more than one expert is allowed, they will usually be required to issue a joint statement (p.655) setting out areas of agreement and disagreement.
- It is vital that forensic psychiatrists and/or psychotherapists who do this work maintain a strict boundary around their expertise and opinion. They may work closely with CAMHS consultants but not comment on CAMHS issues, and in cases involving child physical health, they should not comment on paediatric matters.

Addressing factual issues

It is common for facts to be in dispute in family proceedings. The expert should not take a view as to which of competing narratives is the correct one. Therefore, usually it will be appropriate to give alternative 'conditional' opinions in terms 'if X is accepted then.... , if Y then ...'.

On occasion, parties attempt to use expert psychiatric opinion to prove one particular version of events (e.g. 'Given that the mother has border-line personality disorder, is it not likely that she killed her previous child?'). Psychiatric experts cannot and should not answer such questions.

A note of caution

It will be obvious that these are complex questions with far-reaching consequences. There is no established evidence base for many of the questions (e.g. Does having schizophrenia impact parenting capacity? has not been studied in detail.) Often formulation (p.146) is more helpful than simple diagnosis, and a forensic psychotherapy (p.204) consultation may assist with this.

Most adult and forensic psychiatrists do not have the expertise to advise on parenting ability, which requires training, experience, and systematic observation, and they will not have assessed the parent interacting with the children. Their role is limited to describing the parent's disorder and its potential general implications for parenting or risks to the child.

Practice directions

In addition to the general duties of an expert, experts in family proceedings in E&W are required to satisfy eleven minimum standards, essentially identical to those in the corresponding criminal procedure rules and <u>Practice Direction</u> (p.658), with the following significant additions (shown in Box 22.2).

Box 22.2 Additional specific minimum standards for expert reports to family courts

In expressing an opinion to the court:
- take into consideration all of the material facts including any relevant factors arising from ethnic, cultural, religious, or linguistic contexts at the time the opinion is expressed …
- describe the expert's own professional risk assessment process and process of differential diagnosis, highlighting factual assumptions, deductions from the factual assumptions, and any unusual, contradictory or inconsistent features of the case; and
- indicate whether any proposition in the report is a hypothesis (in particular a controversial hypothesis)

Where there is a range of opinion on any question:
- identify and explain, within the range of opinions, any 'unknown cause', whether arising from the facts of the case (e.g. because there is too little information to form a scientific opinion) or from limited experience or lack of research, peer review, or support in the relevant field of expertise; and
- give reasons for any opinion expressed—the use of a balance sheet approach to the factors that support or undermine an opinion can be of great assistance to the court …

Reports for civil compensation cases

Reports for cases involving psychiatric injury should follow the <u>general advice on report-writing</u> (p.684). Experts are also bound by <u>civil procedure rules</u> (p.658). The expert in a <u>personal injury</u> case (p.640) should only accept instructions relating to mental disorders in relation to which they have expertise. For example, the sequelae of brain injury may be an area in which psychiatrists with general experience have little expertise.

Main issues

- **The presence of a recognised mental illness** will be addressed by reference to whether any psychiatric diagnosis exists. Courts will often expect clinical judgment to be supported by widely used, validated diagnostic procedures or measures.
- **The causal relationship with the act or omission** alleged to have resulted in the psychiatric disorder.
- **Prognosis with or without treatment** in psychiatric and functional terms, relevant to <u>quantum</u> (p.549). This may include giving a view as to the likely <u>capacity to work</u> (p.646), now and in the future.
- **Opinion regarding treatment** including the likelihood of benefit.

Dilemmas

The issue of **causation** of mental disorders is rarely straightforward (and ultimately a legal issue), but can be addressed medically as follows:

- Gaining a very clear and detailed history is the best approach to establishing the apparent relationship between the event and the mental disorder.
- The report should contain details of any pre-existing symptoms, the timing and relationship with new symptoms, and explanations for the relationship between any event and the development of mental disorder, with a clear formulation of any other relevant factors.
- The presence of symptoms relating directly to the event, such as in PTSD re-experiencing symptoms, or evident changes in mental state on discussion of the litigated event, and evidence of avoidance of treatment or legal appointments.
- Any particular psychological significance of the event should be recorded; this may include there having been **priming** events similar to and prior to the index (litigated) event.
- The presence of predisposing factors such as personality structure.
- If there are alternative explanations for the mental disorder these should be recorded, including other life events and the natural history of a pre-existing mental disorder.

Distinguishing an ordinary response from mental disorder can be complex. A clear approach using a specified diagnostic system should be used. There may be <u>controversial diagnostic categories</u> (p.668): the law does not recognise every classifiable disorder as amounting to psychiatric injury.

<u>Malingering</u> (p.118) **or feigning** of symptoms is more likely to arise in cases involving compensation.

- Any symptoms that can be assessed by <u>objective testing</u> (p.130) should be, using recognised instruments, and if necessary involving clinical psychology colleagues.
- Specifically, administer (or ask a psychologist to administer) recognised tests of malingering such as the <u>TOMM</u> or <u>SIRS</u> (p.139) whilst recognising that they do not give definitive answers.
- A detailed history, with use of all available sources of information may be the most helpful way to assess this issue, with consideration of discrepancies, exaggerations, and false claims.
- Lack of cooperation with any assessment should be considered as relevant (although in PTSD it may represent trauma-related avoidance).
- Presence of highly unusual symptoms should be considered suspicious.
- Description of a 'full house' of symptoms may be suspicious.
- Answering 'no' to symptoms that are consistent with the putative diagnosis is less consistent with feigning.
- Observation of inconsistency in physical symptoms (e.g. back pain) said to be causal of mental symptoms (e.g. walking differently when thought to be unobserved).
- Evidence in medical records of somatisation in the past.
- Video surveillance evidence, usually presented as suggestive of feigning.

Reports in clinical negligence cases

There are various situations in which a psychiatrist may be asked to write a report in relation to alleged clinical negligence, either by one party or as a single joint expert (p.653), in relation to:
• reasonable practice and standards of care in psychiatric treatment cases, where the _Bolam_ and _Bolitho_ tests apply (p.550);
• material risks in consent cases (though what the patient would have considered material is now more important than the professionals' view: _Montgomery v Lanarkshire_, p.762);
• whether the breach of the duty of care caused the patient harm; and
• the prognosis for any mental disorder arising from that harm.

Assessment and reporting

Assessment for clinical negligence cases is time-consuming, detailed, and often complex. Where the claimant is alive it will usually include a clinical interview, but many cases are assessed 'on the papers', by way of thorough reading and analysis of the medical records, inquiry documents, and inquest statements and transcripts, and other relevant legal papers. It is important to be certain that you have the expertise to do this.

Always ground any opinion, wherever possible, in published evidence and guidance that you have cited (including evidence that does not support your opinion).

Giving advice after submitting your report

After providing a report, if it is helpful to the side instructing you, then you are likely to be asked later to read through draft documents within the legal 'pleadings'. This is entirely acceptable and ensures that the barrister acting for the claimant or defendant understands fully the nature and effect of your opinion. At a later stage you may be asked to review a medical report and 'pleadings' from the other side.

Pitfalls

• Generally, it is unwise for junior professionals to take on medical negligence cases.
• It is very unwise for a specialist to offer an opinion on a different specialty (e.g. a psychiatrist commenting on psychological treatment).
• Keeping an unbiased approach is difficult. Do not think, 'What would I have done?' Instead think, 'Do I know responsible professionals who would have done as this professional did?'
• Remember that an error of judgment does not automatically amount to a breach of duty of care.
• You should not provide expert evidence in a negligence action in relation to peers or colleagues you know well or with whom you have had a professional relationship. This can be difficult to hold to in complex cases and small subspecialties.
• Expert evidence should address 'What was the process?' (e.g. What steps were taken in deciding not to detain a patient under mental health law who went on to kill themselves?), not 'What does the outcome imply about the process?'

- Absence of good record-keeping is relevant to addressing process, but it is not definitive evidence of bad process; there may be other evidence (e.g. within statements or transcripts or within inquiries or inquests).

Hindsight bias, especially where the outcome has been tragic, must be guarded against; it is easy for an expert to be outraged on behalf of the grieving relatives (or to counter this by defending the doctor who is being criticised).

Safety in balance

It is advisable to balance being instructed for the defence by taking instructions from claimants, and vice versa—though this can be difficult to achieve, given that solicitors tend to act for one class of litigant or the other, and build natural relationships with experts.

Reports in professional regulatory cases

You should have been told by lawyers instructing you the type of proceedings involved and the legal, or other questions you will need to address; if not, as in all clinico-legal practice you must ask.

Issues for expert witnesses

- <u>Fitness to practise</u> proceedings (p.642) commonly arise in parallel with <u>disciplinary</u> (p.557), <u>clinical negligence</u> (p.550), or even criminal proceedings, but must be considered separately on their own merits, even if the facts under consideration overlap substantially: see <u>Bawa-Garba v GMC</u> (p.747).
- In <u>complex cases</u>, you may be unable to advise on <u>causation</u> (p.551), if this means separating out the actions of the subject of the report from those of other team members and other services (being separately assessed).

Independent assessment

- In the UK the <u>Practitioner Performance Advice</u> (formerly the National Clinical Assessment Service) offers 'in-house' assessments of a doctor's performance, without instructing external experts: ask to see their findings, if available.

Mental disorder as explanatory of behaviour

Preparing a report on this within professional regulatory proceedings is perhaps somewhat similar in process to assessing an alleged offender in a criminal legal context because there may be required positing of a link between disorder and behaviour (though it is important not to write 'as if' the proceedings are criminal). A full clinical assessment is required, including in retrospect at times relevant to the allegations, as is a formulation of the individual and their alleged behaviour. Take care to distinguish between the direct effect of any mental disorder upon clinical practice *and* its effect in determining improper conduct.

Reports for employment tribunals

The scope for psychiatric evidence to employment tribunals is limited. Clear instructions should be sought, and the general advice on report-writing (p.684) followed.

An area that is likely to be relevant to the psychiatrist is whether the claimant is suffering from a disability, which is defined as a protected characteristic under equality law (p.556). Other actions may relate to work-related stress, harassment, or bullying.

Which expert?

Occupational physicians may be involved in preparing reports for employment tribunals, and there is a subgroup of psychiatrists who have special expertise in mental health at work. General or forensic psychiatrists may also be asked for reports on their own patients who face employment proceedings, though care must be taken to avoid bias (p.674) in this situation.

Common issues

See Box 22.3.

Box 22.3 Issues when assessing fitness to work
- Workers health and safety risk
- Third-party health and safety risk
- Psychological capacity for work
- Predicted performance and absenteeism
- Any factors that would enable work

- Presence and diagnosis of mental disorder
- Distinguishing ordinary stress from mental disorder
- Does it amount to a relevant 'mental impairment' or disability?
- Assessment of risk of harm to self or others
- Duration of impairment; is it long-term (longer than twelve months)?
- Prognosis and recommended treatment
- Formulation of the relevance of events at work to the mental disorder, including any attempts by the employer to mitigate their effect
- Impact of mental disorder on capacity to work in relation to their whole job, or particular aspects of it
- Recommendations on minimising the impact of work on mental health (e.g. measures to reduce workplace stress, or to match duties to the patient's current functional ability)

Assessment

This involves clinical interview, plus reading all health (including occupational medical) records, the employment record, and any legal papers relating to the action.

Pitfalls

- Confusing psychiatric constructs (p.354) with legal ones (e.g. 'disability')
- Stating an opinion on the ultimate issue (p.664; e.g. discrimination)

Reports for deportation or extradition

Reports may be requested by lawyers acting for people facing deportation or extradition, by the government body handling their case, or by the relevant tribunal or court. Reports are usual where there is known or suspected mental disorder (often because of trauma) or a risk of suicide.

Assessment

- Take care to consider any transcultural issues (p.40).
- There may be other medical reports regarding physical injuries relating to alleged torture, which you should read beforehand.
- An interpreter will be required; if so, extra time may need to be allowed for the assessment.
- As with other types of medico-legal work, there may be a need to consider (and possibly rule out) malingering (p.118) or feigning of symptoms, as there may be strong motivation not to return to a country where mistreatment, discrimination, or torture may be feared.

Report content

The general recommendations for report-writing (p.684) should be followed. You should be cautious about basing your opinion on disputed facts, such as whether the person was tortured; if this or other similar evidence is crucial to your opinion, give a conditional opinion ('if this is the case, then my opinion would be X; if it is not, then Y').

Avoiding pressure

Experts in immigration cases can experience emotional pressure; it is easy to become emotionally involved, based upon one's own sense of natural justice, and to become biased (p.674). Immigration law can appear harsh, but it is not the role of doctors to bend assessments to counter its effects.

Reports concerning deportation or removal

The deportation or removal of mentally disordered people may in some circumstances breach their article 2, 3, and 8 rights (p.516). Consider:
- the impact of news of deportation and of physical removal on the risk of suicide and self-harm;
- their need for treatment, and the likelihood this will be met in the destination country;
- the impact on their mental health (and on ability to reintegrate into society in the destination country) of failure to meet treatment needs; and
- if they are already detained under mental health law, whether repatriation directly to a mental health facility is feasible.

Detention pending deportation

Your report may also need to cover the person's fitness for detention.
- If they have **serious medical or psychiatric disorder**, give your view on whether their disorder could be worsened by the conditions of detention, or whether they are at risk of harm in other ways.
- Consider the availability of treatment in the detention centre.
- Consider recommending transfer to hospital if appropriate.

Additional elements in extradition reports

In addition to the human rights considerations above, extradition can also be blocked or delayed if it would currently be <u>unjust and oppressive</u> (p.558). This term is not clearly defined, and depends on the facts of each individual case, including:

- presence of severe mental disorder, or specific mental disorders related to relevant trauma;
- treatment needs and the impact of not receiving treatment;
- incapacity to resist the impulse to commit suicide
- current risk of suicide, including referencing any recent attempts at suicide, and taking into account the impact of the uncertainty about extradition and trial;
- risk of suicide if extradited (taking into account conditions of detention in the destination country);
- <u>fitness to plead</u> (p.602)[15];
- prognosis in relation to alternative decisions on extradition;
- loss of any protective factors, such as family in the UK or RoI;
- mitigating factors, such as having relatives in the destination country who could support them; and
- the law's focus upon 'incapacity to resist the impulse to commit suicide', driven by its wish to exclude avoidance of extradition based upon 'rational' suicide, or its threat, when faced with extradition, is arguably inconsistent with medical thinking. 'Incapacity' is a legal, and not medical, construct, and many suicides are not impulsive but deliberative. By comparison, a test based upon 'causation', that is, any prospective suicide, or its risk, would be the 'product' of mental disorder, is consistent with medical thinking. Arguably, an expert should therefore resist addressing the 'incapacity to resist suicide' test; in favour of addressing 'whether any prospective suicide would be likely causally to originate in mental disorder', and 'how this might arise'. The court may then wish, for itself, to determine the relevance of such evidence to the 'incapacity' test. Framing evidence in terms of causation will also allow addressing of the level of risk of suicide, in a range of circumstances.

15 In the UK, this has to be assessed based on the E&W fitness criteria, not those of the destination country.

Reports for inquests

If you have been professionally involved in the care of a patient shortly before their death, you are likely to be asked for a statement as a <u>professional
witness</u> (p.652). If not involved, the Coroner or Sheriff (or another interested party, including relatives of the deceased) might also instruct you to
provide an independent <u>expert witness</u> report (p.652).[16]

The information below applies to inquests in E&W, NI, and RoI, and Fatal
Accident Inquiry reports in Scotland. The <u>general advice on report-writing</u>
(p.684) should also be followed.

Special considerations

- You may have a legal,[17] professional or contractual obligation to prepare
  a witness statement if this is requested, and to attend court.
- Be clear about the nature of your involvement and whether you are
  writing a professional witness statement or independent expert report.
  In the latter case, you may give expert opinions if relevant and within
  your area of expertise; in the former, you may only make factual
  statements about what your opinions were at a material time before
  the death.
- A witness statement should be clear and concise, based on the
  contemporaneous records as far as possible, and include all relevant
  information.
- Check whether the court will want you to address any particular
  issues—but even if it does, a synopsis of the relevant psychiatric history
  and the diagnosis should always be included.
- If a detailed and comprehensive account of the psychiatric history
  already exists (e.g. in a recent tribunal report), append it to your witness
  statement rather than recite the information.
- If you think there is the possibility of criticism of your clinical practice,
  consult your defence union and/or your employer as necessary.

Pitfalls in professional witness statements

- Misrepresenting facts, avoiding issues, or deliberately omitting
  information in the hope of avoiding criticism
- Improperly justifying your, or your colleagues' clinical practice—you
  have a duty to be honest
- Giving evidence of matters outside your direct knowledge (except
  where you have made it clear you are reporting on records you
  have read)
- Addressing hypothetical situations
- Speculating about others' actions, opinions, and or motives where you
  have no knowledge of these

16 Your report may be in the form of an independent report for the inquest, or <u>advice to counsel</u>
(p.666) to assist in cross-examination. Depending on the outcome of the inquest, your report (or
a subsequently commissioned report) may lay a foundation for subsequent litigation. Conversely,
if your report was originally written for civil litigation (which an inquest is not), then the coroner
cannot demand to see it, or be required to admit it in evidence. If you are called, you will appear
as the coroner's witness and may have to disclose all communications with the interested party.

17 If a specific notice or summons is issued by the coroner or Sheriff.

Preparation of an expert report

An expert report should be based upon reading all recent clinical records, available witness statements, and relevant earlier records (e.g. that show issues or risks pertinent to the death). It should explain what it appears was known about the patient at the time, and, if relevant, what should have been known and how it should have been interpreted. It may be necessary to read protocols and policy documents from the hospital or prison concerned, or relevant national guidelines. Bear in mind before accepting instructions that you may have to comment on a colleague's practice.

As with any report for legal purposes, expect to be given clear instructions setting out the specific issues you are asked to consider and/or questions you are to answer, including on how to address the required standard of care, and causation (the approach may be different to that in <u>negligence</u>, p.548, e.g.). You may also be asked explicitly to comment on any other matter you think relevant.

You are likely to be the only expert in this inquisitorial setting: where there is a range of alternative yet reasonable opinions, make this clear,

As an expert you may hear witnesses' oral evidence in court after you have written your report based on the documentary evidence. If this leads you to change your opinion on any relevant matter you should inform the court without delay.

Where the death was of a patient in custody, it may be necessary to consider whether the patient was in the correct facility, which may involve reviewing national guidelines on transfer to hospital, as well as considering pressure on hospital beds at the time.

Do not speculate or directly state your view on the *legal* cause of death: your opinion must be founded on factual evidence, and remain within the boundaries of your expertise. Techniques such as 'psychological autopsy' (attempting to infer the deceased's likely mental state at the time from available records) are suitable for research but not sufficiently factual for expert witness evidence.

Reporting without giving oral evidence

Giving oral evidence is not a necessary feature of every medico-legal endeavour. A well-written and sufficiently comprehensive report can avoid the need for oral evidence at all, especially in civil cases, the majority of which are settled occurs out of court.

This should be distinguished from advice to counsel (p.666), where the expert offers assistance which will not become evidence in court.

Reasons for requiring oral evidence

Courts prefer to receive written evidence because it keeps down costs. Examples of when oral evidence is heard include:

- Statute requires it (e.g. before making a restriction order, p.510).
- Parties to the proceedings request it (e.g. in care proceedings, the Local Authority may ask for oral evidence to be heard even though all the other parties are content with written evidence). This is usually because counsel for the interested party considers they may be able to make a point from your evidence, or an opposing barrister may wish to cross examine on aspects of written evidence. It is worth trying to find out what this point is.
- The expert evidence is disputed; either by the parties represented in terms of its legal implications or where there is conflicting expert evidence.
- The report is poorly written and needs further explanation, even though it addresses all the relevant evidence and questions.

Avoiding the need for a hearing

Sometimes, to save court time, judges will ask conflicting experts to meet and provide a joint statement (p.655) setting out areas of agreement and disagreement, which can then be submitted into evidence, without the need for any of the experts to be present.

There may also be occasions where solicitors, counsel, or even judges ask for an opinion on a technical, medical matter, not an opinion on a particular individual. This may be expressed solely as a written opinion. It is important to establish at the outset:

- Exactly what question is being asked?
- How the answer will be used?
- Who will have access to it?
- Could it possibly be used in evidence, and by whom?

As with all forensic activity, it is important to be cautious and circumspect and not to address questions beyond one's expertise. Lawyers and courts, however, may need assistance to know what questions psychiatry can, and cannot, address, and there is an ethical duty (if only as a citizen) to assist legal processes if possible.

Chapter 23

Giving evidence

Giving oral evidence

Much of the advice given in the following pages about giving oral evidence applies to all courts and tribunals, but some specific courts and tribunals are also considered separately.

Giving oral evidence can be a demanding, intimidating, and anxiety-provoking experience for the expert witness. Poor performance can reduce the credibility and cogency of your written report. You must know your evidence and the case well, including relevant legal papers. If you do, and your report is sound, then oral evidence, including cross-examination, should hold no fears; good forensic psychiatrists who know their case will fare well under cross-examination by a barrister whose understanding of psychiatry may well be superficial.

Preparation

Preparation is vital. So:
- Obtain any court dates well in advance and block these out in your diary—arrange potential cover at your usual job.
- Contact the instructing lawyer to check whether there is any new information available.
- Ensure you understand fully the psychiatric and psychological issues you addressed, why and how you did so, and whether any have changed or been added to since you wrote your report.
- Be sure you understand the legal questions to which psychiatric evidence is relevant and how your psychiatric opinion maps onto those questions.
- Read any reports prepared by other experts and consider the implications of differing opinions. Consider which points (if any) you should concede; which not, and why.
- Reread your report, as well as any notes you wrote on the background information you received.
- Think of the arguments or data that go against your opinion, and know how to deal with them, including potentially simply conceding them.
- If the case is complex, consider whether making evidential notes, for example in the form of a 'mind map', will assist you in communicating your opinion, and its justification, to the court (thereby avoiding fumbling through pages of a long report searching for elements of opinion or data, when you should be looking at the jury, or judge); you may sensibly cross-refer particular points to pieces of evidence.
- Alternatively (or in addition), mark up a paper copy of your report with a highlighter pen, with added marginal notes, for ease of reference.
- Ensure you have also marked up all directly relevant papers, including others' reports, past medical records, and legal papers.
- Remember that giving evidence, like teaching, requires skills of communication, simplification, and precis. Prepare with this in mind.
- Psychiatry is abstract and difficult for lay people to comprehend, including juries. Think in advance of concrete analogies that might be helpful in conveying complex concepts or causal relationships, especially before a jury trial.[1]

---

1 It is sensible to build up a body of examples for each diagnosis and mental state symptom or sign and to use those examples that you find juries easily understand.

- Bring all your handwritten notes with you, including original psychometric tests, as you may be asked to refer to them when giving evidence, or the other side may wish to scrutinise them.
- It is essential to have at least a brief discussion with the barrister before giving your evidence, so ask for this if the barrister doesn't ask you first. In a complex case a more formal conference prior to giving evidence will be necessary. Resist having a conference at the courtroom door if you consider this will be inadequate (remember, you understand your evidence and its problems better than the barrister does, and it is you that will be on the spot in the witness box).
- If you are inexperienced, practice with colleagues what you want to say in court during your evidence-in-chief (see below) and how you will respond to what might be asked in cross-examination. Ideally, obtain supervision or mentoring from an experienced senior or colleague.[2]
- If you will be required to give evidence remotely via video link, make sure you will have access to the required IT equipment and that it will be properly configured and working on the day.

On the day

- Dress in clothes you consider appropriately smart, but feel comfortable.
- Ensure you know which court you are attending and how to get there.
- On arrival, you may need to pass through a security scanner.
- Ensure that your mobile phone is silent at all times. You are not allowed to use its phone or camera functions when in the court room.
- Once in court find the court listings sheet to check the hearing time.
- Ensure you meet the instructing lawyer in good time before you are due to give evidence (or to listen to other evidence).
- Ask for the usher, clerks, or other court staff, if you cannot speak to a relevant lawyer, as they will be able to aid you with any questions that you may have about the proceedings.
- You may be required to wait for long periods of time, so bring reading material (or read through materials in the case if you need further time to do this), or a laptop to work on.
- Clarify with the instructing lawyer whether you should sit in court whilst other evidence is given (e.g. by the defendant or by another expert).
- Make notes of relevant parts of oral evidence to which you listen and note its relevance to your psychiatric opinion or legal implications.

Courtroom process

The court will move through a series of court procedures (p.378), starting with **examination-in-chief**, evidence called by the side instructing the expert. The aim is to elicit your psychiatric opinion and its factual and scientific justification, as well as to explore its potential legal implications.[3] Barristers differ in the way they like expert evidence to be adduced. In a criminal trial

---

2 Regular participation in psycho-legal workshops (see Oxford Casebook of Forensic Psychiatry), or equivalent seminars, led by colleagues experienced in giving expert evidence can greatly enhance your skills.

3 In civil litigation, sometimes you do not give oral evidence-in-chief: counsel calling you may simply ask to 'adopt' your report, and hand over to counsel for the other side for cross-examination.

the *traditional approach* arises from how the barrister wishes 'to put their case' overall, and is based upon eliciting points that they consider will resonate with the jury (in a criminal trial): which may result in you being asked a series of short questions. This can be restrictive and make it difficult for you to convey complex points or narrative that you consider medically (and medicolegally) important. The more collaborative approach, which relies on the barrister trusting you,[4] involves asking fewer, more open questions that allow you to deal at greater length with areas of your evidence. In either case the evidence will involve you going through aspects of your report. Doing so in a clear and coherent way that establishes the factual foundations on which your opinion is built will make facing cross-examination that attempts to 'knock down' your opinion far easier.

Cross-examination by the other side will follow. This may be challenging and will usually amount to testing the strength, and attempting to undermine some or all of your evidence (see 'adversarial challenge' below).

Re-examination will follow cross-examination. The counsel that called you will use this to repair any damage they perceive to have been done to their client's case during cross-examination. They/you cannot introduce points not already brought out.

Giving evidence: practicalities

• Be familiar with court etiquette, including standing and nodding when the judge enters or leaves the room, and knowing how to address the judge (you can ask the lawyer or clerk this, or wait to hear how the judge is addressed before you give evidence; see also Table 23.1).

Table 23.1 Titles for addressing the judge in the UK

Justice of the Peace	Sir or Madam; in Scotland, Your Honour
District Judges	Sir or Madam (or Your Worship in NI)
Sheriff (Scotland)	My Lord/Lady
County Court Judge (NI)	Your Honour
Circuit Judges (E&W)	Your Honour
Senior Judges	Your Lordship/Ladyship or My Lord/Lady

In RoI the judge is usually addressed as Judge or The Court.

• The Clerk of the Court will ask whether you wish to swear an oath or affirm: to make a solemn promise that your evidence will be the truth, the whole truth, and nothing but the truth. A selection of holy books will usually be available.
• Use this opportunity to get used to the sound of your own voice and projection.
• You will be asked to state your name, professional address, qualifications and experience.

---

4 Another good reason for ensuring you speak to the barrister before the hearing, to build trust.

- You will be asked about your expertise and experience in general; plus your specific expertise in relation to the current case.
- If you are nervous try to minimise obvious indicators. You may place your hands on the witness box if you wish to avoid wringing your hands anxiously. You are likely to be given water.
- Always look at the jury in a criminal trial or the judge in a civil trial (or when addressed by them in a criminal trial).
- Do not look at counsel, even your own. Counsel ask questions on behalf of the court, and your answers should then be to the court. Being examined, or cross-examined, is not a conversation with counsel. And looking at counsel allows them to use body language to intimidate you during cross-examining. It is not rude not to look at counsel. Focus on a point above the jury, which will assist you to concentrate.
- Make eye contact with the judge and watch their body language if they ask questions, but always watch the judge's pen or typing (out of the corner of your eye as you look towards the jury) to ensure you do not get too far ahead of their note-taking; be ready to slow down and pause at times to allow them to keep up, or catch up.
- In rare cases, you may be examined or cross-examined by a litigant-in-person, possibly the person you have assessed. You should try to confirm this is likely if you are uncertain, so that you are prepared.

Giving evidence: answering and educating

- Speak slowly, clearly, and with as few words as will get over the point you are making; the more words you use the more the risk of contradicting yourself inadvertently, or of creating hostages to fortune in cross-examination.
- In a spirit of educating the court, simplify as you might to students, whilst remaining honest and conveying the essence of the point. Remember that the judge and jurors are not fellow psychiatrists. However, do not lecture or patronise the court.
- During evidence-in-chief and re-examination, be led by the barrister asking you questions. However, if a question is too narrow to allow you to explain the point you wish to convey, give a more wide-ranging answer than the question demands, or ask the judge whether you may expand on what you have said in answering the question.
- Use resonant words and phrases, and vivid examples where appropriate, to assist the court in remembering the points you make. It may be helpful to use concrete analogies to get over the essence of an abstract concept.
- Watch the jury's responses so as to gauge whether they are following you.

Dealing with techniques of adversarial challenge

Many of the difficulties encountered in giving oral evidence originate in the disparities between medical and legal <u>constructs</u> (p.354), the different <u>adversarial</u> and <u>investigative</u> ways medicine and law <u>use information</u> (p.356) to find 'truth'. Familiarity with <u>mapping</u> (p.358) medical concepts onto legal tests will enable you to give high-quality oral evidence and to avoid many pitfalls of cross-examination. Recognise explicitly that challenges to your opinion will be based upon legal adversarial method, and not the medical investigative methods you would normally use in case discussions.

It will help you to understand how the cross-examining barrister wishes to use your evidence within their overall case, which will include their versions of any facts that may be disputed. If the court has not yet adjudicated on these disputed facts, you may need to give a condition opinion ('if the court finds factually X, then my opinion is A; if Y, then it is B').

A common approach in cross-examination is **disaggregation**, or 'death by a thousand cuts': focusing on a small number of the weakest building blocks of your opinion and seeking to undermine or contradict them, whilst ignoring that your opinion is supported by a large number of other mutually reinforcing building blocks. When answering such questions, note the context of your answer each time (i.e. the other mutually supportive building blocks), do not be fazed that the cross-examining barrister tries to resist you doing so. At its most absurd, a barrister may question the validity of individual questions within a psychometric test, so you will need to explain this is scientifically invalid, in that the validity of the test is based on the whole, not on the sum of the validities of the parts.

Asking **yes/no questions** aids the overall adversarial approach, and may be supported by judges on the basis that a barrister must be allowed to ask his questions in any legally acceptable way they may wish. If this prevents you conveying a medically important point, however, ask the judge for assistance, pointing out that, on this point, giving a yes or no answer would mislead the court about the medical evidence.

A **sequence of questions** often builds upon apparently reasonable individual propositions but is designed to lead to an endpoint which contradicts your opinion. Always try to see where a line of the questioning might be headed—not so as to give false answers, but so as to avoid phrasing your answers in ways that could lead to a false endpoint.

A more 'home-grown' difficulty can be created by the expert themselves by failing to explain diagnoses or other medical constructs in a way that jurors and other laypeople can comprehend. Do not hide behind impenetrable DSM or ICD definitions or criteria: find a way to explain the essence of the diagnosis or other concept, perhaps as you would to students. Concrete analogies and examples may help.

General advice on giving evidence under cross-examination

- If a question in cross-examination itself distorts the evidence you are giving, turn to the judge and say so.
- Do not let emotion affect your evidence, and do not see aggressive cross-examination as 'personal': it is merely the means of testing your evidence. If you allow yourself to become angry, you will appear to have lost the argument, and your evidence may be given less weight.
- Be balanced in your answers; do not become defensive or adversarial.
- Concede points validly made against your position.
- Do not be afraid to say you don't know.
- If it becomes apparent that you have made an error or exclusion, either of fact or interpretation, acknowledge the error and apologise to the court at the first opportunity.

- Be careful not to introduce evidence which may be inadmissible in front of the jury: for example, past convictions, or what the sentencing options could be on different convictions. If in doubt about whether something is admissible, don't say it: look towards counsel or the judge with an appropriate facial expression, in the hope they will get the point and intervene to assist you. If necessary, turn to the judge and state that you cannot answer without introducing potentially inadmissible evidence.
- If new admissible evidence is presented to you, consider it, and its impact upon your opinion; you must take it into account even if only recently made available.

After giving evidence

- Do not be upset if your evidence is not accepted—it does not mean that your opinion was necessarily wrong. The court may have translated the evidence into a legal outcome different from that sought by the side that instructed you.
- Ask for a transcript, or oral account, of relevant parts of judge's summing up, in order to know how your evidence was received, including by comparison with that of the other side, and learn for the future.
- Keep all of your papers, at least until you know there will not be a retrial, or appeal possibly followed by a retrial (and at least for the period required by <u>data protection legislation</u>, p.736).

Giving evidence remotely

Since the Covid-19 pandemic, courts have become more willing to allow witness evidence to be given remotely via video link. The experience of doing so, and advice about how best to do so, differs somewhat from when giving evidence in person.

- There is loss of 'theatre' or court atmosphere. It can be more difficult to 'experience' the court and to immerse yourself in the procedure if you are giving evidence from your own clinical office or home study.
- Usually you will not be able to see the jury in a criminal trial, and thereby to gauge whether your evidence is being understood; so as potentially to modify or add to the answers you give. It may help to discuss this with the barrister beforehand, so that they can ask appropriate follow-up questions if necessary.
- You will not be able to watch the judge's pen or typing, so if normally you find yourself having to pause because you have noticed the judge has not kept up, consider speaking more slowly or adding pauses in case they are needed.
- Cross-examining barristers will find it more difficult to use intimidating body language. As a result, the exchanges in a criminal trial may be more intellectual and less theatrical, more similar to appearing in civil proceedings and in the Court of Appeal.

Giving evidence in criminal courts

For general advice see giving evidence in court (p.712), much of which is relevant to criminal courts. The following specific further advice should also assist.

Preparation

- Understand in detail both the psychiatric and the legal questions or issues, and how they relate (e.g. How does the issue of low IQ relate to the defendant's fitness to plead, p.602? How does the defendant's having heard voices relate to diminished responsibility, p.624?).
- Be aware of potential distortions of your evidence that may arise from its presentation within a very restrictive evidential process, and in relation to legal constructs, both of which are highly autopoietic (p.355).
- Think of ways of minimising any likely distortion through the way you frame your evidence-in-chief.
- Be particularly aware of the distinction between your medical opinion and your understanding of the legal implications of your opinion.
- Be clear in your mind where your expertise stops, so as to avoid addressing issues beyond it.
- If the evidence is to be given in front of a jury, or even lay magistrates, plan (with the solicitor or barrister if possible) how you can communicate your evidence most effectively.
- It is normal practice for expert witnesses to sit in court whilst other witnesses (including the defendant) are giving evidence, often in order to know whether the evidence given varies from the statements that are in the case, or to know of new evidence.
- Sitting in court, including listening to other experts' evidence, can also be invaluable in getting to know how it is that each side is 'putting their case', and can assist in preparing for the types of questions you are likely to be asked, particularly in cross-examination.

Giving evidence before a jury

- Ensure that you address all your responses to the jury, or where appropriate the judge. It will help to turn your body towards the judge when answering a question from them.
- Treat the exercise as akin to educating the jury, bearing in mind that jurors will have a wide range of intellectual abilities and life experience. Use simple, nontechnical language; explain jargon if you cannot avoid it; use concrete analogies, since much psychiatry is abstract.
- Criminal law barristers may use adversarial techniques (p.715) and play to the jury; some use emotional techniques rather than calm reason.
- Barristers may also employ unscientific 'folk psychology' which seeks to undermine psychiatric expert evidence per se, sometimes even with the support of their own expert, and/or may attempt to belittle evidence by simplistic approaches, or concentration on emotive words rather than on rational argument. Do not get drawn into this: respond calmly and rationally.

- Offer the jury not only technical diagnosis and formulation but, where appropriate, also offer a narrative, expressed in terms of the mental disorder in relation to the narrative (or competing narratives) of the offence.
- If there is an adjournment during your evidence, you are not permitted to talk to anyone about the case; this rule applies until you have completed your evidence.
- Very rarely the judge may give permission for you to discuss the case with counsel for your side during your evidence, where an issue has arisen which has to be dealt with outside your evidence and cannot be put off until your evidence is finished.
- Often, the jury will be asked to leave whilst there is legal argument. Usually you will not be asked to leave.
- Above all, remain calm and good humoured, and do not become irritated; if cross-examining counsel becomes irritated, this is probably a sign that they are failing to undermine your evidence.
- After giving evidence you may be asked to stay and to sit behind counsel so as to <u>advise on the evidence</u> of another expert (p.666).

Giving evidence in a *voir dire*

Before a jury is empanelled, on occasions there will be a 'trial within a trial', heard before the judge alone, to determine whether, for example, a piece of evidence should be placed before the jury. A *voir dire* (p.383) can also arise within a trial, during which the jury are asked to leave. Sometimes this will address issues to which psychiatric evidence is relevant: for example, the admissibility of a <u>confession</u> (p.608), or where there is concern about the reliability of the police interviews, in relation to alleged <u>suggestibility</u> or <u>compliance</u> (p.160). This may be a different and somewhat calmer experience for the expert, since counsel are unlikely to apply the types of emotional techniques often used in front of juries.

The summing up

Following presentation of all the evidence and closing speeches by counsel for each side, the judge will sum up the case[5]; the jury will then retire to consider their verdict. On their return to the courtroom the chairman of the jury will announce the verdict when asked by the judge. If they cannot reach a unanimous verdict, in some jurisdictions the judge will ask them to determine whether they can reach a verdict on a majority of 10:2. If the verdict is ultimately 'guilty', then pleas in <u>mitigation</u> (p.638) will be heard, and the judge will determine the <u>sentence</u> (p.442), or there may be an adjournment for reports, including psychiatric reports (your report for the trial may well not have dealt with sentencing matters).

5 Ask to read this after the trial, in order to see how your evidence was understood, and contrasted with that of other experts.

Giving evidence to mental health tribunals

Who will be there?

- The judge or president of the tribunal will be an experienced lawyer or (for <u>restricted patients</u>, p.510) a Recorder or equivalent.
- The panel will have a medical member and a third member who may be a lay person or have specialist experience.
- The patient and their legal representative.
- The Responsible Clinician (RC, or RMO) or their deputy if allowed.
- The social worker or other author of the social circumstances report.
- For inpatients, a nurse from the ward.
- Other professionals where relevant, including independent witnesses.
- Family or friends invited by the patient—if the panel consents.
- Occasionally there will be a legal representative for the responsible authority (the hospital's managers), or even justice ministry, if there are contentious legal issues.

Tribunal procedure

- The hearing will be at the hospital where the patient is detained.
- The panel members will sit on one side of a long table, and the parties and witnesses on the other.
- The President will introduce the panel and explain the purpose of the hearing and the procedure it will follow.
- The witnesses will be questioned as shown in box 23.1 below, usually beginning with the RC/RMO, and continuing in the order listed above.
- Witnesses may request to leave after giving evidence, although the tribunal prefers them to remain.
- At the end there will be submissions from the legal representative for the patient and (if there is one) the representative of the hospital.
- All parties will be asked to leave the room whilst the panel deliberate.
- The decision is then delivered orally, and later in writing with reasons.
- The procedure is investigative; though some mental health lawyers question 'adversarially'.

Box 23.1 Procedure for giving evidence at a tribunal

1. The Judge will invite the witness to confirm that their opinion is unchanged from their report, and to describe any changes or updates.
2. The panel members will question the witness (beginning with the medical member for the RC/RMO, and the specialist member for the social worker).
3. The patient's legal representative will question the witness.
4. If the responsible authority is represented at the tribunal, that representative may then question the witness.

Psychiatrists as witnesses

Forensic or other psychiatrists may attend in different capacities:
- As the patient's RC or RMO.
- As an independent expert witness instructed by the patient's solicitor or Ministry of Justice.
- As the representative of the hospital (the responsible authority)—though this is ill-advised; if there is any contentious legal issue, the hospital should obtain its own legal representative.

Preparation

General advice on giving evidence (p.712) should be followed. Reread your report and other records before the hearing. Avoid referring to documents which have not been served during the hearing.

Prepare your answers to obvious questions relating to the **legal criteria** for detention (or for the community order, p.488).
- What is the diagnosis and the important symptoms?
- What is your assessment of risk (p.163)?
- What is your treatment plan and the prognosis?
- Under which of the statutory criteria (p.461) do you justify the compulsory detention or treatment (if you do)?
- How does your evidence show that those criteria are met?

Prepare your answers to **likely questions**, such as:
- Has the situation changed since your report? If so, how?
- What progress has been made?
- What treatment is still needed, and could it be provided in the community? If not, why not?
- Why are compulsory powers needed to give this treatment?
- If the patient is ready for discharge but you are waiting for arrangements to be made (e.g. funding for a hostel), how do you legally justify continued detention? Could the patient safely be cared for elsewhere for a short time (e.g. at a family home) while arrangements are made?
- What is your contingency plan in the event of discharge?
- Who will be responsible for community care, and have they assessed the patient?
- What do you believe would happen (and how would you respond) if, after discharge, the patient stopped treatment, relapsed, or reoffended?

For **restricted patients**, you might also be asked:
- If the relevant minister (p.586) has opposed your recommendation for conditional or absolute discharge (p.513), why do you disagree with their opinion?
- If the tribunal is considering conditional discharge (p.515), what conditions do you recommend and why?

Giving evidence to the Parole Board

Who will be there?

- The chair will be a senior lawyer or a judge.
- If the prisoner has mental health problems, one member will probably be a psychiatrist or psychologist.
- The third member of the panel will be a criminologist, a Probation Officer, or an independent member.
- The prisoner and their representative (a lawyer or a friend/relative[6]).
- A representative for the victim (e.g. Victim Liaison Officer and/or members of their family).
- Other witnesses including probation officers, prison psychologists, or other mental health professionals.

What is it like?

- The hearing will be in a prison (or hospital in the case of a transferred prisoner whom a tribunal has <u>recommended for discharge</u>, p.515).
- There may be a victim statement read at the outset of the hearing, often by a member of the victim's family, if present.
- Each witness will be questioned by the panel.
- Representatives of the prisoner and other parties may question the witness.
- The main focus will be risk. Any issues relating to mental disorder will be geared towards mental disorder as a risk factor.

Psychiatrists as witnesses

A psychiatrist (forensic or otherwise) may attend the parole board in different capacities:

- As a professional witness where the patient has been under their care or they have had some clinical involvement.
- As an expert witness where they are asked to give an opinion on specific issues.

Preparation

The <u>general advice on giving evidence</u> (p.712) should be followed. Reread your report or, if you have not prepared a report, make notes on the person concerned.

- As a professional witness you are highly likely to be asked about your risk assessment. You may be expected to explain some of the science of risk assessment and to give precise explanations of the meaning of summary judgements such as 'low', 'medium', or 'high' risk.
- You are likely to be asked to comment on prognosis and the requirements for treatment.
- Anticipate questions and consider your own involvement critically prior to any hearing, to assist in this process.
- It is not appropriate for psychiatrists to justify detention in a parole hearing in the same way that they may be required to do in a mental health tribunal.

6 Provided the friend/relative is not themselves a prisoner or on licence, or has unspent convictions.

Giving evidence in civil courts and tribunals

See also giving evidence in court (p712). Civil courts have different rules and procedures from criminal courts, including the civil procedure rules (p.658).

- Civil courts (p.372) are usually presided over by a judge sitting alone without a jury.
- A tribunal consists of a panel which is led by a legal chairman (judge or lawyer) and two other members. In employment tribunals (p.705) one member may be from a HR background, and the other may be from a trade union background.

Preparation

You should attend a prehearing conference, to provide you with an opportunity to liaise with other experts and to understand the role of your evidence, and the legal questions. You may be able to discuss the strengths and weaknesses in your report with counsel. You may have already produced a joint statement (p.655) covering areas of agreement and disagreement with other experts.

Procedure in civil courts

The case is brought by a claimant ('plaintiff' in NI or 'pursuer' in Scotland) and defended by a defendant ('defender' in Scotland). The claimant may bring a litigation representative (e.g. a solicitor) with them. Somewhat similar procedures (p.378) to those in criminal trials are broadly followed; however, there are some important differences, outlined below.

General advice

- You will be asked to swear or affirm (p.714) that your evidence will be the truth, the whole truth and nothing but the truth.
- After being asked your name, professional address, qualifications, and experience you will be taken to a copy of your sworn statement or report. You will be provided with a copy in the witness box and will be asked to confirm the contents of your report as your evidence.
- If you have corrections to your report, state them at this point.
- Unlike criminal proceedings, in E&W, your report will usually stand as your examination-in-chief (p.713): so you may not be examined by the side that instructed you but just cross-examined by the other side.
- An expert may be required to give oral evidence without being able to refer to their report. Ensure that you are familiar with its contents in detail.
- You will be subject to cross-examination and may be asked questions by a number of different lawyers representing different parties involved.

Hot-tubbing

Hot-tubbing is the process of hearing expert evidence in civil proceedings concurrently. Experts are sworn in together, and the judge will usually initiate and chair discussion. Legal representatives may ask questions, but cross-examination and re-examination is not permitted. There are variations in the way in which evidence may be taken from experts in a nontraditional form. If you are asked to give evidence in this way, seek clear guidance about the procedure.

At the end of the trial or hearing

At the end of the trial or hearing, the sheriff, judge, or tribunal president will usually retire to consider his judgement and will deliver this in writing later.

Giving evidence at inquests

Who will be there?

- The coroner (or sheriff in Scotland)
- The coroner's officer, who acts as court clerk
- The court usher
- Interested persons, including bereaved family members and if a hospital/care home death, possibly the healthcare regulator
- Legal representatives of the interested persons
- On some occasions outside Scotland, a jury (see p.560 for details)
- Witnesses, including police, pathologists, GPs, and hospital and prison staff
- Members of media organisations

What is it like?

- Coroner's Courts usually sit in shared court buildings or local municipal offices; Fatal Accident Inquiries in Scotland are held in Sheriff Courts.
- The proceedings will be public unless there are national security issues.
- In more lengthy or complex cases an administrative 'preinquest review hearing' may be held some time before the inquest commences.
- A coroner is usually addressed as Sir/Madam, a sheriff as My Lord/Lady.
- The coroner's officer may ask in advance whether you wish to affirm to tell the truth or swear on a holy book when you give your evidence, and may indicate whether you should sit or stand to give evidence.
- Witnesses are examined first by the coroner or sheriff; other interested persons and their representatives may ask questions next; followed by jurors (the coroner may read jurors' questions on their behalf).
- Interested persons or their legal representatives may make submissions on points of law, but not on the facts (or make any closing speech).
- At the end of the evidence in a coroner-only inquest the coroner will state the facts they have found then their conclusions; in a jury inquest they will sum up the evidence, and tell the jury which conclusions are legally open to them before sending them to consider their conclusions.

Psychiatrists as witnesses

A psychiatrist may attend[7] an inquest in different capacities:
- as an ordinary witness of fact to a death;
- as a professional witness (p.652) where you were clinically involved; and
- as an expert witness (p.652) where you are asked to give an opinion on specific issues relevant to the death.

Psychiatrists as interested persons

In some cases, treating psychiatrists may wish to consider asking to be given the status and rights of an 'interested person', where allegations are made that their action or inaction caused or contributed to the death, or where there are other criticisms of the care they provided.

---

7 A coroner can compel you to attend the hearing by serving a witness summons (schedule 5 notice in E&W) but will often assume that as a professional you will attend without a summons. If a summons will assist (e.g. with being permitted time off work from a new employer) you can always ask for one to be served on you.

An interested person is entitled to be notified of the inquest dates; to receive all relevant documents, witness statements, and expert reports; to ask questions of all witnesses; and to be legally represented.

Preparation

You should familiarise yourself with the inquest bundle, the relevant material you are likely to be asked about, and any reports you have submitted. If you are giving evidence because you were clinically involved, review the medical records and think about whether the death puts a new perspective on what you thought at the time; be ready to explain your reasoning, based upon the information available at the time. The court is likely to have access to other internal inquiries and reports relating to the death; if possible, you should obtain and review these.

As a professional witness, you may be asked about:
- Your risk assessment, and about accepted techniques of risk assessment.
- Factors related to suicide risk (e.g. if the person had recently started a new medication, expect questions on any possible link between this and his death).

Your preparation should also include:
- Ensuring you have had a thorough discussion with your employer prior to the hearing if appearing as a professional witness. If your employer is also an 'interested person' at the inquest you may be asked to attend a preinquest meeting with their representatives.
- Considering seeking advice from your medical defence body, especially if you consider that you might be entitled to 'interested person' status in your own right or if there is likely to be any conflict between your own position and that of your employer.
- Anticipating that the bereaved family are likely to be present, be sensitive in the way you express yourself.
- Anticipating questions and considering your own involvement critically prior to the hearing. If there have been shortcomings on your part, think about how you might reflect upon and acknowledge these.
- Preparing for rigorous and searching questions, particularly if as an expert you have been critical of other professionals.

Part VI

Appendices

Appendices

Statutes

Most of the statutes listed on these pages made several changes to the law; some are highly complex, with many different effects. The brief summaries provided here focus on the most important elements of each statute, from the perspective of the handbook. Elements of each Act not relevant to forensic psychiatry are not mentioned.

Statutes

Adult Support and Protection (Scotland) Act 2007 This Act enables people who are unable to care for themselves (p.542) to be removed to a hospital or other place of safety. It also provides a range of measures for safeguarding vulnerable adults (p.179).

Adults with Incapacity (Scotland) Act 2000 This provides ways to help safeguard the welfare and finances of individuals who lack mental capacity (p.522).

Age of Criminal Responsibility (Scotland) Act 2019 This legislation, not yet brought into effect at the time of writing, raises the age of criminal responsibility (p.406) to twelve years, so that children under that age cannot be prosecuted even in exceptional circumstances, and cannot be referred to Children's Hearings because of offending behaviour.

Age of Legal Capacity (Scotland) Act 1991 This sets out that a person under the age of sixteen years has no legal capacity to enter into any transaction, where as a person over age sixteen years has full capacity to enter into any form of agreement. See p.530.

Age of Majority (NI) Act 1969 This Act relates to capacity in children and adolescents, that is those younger than age eighteen years. See p.530.

Assisted Decision-Making (Capacity) Act 2015 RoI This replaced the Lunacy Regulation (Ireland) Act 1871 and established a modern framework of mental capacity law for RoI. See p.522.

Care Act 2014 UK This repealed some remaining parts of the National Assistance Act 1948 (see below), and provided a new framework for social care in England, with some definitions (e.g. the key term 'ordinary residence') and other aspects applicable to Scotland and NI. It also introduced a new framework for safeguarding vulnerable adults in England. The power to remove adults at risk was repealed; only the police now have such powers, under PACE (see p.542). Similar provisions were enacted in Wales by the Social Services and Wellbeing (Wales) Act 2014. See p.568.

Children Act 1989, 2004 E&W 1995 Scotland 2001 RoI. These Acts changed the law in regard to children and introduced the notion of parental responsibility. They simplified child protection legislation and increased the powers of (and also the scrutiny of) child welfare and education departments. See pp.531, 554.

Children's Hearings (Scotland) Act 2011 This updated the law on Children's Hearings (p.386), increasing the rights of children in the system and introducing an advocacy service.

Civic Government (Scotland) Act 1982 This Act modified and simplified the Scottish law relating to acquisitive offences (p.426).

Constitutional Reform Act 2005 UK This removed the judicial functions of the House of Lords and created a Supreme Court (p.372).

Coroners & Justice Act 2009 E&W, NI This Act substantially revised the legal test for diminished responsibility (p.624), and replaced provocation with a new defence of loss of control (p.630).

Courts (Establishment and Constitution) Act 1961 RoI

Courts Service Act 1998 RoI Court of Appeal Act 2014 RoI These Acts established the modern court system in RoI, and provided rules for their management, appeals, and the appointment of judges etc. See p.388.

Crime and Courts Act 2013 UK This established the National Crime Agency. In E&W, it also created a single Family Court to replace the various Family Proceedings Courts and family functions of the county courts and (with a few exceptions) the High Court. Similarly, it replaced the various county courts with a single County Court able to sit in every district.

Crime and Disorder Act 1998 E&W This introduced ASBOs (p.458) and a variety of other community sentences (p.454) and related orders. It also abolished the rule that children between ten and fourteen years old could only be convicted of an offence if they knew what they were doing was wrong (doli incapax, p.406), and established new rules for sentencing children (p.446).

Criminal Evidence (Witness Anonymity) Act 2008 E&W, NI This Act allows the courts to grant protection, most notably anonymity, to vulnerable or intimidated witness where this does not prevent a fair trial. See p.156.

Criminal Justice Act 2003 UK This amended large areas of the law relating to police powers, bail disclosure, allocation of criminal offences, prosecution appeals, hearsay, bad character evidence, sentencing, and release on licence, affecting E&W more than Scotland or NI. The Act replaced <u>automatic life sentences</u> for certain serious offences with <u>IPPs</u> (p.448). It allows offences to be tried by a judge without a jury in cases where there may be threats of interference with jury. It also allows a defendant to be tried twice for the same offence (double jeopardy) if new and compelling evidence has been found. This Act also revised and simplified <u>community sentences</u> (p.454).

Criminal Justice Act (NI) 1966 This created the statutory defence of <u>diminished responsibility</u> (p.624) for NI in terms similar to those in the E&W Homicide Act 1957 (see below). It also decriminalised suicide, clarified the special verdict of not guilty by reason of <u>insanity</u> (p.620), and refined the rules for inferring <u>mens rea</u> (p.402) from behaviour and for criminal liability when <u>intoxicated</u> (pp.614, 616).

Criminal Justice and Immigration Act 2008 E&W, NI Criminal Justice (NI) Order 2008 In E&W, the Act introduced <u>Youth Rehabilitation Orders</u> (p.454) and <u>Violent Offender Orders</u> (p.457), as well as abolishing <u>IPPs</u> (p.449), though made no arrangements for prisoners already subject to them. It also criminalised causing a nuisance on NHS or (in NI) HSS premises. The Order similarly abolished IPPs for NI, but replaced them with ICSs rather than automatic life sentences.

Criminal Justice and Licensing (Scotland) Act 2010 This Act created the <u>Scottish Sentencing Council</u> (p.444), abolished short periods of <u>imprisonment</u> (p.452), created new offences including one of <u>stalking</u> (p.432), revised criminal procedure and <u>rules of evidence</u> (p.382, and replaced common law rules on <u>insanity</u> (p.620) and <u>fitness to plead</u> (insanity in bar of trial, p.602) with new statutory rules.

Criminal Justice and Public Order Act 1994 E&W NI This increased the <u>police power</u> (p.571) to stop and search suspects, and restricted the <u>right to silence</u> (p.572) by allowing courts to draw inferences from it. It also criminalised previous civil <u>torts</u> (p.548), including disruptive trespass, squatting, and unauthorised camping.

Criminal Justice (Public Order) Act 1994 RoI This Act modified the available <u>public order offences</u> (p.424) and changed the law on <u>acquisitive offences</u> (p.426).

Criminal Justice (Theft and Fraud Offences) Act 2001 RoI This is the main statement of the law relating to fraud and other <u>acquisitive offences</u> (p.426).

Criminal Law Act 1967 E&W 1967 NI 1997 RoI These Acts clarified powers of <u>citizen's arrest</u> (p.571) or in RoI police arrest, and what amounts to <u>reasonable force</u> (p.410) in certain situations.

Criminal Law (Insanity) Act 1997, 2006 RoI These Acts provide a statutory definition and restatement of the test for criminal <u>insanity</u> (p.620), changed the plea to not guilty by reason of insanity, introduced a new plea of <u>diminished responsibility</u> (p.624) in cases of murder, and brought in new provisions in relation to a person's <u>fitness to plead</u> (p.604). It amended the law on <u>infanticide</u> (p.414), provided new rules on <u>transferring prisoners to hospital</u> (p.506), and established a new independent Review Board to supervise them.

Criminal Law (Rape) Act 1981 RoI This legislation, and the subsequent Criminal Law (Rape) (Amendment) Act 1990, defined new offences of <u>rape</u> (p.418) and certain other sexual offences.

Criminal Lunatics Act 1800 UK This Act established, for the first time, the principle that mentally disordered offenders found not guilty by reason of <u>insanity</u> (p.620) who pose a risk of harm to the public should be treated compulsorily rather than automatically released. It provided for their indefinite detention in an asylum (or prison). See p.462.

Criminal Procedure (Insanity) Act 1964 E&W This revised the special verdict of not guilty by reason of <u>insanity</u> (p.620), and established procedures for a <u>trial of the facts</u> (p.604) after a finding of unfitness to plead. It also sets out the <u>court orders</u> (p.504) available after a finding of insanity or unfitness to plead. The current version of the Act is the result of amendments by the Criminal Procedure (Insanity and Unfitness to Plead) Act 1991 and Domestic Violence, Crime and Victims Act 2004.

Criminal Procedure (Scotland) Act 1995 This consolidating Act is now the primary source of Scottish criminal procedure. It raised the <u>age of criminal responsibility</u> (p.406), introduced new mental health disposals including the <u>compulsion order</u> (p.500), created the <u>risk assessment order</u> (p.504), and created or revised a number of <u>community sentences</u> (p.454).

Data Protection Acts 1984–2018 UK 1988–2018 RoI These Acts implemented <u>EU law</u> (p.390) on the protection of personal data, and set down many detailed rules on the processing and retention of personally identifiable and <u>confidential</u> (p.320) information.

Domestic Violence Act 2018 RoI This introduced new protections for victims of domestic violence, include safety orders and protection orders prohibiting further acts of violence, and barring orders excluding the alleged perpetrator from the home.

Domestic Violence Crime and Victims Act 2004 E&W This Act focuses on the legal protection and assistance to <u>victims of crime</u> (p.158), particularly domestic violence. It amended the Criminal Procedure (Insanity) Act 1964 (see above) to change the disposals available after a finding of <u>unfitness to plead</u> (p.602), and established new rules for informing victims when <u>restricted patients</u> (p.510) and other patients <u>sentenced to treatment</u> (p.500) are discharged.

Enduring Powers of Attorney (NI) Order 1987 This Act relates to decisions over property and affairs after the donor loses capacity. See <u>powers of attorney</u> (p.538).

Equality Act 2004 RoI 2010 UK These Acts implemented <u>EU law</u> (p.390) updating <u>rules against discrimination</u> (p.556) on the basis of sex, race, and disability, amongst other characteristics. The UK also merged a number of previous bodies into a single Equality Commission.

European Convention on Human Rights Act 2003 RoI This legislation made the <u>European Convention on Human Rights</u> (p.518) directly applicable in Irish courts.

Extradition Acts 2003 UK 1965, 2001 RoI These cover the extradition of people from the UK or RoI to face criminal trial in other countries. See p.558.

Family Law Reform Act 1969 E&W This Act presumes children aged sixteen or seventeen years old to have capacity to consent (p.530) to medical or surgical treatment.

Fraud Act 2006 E&W This Act replaced various previous specific acquisitive offences such as obtaining property by deception with a set of new general offences of fraud (p.427).

Freedom of Information Act 2000 E&W 2014 RoI These acts provide for the release of a variety of nonpersonal information held by public bodies, and for rules under which their release can be blocked in certain circumstances.

Health & Safety at Work etc. Act 1974 UK Health & Welfare at Work Act 2005 RoI These Acts place duties on employers (p.556) to their employees including people with mental disorder, to ensure a safe workplace and safe working practices. There is also a duty to ensure the mental health of employees.

Homicide Act 1957 E&W This was introduced as a partial reform of the common law offence of murder in English law by abolishing the doctrine of constructive malice and reforming the partial defence of provocation (p.630). It introduced the partial defences of diminished responsibility (p.624) and suicide pact (p.412).

Human Rights Act 1998 UK This Act made the European Convention on Human Rights (p.518) directly applicable in British courts, saving the need to appeal to the European Court of Human Rights in Strasbourg. It also requires all public bodies to carry out their duties in ways that conform with the Convention.

Immigration Acts 1971–2006 UK 1999–2010 RoI These complex sets of Acts set out the rules on who can claim British or Irish citizenship, who may enter and remain in either country, who may be granted asylum, and whom the government may legally deport. See p.558.

Justice Acts (NI) 2011–2016 These Acts of the devolved NI Assembly followed similar legislation in E&W (e.g. CJIA2008) and brought in conditional cautions, live links, and violent offences prevention orders, amongst other measures.

Legal Aid, Sentencing and Punishment of Offenders Act 2012 E&W This abolished Custody Plus and intermittent custody, extended community sentencing options, and reintroduced automatic life sentences for certain serious or repeat offences. See p.448.

Life Sentences (NI) Order 2001 This Order provides for the release and recall of offenders serving a life sentence (p.448) in NI. It also makes changes to the way such sentences and sentences of detention at the Secretary of State's pleasure are made in court.

Lunacy Acts 1845–1891 UK These Acts, and the associated County Asylums Act 1888 and Trial of Lunatics Act 1883, established a network of asylums across E&W, Scotland, and Ireland; defined rules for admission, transfer, leave, and discharge; and instituted a system of inspection by Commissioners who could order minimum standards of treatment and the release of patients. See p.462.

Mental Capacity Act 2005 E&W This provides a framework to empower and protect adults who lack capacity (p.522) to make decisions for themselves on medical treatment and other matters. It also enables people to plan ahead for when they may lack capacity, such as by making advance statements (p.536).

Mental Capacity Act (NI) 2016 This Act, not yet in force at the time of writing, unifies mental health and mental capacity law in a single, comprehensive capacity-based framework. Its guiding principles, set out at the start of the Act, are respect for autonomy, justice, beneficence, and nonmaleficence (see p.287)—compare the existing principles of mental health laws (p.466) and principles of mental capacity law (p.522). It is a major international innovation, requiring many changes to practice (which have been delayed by the suspension of the devolved government in NI for several years).

Mental Deficiency and Lunacy (Scotland) Act 1913 Mental Deficiency Act 1913 E&W These Acts set up specific institutions for the care and control of people with learning disability, with a Board of Control to inspect them. See p.462.

Mental Health Act 1983 E&W This Act, which was heavily modified by the Mental Health Act 2007 in particular, is the primary mental health law (p.461) in E&W. It deals with the detention in hospital of people with mental disorders, as well as other compulsory measures including guardianship and supervised community treatment (p.488). It sets out the criteria (p.470) that must be met before compulsory measures can be taken, as well as protections and safeguards for patients. It also introduced the deprivation of liberty safeguards (DoLS, p.532) for patients lacking capacity.

Mental Health Act 2001 RoI This is the primary Irish mental health law (p.461), and covers the circumstances in which patients may be admitted to hospital for mental health treatment against their will. The Mental Health Commission is the statutory independent body which oversees the Acts implementation and use.

Mental Health (Care & Treatment) (Scotland) Act 2003 This Act enables medical professionals to detain and treat people against their will; it is Scotland's primary mental health law. Unlike the equivalents in E&W and RoI (but to a lesser extent than under the MCANI), the main ground for detention of people with mental disorder is their lack of capacity (p.466).

Mental Health (NI) Order 1986 This Order is still, at the time of writing, the primary mental health legislation (p.461) for NI, and it contains provisions on unfitness to plead (p.602) and insanity (p.620). After the MCANI comes fully into effect, the MHNIO will be largely repealed for adults, but will cover treatment of children until new children's legislation is enacted.

Mental Treatment Acts 1930 E&W 1932 NI 1945 RoI These Acts permitted voluntary admission to, and outpatient treatment within, psychiatric hospitals. The RoI Act went much further and abolished the need for judicial orders for admission. See p.462.

Modern Slavery Act 2015 E&W Human Trafficking and Exploitation (Scotland / CJSA NI) Acts 2015 Criminal Law (Human Trafficking) Act 2008 RoI These Acts criminalise new forms of slavery, servitude, and forced or compulsory labour and human trafficking, and seek to protect victims. They can be used to prosecute an adult for the exploitation of children and as a defence for an exploited young person charged with a crime. See p.436.

National Assistance Act 1948 E&W This Act formally abolished the Poor Laws (p.462), and provided basic social welfare for people who were not eligible to receive services because they did not pay National Insurance contributions (e.g. the homeless, unmarried mothers, and the severely disabled). It included a power to move unwilling people unable to care for themselves (p.542) to a hospital or nursing home, but this power was abolished by the Care Act 2014.

Non-Fatal Offences Against the Person Act 1997 RoI This is the principal Act that defines the offences of assault (p.416) that does not amount to homicide.

Offences against the Person Act 1861 E&W, NI This is one of a group of Acts sometimes referred to as the criminal law consolidation Acts of 1861. It is the foundation for prosecuting assault (p.416), short of murder, in the courts of E&W and NI.

Parole Act 2019 RoI This revised and updated the law relating to remission of prison sentences, parole for longer sentences, and the rules of the Parole Board.

Police and Criminal Evidence Act 1984 E&W Order 1989 NI Criminal Justice (Scotland) Act 2016 These and the associated codes of practice provide the core framework of police powers (p.570) and safeguards around stop and search, arrest, detention, investigation, identification, and interviewing suspects. Their aim is to achieve a proper balance between the powers of the police and the rights and freedoms of the public.

Powers of Attorney Act 1996 RoI This Act relates to decisions over property, money, and personal care after the donor loses capacity. See powers of attorney (p.538).

Prisoners and Criminal Proceedings (Scotland) Act 1993 This is the legislation that relates to detention, transfer (except to hospital) and release of imprisoned offenders (p.583) in Scotland.

Probation of Offenders Act 1907 E&W, NI and RoI This Act gave judges the discretion to dismiss a charge against a defendant after a summary trial (p.398) even when the court is of the opinion that it is proved, or to conditionally discharge a defendant (whether charged on an indictment or summarily). The judge could also dismiss a case under the Act on condition that the defendant pay a contribution to charity, or repay costs arising from his actions, or if the case was seen as trivial. The Act established a system of probation of offenders (p.584) that continues today in modified form.

Public Order Act 1986 E&W Order 1987 NI This Act and Order respectively created a new set of public order offences (p.424), replacing the common law offences of riot, unlawful assembly, and affray that had by then become confused.

Sexual Offences Act 2003 E&W 2009 Scotland Order 2008 NI These Acts and this Order each consolidated and replaced the older common law and statutory sexual offences (p.418), redefining the offences more clearly and explicitly. Several new offences were created in some cases, such as nonconsensual voyeurism, assault by penetration, penetration of any part of a corpse, and causing a child to watch a sexual act. *Rape* was redefined to include male rape in Scotland. The law was also amended to make it clear that only a reasonable and genuine mistaken belief that the other party consented could be a defence to rape.

Social Services and Wellbeing (Wales) Act 2014 This Act, passed in Wales around the same time as the Care Act 2014 in England, provided a similar framework for social care and safeguarding to that adopted in England.

Terrorism Acts 2000, 2006 UK Criminal Justice (Terrorist Offences) Act 2005 RoI These Acts extend existing offences, and create new ones, relating to acts done for terrorist purposes (e.g. overthrowing the government or intimidating the population). See p.430.

Theft Acts 1968, 1978 E&W 1969 NI These Acts replaced the over-complicated and confusing common law offences of larceny with a new set of theft offences (p.426).

Vagrancy Acts 1349–1898 UK These laws, beginning with the Ordinance of Labourers 1349, were first introduced to increase the supply of workers after the Black Death (bubonic plague) killed many; later their focus was the large numbers of soldiers and others returning after overseas wars, who were often homeless and out of work. They criminalised idleness, homelessness, and begging. They later provided for vagrants to be sent to their home parish to receive relief under the Poor Laws. See p.462.

Legal cases

Selected important cases referred to in the text of the handbook are listed below and summarised briefly on the following pages. In these summaries, we have focused on the elements most relevant to the topic in the handbook that refers to the case. With a few cases, this means that the summary we have given might not reflect other significant aspects of the judgment. Other cases referred to, but not listed below or summarised, are given their full citation within the text, in order to allow the reader to research them.

Cases

ABC v St George's Healthcare NHST & others [2020] EWHC 455 p.745

Assoc Provincial Picture Houses v Wednesbury Corp [1948] KB 223 p.770

Attorney General v Whelan [1934] IR 518 p.746

Attorney-General's Reference (No. 2 of 1992) [1993] 3 WLR 982 p.746

Austin v Commissioner of Police of the Metropolis [2009] AC 564 p.746

Bailey v Ministry of Defence [2008] EWCA Civ 883 p.747

Bawa-Garba v GMC [2018] EWCA Civ 1879 p.747

Black v Forsey [1988] SC (HL) 28 p.748

Bolam v Friern Hospital Management Committee [1957] 1 WLR 583 p.748

Bolitho v Hackney Health Authority [1998] AC 232 p.748

Bratty v Attorney-General for Northern Ireland [1963] 1 AC 386 p.749

Caparo Industries PLC v Dickman [1990] 2 AC 605 p.751

Clunis v UK [1998] ECHR 116 p.751

Darnley v Croydon Health Services NHS Trust [2018] UKSC 50 p.752

Donoghue v Stevenson [1932] UKHL 100 p.753

Dooley v Cammell Laird [1951] 1 Lloyd's Rep 271 p.753

DPP v Camplin [1978] UKHL 2 p.750

DPP v Majewski [1977] AC 443 p.761

DPP v Morgan [1976] AC 182 p.753

Drury v HM Advocate [2001] SCCR 583 p.754

Edwards v UK [2002] ECHR 46477/99 p.754

F v West Berkshire Health Authority [1989] 2 AC 1 p.755

Freeman v Home Office [1984] 1 AllER 1036 p.756

Galbraith v HM Advocate (2002) JC 1 p.756

Gillick v West Norfolk and Wisbech AHA [1985] 3 All ER 402 p.756

Gillon v HM Advocate [2007] SC(JC) 24 p.757

Hertfordshire County Council v AB [2018] EWHC 3103 p.745

Hirst v UK (No.2) [2009] ECHR 2260 p.757

HL v UK [2004] 40 EHRR 761 p.758

HM Advocate v Savage (1923) JC 49 p.767

HM Attorney-General for Jersey v Holley [2005] UKPC 23 p.758

Home Office v Dorset Yacht Co [1974] 2 AllER 294 p.758

In re M and R (Child abuse: evidence) [1996] 2 FLR 195 p.761

K v Secretary of State for the Home Dept [2002] EWCA Civ 775 p.759

Kennedy v Cordia (Services) LLP [2016] UKSC 6 p.759

Kumar v General Medical Council [2012] EWHC 2688 (Admin) p.760

Lewisham London Borough Council v Malcolm [2008] UKHL 43 p.760

Loake v CPS [2017] EWHC 2855 p.761

R v A This case involved a sexual encounter between two people with learning disability. The defendant received a supervision order (p.504) after being found unfit to plead (p.602) and to have done the acts associated with sexual assault, the acts being deemed nonconsensual because the alleged victim lacked mental capacity on the balance of proof. The Court of Appeal ruled that the wrong standard of proof (p.380) was applied: the prosecution should have been required to prove beyond reasonable doubt that the alleged victim lacked capacity and therefore could not have consented, and Mr A was therefore acquitted. See p.522. *R v A(G)* [2014] EWCA Crim 299.

AB Mr AB was a high-risk sexual offender with a mild learning disability; he had mental capacity to make relevant decisions. In response to the Supreme Court decision in *MM* (see below), Hertfordshire County Council applied to the High Court for permission to follow a care plan depriving AB of his liberty (with his capacitous consent, albeit arguably subject to coercion as the alternative was detention in hospital). The High Court declared the care plan lawful under its inherent jurisdiction, confirming (contrary to guidance from the MoJ) that such applications can be made in future cases involving patients with capacity. See p.532. *Hertfordshire County Council v AB* [2018] EWHC 3103.

ABC v St George's ABC's father, suffering from psychotic depression related to undiagnosed Huntington's disease, killed her mother. The hospitals caring for him later made the diagnosis of Huntington's disease, and wanted to inform his daughters, but he refused consent. He and ABC both took part in family therapy, where again the diagnosis was not disclosed. She only learnt of the autosomal dominant hereditary condition a year afterwards, by when she had had her first child; she later discovered that she had inherited the gene, and there was a 50% chance she had passed it on to her child. She sued the hospitals involved, claiming that they had had a duty to disclose the information to her in time for her to consider terminating the pregnancy. The High Court, rehearing the case after a successful appeal against its original dismissal, considered analogies with cases involving breach of confidentiality regarding child sexual abuse, and duties owed to women who became pregnant after their partners had negligently ineffective vasectomies. It found that, because the second hospital had a relationship 'of close proximity' with the claimant (because of the family therapy and her frequent involvement in her father's care), it had a duty to balance her interests against her father's in considering whether to breach her father's confidentiality and disclose the diagnosis to her. However, it had not breached that duty: since it had conducted a balancing exercise, via its clinical ethics committee, and its decision not to disclose was also not illogical, and was supported by a responsible body of medical opinion.

See p.550. *ABC v St George's Healthcare NHS Trust, South West London & St George's Mental Health NHS Trust and Sussex Partnership NHSFT* [2020] EWHC 455.

A-G's ref The defendant had killed two people by driving his lorry into parked cars on the side of the motorway. He claimed to be in an automatic state caused by 'repetitive visual stimulus experienced on long journeys on straight flat roads'. The trial court accepted the defence of automatism; the Attorney-General appealed, and the Court of Appeal ruled that, on the medical evidence, the defendant had partial control over his actions and the defence of automatism therefore did not apply, stating, 'the defence of automatism requires that there was a total destruction of voluntary control on the defendant's part'. See p.612. *Attorney-General's Reference (No. 2 of 1992)* [1993] 3 WLR 982.

A-G v Whelan Whelan knowingly <u>received stolen goods</u> (p.427), and was convicted despite the jury accepting he had acted under <u>duress</u> (p.634) from Farnon, who was known to carry a revolver. The Court of Criminal Appeal overturned the conviction, and set down the test for duress in RoI. See p.634. *Attorney General v Whelan* [1934] IR 518.

R v Ahluwalia The defendant was a woman in an arranged marriage who had suffered years of abuse and violence from her husband. One evening, after an argument in which he threatened to beat her in the morning, she set him alight in his sleep, killing him. She pleaded <u>provocation</u> (p.630) but was convicted of murder on the ground that the time that elapsed between the argument and the killing meant that her loss of self-control, if any, had not been 'sudden and temporary'. This was upheld by the House of Lords, but a retrial was ordered to allow her to claim <u>diminished responsibility</u> (p.624) on the grounds that she suffered from 'battered woman syndrome', a form of <u>PTSD</u> (p.96); her conviction was later reduced to manslaughter on these grounds. The law was later changed by statute to remove the need for 'sudden' loss of control: see p.632. *R v Ahluwalia* [1992] 4 AllER 889.

R (Ashworth Hospital) v MHRT H had been detained at Ashworth high-security hospital since 1994, having been transferred after seriously assaulting a junior doctor at a medium secure unit. A tribunal discharged him on the ground that he had recovered from schizophrenia, despite opposition from the hospital and the local services, and despite the lack of any after-care arrangements; it considered adjourning but said that it did not believe Ashworth Hospital would make the necessary arrangements. The RMO redetained him, and the hospital applied for judicial review of the tribunal's decision. The decision was ruled unlawful because it was *Wednesbury* unreasonable not to adjourn and because the tribunal had not given adequate reasons for its decision. The redetention was also held to be unlawful: the hospital should instead have applied to the High Court for a stay of the tribunal's decision. See p.375. *R (Ashworth Hospital) v Mental Health Review Tribunal; R (on the application of H) v Ashworth Hospital Authority and others* [2002] EWCA Civ 923.

Austin Austin and thousands of others were kept by police ('kettled') for several hours in one group of streets following a demonstration. He argued that this was an unlawful detention; the House of Lords ruled that, even though article 5 did not include 'public safety or the protection of public order' amongst the legitimate purposes of detention, because the police had reasonable grounds to believe that a breach of the peace was imminent, their actions represented a reasonable balance between the article 2 right to life of potential victims of 'mob violence', and the right to liberty of the protestors. Brief detentions for crowd control purposes are not deprivations of liberty provided they are not arbitrary, are resorted to in good faith, and are proportionate and enforced for no longer than necessary. See p.424. *Austin v Commissioner of Police of the Metropolis* [2009] AC 564.

Miss B was tetraplegic and could only live on a mechanical ventilator. She regarded her quality of life as unacceptably low, and requested that the ventilator be disconnected. Her doctors would not agree, but she applied to the <u>High Court</u> (p.372), which ruled that she had the right to refuse ventilation, even though she would die as a result. See p.336. *Re B (Adult: Refusal of treatment)* [2002] 2 FCR 1.

Bailey v MoD Miss Bailey was treated for gallstones at an MoD hospital; she bled during the ERCP procedure and received inadequate after-care, but also contracted pancreatitis (a recognised nonnegligent complication of ERCPs). She was transferred to a nearby NHS hospital, where after ten days of successful intensive care, she drank lemonade, vomited and (being too weak to cough adequately) aspirated her vomit, then suffered a cardiac arrest and hypoxic brain damage. In her subsequent claim for clinical negligence, the court could not establish whether it was more likely than not that the weakness would have occurred 'but for' the MoD hospital's poor care (because the pancreatitis could also have caused such weakness). The court ruled that the MoD was still liable because the MoD's breach of duty 'materially contributed' to the weakness. See p.551. *Bailey v Ministry of Defence* [2008] EWCA Civ 883.

Bawa-Garba v GMC Dr Bawa-Garba was a higher trainee in paediatrics. She had just returned from maternity leave to a job covering a children's assessment unit. She was responsible for the care of a young boy whose streptococcal pneumonia and sepsis the unit failed to diagnose; he died within a day. She was convicted of <u>gross negligence manslaughter</u> (p.414), but an investigation demonstrated that her own failings were compounded by the lack of support from her superiors and the system within which she had worked. The MPTS found her fitness to practise only temporarily impaired, and suspended her for a year; the GMC appealed to the High Court, which agreed she should have been erased from the register because of the criminal conviction and because the jury's findings precluded it taking into account the systemic failures. The Court of Appeal overturned this, ruling that there should have been no presumption of any particular professional sanction following the conviction, and that a criminal jury's findings did not constrain the evidence that could be considered by the MPTS; it reinstated the suspension. See p.704. *Bawa-Garba v GMC* [2018] EWCA Civ 1879.

R v Bentley Derek Bentley was a nineteen year old who had twice suffered serious head injuries and had low IQ. He and a sixteen year old, Christopher Craig, were caught by the police after breaking into a warehouse. Bentley allegedly shouted, 'Let him have it, Chris', after which Craig shot a police officer, wounding him. Bentley was arrested, and shortly afterwards another officer was shot and killed (by Craig, it was alleged). Craig was convicted of <u>murder</u> (p.414), but as a child, received an <u>indeterminate</u>

sentence (p.448) and was released ten years later. Bentley was also convicted on the basis of joint enterprise (p.408), the key evidence being his alleged shout, which implied that he knew Craig had a gun. As an adult, he was sentenced to death. The case generated great public unease, and Bentley received a posthumous pardon in 1993, with his conviction formally being quashed several years later. See p.408. *R v Bentley* (1952, unreported); *R v Bentley (Deceased)* [2001] 1 CrAppR 307.

Black v Forsey Dr Forsey was a Scottish junior doctor who detained Mr Black using a second assessment section (p.474) on the instructions of her consultant, despite this being illegal under Scottish mental health law at the time. The hospital claimed that, although the purported section was unlawful, it had a common law power to detain Mr Black, nevertheless. The court confirmed the existence of a common law power to detain 'a person of unsound mind who is a danger to himself or others', 'in a situation of necessity', but held that this could only apply to a private individual, not to a hospital or other authority that can detain patients under mental health law. See p.542. *Black v Forsey* [1988] SC (HL) 28.

R v Blackman Sergeant Blackman deliberately killed an Afghan insurgent, with his clear intention and motive for doing so captured on a head camera. His conviction for murder by a Court-Martial was substituted in the Court of Appeal with diminished responsibility manslaughter, on the unanimous evidence of doctors that he had suffered from an 'adjustment disorder'. This was despite there being no pathognomic diagnostic criteria (p.627) for the condition, or any reliable way other than via clinical judgment, of distinguishing 'abnormal' from 'normal' reactions to stress. See p.669. *R v Blackman* [2017] EWCA Crim 190.

Bolam Mr Bolam was a patient at a mental hospital. He agreed to undergo ECT (p.198), at a time when the risk of mortality with muscle relaxants was widely believed to outweigh the benefits, and the use of restraints was thought to increase the risk of injury. He suffered a fractured acetabulum and sued, claiming negligence. The claim was dismissed, on the grounds that the doctors at the hospital had followed a practice accepted as proper by a responsible body of medical opinion. See p.550. *Bolam v Friern Hospital Management Committee* [1957] 1 WLR 583.

Bolitho A two-year-old child suffered three bouts of respiratory difficulty, during the third of which he had a cardiac arrest and sustained brain damage. The parents claimed negligence because no doctor had attended, and the child had not been prophylactically intubated after the earlier respiratory difficulty. The claim was dismissed, and this was upheld on appeal by the House of Lords, as a responsible body of paediatric opinion held that such intubation would have been inappropriate. However, the House of Lords ruled that if the body of opinion 'was incapable of withstanding logical analysis', it would not be a defence to negligence. See p.550. *Bolitho v Hackney Health Authority* [1998] AC 232.

Bournewood In this case, a forty-eight-year-old man with severe autism who frequently harmed himself was admitted informally to hospital after becoming very agitated at a day centre. He lacked the relevant capacity, but did not express a refusal of treatment. The RMO (p.468) indicated that she would detain him if he tried to leave, for his own safety. His carers sued on his behalf, claiming false imprisonment (p.436). The House of

Lords found that he was lawfully detained, but suggested that Parliament review such situations. The case was then taken to the European Court of Human Rights, where it was known as *HL v UK* (see below). See p.334. *R v Bournewood Community & Mental Health NHS Trust, ex parte L* [1999] 1 AC 458.

R v Bowen Bowen was convicted of fraud offences, despite claiming that he had acted under threats that his family would be petrol-bombed if he did not commit the offences. He appealed on the ground that, although a reasonable person would not have experienced <u>duress</u> (p.634), his low IQ and suggestibility should have been taken into account. The appeal was dismissed because a medical diagnosis was necessary in order to underpin 'lack of reasonable fortitude'. See p.634. *R v Bowen* [1996] 2 CrAppR 157.

R v Brady Brady was a patient at Ashworth Hospital with a severe personality disorder. He sought to have part of his tribunal heard in public, apparently in order to publicise his case against detention (while keeping medical evidence confidential). The hospital applied for judicial review of the tribunal's preliminary decision to allow a partially public hearing. In a judgment that overturned this decision, the High Court accepted in principle the argument that Brady might lack <u>capacity</u> (p.522) to request a public hearing, on the ground that his desire to manipulate others distorted his process of weighing information in the balance. See p.522. *R (Mersey Care NHS Trust) v MHRT (Brady and another, interested parties)* [2005] 2 AllER 820.

Brady v Ashworth Brady (as in the case above) wished to be allowed to starve himself to death. Despite the fact that he retained the relevant mental capacity, the High Court ruled that it was lawful for the hospital to force feed him, as this was 'reasonably administered as part of the medical treatment given for the mental disorder from which [he] was suffering' and not a treatment that required a second opinion or consent under part IV of the Mental Health Act. See p.482. *R (Brady) v Ashworth Hospital Authority* [2000] Lloyds Med R 355.

Bratty v A-GNI Bratty was convicted of strangling an eighteen-year-old woman. He had psychomotor epilepsy, and had claimed (amongst other defences) that he had suffered an automatism. The House of Lords held that there were two types of automatism, insane and noninsane, that an insane automatism could only be caused by a disease of the mind, and that 'any mental disorder which has manifested itself in violence and is prone to recur is a disease of the mind'. See p.612. *Bratty v Attorney-General for Northern Ireland* [1963] 1 AC 386.

R v Brennan The long-established principle that juries and not experts should determine the outcome of criminal cases was held to be modified by the requirement that juries must decide cases rationally on uncontested expert evidence. Hence, in a murder trial where there was uncontested medical evidence supporting the partial defence of diminished responsibility, the judge could correctly withdraw the charge of murder from consideration by the jury. See p.624. *R v Brennan* [2014] EWCA Crim 2387.

R v Brown This case concerned the prosecution of sixteen men for various assaults and related offences, based on acts of consensual sado-masochistic violence (e.g. cutting a penis with a scalpel, having nailed it to a board through a foreskin piercing). The House of Lords ruled three to two that consent was immaterial when the violence was 'inflicted for the indulgence of cruelty', explicitly noting that it was prioritising the views of a majority in society over individual freedoms. The ECtHR unanimously found that the judgment did not breach the individuals' right to private life, on the ground that States could balance public health and wellbeing against control over individual citizens' lives. See p.48. *R v Brown* [1993] 2 All ER 75; *Laskey, Jaggard & Brown v UK* [1997] ECHR 4.

R v Bunch The defendant killed the victim in front of her husband after her relationship with Bunch had ended. Bunch claimed that he was a heavy drinker and had no recollection of the killing and therefore was entitled to a defence of diminished responsibility. A consultant psychiatrist opined that he was not physically dependant on alcohol, had not been suffering from a mental disorder at the time of the killing and there was no abnormality of his mental functioning. The judge refused to leave the partial defence of diminished responsibility to the jury. The Court of Appeal upheld the conviction, stating that medical evidence for all aspects of the defence is required for it to succeed. See p.624. *R v Bunch* [2013] EWCA Crim 2498.

R v Burgess The defendant caused GBH whilst sleepwalking. The High Court ruled on appeal that the sleepwalking, albeit transient, was still a disease of the mind (and therefore an insane automatism) because it was 'due to an internal factor ... had manifested itself in violence and might recur'. See p.612. *R v Burgess* [1991] 2 QB 93.

R v Byrne Byrne strangled a young woman and mutilated her corpse. There was evidence that from an early age he had been subject to perverse violent desires and that the impulse or urge associated with these desires was stronger than normal. The Court of Appeal ruled that the term *abnormality of mind* in relation to diminished responsibility should be taken to mean 'the mind's activities in all its aspects, not only the perception of physical acts and matters; and also the ability to form a rational judgment whether an act is right or wrong and to exercise will-power to control physical acts in accordance with that rational judgment'. See p.624. *R v Byrne* [1960] 2 QB 396.

Re C concerned a patient with schizophrenia detained long term in a high secure hospital. He had gangrene in his leg and was advised to have an amputation, but refused. The Court ruled that he retained his capacity to refuse surgical treatment even though his delusions included the belief that he was an expert in surgery because his decision was not directly based upon his delusions. (In the event he recovered without surgery.) The ruling established the common law definition of mental capacity which still apply in NI, and which was effectively adopted in the Mental Capacity Act 2005. See p.336. *Re C (Adult: Refusal of Treatment)* [1994] 2 FCR 151.

Caldwell set fire to a hotel where he had been employed, because of a grudge against the proprietor; he was so drunk that he did not consider the risk that anyone's life might be endangered. The House of Lords upheld his conviction on the ground that a reasonable person would have considered the risk, undermining the subjective nature of recklessness. It was overturned twenty-two years later by *R v G*, below. See p.404. *Metropolitan Police Commissioner v Caldwell* [1982] AC 341.

DPP v Camplin The defendant, at the age of fifteen, killed a man by hitting him on the head with a heavy pan. He claimed that the victim had forcibly raped him and then taunted him (i.e. that he had been provoked). The jury was instructed to decide whether the reasonable person (i.e. an adult) would have done so, not a 'reasonable boy', and convicted him. The House of Lords ruled that the trial judge had misdirected the jury, and that they should have been allowed to take his age into account (whilst still retaining an 'objective' test). See p.631. *DPP v Camplin* [1978] UKHL 2.

Caparo v Dickman Caparo bought a struggling company, Fidelity, intending to make a profit. However, when it gained control, it realised Fidelity was in a far poorer condition that its accounts had revealed, meaning Caparo would make a loss. Caparo sued for negligence in the production of the accounts. The House of Lords ruled that Caparo was not owed a duty of care by the accountant Dickman, who prepared Fidelity's accounts. It laid down the 'threefold test' of a duty of care in negligence cases. See p.549. *Caparo Industries PLC v Dickman* [1990] 2 AC 605.

R v Chan Wing-Siu Chan was found guilty of murder after his co-defendant used a knife (that Mr Chan knew he was carrying) to kill someone in a failed debt collection. Although Chan did not intend this to happen, it was held that foreseeing that it might happen was sufficient to convict him of murder, under the principle of joint enterprise or 'parasitic accessory liability'. This principle was later overturned by *R v Jogee* (see p.408.); *R v Chan Wing-Siu* [1985] AC 168.

Cheshire West This pair of cases involved a man with cerebral palsy (*P v Cheshire West*) and two sisters with learning disability (*P & Q v Surrey*). All lived in homes where they were (or would be) restrained if they tried to leave without an escort. The Court of Appeal had ruled that on balance these were not deprivations of liberty, but the Supreme Court stated that they were, laying down the 'acid test' of being under complete supervision and control and not free to leave. Adding that it was irrelevant that the person might not object, that the setting might seem very normal and family oriented, and the purpose might be entirely benevolent. See p.532. *P v Cheshire West & Chester Council; P & Q v Surrey County Council* [2014] UKSC 19.

R v Clinton Clinton killed his wife because of her sexual infidelity. He was convicted of murder and arson. The jury had only considered the defence of 'diminished responsibility', the judge having ruled that there was insufficient evidence of 'loss of control', because the statute explicitly excluded sexual infidelity as a 'qualifying trigger'. Clinton successfully appealed, because sexual infidelity was not the only potential trigger, and sexual infidelity should be taken into account where it is integral to the facts as a whole. See p.631. *R v Clinton* [2012] EWCA Crim 2.

Clunis Christopher Clunis had schizophrenia, and was often violent when psychotic; his condition responded well to antipsychotics when detained in hospital, but after discharge he invariably defaulted from treatment, and avoided contact with community mental health staff. Eventually he killed a stranger, Jonathan Zito, on a tube station platform because of a persecutory delusion that Mr Zito was about to attack him. He was convicted of manslaughter on the grounds of diminished responsibility (p.624). Following the Ritchie Report (p.782), he sued one of the responsible health authorities over the standard of care he had received. His case was dismissed by the Court of Appeal and the European Court of Human Rights on the ground that he bore primary responsibility for his own criminal acts. See p.553. *R v Clunis* (unreported); *Clunis v UK* [1998] ECHR 116.

R v Coley In this case the Court of Appeal considered three related appeals against conviction: Coley's for attempted murder after stabbing his neighbour whilst intoxicated with cannabis (his defence had been that he had experienced temporary insanity, causing him to confuse reality for a computer game); McPhee's for <u>GBH with intent</u> (p.416) after stabbing a stranger having ingested alcohol and temazepam; and Harris' for <u>arson recklessly endangering life</u> (p.422) during a period of alcohol-induced hallucinosis (in which he claimed he was unaware that others might be endangered). The Court of Appeal upheld all three convictions, holding that insanity and sane automatism are not available in cases of voluntary intoxication. See p.618. *R v Coley & Ors [2013] EWCA Crim 223.*

R v Crozier Crozier attacked his sister with an axe; he pleaded guilty to attempted murder. A psychiatrist instructed by the defence found that he exhibited legally <u>psychopathic disorder</u> (p.90) and recommended detention in <u>high security</u> (p.258). The report was not submitted, and the court passed a sentence of nine-years' imprisonment; the psychiatrist (who had arrived to give evidence) gave the report to the prosecution counsel, who successfully applied to vary the sentence to a <u>hospital order with restrictions</u> (p.510). Crozier appealed, claiming a <u>breach of confidentiality</u> (p.307); this was dismissed, on the ground that the public interest in the disclosure of the report outweighed the patient's right to confidentiality. See p.307. *R v Crozier* [1991] CrimLR 138.

Darnley v Croydon Darnley suffered a head injury and booked in at A&E, where the receptionist told him the wait would be four to five hours; feeling too unwell to sit for that long, he returned home. He later deteriorated and suffered brain damage. Had he been told, correctly, that because of his head injury he would be seen within thirty minutes, he would have remained, and the brain damage would probably not have occurred. The Supreme Court ruled that the hospital's duty of care included taking reasonable care not to provide misleading advice that could reasonably foreseeably lead to him not receiving treatment. The receptionist was not a professional, and therefore *Bolam* was not directly relevant; instead, the standard was that of an averagely competent and well-informed person performing the functions of an A&E receptionist. See p.550. *Darnley v Croydon Health Services NHS Trust* [2018] UKSC 50.

South Africa v Dewani Dewani was charged in South Africa with the murder of his wife on their honeymoon there, by paying others to shoot her, which happened while he was in the car with her. He absconded to the UK, where he was diagnosed with severe PTSD. At his extradition hearing, the court considered whether it would breach his ECHR article 2 and 3 rights to extradite him; extradition being 'unjust and oppressive', given he was unfit to plead, and given his mental condition, and the attendant risk of suicide, whilst taking into account the prison or hospital conditions likely in South Africa. On a second appeal, the court allowed extradition based upon an undertaking from the South African government that he would receive adequate treatment and safeguarding, and that he would be returned to the UK if his unfitness continued beyond a year. (He was eventually released in South Africa after the trial court ruled there was no case to answer.)

See p.649. *Republic of South Africa v Dewani* [2012] EWHC 842; [2014] 1 WLR 3220.

R v Dietschmann Dietschmann killed a man whilst under the influence of alcohol. He believed the victim had insulted his dead aunt. At trial psychiatrists agreed that he was suffering from an 'abnormality of mind' for the purposes of 'diminished responsibility': specifically a delayed grief reaction or adjustment disorder. The trial judge directed the jury to consider whether if he had not consumed alcohol he would still have killed. On appeal it was held that the underlying condition was the relevant issue, not whether he would have killed if not intoxicated. See p.618. *R v Dietschmann* [2003] UKHL 10.

R v Dix Dix shot a friend 'to put her out of her misery'. He later claimed 'diminished responsibility' on the basis of his odd behaviour and claims after the killing. The trial judge and Court of Appeal ruled that the defence required medical evidence, not merely ordinary evidence, no matter how odd the behaviour. See p.625. *R v Dix* [1982] CrimLR 302.

Donoghue v Stevenson Donoghue drank some ginger beer bought for her by her friend. They later realised the bottle contained the decomposing remains of a snail. Donoghue suffered gastroenteritis. She claimed £500 damages from Stevenson, the manufacturer. The House of Lords ruled that Stevenson owed her a duty of care even though she had not purchased the drink: the manufacturer ought to have had the ultimate consumer, not merely the purchaser, in mind. The case laid the foundations of the modern law of <u>negligence</u> (p.548). *Donoghue v Stevenson* [1932] UKHL 100.

Dooley v Cammell Laird The plaintiff was a crane driver whose employer had fitted his crane with a defective rope; the rope snapped, dropping the load into the hold of a ship where the driver's fellow employees were working. Dooley received compensation for the psychiatric illness he suffered because of his fears for their safety, even though in fact they were not injured; the court held he was an 'involuntary participant' in the creation of the dangerous situation. See p.640. *Dooley v Cammell Laird* [1951] 1 Lloyd's Rep 271.

R v Dowds The appellant argued that voluntary acute intoxication (uncomplicated by any alcoholism or dependence) was sufficient for the partial defence of diminished responsibility under the amended Homicide Act in E&W and NI because it is a 'recognised medical condition'. The Court of Appeal held that the wording of the new Act must be interpreted in the light of the substantial body of case law that voluntary intoxication could not form the basis of a defence alone, and therefore that the presence of a recognised medical condition is necessary, but not always sufficient, for diminished responsibility. See p.618. *R v Dowds* [2012] EWCA Crim 281.

DPP v Morgan The defendant invited three younger men to his house for sex with his wife, telling them that she was 'kinky' and would only pretend to resist. In fact she did not consent, and was raped by all four men. They were convicted on the ground that they had no sufficient reason to believe that she consented. The Court of Appeal ruled that the test was subjective, and that a genuine mistaken belief prevented conviction for rape (but also upheld the conviction on the ground that the defendants did not have such genuine beliefs). The law was later changed to overturn this precedent. See pp.404, 412. *DPP v Morgan* [1976] AC 182.

Drury v HM Advocate This controversial case concerned a man who killed his wife with a hammer after discovering her affair. The Court of Criminal Appeal redefined murder as requiring 'wicked intent' or 'wicked recklessness', such that provocation (if the violence was in proportion to it) made the intent no longer wicked. Conversely, a provoked defendant who used excessive violence could still be convicted of murder. This conflicts with other principles of the provocation defence. See p.630. *Drury v HM Advocate* [2001] SCCR 583.

R v Duffy Duffy was the victim of repeated domestic violence by her husband, who had refused to allow her to leave with their child. Seeing no alternative, she later killed him with a hatchet while he slept. The Court of Criminal Appeal upheld the trial judge's direction that provocation (p.630) required a 'sudden and temporary loss of self-control'. This rule was later changed in E&W under the new statutory defence of 'loss of control' (p.630), but it remains the law in RoI. See p.630. *R v Duffy* [1949] 1 AllER 932.

R v Edwards Like the complainants in *Vowles* (below) the four appellants (in different cases) had been sentenced to IPPs, three with hybrid orders; all claimed that they should have received restricted hospital orders instead. The Court of Appeal clarified its guidance to judges in *Vowles*: there is no default sentence of imprisonment, but if the criteria for a hospital order are met, the judge must consider, alongside the psychiatric opinions, the extents to which: the offender needs treatment; the offence was attributable to their mental disorder; punishment is required; and the public needs to be protected (including by the regime for deciding on release and subsequent management). If there is mental disorder, the offence is significantly attributable to it, and treatment is available, it must *first* consider a hybrid order. Only if that is inappropriate (or unavailable because the defendant is younger than twenty-one years old), can it then consider a hospital order. It added that, even if the criteria are met, a sentence of imprisonment followed by transfer might still be appropriate, and very clear evidence is required to make an interim, rather than final, hospital order. See p.504. *R v Edwards and Knapper and Payne and Langley* [2018] EWCA Crim 595.

Edwards v UK Edwards was kicked to death by his cellmate, who was violent and mentally unwell. The cell call button did not work, and the prison had failed to assess the cellmate's mental disorder or risk of harm properly, or to care for Mr Edwards appropriately. The ECtHR ruled that this was a breach of the UK's article 2 duty to protect the life of Edwards whilst in custody. See p.516. *Edwards v UK* [2002] ECHR 46477/99.

W v Egdell W was a patient detained in a high secure hospital after shooting and killing or wounding seven people. He applied to a mental health tribunal, seeking transfer to a medium secure unit. His solicitor commissioned an independent psychiatric report, which strongly opposed transfer and commented on his continued interest in firearms and explosives. W then withdrew his application. The independent psychiatrist, Dr Egdell, was concerned that the treating hospital lacked key information and disclosed his report to the hospital, breaching W's confidentiality. The Court held that Dr Egdell did owe W a duty of confidentiality, but that the breach of it was justified by the public interest in preventing further very serious offending by W since there was a 'significant risk of serious harm' (see p.307). *W v Egdell* [1990] 1 AllER 835.

R v Emery The defendant, a teenage mother, was acquitted of assaulting her eleven-month-old daughter (but convicted of failing to protect her from multiple, ultimately fatal, assaults by the father). The acquittal was partly based on evidence from psychologists that Emery suffered from 'battered woman syndrome' and behaved as she did because of 'learned helplessness'. The Court of Appeal upheld the trial judge's admission of this evidence, even though it was not evidence of a recognised mental disorder, because it was 'complex and not known by the public at large'. See p.656. *R v Emery* [1993] 14 CrAppR(S) 394.

R v Erskine Erskine had been convicted of a series of murders of elderly people in 1988, many of whom he had also sexually assaulted. His behaviour after arrest was bizarre, and it was later accepted that there would have been grounds for a plea of <u>diminished responsibility</u> (p.624), based upon his schizophrenia. However, at the time he did not allow this plea to be put forward because of his beliefs arising from his mental illness. The Court of Appeal rejected the contention that Erskine would have been 'unfit to plead' at the original trial, ruling that a defendant is not unfit 'merely because he will not accept ... eminently sensible advice from his legal advisors'. However, it went on to substitute a verdict of manslaughter on the grounds of diminished responsibility 'in the interests of justice'. See p.603. *R v Erskine* [2009] EWCA Crim 1425.

Evans v Attorney-General This case concerned a campaign by the *Guardian* newspaper to publish letters written by the Prince of Wales to various government departments, expressing his opinions. Evans, a journalist at the newspaper, requested disclosure of the letters under the <u>Freedom of Information Act 2000</u> (p.737); the departments refused, citing exceptions allowed under the Act, and were backed by the Information Commissioner. Evans appealed to the Upper Tribunal (a body equivalent in seniority to the High Court) and won, but the Attorney General then issued an 'executive override' certificate under the Act blocking the implementation of the Tribunal's decision. Evans sought judicial review of the certificate, and the Supreme Court ultimately ruled that, because the relevant provision of the Act broke the constitutional principle that the executive is bound by decisions of the court, it could only be given effect where it was 'crystal clear' that Parliament had intended what was claimed. It went on to find that the wording of the Act did not clearly cover the situation faced by the Attorney General, and therefore that he did not have 'reasonable grounds' for believing, in essence, that the tribunal judgement had been wrong. It ordered the disclosure of the letters. See p.363. *R (Evans) and another v Attorney General* [2015] UKSC 21.

F v West Berkshire F was a thirty-six-year-old woman with severe learning disability who lived permanently in a mental hospital. Her mother was concerned about the risk of her becoming pregnant (she had started a relationship with a male patient) and requested a court declaration that she could lawfully be sterilised. The House of Lords ruled that the operation would be in her best interests and could proceed. Lord Goff also recognised the relevance of any 'advance statement' made by a patient who later lost capacity. See p.537. *F v West Berkshire Health Authority* [1989] 2 AC 1.

NHS v FG FG suffered from schizoaffective disorder and lacked capacity to make decisions relating to her antenatal and postnatal care, her own welfare, or that of her unborn baby, or to litigation involving her. She was at high risk of harming herself and her baby because of her persecutory delusion that staff were trying to murder them both. Exceptionally, while she remained pregnant, the Court of Protection ruled (balancing her best interests with those of her unborn child) that she should not be notified of the proceedings concerning her, and that the media should be barred from reporting the case at that time. The acute and psychiatric hospital trusts proposed to deliver her baby (potentially performing a Caesarean section against her will if necessary), and the social services authority proposed to remove the child at birth. The Court found that the intrusion on her liberty this involved, including the likely need for force in circumstances amounting to a (perhaps brief) deprivation of liberty, was of a degree that could only be authorised by a court, and not under schedule A1 of the MCA (the <u>DoLS</u>, p.532). It made an order authorising the proposed care plan. In the event Ms FG co-operated with the delivery and the baby was born healthy without any deprivation of liberty. The Court issued guidance on when court orders would be necessary in future. *NHS Trust and others v FG* [2014] EWCOP 30.

Freeman v Home Office Freeman was a life sentence prisoner with personality disorder and intermittent depression, who was administered antipsychotic drugs in Wakefield Prison. He later sued, claiming that his apparent consent was not valid because, amongst other reasons, the administering Prison Medical Officer was acting as a disciplinary agent of the prison rather than as a doctor. The Court of Appeal ruled that prisoners were capable of giving or withholding consent, notwithstanding the disciplinary nature of staff. See p.482. *Freeman v Home Office* [1984] 1 AllER 1036.

R v G This case was similar on the facts to *Caldwell* (above). Two young boys, out camping, entered a disused building and set fire to some newspapers, thinking they would extinguish it themselves. The fire spread and damaged nearby shops. The boys were initially convicted because a reasonable person would have recognised the risk of the fire spreading, but the conviction was overturned by the House of Lords on appeal, which returned recklessness to its original subjective definition. See p.404. *R v G and another* [2004] 1 AC 1034.

Galbraith v HM Advocate Galbraith killed her husband and was convicted of murder. She appealed her conviction on the grounds that she was abused for many years by the deceased and was suffering from a form of PTSD. The court ruled that the test in *HM Advocate v Savage* (below) should not be interpreted narrowly: diminished responsibility required some form of 'abnormality of mind' sufficient to have a substantial effect on a person's mind and in relation to his act, but it was not necessary to prove that the accused's mental state bordered on insanity. See p.624. *Galbraith v HM Advocate* (2002) JC 1.

Gillick A mother sought a declaration that a Department of Health guideline allowing doctors to prescribe contraception to under sixteen year olds was unlawful. The House of Lords ruled that it was lawful, and that a child younger than sixteen could consent to treatment in her own right if she has 'sufficient understanding and intelligence to understand fully what is proposed'. See p.530. *Gillick v West Norfolk and Wisbech Area Health Authority* [1985] 3 All ER 402.

Gillon v HM Advocate Gillon did not dispute that he had killed the victim by repeatedly hitting him on the head with a spade, but claimed that the victim had provoked him by first attacking him with the spade. The Appeal Court reaffirmed the rule in *Robertson v HM Advocate* (below) that the violence must be proportionate to the provocation, and rejected an alternative rule based on what an ordinary person might do. See p.630. *Gillon v HM Advocate* [2007] SC(JC) 24.

R v Golds The Supreme Court stated that, in E&W and NI, the new 2009 law on diminished responsibility (see p.624) had swept away the rule from *R v Lloyd* that 'substantial' within the defence meant 'less than total, more than trivial'. The word is to be understood in the ordinary sense, and no direction to the jury is required, unless counsel have introduced some meaning of their own, in which case the judge should direct the jury that *substantial* means 'not just more than trivial', but a 'weighty' impairment. *R v Golds* [2016] UKSC 61.

R v Gotts Gotts was charged with attempted murder. He claimed duress, having been ordered by his father to kill his mother. The trial judge ruled that duress was not available as a defence to attempted murder. The trial judge's direction was upheld on appeal. See p.634. *R v Gotts* [1992] 2 WLR 878.

R v Hardie Hardie lived with a woman at her flat. Their relationship broke down and she asked him to leave. As a result of being upset he took a quantity of diazepam, making him voluntarily intoxicated (p.616), in which state he started a fire in the flat. The judge at his trial for arson directed that the self-administration of the drug was irrelevant, but this was overturned on appeal. The jury should have been directed to consider whether taking the drug did negate *mens rea*, and if it did, whether taking it was reckless (p.403). See p.616. *R v Hardie* [1985] 3 AllER 848.

R v Hasan Hasan was convicted of an aggravated burglary. He had claimed that he had acted under duress (p.634), having been threatened by another person (who had boasted of murdering others) that if he did not commit the burglary he and his family would be harmed. The House of Lords upheld the conviction and set down the requirements of the defence of duress by threats. See p.634. *R v Hasan* [2005] UKHL 22.

R v Hennessy Hennessy had diabetes, and not having taken insulin for several days, experienced a hyperglycaemic episode in which he took, and drove off in a car. He claimed having been in an automatism; the trial judge ruled that as it was due to an intrinsic cause, the disease of diabetes, the only available defence was insanity. The Court of Appeal ruled that the trial judge was correct, and moreover that stress, anxiety, and depression, while perhaps 'external', lacked the 'feature of novelty or accident' required of causes of noninsane automatism. See p.612. *R v Hennessy* [1989] EWCA Crim 1.

Hirst Hirst, who was serving a sentence of imprisonment for manslaughter, challenged the law that prevented him from voting in elections. The court held that the law contravened article 3 of the first protocol to the ECHR (see p.518), which requires the 'free expression of the opinion of the people', a right extended to 'everyone within [the] jurisdiction' by article 1. After twelve years of refusal, the UK agreed to amend the law to allow some but not all prisoners to vote, which was accepted as complying with the ruling. See p.541. *Hirst v UK (No.2)* [2009] ECHR 2260.

HL v UK This was the continuation of the *Bournewood* case (above) at the European Court of Human Rights (p.390). The court found, contrary to the decision of the House of Lords in the UK, that the lack of procedural safeguards in detaining HL, and the lack of access to a tribunal, made his detention unlawful. It stated that the three minimum conditions for lawful detention of a person of 'unsound mind' were that the mental disorder must be reliably diagnosed, of a kind or degree warranting detention, and persistently present; and it must be under clearly defined ('precise') law incorporating 'adequate legal protections and ... fair and proper procedures'. The government responded by inserting the DoLS into the Mental Capacity Act 2005. See p.532. *HL v UK* [2004] 40 EHRR 761.

Holley Holley killed his alcoholic girlfriend with an axe whilst himself drunk. He claimed provocation, stating that she had taunted him about having an affair and about his alcoholism. There was disagreement at his various trials about whether he was voluntarily intoxicated (p.616), including concerning whether he suffered from personality disorder that made it difficult for him to control his drinking, as well as making him sensitive to being taunted about his alcoholism. The Privy Council (p.391) reversed the decision of the House of Lords in *Morgan Smith* (below), and stated that the law required the reasonable person test to be a purely objective test in regard to any violent reaction, meaning that none of the special characteristics of the defendant could be taken into account in that regard. However, his sensitivity to being taunted by the victim as 'an alcoholic' was relevant to the defence. The Coroners and Justice Act 2009 similarly allows 'circumstances' to be relevant to a defendant's 'sensitivity' but still not to his propensity for violence. *Attorney General for Jersey v Holley* [2005] 3 WLR 29See p.631.

Home Office v Dorset Yacht Co A group of detainees at a Borstal (a type of youth detention centre) were working in a harbour under the direction of prison officers. They absconded with a yacht which they crashed into another boat, damaging it. The owners of the second yacht sued for damages. The court upheld their claim, stating that the prison officers had failed to exercise proper control over the detainees and that the detainees' behaviour, and the consequent damage, was of a kind that was reasonably foreseeable if they were not properly controlled. See p.552. *Home Office v Dorset Yacht Co* [1974] 2 AllER 294.

R v Jason Cann The defendant had paranoid schizophrenia and was detained in hospital. He killed a nurse whom he believed, because of delusions, intended to rape him. Appealing against conviction for manslaughter on the grounds of diminished responsibility (p.624), he claimed that he should have been allowed to plead self-defence (p.410). The Court of Appeal rejected this, ruling that the test of reasonable force was entirely objective, and his delusions were irrelevant. See p.410. *R v Jason Cann* [2005] EWCA 2264.

R v Jogee Jogee was convicted of murder for shouting generally encouraging words from outside a property to a co-defendant who killed a person inside. Jogee did not intend this outcome despite its foreseeability. In a separate case, also from Jamaica, Ruddock was convicted of murder after his accomplice slit the throat of a man during a failed robbery. They both appealed, ultimately to the UK Supreme Court, which ruled unanimously that foresight of their co-defendant's actions was not sufficient: also required was proof of intent to assist or encourage the co-defendant to act with the intent relevant to the crime, along with any knowledge necessary to make the co-defendant's acts criminal. See p.408. *R v Jogee* [2016] UKSC 8.

R v Joyce A man with paranoid schizophrenia and a habitual drug user became intoxicated whilst in a psychotic episode and stabbed someone to death; he was convicted of murder. The Court of Appeal ruled that someone with schizophrenia may plead diminished responsibility where voluntary intoxication triggers the psychotic state, provided the 'abnormality of mental functioning' (the psychosis) arose from a 'recognised medical condition' (schizophrenia), which then substantially impaired his responsibility, even if the medical condition would not have substantially impaired responsibility in the absence of drug or alcohol *dependence*. However, if there would have been no substantial impairment of responsibility without the voluntary intoxication, the defence will fail. See p.618. *R v Joyce* [2017] EWCA Crim 647.

K v Home Office The Home Office had issued a deportation order against Mr M, a Kenyan convicted of a sexual offence and burglary; however, it was not carried out, and he went on to rape Ms K. She sued the Home Office for the harm she had suffered from the rape, but her claim was dismissed on the ground that there was no proximity (p.549) between her (an, at the time, unidentified member of the public) and the Home Office. See p.553. *K v Secretary of State for the Home Department* [2002] EWCA Civ 775.

R v Kemp Kemp, who had assaulted his wife, suffered from arteriosclerosis. Transient cerebral ischaemia had caused a temporary 'lapse of consciousness' during which he attacked his wife. It was held that this amounted to an 'insane automatism', despite the temporary nature of the 'lapse', because arteriosclerosis was a disease affecting the mind. It does not matter whether the disease concerned has a physical or mental origin. See p.612. *R v Kemp* [1957] 1 QB 399].

Kennedy v Cordia A seminal case defining expertise not by status (e.g. being on a particular GMC Specialist Register) but by 'study or experience'. See p.654. *Kennedy v Cordia (Services) LLP* [2016] UKSC 6.

R v Khan Khan bludgeoned his roommate to death with a cricket bat. He claimed diminished responsibility, with psychiatric evidence in support, but was convicted of murder. He appealed, claiming that the judge should have directed the jury that they should accept the plea of diminished responsibility based upon the expert evidence presented. The Court of Appeal upheld the conviction, ruling that the issue was for the jury to decide. See p.624. *R v Khan* [2009] EWCA 1569.

R v Kimber The defendant was charged with indecent assault of a female patient in a mental hospital. He claimed that she had known what he was doing and had consented. The trial judge told the jury that the sole issue was whether the victim had truly consented or not. The Court of Appeal held that the judge had erred, and that a mistaken belief that consent had been given would lead to acquittal. (However, it upheld the conviction on the ground that the defendant lacked any such mistaken belief.) See p.412. *R v Kimber* [1983] 1 WLR 1118.

R v Kingston Kingston was charged with <u>indecently assaulting</u> (p.419) a fifteen-year-old boy. He contended that he had been drugged by a co-defendant (with triazolam, a benzodiazepine) and that he would not have acted as he had done if he had not been drugged. The jury were directed that if he was found to have had <u>intent</u> (p.402) then the fact he was drugged was not relevant; that acquittal would require that the <u>involuntary intoxication</u> (p.614) had made him <u>incapable of forming intent</u> (p.610). The jury found that the photographs and audiotapes of Kingston's behaviour in assaulting the boy demonstrated that he must have intended assault at the time, notwithstanding his intoxication. This was upheld at appeal. See p.614. *R v Kingston* [1994] 3 WLR 519).

Kumar v GMC Dr Kumar, a consultant psychiatrist, appealed against the decision of a Fitness to Practise Panel of the GMC to suspend him from the register. The Panel found that his fitness to practice was impaired by virtue of misconduct relating to evidence he gave as an expert witness for the defence in a murder trial in 2009, and suspended him in relation to all clinical practice. Emphasising that 'there is expertise in being an expert witness' and that a doctor may be disciplined solely in respect of poor expert witness practice, the court upheld the ruling 'to reaffirm to the public and practitioners the standards of conduct expected from them'. See p.655. *Kumar v General Medical Council* [2012] EWHC 2688 (Admin).

Laporte This case concerned protestors demonstrating against the Iraq War, who were arrested for breach of the peace. The House of Lords made it clear that not only police officers, but all citizens could arrest people to prevent a breach of the peace (i.e. the use or threat of violence). See p.543. *R (on the application of Laporte) v Chief Constable of Gloucestershire* [2006] UKHL 55.

Lewisham v Malcolm Malcolm had sublet his council flat, in breach of his tenancy agreement. He had schizophrenia (although the council did not know this) and had not been taking his medication. Lewisham sought an order for possession (i.e. to evict him), and was granted one; Malcolm appealed. The House of Lords eventually dismissed his appeal, stating that because the council had treated him in exactly the same way as it would have treated anyone else, there was no discrimination. This precedent was overturned by the Equality Act 2010, which provided for cases in which a consequence of a disability made it more difficult for someone to comply with a requirement. See p.556. *Lewisham London Borough Council v Malcolm* [2008] UKHL 43.

R v Lindo This case followed *R v Dowds* (which related to alcohol intoxication). The Court of Appeal confirmed that a psychotic state induced by voluntary drug intoxication, while it might be a medical condition recognised by doctors, did not *legally* amount to a 'recognised medical condition' for s52 Coroners and Justice Act 2009. See p.618. *R v Lindo* [2016] EWCA Crim 1940.

R v Lloyd Lloyd strangled his wife to death. On trial for murder, there was psychiatric evidence that he suffered from an 'abnormality of mind' due to depression, but none of the psychiatrists thought that this would have 'significantly' affected his mental responsibility for the killing. The trial judge ruled that 'substantial' meant 'less than total, but more than trivial or minimal', and the jury convicted him of murder. The trial judge's direction was approved by the Court of Appeal. See p.625. *R v Lloyd* [1967] 1 QB 175. But see now *R v Golds* (above).

R v Loake Loake was convicted of harassment after sending her estranged husband many unwanted text messages, her defence of insanity having failed. It was not clear to the Court whether this defence was available for harassment and the matter was referred to the Court of Appeal. They did not overturn Loake's conviction but did clarify that an insanity defence could be offered for any crime in both the Magistrate's and the Crown court. See p.620. *Loake v CPS* [2017] EWHC 2855.

In re M & R A local authority applied to take four children into care, alleging their mother had sexually abused them. The judge in the family court accepted that there was 'a real possibility' that the abuse had occurred, but that it had not been <u>proved</u> (p.381) to the requisite standard under the Children Act 1989 (that the judge was 'satisfied' the abuse had occurred), and refused a full care order (but made interim care orders on the grounds that there was 'reasonable cause to believe' the abuse had occurred). Although the Court of Appeal dismissed the local authority's appeal, it ruled that the judge could admit evidence from child psychiatrists as to the reliability of the child witnesses. See p.657. *In re M and R (Child abuse: evidence)* [1996] 2 FLR 195.

R v M (John) The defendant had been convicted on several counts of sexually abusing his granddaughter, and appealed on the ground that the jury would have found him unfit to plead because of anterograde amnesia, if the trial judge had not 'set the bar too low' in the way he described the *Pritchard* test of fitness to plead. The Court of Appeal dismissed the appeal, and restated the test in clear language. See p.602. *R v M (John)* [2003] EWCA Crim 3452.

DPP v Majewski Majewski had used large quantities of alcohol and drugs over forty-eight hours, and then assaulted several people, including police officers. His convictions for assault were upheld by the House of Lords, despite the lack of evidence of specific intent to assault, or recklessness as to the risk of assaulting others. The House of Lords confirmed that <u>voluntary intoxication</u> (p.616) is no defence for offences of <u>basic intent</u> (p.403), although it may be for offences of <u>specific intent</u> (p.403). The rule that a person may be deemed to intend or foresee the 'natural and probable consequences' of their acts enabled the trial jury to conclude that the defendant would have foreseen that he might commit assault while drunk, and was therefore <u>reckless</u> (p.403). See p.616. *DPP v Majewski* [1977] AC 443.

R v Martin Martin was disqualified from driving. His wife's son was late for work; she threatened suicide if he did not drive him to work. He was caught and convicted of driving while disqualified. He appealed on the ground of necessity, supported by medical evidence that she was likely to have attempted suicide if he refused to drive. His conviction was quashed on the ground that the jury should have been allowed to consider whether the facts supported <u>duress of circumstances</u> (p.634); in the judgment, the House of Lords set out the requirements of the defence. See p.634. *R v Martin* [1989] 1 AllER 652.

R v Martin (Anthony) The defendant had been convicted of murder for shooting a burglar who broke into his isolated farmhouse at night; his claim of self-defence having been rejected. He had paranoid personality disorder and depression, and appealed on the ground that his symptoms made him perceive more threat from the burglar than a reasonable person would, and that the force used was therefore reasonable. The court held that this was not relevant to the objective test of whether a reasonable person would have used that degree of force in what the defendant believed to be the circumstances. Instead, he was convicted of manslaughter on the grounds of <u>diminished responsibility</u> (p.624). See p.411. *R v Martin (Anthony)* [2002] 1 CrAppR 27.

R v Marcantonio Marcantonio was convicted of burglary. He appealed on the basis of psychiatric evidence that, although he recalled committing the burglary (and had pleaded guilty), his cognitive impairment was such that he could not follow the court proceedings. Although the expert evidence was not accepted at the Court of Appeal, their judgment made plain that fitness to plead cannot be separated into different components. If the defendant is later found unfit to stand trial, then the entire matter must be treated as if he had not been fit to enter a plea at the outset of the trial. The Court of Appeal also held that the test of fitness is determined by the court itself, not the expert witnesses, and that it is proper for the court to give its own judgment even if this is contrary to the unanimous opinion of psychiatrists. See p.602. *R v Marcantonio* [2016] EWCA Crim 14.

MM and PJ These cases involved two patients who were subject to conditions of living in the community that amounted to a deprivation of liberty; in MM's case after <u>conditional discharge</u> (p.511), in PJ's under a <u>Community Treatment Order</u> (p.488). The conditions required residence at a place they would not usually be allowed to leave without an escort; both patients had capacity and consented to the arrangements. The Supreme Court ruled that such conditions would breach the patient's rights to liberty under article 5 of the <u>ECHR</u> (p.518) and that the tribunal and the RC had no power to make orders with such conditions. See p.511. *Secretary of State for Justice v MM* [2018] UKSC 60; *Welsh Ministers v PJ* [2018] UKSC 66.

R v Mohan Dr Mohan, a paediatrician, was charged with sexually assaulting four teenage patients. In a <u>voir dire</u> (p.383), psychiatric '<u>profiling</u>' (p.576) evidence that the assaults were probably committed by someone with characteristics Dr Mohan lacked (e.g. psychopathy) was ruled inadmissible because it was not sufficiently relevant; addressed the <u>ultimate issue</u> (p.664); and was unreliable, given the poor evidence base for such profiling. See p.657. *R v Mohan* [1994] 2 SCR 9.

Montgomery v Lanarkshire Mrs Montgomery was pregnant, and knew that she was at particularly high risk of having a large baby who would not easily be delivered vaginally. Her obstetrician advised against a Caesarean section, but did not mention the risk of the baby suffering limb paralysis due to shoulder dystocia with vaginal delivery, because that was not her routine practice (a practice with which a responsible body of medical opinion agreed). The Supreme Court ruled that this was insufficient: the test was whether, in the circumstances, a reasonable person in the patient's position would be likely to attach significance to the risk, or the doctor was (or should reasonably have been) aware that the particular patient would do so. See p.702. *Montgomery v Lanarkshire Health Board* [2015] SC 11.

R v Morgan Smith The defendant fatally stabbed a man whom he believed had stolen his carpentry tools. He claimed provocation (p.630), based upon a diagnosis of depression. The trial judge, in directing the jury, limited the scope for them to take his depression into account in determining what the reasonable person would have done. The House of Lords allowed an appeal, ruling that the reasonable person should have been deemed to have depression, like the defendant. This case was the high-water mark of the subjective form of the reasonable person test. See p.630. *R v Smith* (Morgan) [2001] 1 AC 146.

Moss v Howdle Moss was driving on the motorway when his passenger suddenly cried out and was clearly in severe pain. Moss broke the speed limit in order to get to the nearest service station quickly, where he could assist his passenger. He appealed against conviction for breach of the speed limit, claiming that the circumstances amounted to necessity (p.634). The High Court of Justiciary set down the rules for the defence, and concluded that it did not apply because Moss could have stopped at the side of the motorway rather than breaking the speed limit to get to a service station. See p.634. *Moss v Howdle* [1997] SCCR 215.

Munjaz Munjaz was a patient at Ashworth high secure hospital (p.258) who had been repeatedly secluded for long periods. The hospital's seclusion policy was found to be unlawful because it provided for substantially fewer reviews than the MHA Code of Practice; a revised policy with more reviews, but still fewer than in the Code, was upheld on appeal to the House of Lords. At an earlier stage of the case, the Court of Appeal had ruled that, separate from the MHA, there is a general common law power to take 'reasonably necessary' and 'proportionate' steps to prevent significant harm, even from people retaining capacity; that this included a power to seclude patients (insofar as it applied to actions by public authorities and their staff, this was overturned by *Sessay*). See p.542. *Munjaz v. Ashworth* [2005] UKHL 58; *Munjaz v Mersey Care NHS Trust* [2003] EWCA Civ 1036.

R v O'Brien O'Brien and his co-defendants robbed and seriously assaulted a man, who died five days later. All three were convicted of murder, largely on the evidence of their co-defendant Hall, and sentenced to custody for life (p.448), as they were under twenty-one years old. Some years later, the Criminal Cases Review Commission (p.567) referred the case to the Court of Appeal on the ground that Hall had a high level of compliance (p.160)—but no diagnosed mental disorder—that predisposed him to lie and fantasise, casting doubt on the convictions. The court ruled that such expert evidence could be admitted even in the absence of a diagnosis, because it showed 'a very significant deviation from the norm'. See p.657. *R v O'Brien, Hall & Sherwood* [2000] EWCA Crim 3.

R v Orr Orr was convicted of being concerned in a money laundering arrangement. He became unwell in the course of the trial and lost his ability to participate. The trial judge decided that, although he became unfit to be cross-examined, he had been fit to give evidence-in-chief. He directed the jury accordingly. When Orr appealed to the Court of Appeal it was held that, although this had not disadvantaged Orr, the way fitness was dealt with was incorrect. Fitness to plead cannot be determined by reference to only part of the trial process. See p.602. *R v Orr [2016] EWCA Crim 889*.

Osman v UK Osman was shot and killed by his son's former teacher. The teacher had made threats and vandalised the son's family home; this having been reported to the police, who tried to arrest him but could not find him. The son and widow's claim that the police had been negligent was dismissed. The ECtHR affirmed that the State (and therefore the police) did have a positive duty to protect Osman's life, but found that the police had taken reasonable steps and had not breached that duty. The UK was required to provide an effective remedy for negligence that did breach this duty, and a blanket ban on negligence cases against the police breached article 6. See p.516. *Osman v UK [1998] ECHR 23452/94*.

R v Oye Where a defendant suffering from an insane delusion that he was being attacked or threatened reacted violently, using force that was reasonable in the circumstances as he perceived them to be, he was not entitled to an acquittal based on self-defence. An insane person could not set the standards of reasonableness as to the degree of force used by reference to his own insanity. See p.411. *R v Oye [2013] EWCA Crim 1725*.

Page v Smith Page was involved in a moderately severe car accident caused by Smith's negligent driving. Nobody was physically injured, but Page later suffered a recurrence of <u>chronic fatigue syndrome</u> (p.101). The House of Lords held that Page was a primary victim, and that Smith owed a duty of care to avoid causing injury, including psychiatric illness, since it was reasonably foreseeable that he might suffer some form of injury (in this case physical injury): there was no need for the specific harm caused to be foreseeable. See p.640. *Page v Smith [1996] AC 155*.

Palmer v Tees Palmer's three-year-old daughter had been abducted, raped, and murdered by a man. He had been in psychiatric hospitals on various occasions after suicide attempts, and had allegedly disclosed fantasies about sexually abusing and killing young children. Palmer sued the health authority for the trauma she had suffered, but the claim was dismissed because there was insufficient <u>proximity</u> (p.552) between her and the hospital. The judges noted that, even if the man's actions had been found to be reasonably foreseeable, there was no treatment the hospital could have given that would have protected the claimant's daughter, nor was she identifiable in advance as someone who could have been warned. See p.553. *Palmer (administratrix of the estate of Palmer) v Tees Health Authority [1999] AllER 722*.

PBU v Tribunal PBU and NJE were both detained in mental hospitals in Victoria, Australia, and were treated compulsorily with ECT. Both were found to lack mental capacity to consent on the ground that they did not accept their diagnoses (there was some criticism of staff efforts to engage with patients to reach agreement on these points). The Supreme Court of Victoria ruled that lower tribunals were wrong to find that this amounted to being unable to 'use or weigh information', the relevant part of the capacity definition. See p.522. *PBU and NJE v Mental Health Tribunal [2018] VSC 564*.

R v Podola Podola was charged with murder. He claimed that he was suffering from hysterical amnesia rendering him unfit to plead and was insane at the material time. The court ruled that amnesia for the offence could not amount to unfitness to plead because a defendant might still be able to understand the trial process (and that Mr Podola was able to do so). It also emphasised that where the defence raised a defence of insanity and this is contested by the prosecution, the burden of proof is on the defence. See p.602. *R v Podola* [1960] 1 QB 325.

Pora Pora confessed to raping and murdering a female victim. He had experienced foetal alcohol syndrome, which had left him with executive dysfunction. He was twice convicted. He appealed twice, claiming his confessions were unreliable, and that evidence suggesting another perpetrator should have been admitted. The court stated that evidence from an expert who had addressed the ultimate issue could not be admitted; nevertheless, it ruled that the confessions were unreliable and quashed the convictions. See p.609. *Pora v The Queen* [2015] UKPC 9.

Powell v UK The Powells' son Robert died from Addison's disease, which several doctors had negligently failed to treat despite suspecting its presence; they then sought to cover up their failure by falsifying records, and the Powells' attempts to seek justice were frustrated by collusion amongst the local Welsh authorities and the doctors, who were senior figures in their community. The ECtHR ruled that the UK had discharged its obligation to protect Robert's life when in NHS care by instituting a system for regulating care standards, and negligence of individual doctors in falling below those standards and their subsequent collusion did not mean the State had breached its article 2 duty. See p.516. *Powell v United Kingdom* [2000] 30 EHRR CD 362.

R v Pritchard Pritchard was a person of sound mind who was charged with bestiality. He could not easily communicate with others because he was both deaf and mute. The trial judge stated the rules for the jury to follow in deciding whether he was fit to plead (p.602). *R v Pritchard* [1836] 7 CP 303.

R v Quick Quick was a nurse at a mental hospital in Somerset. He and a co-defendant were charged with assaulting a patient. Quick had diabetes, and that morning he had taken insulin but then drunk spirits and eaten too little food, resulting in hypoglycaemia. The High Court allowed his appeal against conviction, holding that a 'transitory effect … of some external factor' could not be a 'disease of the mind' (and therefore could not amount to insanity), but that it could be an 'automatism'. See p.612. *R v Quick* [1973] 1 QB 910.

R v Rabey Rabey was a student who had unreciprocated feelings for a fellow student. He found a note amongst her books in which she described him as one of 'a bunch of nothings'. He felt 'hurt and angry' and entered a dissociative state in which he hit her on the head with a rock and then strangled her. At trial, he was acquitted on the ground of noninsane automatism. The Supreme Court of Canada ruled that the dissociation was internal to the mind and could therefore only amount to an insane automatism; in that the 'ordinary stresses and disappointments of life'" do not amount to a 'psychological blow' that would make the automatism noninsane. A retrial was ordered. See p.612. *R v Rabey* [1980] SCR 513.

Rabone Rabone was an informal patient receiving treatment for psychotic depression following a suicide attempt. While on home leave, she hanged herself. The Trust admitted that it had been negligent in allowing her home unsupervised, against her parents' wishes, when it knew she was at high risk of suicide. The Supreme Court held that the operational duty from *Savage v SEPT* (see below) to protect such patients applies even to informal patients, at least if it is clear that they would have been detained had they withdrawn consent to admission and treatment. It found that the Trust had breached Rabone's article 2 right to life. See p.516. *Rabone and another v Pennine Care NHSFT* [2012] UKSC 2.

R v Rejmanski, Gassman Rejmanski kicked a housemate to death when drunk, in an argument over missing food. He suffered from prior PTSD and claimed <u>loss of control</u> (p.630), but was convicted of murder. Gassman, <u>encouraged</u> (p.408) by her sister, stabbed and killed an acquaintance who had headbutted her. She suffered from EUPD and claimed loss of control but was convicted of murder. The Court of Appeal ruled that, in both cases, the mental disorders could not be taken into account because they were only relevant to the defendants' general capacity for tolerance and self-restraint, for which the statute sets an objective standard. See p.630. *R v Rejmanski; R v Gassman and another* [2017] EWCA Crim 2061.

RM v St Andrew's M had epilepsy, organic personality disorder, and organic delusional disorder, and he refused to accept anticonvulsants or other medication. He improved with covert medication, but he angrily stopped it when he learnt of this at a tribunal hearing. He deteriorated, requiring restraint and seclusion (and was at risk of sudden death from a seizure). Covert medication was later restarted. At his next hearing, the hospital applied to prevent disclosure of the covert medication (though his solicitor was allowed to know). The tribunal held that disclosure would cause serious harm and that concealment was proportionate. RM's solicitor appealed to the Upper Tribunal, which ruled that the covert medication was central to his case for release and had to be disclosed, despite the consequences. See p.323. *RM v St Andrew's Healthcare* [2010] UKUT 119.

Robertson v HM Advocate Robertson killed a man who made homosexual advances towards him and threatened him with a knife. He claimed <u>provocation</u> (p.630). The High Court of Justiciary refused his appeal against conviction for murder, holding that provocation required not only a loss of self-control but also a reasonably proportionate relationship between the provocation and the reaction to it. See p.630. *Robertson v HM Advocate* [1994] SC(JC) 245.

R v Roberts Roberts made a confession to a shopkeeper that he had stolen an item from their shop. The confession was not admissible in the court because the shopkeeper had lied to Roberts, promising not to call the police if a confession was made. See p.382. *R v Roberts* [2011] EWCA Crim 2974.

R v Robertson The defendant was charged with murder, but before the case began, the prosecution raised the issue of his <u>fitness to plead</u> (p.602), claiming that he was unable 'properly' to instruct counsel or defend himself. The medical evidence was that he could understand the relevant requirements; but, because of his 'persecution mania', might make unwise decisions or fail to defend himself 'properly'. In the Crown Court he was found unfit, but this finding was quashed by the Court of Appeal, which ruled that the fact that he might not act 'in his own best interests' was insufficient to render him unfit. The fact that the issue was raised by the prosecution and opposed by the defendant might have been significant in this controversial ruling. See p.602. *R v Robertson* [1968] 3 AllER 557.

R v Robinson A fifteen-year-old girl with learning disability was allegedly raped by her stepfather. The trial judge allowed a psychologist to give evidence that she was not particularly suggestible or likely to fantasise. On appeal, the conviction was quashed on the ground that there had been no claim that the victim was suggestible or liable to fantasise, and that therefore the psychologist's evidence amounted to an attempt by the prosecution to improve the perceived reliability of their witness's evidence. See p.657. *R v Robinson* [1994] 3 AllER 346.

R v Sanderson Sanderson was convicted of murdering his girlfriend after hitting her over a hundred times with a wooden stave. At trial Sanderson was described by the defence expert as having had a paranoid psychosis exacerbated by drug use; but as having paranoia due to drug use by the prosecution psychiatrist. The judge directed that paranoid psychosis and functional mental illness could amount to 'abnormality of mind', within 'diminished responsibility', but not drug-induced paranoia alone unless it had caused brain disease or injury. (Mr Sanderson successfully appealed against his conviction, but the rule stood.) See p.625. *R v Sanderson* (1994) 98 Cr.App.R 325.

Savage v SEPT Savage was detained in hospital under s3 MHA, suffering from paranoid schizophrenia. Three months later, she absconded from the hospital and jumped under a train, killing herself. The House of Lords confirmed that article 2 was relevant, and that if the subsequent trial showed that the NHS Trust was aware of a 'real and immediate risk to life' from self-harm, it had an operational duty to do 'all it reasonably could' to safeguard Savage specifically, over and above its general duty to have systems of safeguarding in place. (The subsequent trial found that her daughter could be regarded as a 'victim' of her mother's death under the relevant law, and declared that the Trust had indeed breached its article 2 obligation to her mother.) See p.516. *Savage v South Essex Partnership NHSFT* [2008] UKHL 74.

HM Advocate v Savage Savage was charged with murdering Jemima Grierson by cutting her throat. It was argued that, because of his mental condition, the verdict should be culpable homicide and not murder. The judgement led to the view that there must be aberration or weakness of mind; some form of mental unsoundness; a state of mind which is bordering on, though not amounting to, insanity; and that there must be a mind so affected that responsibility is diminished. This test was later replaced by *Galbraith v HM Advocate* (above). See p.624. *HM Advocate v Savage* (1923) JC 49.

Sessay Sessay had been removed unlawfully from her home by police, who wrongly believed that they had the power to take her under s5 of the MCA. She remained unlawfully detained in the hospital's s136 suite for a period of time (the hospital staff mistakenly believing that she had been detained by police under s136) until she was lawfully detained under s2. The hospital took thirteen hours to arrange detention under s2, which was found excessive; had there been no 'undue delay', her detention pending completion of s2 would have been lawful. Sessay was compensated for false imprisonment by the police and (for the thirteen hours) by the hospital. See p.542. *R (Sessay) v South London & Maudsley NHSFT and another* [2011] EWHC 2617.

SLL v Priory SLL was convicted of arson and received a restricted hospital order. Whilst in a secure hospital, he was charged with violent disorder and remanded to prison. While in prison, a tribunal reviewed his restriction order and ordered conditional discharge without conditions, thereby facilitating prosecution and imprisonment if he was convicted but allowing the possibility of a future recall. Mr L appealed, claiming he should have been absolutely discharged. The Upper Tribunal ruled that the first tribunal had erred in law by failing to properly consider whether liability to recall was appropriate, in part because it had not adequately considered the treatment that would be available in hospital. It noted that to be 'appropriate', treatment had to have 'a realistic prospect of therapeutic benefit'. See p.341. *SLL v Priory Health Care and SS for Justice* [2019] UKUT 323 (AAC).

R v Stephenson The defendant had schizophrenia. One night, he went to sleep in a haystack, having made a small fire in order to keep warm. The haystack erupted into fire. Medical evidence suggested that, because of his disorder, he was unable to foresee the fire as a possible consequence of his actions. His conviction was overturned by the Court of Appeal, which held that what was required for recklessness (p.403) was actual foresight. The fact that a reasonable person would have foreseen the risk of fire was not relevant. See p.403. *R v Stephenson* [1979] QB 695.

R v Stewart Stewart had alcohol dependence syndrome. He was homeless and killed another man. One of the psychiatrists at trial gave evidence that drinking in the context of alcohol dependence syndrome could never be involuntary: 'there is always some degree of choice'. Stewart appealed twice but his conviction was upheld because the jury had had the option of rejecting the evidence of the psychiatrist. The first appeal set the current legal rule on dependence and involuntary intoxication (p.614). *R v Stewart* [2009] EWCA Crim 593; [2010] EWCA Crim 2159.

Storck Storck was repeatedly confined to psychiatric hospitals at her father's insistence between 1974 and 1992 without her consent and without the necessary judicial orders. When she was a child this had been lawful, on the basis of her father's consent alone. The ECtHR ruled that the continuation of her detention as an adult was unlawful; noting that, for a deprivation of liberty to have occurred, it must be 'for a not negligible length of time'; where a few hours is negligible if it is the time 'strictly necessary to accomplish certain formalities'. See p.516. *Storck v Germany* [2005] 43 EHRR 96.

R v Sullivan Sullivan seriously assaulted a man whilst suffering an epileptic fit. The House of Lords upheld the trial judge's ruling that epilepsy was a 'disease of the mind', and that, in this case, the fit had rendered Sullivan insane at the time of the assault. (The defendant had changed his plea to guilty to avoid the then-automatic hospital order with restrictions, p.510 for a verdict of not guilty by reason of insanity, p.620.) See p.612. *R v Sullivan* [1984] 1 AC 156.

Sunderland v South Tyneside SF was detained under s3 and placed under s117 by Leeds services in accommodation in Sunderland, where she was studying. She was then voluntarily admitted to a hospital in South Tyneside. Her place on the course and her student accommodation were withdrawn after admission, and some weeks later her informal admission became a compulsory one under s3. The case centred on which local authority would be responsible for her after-care when she was discharged again. The Court of Appeal defined 'ordinary residence' as the place where a person eats and sleeps, provided it is voluntarily accepted by them, whatever the reason for their being there. This meant that, once the accommodation was withdrawn, SF was 'ordinarily resident' at the hospital in which (at that time) she was a voluntary patient, and South Tyneside was therefore responsible for her after-care. See p.492. *R (on the application of Sunderland City Council) v South Tyneside Council (SF, Leeds City Council: Interested Parties)* [2012] EWCA Civ 1232.

Surrey v McManus The council's social services department was in contact with a man who went on to sexually abuse three McManus children. They later sued the council. The claim for negligence was struck out on the ground that the council could not reasonably have known the children were at risk and therefore did not owe them a <u>duty of care</u> (p.548). See p.553. *Surrey County Council v McManus and others* [2001] EWCA 691.

R v T The defendant was raped and suffered PTSD. Three days afterwards, she stabbed a victim, while in a dissociative state, who she misperceived as intending her harm, and reaching into her car to take her bag. The Crown Court ruled that the defence of noninsane automatism was available because the earlier rape had been a severe external psychological blow, so that the dissociative state had not been solely 'inherent' to her. (However, the jury did not accept the defence, and convicted her.) See p.612. *R v T* [1990] CrimLR 256.

R v Tandy Tandy, an alcoholic, strangled her daughter after drinking most of a bottle of vodka. The judge directed the jury to decide whether she suffered from an 'abnormality of mind' or whether her abnormality was due to her voluntary drunkenness. She was convicted and appealed. Her conviction was upheld, three conditions being necessary for diminished responsibility where there was intoxication: that the defendant had 'an abnormality of mind'; 'that this was induced by the disease of alcoholism'; and there was 'an irresistible impulse to take the first drink (or drugs) of the day', so that ingestion was involuntary. If chronic brain damage had occurred, then this could in itself be an 'abnormality of mind'. See p.625. *R v Tandy* [1989] 1 WLR 350.

Tarasoff Poddar, a student at the University of California, became friends with Tatiana Tarasoff. He misinterpreted her kiss on New Year's Eve, and became resentful when she rebuffed him subsequently. He began stalking her. He saw a psychologist, and revealed his intent to kill her. The psychologist arranged for the campus police to detain him for psychiatric assessment, but he was thought to be rational and was released. He stopped seeing the psychologist and no further action was taken. He went on to kill Tatiana. Her family sued the university, and the court found in their favour, ruling that a mental health professional has a duty to protect third parties who may be harmed by their patient. See p.553. *Tarasoff v Regents of the University of California* 17 Cal 3d 425.

R v Toner Toner had been fasting for a prolonged period, broke his fast, and went on to strangle his wife. He was charged with attempted murder. Medical evidence on the effect of the fasting, and of breaking, it was excluded by the trial judge. A retrial was ordered by the Court of Appeal on the ground that the jury should have heard the evidence, because Toner was not simply an ordinary person; he was affected by a medical condition. See p.657. *R v Toner* [1991] 93 CrAppR 382.

R v Turner Turner killed his girlfriend with a hammer after she had taunted him about her having an affair. There was no evidence of mental disorder, but the defence attempted to introduce psychiatric evidence that he had felt a 'deep emotional relationship' with his girlfriend that had been shattered in what might amount to <u>provocation</u> (p.630). The court ruled the evidence inadmissible because it dealt with matters within the jury's 'common knowledge and experience'. See p.656. *R v Turner* [1975] QB 834.

Vowles Vowles, and five other mentally disordered offenders, had all received indeterminate prison sentences followed by transfer directions, and sought to have sentences of restricted hospital orders substituted; Ms Vowles also sought judicial review of the Parole Board's delay in hearing her case following the tribunal's determination that she would have been conditionally discharged if on a <u>restriction order</u> (p.510). The Court of Appeal ruled that requiring separate tribunal and Parole Board hearings was compatible with the ECHR; that the delay she suffered did not amount to a breach of article 5(4); and that judges must consider 'hybrid orders' whenever the criteria for a hospital order are met. It issued detailed guidance, now clarified by *Edwards* (see above). *R (Vowles) v Secretary of State for Justice* [2015] EWCA Civ 56.

Wednesbury A cinema chain challenged the local council's power to impose sweeping conditions on Sunday opening. It lost its case, because of the very wide powers granted to the council under the relevant legislation, but the case was notable because the Court of Appeal laid down the grounds for judicial review of administrative decisions: taking inappropriate matters into account, ignoring appropriate matters, or unreasonableness. The test of unreasonableness was stated vividly by Lord Diplock in *Council of Civil Service Unions v Minister for the Civil Service* [1983] UKHL 6 as a decision 'so outrageous in its defiance of logic or accepted moral standards that no sensible person who had applied his mind to the question to be decided could have arrived at it'. See p.374. *Associated Provincial Picture Houses Ltd v Wednesbury Corporation* [1948] 1 KB 223.

R v Weightman In this complex case a defendant suspected of having histrionic personality traits (but not necessarily a personality disorder) was charged with killing her two-year-old daughter. She had confessed the murder (which had initially been thought by the coroner to be accidental asphyxiation) to her husband, probation officer, and police. At her trial, she did not plead 'diminished responsibility' or 'insanity'. The judge refused an application to call evidence from a psychiatrist who had attended the police interviews. The Court of Appeal upheld her conviction, ruling that expert psychiatric evidence was inadmissible when its effective purpose was to tell the court how a person without mental disorder would 'react to the stresses and strains of life'. See p.656. *R v Weightman* [1990] 92 CrAppR 291.

Whetstone v MPS Whetstone was a dentist who engaged the services of an associate, Mr Sudworth. The contract between them suggested that Mr Sudworth was self-employed, but it entitled Whetstone to exercise such tight control that it was deemed 'akin to employment'. Whetstone was therefore vicariously liable for Mr Sudworth's negligent treatment. See p.551. *Whetstone v Medical Protection Society* [2014] EWHC 1024.

R v Windle Windle married an older woman who was believed to suffer from mental disorder, who repeatedly threatened suicide. He became obsessed with this and discussed it continually with his workmates, one of whom, exasperated, eventually suggested giving her 'a dozen aspirin'. He gave her a hundred, causing her death. He was diagnosed with folie à deux (p.74), but not found insane because he knew he was 'doing an act which *the law* forbade'. The Court of Criminal Appeal held that the fact that he believed he was not doing anything *morally* wrong was irrelevant. See p.620. *R v Windle* [1952] 2 QB 826.

Winterwerp Winterwerp complained that, while he was detained in hospital in the Netherlands for treatment of schizophrenia (initially under an emergency procedure), he was unable to manage his property, meaning that his legal right to do this had been taken away without an appropriate judicial procedure. The ECtHR found that detention for mental disorder is only lawful under article 5(1) only if there is supportive objective medical evidence, but that emergency procedures were nevertheless lawful in principle and represented a temporary exemption to the requirement for such evidence. However, as Dutch law at the time did not require the patient to be notified of review proceedings, nor to be given an opportunity to argue their case, and allowed prosecutors to dismiss applications for release without a court hearing, Winterwerp's article 5(4) and 6(1) rights had been breached. The Dutch government replaced the 1884 mental health law with the Psychiatric Hospitals (Committal) Act [BOPZ in Dutch] to comply with the ECHR. See p.516. *Winterwerp v The Netherlands* [1979] 2 EHRR 387.

R v Wood Wood was an excessive drinker who went to the flat of an acquaintance after consuming large amounts of alcohol. He claimed that he fell asleep and awoke to find the victim trying to perform oral sex on him. He killed him using a meat cleaver. At trial two psychiatrists concluded that he had alcohol dependence syndrome. The trial judge applied *Tandy* (above): asserting that 'diminished responsibility' was only available if the drinking was truly involuntary, not merely the result of a craving. The Court of Appeal overruled this, modifying the rule such that, if there was severe craving, the question whether it was sufficient to make drinking 'involuntary' was a factual question for the jury. See p.625. *R v Wood* [2008] EWCA Crim 1305.

Worboys The defendant, a taxi driver, raped or sexually assaulted a large number of women by persuading them to take 'spiked' drinks (he was convicted of twenty-three offences, but investigations and reports suggested the true number of victims was well over a hundred). Ten years after his initial convictions, the Parole Board proposed to release him on licence, based on what was later considered to be a flawed risk assessment that ignored postconviction evidence from women not involved in the original trials. This led to a public outcry and judicial review proceedings, which ultimately concluded that the Parole Board had been *Wednesbury* unreasonable in failing to consider the postconviction evidence. The case was reheard by a new Board, which rejected his application for release. See p.582. *R (DSD & NBV; the Mayor of London; and News Group Newspapers Ltd) v The Parole Board of E&W, Secretary of State for Justice; and John Radford (formerly Worboys)* [2018] EWHC 694 (Admin).

Miller v Prime Minister Ms Miller in England and Ms Cherry and colleagues in Scotland sued the government for advising the Queen to prorogue (suspend) Parliament for an exceptionally long period of five weeks, at a time when Parliament and the government were in dispute about an issue of national controversy, close to an important deadline (leaving the European Union by 31st October 2019). They claimed that the Prime Minister's advice to the Queen was unlawful for being based on personal political interest rather than the national interest, and they sought judicial review. The High Court in England had found that this was a political question that the court could not review; the Court of Session in Scotland had found that the issue *was* justiciable. The Supreme Court confirmed that the actions of the Queen could not be judicially reviewed, but that the Prime Minister's advice could be. It ruled that advice to "the monarch to prorogue Parliament … will be unlawful if the prorogation has the effect of frustrating or preventing, without reasonable justification, the ability of Parliament to… legislat[e] and … supervis[e] … the executive.", and held that on the evidence before it could not "conclude … that there was any reason—let alone a good reason—to advise" the Queen to prorogue for such a long period as five weeks, and therefore the advice was unlawful. It declined to consider the Prime Minister's actual or alleged motives for advising the Queen to prorogue Parliament. It further ruled that because the advice on which it was based was unlawful, the prorogation proclamation was "unlawful, null and of no effect", and Parliament therefore continued in session. See pp. 362,364. *R (Miller) v The Prime Minister; Cherry and others v Advocate General for Scotland* [2019] UKSC 41.

R (McCann) v Manchester The three teenage McCann brothers were alleged to have caused significant distress in their local community through their antisocial behaviour. A magistrate accepted on the balance of probabilities that they had done so, and issued ASBOs preventing them using insulting, offensive, threatening or abusive language or behaviour in any public place in Manchester, threatening or using violence or causing criminal damage, or entering the Beswick area of the city. If they breached the ASBO, they could each be prosecuted criminally. Their mother sought judicial review on their behalf. The Court of Appeal upheld the orders, on the basis that the intention of the statute was clear, and the civil proceedings for making the ASBO could be distinguished from criminal proceedings for its breach. See pp. 457,458. *R (McCann and others) v Manchester Crown Court and the Chief Constable of Greater Manchester* [2001] EWCA Civ 281.

Ethical codes

The following pages reproduce extracts from <u>ethical codes</u> and <u>professional guidelines</u> (p.294) of particular relevance to forensic psychiatrists, as well as to those who may adjudicate or comment upon their practice.

General Medical Council

Good Medical Practice (2020)

- 7: You must be competent in all aspects of your work, including management, research, and teaching.
- 8: You must keep your professional knowledge and skills up to date.
- 9: You must regularly take part in activities that maintain and develop your competence and performance.
- 12: You must keep up to date with, and follow, the law, our guidance, and other regulations relevant to your work.
- 13: You must take steps to monitor and improve the quality of your work.
- 14: You must recognise and work within the limits of your competence.
- 65: You must make sure that your conduct justifies your patients' trust in you and the public's trust in the profession.
- 66: You must always be honest about your experience, qualifications, and current role.
- 69: When communicating publicly, including speaking to or writing in the media, you must maintain patient confidentiality. You should remember when using social media that communications intended for friends or family may become more widely available.
- 71: You must be honest and trustworthy when writing reports, and when completing or signing forms, reports, and other documents. You must make sure that any documents you write or sign are not false or misleading. You must take reasonable steps to check the information is correct. You must not deliberately leave out relevant information.
- 72: You must be honest and trustworthy when giving evidence to courts or tribunals. You must make sure that any evidence you give or documents you write or sign are not false or misleading.
- 73: You must cooperate with formal inquiries and complaints procedures and must offer all relevant information while following GMC guidance on confidentiality.
- 74: You must make clear the limits of your competence and knowledge when giving evidence or acting as a witness.

Royal College of Psychiatrists Good Psychiatric Practice Code of Ethics (2014)

1 Psychiatrists shall respect the essential humanity and dignity of every patient.
2 Psychiatrists shall not exploit patients' vulnerability.
3 Psychiatrists shall provide the best attainable psychiatric care for their patients.
4 Psychiatrists shall maintain the confidentiality of patients and their families.

5 Psychiatrists shall seek valid consent from their patients before undertaking any procedure or treatment.
6 Psychiatrists shall ensure patients and their carers can make the best available choices about treatment.
7 Psychiatrists shall not misuse their professional knowledge and skills, whether for personal gain or to cause harm to others.
8 Psychiatrists shall comply with ethical principles embodied in national and international guidelines governing research.
9 Psychiatrists shall continue to develop, maintain, and share their professional knowledge and skills with medical colleagues, trainees, and students, as well as with other relevant health professionals and patients and their families.
10 Psychiatrists have a duty to attend to the mental health and wellbeing of their colleagues, including trainees and students.
11 Psychiatrists shall maintain the integrity of the medical profession.
12 Psychiatrists shall work to improve mental health services and promote community awareness of mental illness and its treatment and prevention, and reduce the effects of stigma and discrimination.

Good Psychiatric Practice: Confidentiality and Information-Sharing

• Express consent should be sought where sharing of information outside the healthcare team is anticipated.
• Competent refusals made before death should be respected after death unless there are overriding circumstances.
• Information should not be shared within interagency teams without consent.
• At CPA meetings, the psychiatrist's duty of confidentiality must be acknowledged and respected if information is to be shared.
• If non–team members are to be involved in your patient's care (including attending team meetings), you should discuss it with the patient.
• If you attend a meeting arranged by an outside agency, consider and record your decisions about disclosure to them. Remember, the agency to which you disclose information may apply standards of confidentiality different from your own.
• In situations with dual obligations you must be clear in explaining your role to your patient, and in seeking consent.
• For court proceedings, you do not have to disclose in the absence of a court order unless you have consent or there are grounds to override refusal.
• It is sometimes justifiable for a psychiatrist to pass on patient information without consent or statutory authority. Such situations include:
  • where death or serious harm may occur to a third party, whether or not a criminal offence (e.g. disclosure of threat of serious harm to a named person, on the expectation that this would prevent the harm);
  • when a disclosure may assist in the prevention, detection, or prosecution of a serious crime, especially crimes against the person, or conversely in situations where it is necessary to the defence of a case to ensure that there is no miscarriage of justice;

- where the patient is a health professional, and the psychiatrist has concerns over that person's fitness to practise;
- where a psychiatrist has concerns over a patient's fitness to drive; and
- where a psychiatrist has concerns over a patient's fitness to hold a firearms licence.

- When deciding to disclose you must take a wide range of factors into account. You must communicate with your patient; it is advisable to discuss the proposed disclosure with appropriate colleagues or organisations.
- You have a duty to cooperate with MAPPA. You do not have an obligation to disclose. Public interest will be an important factor for your consideration.
- You should normally seek written consent before drafting a report. However, where there is a statutory obligation or there are overriding considerations, consent is not required. Remember to make your role clear to the patient when seeking consent, and disclose only the necessary information.

Royal College of Psychiatrists CR193 Expert Evidence to Courts and Tribunals (2021)

This includes advice:

- The administration of justice depends on the willingness of psychiatrists to play their part in offering expert assistance ... (and) to the highest professional and ethical standards.
- It is important to keep abreast of developments in statute and case law and, where appropriate, to take account of ... legal advice as to the significance of such developments.
- The expert witness must comply with a number of duties, some common to all expert witnesses and some specific to certain courts and jurisdictions.
- Expert witnesses who provide training and supervision have additional duties, as do those they train or supervise.
- Expert testimony, or expert evidence, is information which is relevant, likely to be outside of the experience of a judge or jury, based on a reliable body of knowledge or experience, or for which there is a sufficiently reliable scientific basis for the evidence to be admitted.
- Whether or not a psychiatrist has the appropriate or relevant expertise for a particular case is initially for the parties, and ultimately for the court or tribunal, to decide; but in making this ultimate decision, the court or tribunal has to be able to rely upon information provided by the expert.
- There is a duty on psychiatrists who give expert testimony to ensure that such work is included in their appraisal for revalidation.
- Other than exceptionally, psychiatrists who provide expert evidence, even in cases where there is no clinical contact in the form of history-taking and examination, should hold a licence to practise.
- Specialist forensic psychiatry trainees are required, as a core part of their training, to acquire knowledge and skills concerning law and the interface of law and psychiatry.

- Psychiatrists have a duty not to give evidence or opinion on matters outside their areas or fields of expertise.
- It is the duty of any psychiatrist to assist the court to 'effect' justice and never to seek to 'affect' it; which means being able to reflect upon how their own values, and other sources of bias, might influence the opinions they give.
- Psychiatrists will likely need to decline instructions in cases where they have competing or conflicting interests.
- Where people involved in legal actions are adversely affected by experts who cause delays, those experts may be at risk of financial penalties, such as a wasted costs order.
- It is generally inadvisable for the treating clinician to provide expert testimony within litigation involving their patient, although there are exceptions.
- The first, or overriding duty of the expert is to the court and to the administration of justice, but psychiatrists should not ignore their ordinary clinical ethical duties as doctors when evaluating individuals for the courts.
- Psychiatrists may occasionally be asked to prepare reports without consulting with, or otherwise directly assessing, the subject of the report, but such a report should not usually be prepared without either the consent of the subject of the report or the agreement of the parties to the litigation or an order from the court.
- In some circumstances a psychiatrist may be asked ... to offer a critique of, or commentary upon, the report of another expert, in the role of 'expert advisor'; this should not be confused with providing an independent opinion to the court.
- Similarly, a psychiatrist in a criminal case may be provided with a defence psychiatric report and asked to comment upon it in order to inform a charging decision or to assist as to a defence that is raised; and, again, this should not be confused with providing an independent opinion to the court.
- In order to base an opinion as to diagnosis upon subjective symptoms, the expert has to assess the worth of the evidence overall, so that multiple primary sources of information, independent of the individual assessed, are essential.
- It is for the court to determine the ultimate issue of culpability and subsequent need for punishment, not the expert; although the expert may offer expert advice on the causal relevance of the defendant's mental disorder in determining commission of the index offence.
- It is ethically problematic for experts explicitly to recommend a <u>s45A hybrid order</u> (p.670) because this amounts to recommending punishment; this is distinct from giving expert evidence concerning the therapeutic or public safety implications of such an order.
- Experts must liaise with local mental health services when making medical recommendations.
- Psychiatrists giving evidence in the family courts need to be able to show that they have the necessary particular training and expertise in this complex field.

- An expert who uses a published psychometric test or instrument or tool, such as a risk assessment, should be prepared to be cross-examined on its validity and reliability ... by a cross-examiner who is assisted by an expert who is qualified to administer the test, instrument, or tool, and/or is familiar with the literature relating to that instrument.
- Experts should strive to respect the normal duties of confidentiality, which should include proper procedures for the secure storage of documents and records.
- Other than exceptionally, reports should not be disclosed without the subject's consent and/or consent of their legal representatives, or unless directed by a court, or where there is an overriding public interest in disclosure.
- Experts who engage with, or come across, erring experts in litigation are probably best able to expose and delineate their shortcomings and misdemeanours, and they do a disservice to their profession if they turn a blind eye and do nothing.
- Any complaint against another expert should be conciliatory, constructive, and respectful.
- Psychiatrists concerned about potentially having a negative effect on litigants may choose to withdraw from particular classes of expert witness work, but this may leave the courts increasingly reliant on a pool of experts who appear to favour less therapeutic approaches, thus distorting the range of expert opinion available to the court.
- When courts require assistance in novel areas, it is better for them to be assisted by provisional or qualified, even heavily qualified, opinions and to understand the limitations, inadequacies, and weaknesses of research and guidance than to have no assistance at all.

American Academy of Psychiatry and the Law

Ethical Guidelines for the Practice of Forensic Psychiatry

... Forensic psychiatrists practice at the interface of law and psychiatry, each of which has developed its own institutions, policies, procedures, values, and vocabulary. As a consequence, the practice of forensic psychiatry entails inherent potentials for complications, conflicts, misunderstandings, and abuses.

Psychiatrists in a forensic role are called upon to practice in a manner that balances competing duties to the individual and to society. In doing so, they should be bound by underlying ethical principles of respect for persons, honesty, justice, and social responsibility. However, when a treatment relationship exists, such as in correctional settings, the usual physician-patient duties apply.

Confidentiality

... Psychiatrists should maintain confidentiality to the extent possible, given the legal context. Special attention should be paid to the evaluee's understanding of medical confidentiality. A forensic evaluation requires notice to the evaluee and to collateral sources of reasonably anticipated limitations on confidentiality. Information or reports derived from a forensic evaluation are subject to the rules of confidentiality that apply to the particular evaluation, and any disclosure should be restricted accordingly ... Psychiatrists should indicate for whom they are conducting the examination and what they will do with the information obtained. At the beginning of a forensic evaluation, care should be taken to explicitly inform the evaluee that the psychiatrist is not the evaluee's 'doctor'. Psychiatrists have a continuing obligation to be sensitive to the fact that although a warning has been given, the evaluee may develop the belief that there is a treatment relationship....

Consent

At the outset of a face-to-face evaluation, notice should be given to the evaluee of the nature and purpose of the evaluation and the limits of its confidentiality. The informed consent of the person undergoing the forensic evaluation should be obtained when necessary and feasible. If the evaluee is not competent to give consent, the evaluator should follow the appropriate laws of the jurisdiction....

It is important to appreciate that in particular situations, such as court-ordered evaluations for competency to stand trial or involuntary commitment, neither assent nor informed consent is required. In such cases, psychiatrists should inform the evaluee that if the evaluee refuses to participate in the evaluation, this fact may be included in any report or testimony. If the evaluee does not appear capable of understanding the information provided regarding the evaluation, this impression should also be included in any report and, when feasible, in testimony.

Absent a court order, psychiatrists should not perform forensic evaluations for the prosecution or the government on persons who have not consulted with legal counsel when such persons are: known to be charged [or] under investigation....

Consent to treatment in a jail or prison or in other criminal justice settings is different from consent for a forensic evaluation. Psychiatrists providing treatment in such settings should be familiar with the jurisdiction's regulations governing patients' rights regarding treatment.

Honesty and striving for objectivity

When psychiatrists function as experts within the legal process, they should adhere to the principle of honesty and should strive for objectivity [despite being] retained by one party to a civil or criminal matter....

Psychiatrists practicing in a forensic role enhance the honesty and objectivity of their work by basing their forensic opinions, forensic reports, and forensic testimony on all available data. They communicate the honesty of their work, efforts to attain objectivity, and the soundness of their clinical opinion, by distinguishing, to the extent possible, between verified and unverified information as well as among clinical 'facts', 'inferences', and 'impressions'.

Psychiatrists should not distort their opinion in the service of the retaining party. Honesty, objectivity, and the adequacy of the clinical evaluation may be called into question when an expert opinion is offered without a personal examination....

In custody cases, honesty and objectivity require that all parties be interviewed, if possible, before an opinion is rendered. When this is not possible, or is not done for any reason, this should be clearly indicated in the forensic psychiatrist's report and testimony. If one parent has not been interviewed, even after deliberate effort, it may be inappropriate to comment on that parent's fitness as a parent. Any comments on the fitness of a parent who has not been interviewed should be qualified and the data for the opinion clearly indicated.

Contingency fees undermine honesty and efforts to attain objectivity and should not be accepted. Retainer fees, however, do not create the same problems in regard to honesty and efforts to attain objectivity and, therefore, may be accepted.

Psychiatrists who take on a forensic role for patients they are treating may adversely affect the therapeutic relationship with them. Forensic evaluations usually require interviewing corroborative sources, exposing information to public scrutiny, or subjecting evaluees and the treatment itself to potentially damaging cross-examination. The forensic evaluation and the credibility of the practitioner may also be undermined by conflicts inherent in the differing clinical and forensic roles. Treating psychiatrists should therefore generally avoid acting as an expert witness for their patients or performing evaluations of their patients for legal purposes.

Treating psychiatrists appearing as 'fact' witnesses should be sensitive to the unnecessary disclosure of private information or the possible misinterpretation of testimony as 'expert' opinion. In situations when the dual role is required or unavoidable (such as Workers' Compensation, disability evaluations, civil commitment, or guardianship hearings), sensitivity to differences between clinical and legal obligations remains important....

Qualifications

Expertise in the practice of forensic psychiatry should be claimed only in areas of actual knowledge, skills, training, and experience.

When providing expert opinion, reports, and testimony, psychiatrists should present their qualifications accurately and precisely....

World Psychiatric Association Declaration of Madrid

Psychiatry is a medical discipline concerned with the prevention of mental disorders in the population, the provision of the best possible treatment for mental disorders, the rehabilitation of individuals suffering from mental illness, and the promotion of mental health. Psychiatrists serve patients by providing the best therapy available consistent with accepted scientific knowledge and ethical principles. Psychiatrists should devise therapeutic interventions that are **least restrictive** to the freedom of the patient and seek advice in areas of their work about which they do not have primary expertise. While doing so, psychiatrists should be aware of and concerned with the **equitable allocation** of health resources.

It is the duty of psychiatrists to keep abreast of **scientific developments** of the specialty and to convey updated knowledge to others. Psychiatrists trained in research should seek to advance the scientific frontiers of psychiatry.

The patient should be accepted as a partner by right in the therapeutic process. The psychiatrist-patient relationship must be based on mutual trust and respect to allow the patient to make free and informed decisions. It is the duty of psychiatrists to provide the patient with all **relevant information** so as to empower the patient to come to a rational decision according to personal values and preferences.

When the patient is gravely disabled, incapacitated, and/or incompetent to exercise proper judgment because of a mental disorder, the psychiatrists should consult with the family and, if appropriate, seek legal counsel, to safeguard the human dignity and the legal rights of the patient. **No treatment should be provided against the patient's will**, unless withholding treatment would endanger the life of the patient and/or the life of others. Treatment must always be in the **best interest** of the patient.

When psychiatrists are requested to assess a person, it is their duty first to inform and advise the person being assessed about the purpose of the intervention, the use of the findings, and the possible repercussions of the assessment. This is particularly important when psychiatrists are involved in third-party situations.

Information obtained in the therapeutic relationship is private to the patient and should be **kept in confidence** and used, only and exclusively, for the purpose of improving the mental health of the patient. Psychiatrists are prohibited from making use of such information for personal reasons, or personal benefit. Breach of confidentiality may only be appropriate when required by law (as in obligatory reporting of child abuse) or when serious physical or mental harm to the patient or to a third person would ensue if confidentiality were maintained; whenever possible, psychiatrists should first advise the patient about the action to be taken....

Important inquiries and reports

Barrett Inquiry Also known as the **Robinson inquiry** (after its chair), this inquired into the circumstances that led to a recently readmitted (but not <u>recalled</u>, p.589) medium secure psychiatric patient, John Barrett, being allowed brief <u>leave</u> (p.486) from the unit, during which he stabbed a member of the public to death. The consultant forensic psychiatrist involved was heavily criticised in the inquiry report, also by her Trust, for prioritising the working relationship with the patient over acting on risk concerns raised by some members of the clinical team. She was effectively exonerated in litigation she took against her Trust employer.

Bennett Inquiry An inquiry into the death of David 'Rocky' Bennett in a psychiatric unit, after a fatal incident during which he was restrained in the prone position, with staff pressing down on his back. The inquiry found that misunderstanding of, or discrimination against, Mr Bennett because of his Afro-Caribbean background was a contributory factor, and recommended employment of a greater proportion of staff from black and minority ethnic (BME) groups.

Blom-Cooper Inquiry The first of the two inquiries into Ashworth Hospital, this 1992 inquiry examined conditions at the hospital; in particular concerning two patient deaths (one by suicide) and the abuse of two others. It found serious deficiencies in standards of care. Seven staff members were disciplined and/or charged as a result.

Bradley Report This 2009 report focused on people with mental disorder and learning disability in the criminal justice system, as had parts of the Reed Report twenty years earlier. It recommended a wide range of measures to improve detection and treatment of mental disorder within the CJS and to facilitate transfer to hospital if needed. It required substantial additional resources and therefore, at the time of writing, has not been fully implemented.

Butler Inquiry An influential 1974 report, of the Committee on Mentally Abnormal Offenders, set up after a patient released from Broadmoor, Graham Young, committed murder. It recommended (amongst other things) the creation of <u>Regional Secure Units</u> (p.258).

The Falling Shadow This inquiry related to the killing of Georgina Robinson, an occupational therapist, by Andrew Robinson in 1993. The inquiry was published as a book (under this title) by its chair, Louis Blom-Cooper QC. Andrew Robinson had a long history of mental illness and had been admitted to a high-security hospital following a previous offence. The report was highly critical of aspects of his clinical care, including the failure to observe the legal requirements for leave relating to detained patients. There was a specific recommendation to extend the powers of compulsory treatment to patients in the community, which (with the Ritchie Report) resulted in the introduction of 'supervised discharge' in 1995 (a precursor to the <u>Community Treatment Order</u>, p.488).

Fallon Inquiry Extradition A second inquiry, in 1996, (after the Blom-Cooper Inquiry) into <u>Ashworth Hospital</u> (p.258), specifically into the Personality Disorder Unit. It found that security policies were ignored; pornography was widely available; and a child visitor was groomed for paedophile abuse. It recommended that the hospital close, although this did not happen.

Second Report of the 2014–15 Session of the House of Lords Select Committee on Extradition Law and Practice. This found that legally required 'assurances' given of adequate safeguarding and treatment in requesting countries within extradition proceedings were, in practice, highly unreliable and incapable of being 'policed'. Since courts in extradition cases in the UK and RoI frequently invoke such assurances in permitting extradition (see e.g. _Dewani_, p.752), this is a major flaw.

Glancy Report This 1974 Report of the Working Party on Security in NHS Psychiatric Hospitals recommended that psychiatric hospitals establish secure wards for patients (whether offenders or not) whose behaviour could not be safely managed on open wards.

Lukewarm Luke Inquiry This concerned the killing of Susan Milner by Michael Folkes in 1994 (he later changed his name to Lukewarm Luke). Mr Folkes was under the care of a forensic psychiatric community service, following discharge by a tribunal against medical and Home Office advice, with a condition to take antipsychotic medication. He subsequently stopped taking depot medication in favour of oral medication and, at the time of the killing, was not taking anything. He had presented to hospital the day before the killing. Criticism focused on communication between members of the clinical team and the decision to allow him to stop depot medication. There was also criticism of the decision not to discharge him to a staffed hostel.

Michael Stone Inquiry Michael Stone had a severe personality disorder (p.78) and misused substances. In 1996, he committed a very high-profile multiple murder, of Lin Russell and her daughter Megan (her other daughter Josie was seriously injured, but survived). Despite the Inquiry's finding that mental health and probation services had done everything that could reasonably have been done to help Mr Stone (with some minor criticisms), the case was one used by the then New Labour government in support of both its programme of detention of 'dangerous' people with severe personality disorder (DSPD, p.15) and effective abolition of the legal 'treatability' requirement via the Mental Health (Amendment) Act 2007.

National Confidential Inquiry into Suicide and Safety in Mental Health (NCISS), (p.599), is a research project funded by the Scottish Government and the English and Northern Irish Departments of Health. All incidences of suicide by people in contact with mental health services in the UK are examined (homicides having been removed from its remit). A variety of research studies have been published since the Inquiry was founded.

ONS studies A series of studies carried out by the Office of National Statistics and, before that, the Office of Population Censuses and Surveys, of the epidemiology of psychiatric conditions. One key study in 1997 of over 3,000 prisoners established the prevalence of psychosis in prison as 7%–14%, and all mental disorders as 90%.

Reed Report This report, produced by the Department of Health in 1992, into services for mentally disordered offenders contained multiple recommendations, with a general theme that the care provided to mentally disordered offenders should be equivalent to that available to other patients. There were also significant recommendations relating to multiagency working.

Ritchie Report An inquiry into the killing of Jonathan Zito by Christopher Clunis (p.751), a man with paranoid schizophrenia who had repeatedly defaulted from treatment, in 1992. The report highlighted numerous failings of community care services in London, and recommended better quality risk assessment (p.163); a change of professional culture, including interagency working across boundaries; more resources; more hostels; a form of compulsory community treatment (p.488); and special services for patients who were difficult to follow up.

Sentencing Council Guidelines for Offenders with Mental Disorders, Developmental Disorders or Neurological Impairments. Not strictly a report, this advises how judges should utilise knowledge of a defendant's mental disorder, as well as its role in the commission of the index offence, in determining whether the defendant should receive a mental health disposal, and if the latter, what sentence. It arose partly out of cases such as *Vowles* and *Edwards* (pp.754, 770), in which the Court of Appeal posed questions to expert psychiatric witnesses about defendant's 'dangerousness' (p.672) and degree of culpability (p.354). This challenged medical ethics, which might allow expert comment on causation of the offence and on risk assessment, but not culpability or dangerousness. The guideline sets out suggested questions that courts may properly pose to experts which avoid these problems.

Shipman, Ayling, Ledward, Neale and Kerr-Haslam Inquiries These concerned a series of grave breaches of trust by doctors: GP Clifford Ayling indecently assaulted his patients; gynaecologists Rodney Ledward and Richard Neale carried out dangerous operations with poor postoperative care resulting in unnecessary deaths; Neale moved from one hospital and country to another to avoid investigation; psychiatrists William Kerr and Michael Haslam indecently assaulted vulnerable patients; and most notoriously, GP Harold Shipman murdered over 200 elderly patients. They resulted in a series of reforms of regulation of the medical profession in the UK, requiring amongst other things revalidation (p.552) every five years of doctors' professional registration based upon annual appraisal.

Tilt Report This report into the level of security (p.190) at the three English high-security hospitals (p.258) was commissioned to comply with a recommendation of the Fallon inquiry (above). It recommended that external physical and procedural security at the hospitals should be increased, to allow a reduction in internal procedural security measures (e.g. internal escorting within the site), and that long-term medium secure facilities should be developed for patients whose slow progress and risk to others prevented movement through the usual medium secure system to the community, but who no longer warranted high security.

Wessely Report The Independent Review of the Mental Health Act 2018 was commissioned by the UK government because of concerns about rising rates of civil detention and compulsory treatment, and the disproportionate use of compulsory powers on people from certain BME backgrounds in E&W (see p.40). It made 154 recommendations, set out four new principles to be included in law ('choice' and 'autonomy', 'least restriction', 'therapeutic benefit', and 'treating the person as an individual'), and strongly hinted that mental health law should become more closely aligned with mental capacity law (and perhaps even 'fused' with it) in future, depending on the experience of implementing the MCANI in NI (see also Richardson Report above). At the time of writing, the government has published a draft Bill that would implement many of its recommendations.

Mental health law: quick reference

This appendix shows the pages on which each important aspect of mental health law is covered. The pages on which other Acts are covered are listed in the appendix on <u>statutes</u> (p.732).

See Box A.1 for mental health law statutes in each jurisdiction.

Box A.1 Mental health law statutes in each jurisdiction

E&W	Mental Health Act 1983
Scotland	Mental Health Care and Treatment Act 2003 and
	Criminal Procedure (Scotland) Act 1995 (prefixed by C)
NI:O	Mental Health (Northern Ireland) Order 1986
NI:C	Mental Capacity Act (Northern Ireland) 2016
RoI	Mental Health Act 2001 and
	Criminal Law (Insanity) Act 2006 (prefixed by C)

E&W	Scotland	NI:O	NI:C	RoI	Provision	Page
				C4,5	Committal for examination/treatment	498
2		4	Sch2	9	Civil admission for assessment	474
				12	Removal by police officer	494
3			Sch1	15	Civil admission for treatment	478
				C15	Transfer of prisoner	506
4			Sch2		Emergency civil admission	476
5	7		Sch2	23	Emergency detention of inpatient	476
7			Sch1		Guardianship	488
	12				Civil detention for treatment	478
17	15	25,27		26	Leave from hospital	487
17A			Sch1		Community treatment order	488
	18				Guardianship	488
	25-27		16-23		After-care	493

Index

For the benefit of digital users, indexed terms that span two pages (e.g., 52–53) may, on occasion, appear on only one of those pages.
Tables and boxes are indicated by t and b following the page number